Principles and Practice of
PEDODONTICS

Principles and Practice of
PEDODONTICS

Third Edition

Editor

Arathi Rao MDS
Professor and Head
Department of Pedodontics and Preventive Dentistry
Manipal College of Dental Sciences, Manipal University
Mangalore, Karnataka, India
e-mail: arathi_rao@hotmail.com

Foreword
V Surendra Shetty

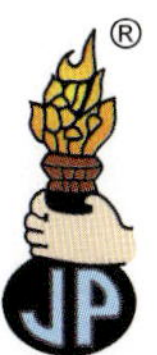

JAYPEE BROTHERS MEDICAL PUBLISHERS (P) LTD

New Delhi • Panama City • London

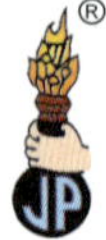 **Jaypee Brothers Medical Publishers (P) Ltd.**

Headquarter
Jaypee Brothers Medical Publishers (P) Ltd
4838/24, Ansari Road, Daryaganj
New Delhi 110 002, India
Phone: +91-11-43574357
Fax: +91-11-43574314
Email: jaypee@jaypeebrothers.com

Overseas Offices
J.P. Medical Ltd.
83 Victoria Street, London
SW1H 0HW (UK)
Phone: +44-2031708910
Fax: +02-03-0086180
Email: info@jpmedpub.com

Jaypee-Highlights Medical Publishers Inc.
City of Knowledge, Bld. 237, Clayton
Panama City, Panama
Phone: + 507-301-0496
Fax: + 507-301-0499
Email: cservice@jphmedical.com

Website: www.jaypeebrothers.com
Website: www.jaypeedigital.com

© 2012, Jaypee Brothers Medical Publishers

Inquiries for bulk sales may be solicited at: jaypee@jaypeebrothers.com

This book has been published in good faith that the contents provided by the contributors contained herein are original, and is intended for educational purposes only. While every effort is made to ensure accuracy of information, the publisher and the editor specifically disclaim any damage, liability, or loss incurred, directly or indirectly, from the use or application of any of the contents of this work. If not specifically stated, all figures and tables are courtesy of the editor. Where appropriate, the readers should consult with a specialist or contact the manufacturer of the drug or device.

Principles and Practices of Pedodontics

First Edition: 2006
Second Edition: 2008
Third Edition: **2012**

ISBN: 978-93-5025-891-0

Printed at Replika Press Pvt. Ltd.

Contributors

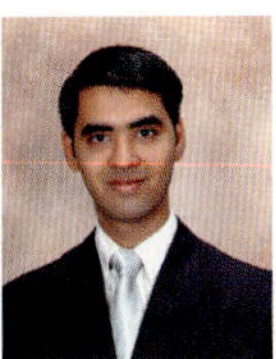

Ashwin Rao MDS
Associate Professor
Department of Pedodontics and
Preventive Dentistry
Manipal College of Dental Sciences
Manipal University
Mangalore, Karnataka, India

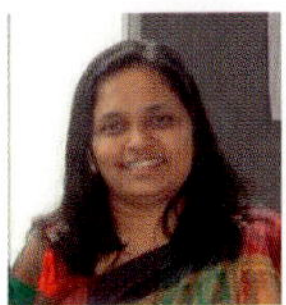

Ashwini Rao MDS
Professor and Head
Department of Community and
Preventive Dentistry
Manipal College of Dental Sciences
Manipal University
Mangalore, Karnataka, India

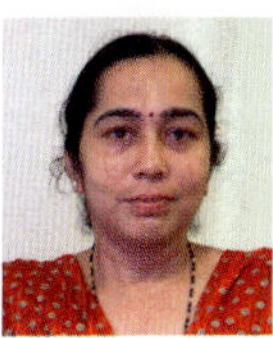

Ramya Shenoy MDS
Reader
Department of Community and
Preventive Dentistry
Manipal College of Dental Sciences
Manipal University
Mangalore, Karnataka, India

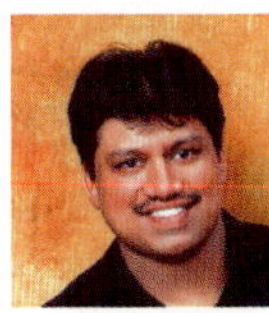

Sumanth KN MDS
Professor and Head
Department of Oral Medicine and Radiology
Thai Moogambigai Dental College and Hospital
Dr MGR University
Chennai, Tamil Nadu, India

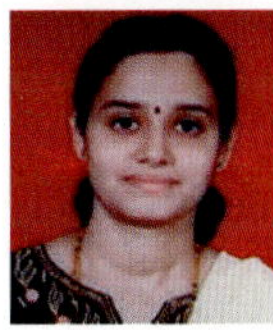

Suprabha BS MDS
Associate Professor
Department of Pedodontics and
Preventive Dentistry
Manipal College of Dental Sciences
Manipal University
Mangalore, Karnataka, India

Foreword

I am extremely pleased to write the foreword for the third edition of the book titled *Principles and Practice of Pedodontics* by Dr Arathi Rao. I have seen the book grow from its first edition to the present edition. The previous editions of this book have done extremely well and have fulfilled the need for a concise and comprehensive book, as reflected by its enormous popularity.

Dr Arathi Rao is an extremely focused and goal-oriented professional. She is committed to her specialty and department. Her concern for children and their health has made her achieve, what she is today as both an academician and a clinician. She is very innovative, always ready with new ideas and definitely this quality will help her achieve higher levels in her career.

The second edition was a brilliant upgrade. The present edition is definitely a class ahead. I would like to congratulate the author for bringing out the present edition and wish her good success in all her endeavors.

V Surendra Shetty MDS
Dean
Manipal College of Dental Sciences
Mangalore, Karnataka, India

Preface to the Third Edition

Progress in information and research is non-stoppable neither my addition of new information to the previous editions of my book. Pulp Therapy and Preventive Dentistry are two divisions of Pedodontic Practice that have been expanding in great speed. Newer additions in the Pulp Therapy chapter have been techniques like use of MTA (Mineral Trioxide Aggregate), Apical Plug Placement, Regeneration, etc.

Preventive Dentistry is the most revolutionized branch of Pediatric Dentistry. Newer concepts of management, such as Caries Risk Assessment, Dental Home, Anticipatory Guidance, etc. have been included.

Child Psychology has always been a difficult chapter to understand. In the present edition, I have enriched this topic and have tried to make it easy-to-understand and interesting.

The presentation of the chapters have been modified and merged into different sections for easy understanding. Questions are added at the end of each chapter. I believe this will help the students to evaluate themselves. And those with extra thirst for information can benefit from the References and Further Reading at the end of each chapter.

Arathi Rao

Preface to the First Edition

Pedodontics has always been a subject which is interesting but very vast. It is very difficult to find a book that is complete and suited for the undergraduate students, which is comprehensive, yet easy to understand. I have tried to cover all the topics in compliance with the syllabus of various universities in a very easy-to-understand way with adequate illustrations. Some extra useful information is given in separate boxes which makes it easy to read and remember. This book is aimed at helping the undergraduate students to have a better knowledge of pedodontics and to reproduce the same during the examinations.

I would request the readers to send their valuable suggestions and advice to me.

Arathi Rao

Acknowledgments

Thanks to all the students all over the country and abroad for appreciating the previous editions of the book.

Three people to whom I vow what I am today are—my parents Dr (Prof) K Nagesh Rao and Mrs Usha N Rao, and my dear guide Dr Subrato Sarkar.

The affection and support given to me by my family is heartening.

Last but not least for whom my whole life is dedicated, Arjun my wonderful son, without whom there is no meaning to my life.

Contents

Introduction

INTRODUCTION

A young child is definitely more than just a miniature adult. Managing and convincing a child as a patient for any dental procedure requires extra effort. Pedodontics is a specialized subject that deals with the management of oral and dental problems in children. Pedodontists are specialists who have mastered these skills and are in a position to manage children. It is a challenging venture where only few dare to go.

Pediatric dentistry as it is also referred to, in the beginning was mainly concerned with extraction and restorations. The trend in pedodontic practice has changed from extractions to preservation, concentrating on minimal invasion.

Pedodontists are in an excellent position to alter the growth pattern and improve the resistance to diseases, as he or she deals with children during their formative periods.

DEFINITION

According to Stewart, Barber, Troutman and Wei (1982)[1]–

"Pediatric dentistry is the practice and teaching of comprehensive preventive and therapeutic oral health care of child from birth through adolescence. It is constructed to include care for special patients who demonstrate mental, physical or emotional problems."

According to the American Academy of Pediatric Dentistry (AAPD) and Approved by the Council on Dental Education, American Dental Association (1995) –

"Pediatric dentistry is an age-defined specialty that provides both primary and specialty, comprehensive, preventive and therapeutic oral health care for infants and children through adolescence including those with special health care needs."

It, therefore, emphasizes the importance of initiating professional oral health intervention in infancy and continuing through adolescence and beyond.

- First textbook describing the dental problems and management for children was published in the year 1924.
- The American Society for the Promotion of Dentistry for Children was established at Detroit in the year 1927. The name was later changed to American Society of Dentistry for children in the year 1940.
- The American Academy of Pedodontics was started in the year 1947 and later in the year 1984 was changed to American Academy of Pediatric Dentistry.

List of pedodontic and related journals

1. Journal of Indian Society of Pedodontics and Preventive Dentistry
2. Journal of Dentistry for Children
3. International Journal of Pediatric Dentistry
4. Journal of Clinical Pediatric Dentistry
5. Journal of Dental Traumatology
6. Fluorides
7. Journal of Canadian Dental Association
8. Journal of American Dental Association
9. Journal of Dental Research
10. Quintessence International
11. British Dental Journal
12. European Journal of Oral Sciences
13. Endodontology

List of some of the pedodontic associations

1. Indian Society of Pedodontic and Preventive Dentistry (ISPPD)
2. American Academy of Pediatric Dentistry (AAPD)
3. British Society of Pediatric Dentistry (BSPD)
4. International Association of Pediatric Dentistry (IAPD)

PEDODONTICS IN INDIA

1. First dental college began as "Calcutta Dental College and Hospital in the year 1920, by Dr R Ahmed which was later renamed as Dr R Ahmed Dental College and Hospital. He is called as the 'The Grand Old Man of Dentistry in India'.
2. Initially, pedodontics as a subject, was combined with orthodontics and only in the year 1978 was introduced as a separate subject for undergraduates.
3. Pedodontics became a separate specialty much before it was introduced as a separate subject for the undergraduates in the year 1950 at Government Dental College, Amritsar.
4. Indian Society of Pedodontics and Preventive Dentistry began functioning in the year 1979.
5. November 14th was declared as the 'Pedodontists Day' by the Indian Society of Pedodontics and Preventive Dentistry at their annual meeting in 2010.

AIMS AND OBJECTIVES OF PEDODONTIC PRACTICE

1. The services rendered to the child must be focused from the point what is best for the child at that moment and also for the adult into whom the child will eventually grow.
2. The child should be treated as a whole. Effort must be made for the general and oral health to be in accordance with each other.
3. Prevention of oral diseases must be the prime motive and should begin if possible from before the birth, directing the expectant mothers.
4. Educating parents regarding importance of deciduous teeth, dental treatment and preservation of teeth.
5. Developing dentition and jaws should be observed regularly so that any developing malocclusion can be intervened at the right time.
6. Relief of pain and sepsis forms one of the main theme of a care provider.
7. To achieve and maintain esthetics.
8. Improving personal information data bank is very important and can be done thorough updating of both clinical and theoretical knowledge on a regular basis.

SCOPE OF PEDODONTICS

1. Pedodontics encompasses a variety of disciplines, techniques, procedures and skills, all which are aimed, adapted and targeted to achieve healthy oral health to children.
2. Pediatric dentistry is an age specific specialty. It is not just a technique or disease specific specialty and thus covers a wide range of treatment procedures that can be provided to a child patient.
3. Since it deals with children, pedodontists are in an excellent position to monitor growth and accordingly deal with the arising problems.
4. Pediatric dentists have extended services to fulfill the needs of the special child, including physically, medically and mentally handicapped.
5. They also form team members in the management of cleft lip and palate patients.

SPECIFIC DIFFERENCES BETWEEN CHILD AND ADULT PATIENTS

Child is in a dynamic state of growth and development and is thus a changing person. The differences between a child and an adult are obvious. But there also exists significant difference between a 2-year and a 13-year-old child. Therefore, a child is unique and different at each stage of his or her pediatric life.

Three general areas in which pediatric patients are unique compared to the adults are:
1. Physiologic and anatomic differences
2. Pharmacokinetics
3. Emotional differences

Physiologic and Anatomic Differences[2-5]

These differences can be discussed based on body size, body fluids, respiratory system, cardiovascular system and the urinary system.

Body Size

i. Less amount of drug is needed to reach an effective plasma level but less is also needed to produce toxicity in children due to small body size.
ii. Height and weight of children are less than that of adults; their proportions also differ from adults.
iii. Ratio of body surface area (BSA) to body weight is about seven times greater for neonates than for adults. Many physiologic functions are proportional to BSA, which may be the reasons why some professionals advocate the use of body surface area to calculate drug dose.
iv. Smaller the patient, the higher is the basal metabolic rate, oxygen consumption and fluid requirement per hour.

> Child's weight increases by about 20 times from birth to adulthood and height increases only about 3½ times.

Body Fluids

i. Children have larger volume of total body water (TBW). Child's TBW is 80% of body weight and that of an adult's is 50-60%. This has direct bearing on pharmacokinetics of water soluble medications. Because these drugs are distributed to a relatively larger volume once absorbed, a larger dose is necessary to achieve therapeutic effect in a small child.
ii. Total body fat also varies: Fat content in a premature infant is about 1% of the body weight, whereas a full-term infant's body fat is about 16% of the body weight. In a one year old it forms 22% of body weight, four year old 12% and in 10-11 years it forms 18-20% of body weight.

   The child with the smaller percentage of body fat thus requires a smaller dose of a lipid soluble drug. Lipid soluble drugs such as barbiturates and diazepam may require higher dosage in an obese child as most of it will be distributed to fat tissues, therefore, decreasing their effective plasma levels.

Respiratory System

i. Relatively large head, narrow nasal passage, smaller diameter of glottis and trachea predisposes the child to increased risk of airway obstruction. Tongue is proportionally larger, larger mass of lymphoid tissues, more copious secretions and loose glottic areolar tissue further compromises the airway. This makes it difficult to manage the child during sedation, general anesthesia or respiratory emergency.
ii. In a child smaller bony thorax and soft sternum provide a less stable base for the ribs and intercostal muscles. Ribs are more horizontal than in adults and do not allow as much chest expansion as do the more vertically curved adult ribs.
iii. A child cannot compensate as readily as an adult by increasing ventilatory volumes by increasing chest expansion. So a child is more dependent on the diaphragm as the primary muscle of respiration. Thus care should be taken not to impede diaphragm movement, which might occur when the child is made to lie supine or with head low because the abdominal contents will place gravitational forces on the diaphragm.
iv. Respiratory rate of the child is higher due to higher metabolic rate.
v. Basal metabolic rate (BMR) in children is double that of an adult thus requiring greater oxygen consumption and carbon dioxide production.

> **Respiration rate**
>
> Newborn—30-60/min
> 1 year—20-35/min
> 5-year—20-25 /min
> 15-year—15-20 /min
> Adult—12-20/min

Cardiovascular System

i. Relative blood volume in children is greatest at birth and decreases with age.

   In a newborn, it is 85 ml/kg and in adult it is 70 ml/kg.
ii. Heart rate is highest in infants.
iii. Parasympathetic tone (vagal) is more pronounced in infants due to immaturity of sympathetic nervous system. Any vagal stimulation may cause a decrease in heart rate, as seen with manipulation of the airway (endotracheal intubation), bladder distension and pressure on eyes. For these reasons children undergoing treatment under general anesthesia should be given parasympathetic blockers such as atropine.
iv. In a newborn, peripheral circulation is very much poorly developed. This is important as uptake of intramuscular injections are low.

v. About 40% of the cardiac output in children contributes to the cerebral blood flow, compared to only about 29% in adult.

Heart rate

Newborn—115-170/min
1 year—90-135/min
5-year—80-120 /min
15-year—70-100 /min
Adult—70/min

Systolic blood pressure

Newborn—60-75 mm/Hg
1 year—96 mm/Hg
5-year—100 mm/Hg
15-year—120 mm/Hg
Adult—120-125 mm/Hg

Urinary System

i. Level of urine concentration by the kidneys is very much low in neonates. Therefore, infants require more free water per day. Infant and young child may become rapidly dehydrated.

ii. Glomerular filteration rate (GFR) of an infant is 30-50% of an adult which may be due to less mature glomeruli and lower blood pressure. So drugs that are excreted primarily by glomerular filtration have longer half lives (up to 50% longer) in a child. Example of such drugs are aminoglycoside antibiotics, digoxin and curare. GFR reaches adult level by 3-6 months.

iii. Tubular reabsorption and tubular secretion also vary and mature to adult levels during the first few months of life.

Pharmacokinetics[6-8]

It is a dynamic process of drug turnover in the body, which includes absorption, distribution, biotrans-formation and elimination. It determines a drug plasma concentration, duration of action and its effectiveness and toxicity.

Factors affecting kinetics of drug

Dose and form of the drug, plasma protein binding, ionization, lipid solubility, rate of metabolism and volume of distribution.

Uptake of the Drug and Absorption

i. Pulmonary uptake of nitrous oxide is more rapid in infants due to higher cardiac output, good alveolar ventilation and higher percentage of richly perfused visceral tissues.

ii. Topical medications are absorbed more rapidly and completely in children, due to greater permeability and relatively inactive sebaceous glands.

iii. Gastric emptying time in a newborn is 6-8 hours compared to 2 hours in an older child and adult. Younger children have a lower gastric pH, promoting greater absorption of weakly acidic drugs such as penicillin, while delaying absorption of weakly basic drugs such as diazepam and theophyllin. Irregular peristalsis slows down the transit time in the bowel in young infants causing net effect of slower drug absorption. Active transport mechanisms in the bowel mucosa aiding in drug absorption are deficient in infants.

Drug Distribution

i. Neonates and infants have decreased plasma protein concentration especially albumin. This reduces the binding sites of the drug and they remain unbound or in the free form making it available to produce its pharmacological effect. Drugs that are highly protein bound, displace other protein bound drugs. Compounds like bilirubin, sulfonamides, vitamin K are known to displace protein bound bilirubin leading to hyperbilirubinemia and resultant kernicterus (brain damage).

ii. Drugs penetrate blood brain barrier more easily in children than in adults, due to lack of myelination of the nervous tissue and greater membrane permeability. This can be advantages, when it is needed for the antibiotics to reach the CNS, but may be disadvantages owing to the greater sensitivity to CNS depressant like narcotics.

iii. Children require higher concentration of inhalation anesthetics due to decreased receptor site sensitivity to drug. This sensitivity changes with the child's development. Other than this notable exception, children are more sensitive and are, therefore, more prone to drug toxicity.

Drug Metabolism

i. In children, liver enzyme production that is responsible for biotransformation of drugs may be almost absent, reduced or even overproduced at various stages of development.

ii. Poor oxidative rates in infants result in prolonged effects of diazepam, phenytoin and other drugs.

iii. Poor conjugation results in prolonged effects of amphetamines and phenacetin.

iv. Low levels of glucuronyl transferase in newborn, results in an inability to detoxify the antibiotic chloramphenicol, sulfisoxazole, morphine and steroids and thus increasing their sensitivity. Glucoronyl transferase reaches normal levels by 1 month of age.

v. Psuedocholinesterase levels are only 60% of normal for several months after birth.

Drug Excretion

At birth, the ability of the kidneys to clear drugs and concentrate urine is greatly reduced leading to prolongation of the effects of drug that are primarily excreted by the kidneys such as ampicillin, etc.

Emotional Differences

a. The major difference between the treatment of children and an adult is the treatment relationship. Treatment relationship between the dentist and the adult patient is one to one whereas in case of a child patient there is a one to two relationship, with the child being the focus of attention of the dentist as well as the parent. This is represented by the pedodontic treatment triangle as given by Wright[9] (Figs 1.1 and 1.2). The child occupies the apex of the triangle and is the focus of attention of both the dentist and the parent. All the three are interrelated and the arrows denote that the communication is reciprocal. Recently society has been added, meaning that the influence of the society on the child has to be considered affecting the treatment modalities.

b. Children exhibit a fear of the unknown.

c. They do not know to rationalize.

d. Behavior management modalities differ, depending on the age and understanding.

e. Children have less concentration time. Therefore, treatment time should be restricted to not more than 20-30 minutes.

f. Treatment appointments should be preferably given during the morning time and avoided during their nap time.

g. Adult patient seeks treatment by his own will, but the child patient visits the dentist usually by the will of his parents.

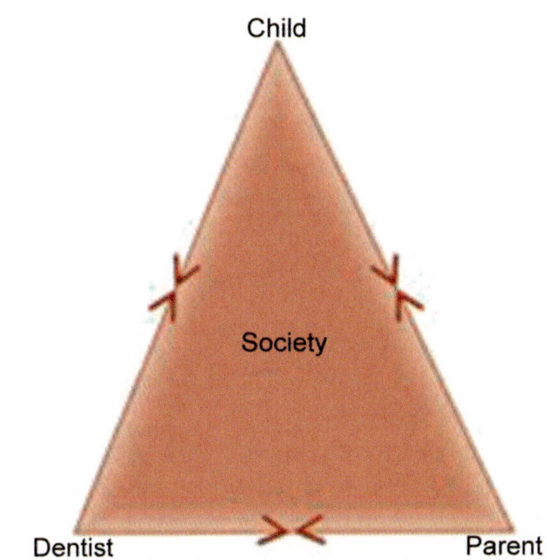

Fig. 1.1: The pedodontic treatment triangle

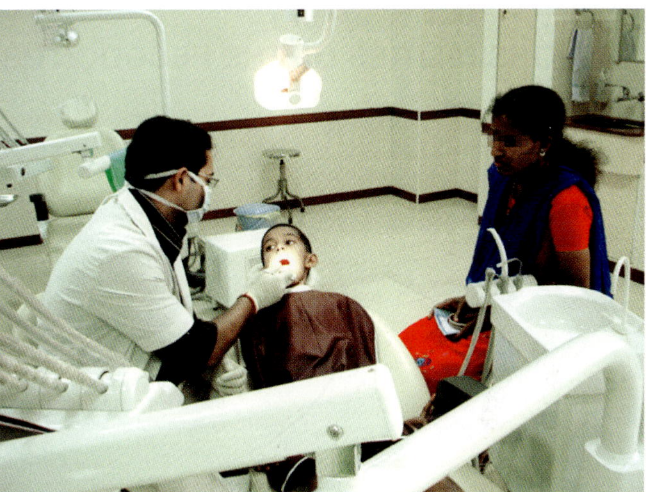

Fig. 1.2: Operatory area where the positioning of the child, operator and the parent resembles triangle and helps in proper communication

General principles of pediatric pharmacology

1. The metric system, rather than apothecary system should be used to determine dosage. Instead of 1 tbsp, 15 ml is preferred.

2. Younger the patient, the more atypical the therapeutic and toxicological response to drug therapy.

3. In older patients the depth of anesthesia is more profound compared to the younger children.

4. Respiratory alkalosis, the initial stage of salicylate intoxication seen in older children and adults is rare or short lived in infants.

5. Immaturity in blood-brain barrier or differences in enzymatic degradation of drugs may account for age dependent variations in response.

Contd...

Contd...

6. The younger the child, the more atypical is the disease manifestations.
7. In infants seizures are characterized only by limpness or apnea. Motor seizures appear as limited tonic stiffening or partial movement of the face and limbs.
8. True petit mal epilepsy is rare before 2 years and after 20 years.
9. Prolonged therapy with agents that affect the endocrine system retards the growth. Large doses of corticosteroids retard growth.
10. Excessive use of syrups and elixers containing sugar, damage teeth and should be avoided especially at night.
11. During nitrous oxide sedation, oxygen supply should be maintained at least at 20% and not less.
12. Allergenicity is greatest during childhood in less than 15 years of age.
13. Tetracycline should be used sparingly and preferably not used in children less than 8-year-old.
14. Dosage rules such as Young's, Cowling's, Catzel's or Clark's rule should be followed. For anesthesia Young's or Clarke's rule is used.

Young's Formula:

$$= \frac{Age \times Adult\ Dose}{Age + 12}$$

Clarke's Formula:

$$= \frac{Body\ Wt.\ (lb) \times Adult\ Dose}{150}$$

RESPONSIBILITIES OF THE PEDODONTIST

REFERENCES

1. Stewart RE, Barber TK, Troutman KC, Wei SHY. Pediatric dentistry, CV Mosby Co 1982.
2. Howry LB, Bindler RM, Tso Y. Physiologic considerations in pediatric medications. Philadelphia, JB Lippincott Co. 1981;3-17.
3. Campbell RL, Weiner M, Stewart LM. General anesthesia for the pediatric patient. J Oral Maxillofacial Surg 1982; 40:497-506.
4. Crawford JD, et al. Simplification of drug dosage calculation by applications of the surface area principle. Pediatrics 1950;5:783-9.
5. Johnson TR. Moore WM, Jeffries JE. Children are different: Developmental Physiology. Columbus, Ohio, Ross Laboratories 1978.
6. Salanitre E, Rockow H. The pulmonary exchange of nitrous oxide and halothane in infants and children. Anesthesiology 1969;30:388.
7. Morselli P. Clinical pharmacokinetics in neonates. Clin Pharmacokinet 1976;1:81-98.
8. Anderson JA. Physiologic principles in pediatric dentistry, in Pinkham's pediatric dentistry infancy through adolescence, WB Saunders 1994.
9. Wright GZ, Stigers JI. Nonpharmacologic management of children's behaviors. Dentistry for the child and adolescent, 9th Ed, Elsevier Mosby 2011;27-40.

FURTHER READING

1. American Academy of Pediatric Dentistry Council on Clinical Affairs. Policy on the role of pediatric dentists as both primary and specialty care providers. Pediatr Dent 2005-2006;27(7 Reference Manual):60
2. American Academy of Pediatric Dentistry Council on Clinical Affairs. Policy on the ethics of failure to treat or refer. Pediatr Dent 2005-2006;27(7 Reference Manual):61.
3. Brennan DS, Spencer AJ. The role of dentist, practice and patient factors in the provision of dental services. Community Dent Oral Epidemiol 2005;33(3):181-95.

4. Goldman HM, Guernsey LH. The role of the dental specialist in the hospital. Dent Clin North Am 1975; 19(4):665-74.
5. Jessee SA. Risk factors as determinants of dental neglect in children. ASDC J Dent Child 1998;65(1):17-20.
6. Konig KG. The role of the dentist in prevention of dental disease. Int Dent J 1974;24(4):443-7.
7. Mouradian WE. Ethical principles and the delivery of children's oral health care. Ambul Pediatr 2002;2(2 Suppl):162-8.
8. Nainar SM. Pediatric dental practice: reconstruction or dis-intermediation. ASDC J Dent Child 2000;67(2):107-11, 82.
9. Pinkham JR. An analysis of the phenomenon of increased parental participation during the child's dental experience. ASDC J Dent Child 1991;58(6):458-63.
10. Rich JP 3rd, Straffon L, Inglehart MR. General dentists and pediatric dental patients: the role of dental education. J Dent Educ 2006;70(12):1308-15.
11. Ryan KJ. The role of the voluntary dental association and the private practitioner. J Dent Child 1967;34(2):74-9.

QUESTIONS

1. Give the American Academy of Pediatric Dentistry (AAPD) definition of Pediatric Dentistry.
2. What are the aims and objectives of pedodontic practice?
3. Explain the scope of pedodontics.
4. Give the specific differences between child and adult patients.
5. Explain the physiologic and anatomic differences.
6. Write in detail the uptake of the drug and absorption and distribution in children.
7. Explain the emotional differences between a child and an adult.
8. What is a pedodontic treatment triangle?
9. Give the general principles of pediatric pharmacology.

Morphology of Deciduous Teeth

INTRODUCTION

Studying tooth morphology includes understanding the shape, configuration and parts of a tooth. It is very important for clinical application during performing various procedures. Cavity preparations must conform to the thickness of enamel and dentin, keeping in mind the location and size of the pulp. Restoration of natural contours and morphology of deciduous teeth is needed for function, which can be achieved only with a good knowledge of tooth morphology.

DIFFERENCES BETWEEN A DECIDUOUS TOOTH AND A PERMANENT TOOTH (FIG. 2.1)

Features of a Deciduous Crown

1. The crown of the deciduous tooth is shorter than the permanent tooth.
2. The occlusal table of a deciduous tooth is narrower labiolingually than is the permanent tooth.
3. The deciduous tooth is constricted in the cervical portion of the crown.
4. The enamel and dentin layers are thinner in the deciduous tooth.
5. The enamel rods in the gingival third extend in a slightly occlusal direction from the dentinoenamel junction in deciduous teeth but extend slightly apically in the permanent dentition.
6. The contact areas between the deciduous molars are very broad and flat.
7. The color of the deciduous tooth is lighter than permanent teeth. The refractive index of milk is

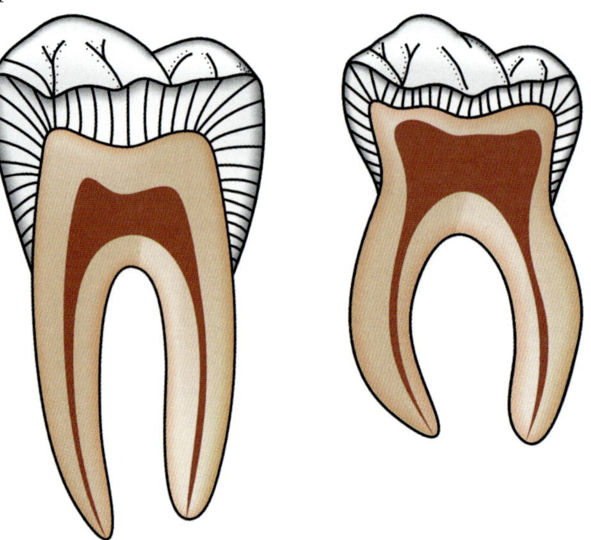

Fig. 2.1: Longitudinal section of a permanent and deciduous tooth

similar to deciduous tooth enamel. Hence the teeth are termed as milk tooth.

Features of a Deciduous Pulp

1. The pulp of the deciduous tooth is larger than that of the permanent tooth in relation to the crown size.
2. The pulp horns of the deciduous tooth (especially the mesial horns) are closer to the outer surface of the tooth than are those of the permanent tooth.
3. The mandibular molar has larger pulp chambers than does the maxillary molar in the deciduous tooth.
4. The form of the pulp chamber of the deciduous tooth follows the surface of the crown.
5. Usually there is a pulp horn under each cusp.
6. Thin and slender roots pulp canals, thin pulp canals.
7. Accessory canals extend from floor of the pulpal chamber to the furcation or interradicular area.
8. Increased blood supply, due to which the deciduous pulp exhibits typical inflammatory response.
9. Responds by inflammatory process, resulting in increased internal resorption.
10. Reduced sensitivity to pain—due to less number of nerve fibers.
11. Increased reparative dentin formation.
12. Poor localization of infection and inflammation.
13. Multiple ramification, making complete debridement impossible.
14. Ribbon shaped root canal (hour glass appearance) that is narrower mesiodistally, discourages gross enlargement of the canal.

Features of a Deciduous Root

1. The root of the deciduous anterior tooth is narrower mesiodistally than is that of the permanent anterior tooth.
2. The roots of the posterior deciduous tooth are longer and more slender in relation to crown size than are those of the permanent tooth.
3. The roots of the deciduous molar flare more as they approach the apex (which affords the necessary room for the development of the permanent tooth buds) than do the permanent molar roots.

MORPHOLOGY OF INDIVIDUAL DECIDUOUS TEETH

Maxillary Incisors (Figs 2.2 and 2.3)
- The maxillary central and lateral incisors usually erupt by 7-8 months of age.

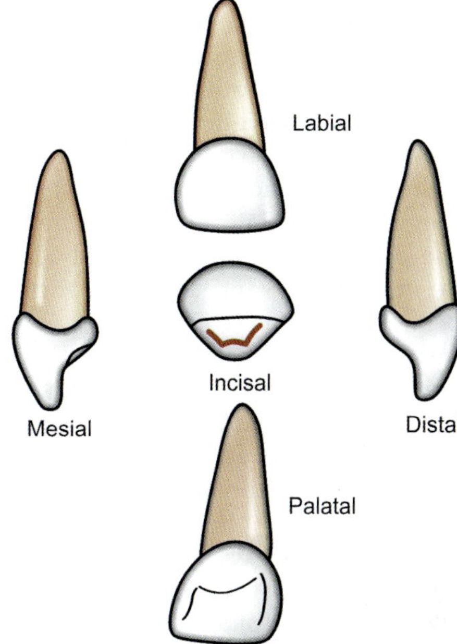

Fig. 2.2: Maxillary central incisor

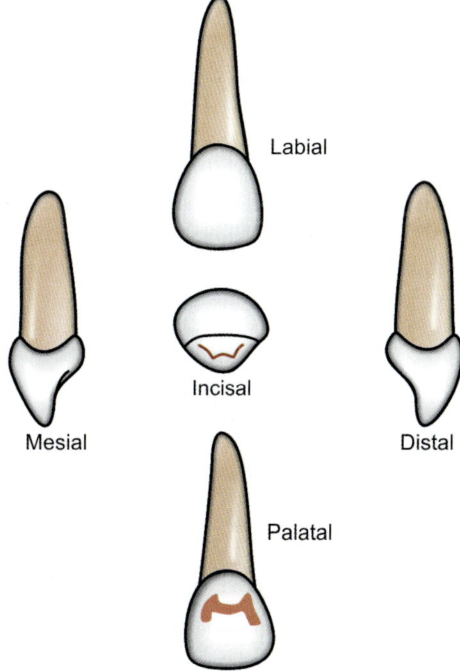

Fig. 2.3: Maxillary lateral incisor

- The deciduous maxillary central incisor is unique in that it is the only tooth in the human dentition that has a greater mesiodistal dimension than crown height.
- The contact points with adjacent teeth are broad, extending from the incisal one-third to the gingival one-third.

- Labial surface is flat.
- There is a prominent lingual cingulum.
- The root is conical and roughly two and a half times as long as the crown height.
- Anatomy of the pulp: The central incisor has two or three small projections (pulp horns) toward the incisal edge. The mesial pulp horn is most prominent. The pulp horn is approximately 2.3-2.4 mm from the incisal edge and about 1.2 mm from the dentinoenamel junction (DEJ).
- The maxillary lateral incisor is smaller than the maxillary central incisor. The distal incisal aspect is rounded. The crown and root are more conical. The pulp chamber is smaller and is about 2.6 mm from the incisal edge and approximately 0.9 mm from the DEJ.

Mandibular Incisors (Figs 2.4 and 2.5)

- These teeth are the first to erupt into the oral cavity at about 6 to 7 months of age.
- The mandibular central incisor is almost flat when viewed from the labial aspect.
- There are no developmental grooves or mamelons.
- The crown is one-third the length of the root with a cingulum on the lingual surface.
- The root is long and cylindrical.
- Anatomy of the pulp: The pulp canal follows the outline form of the surface topography of the primary mandibular central and lateral incisors. The pulp is approximately 2.6 mm from the incisal edge in the primary central incisor. The pulp of the mandibular lateral incisor has similar dimensions but is somewhat smaller.

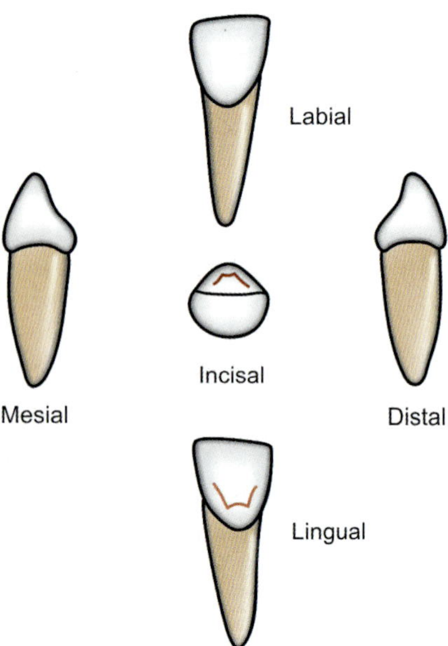

Fig. 2.4: Mandibular central incisor

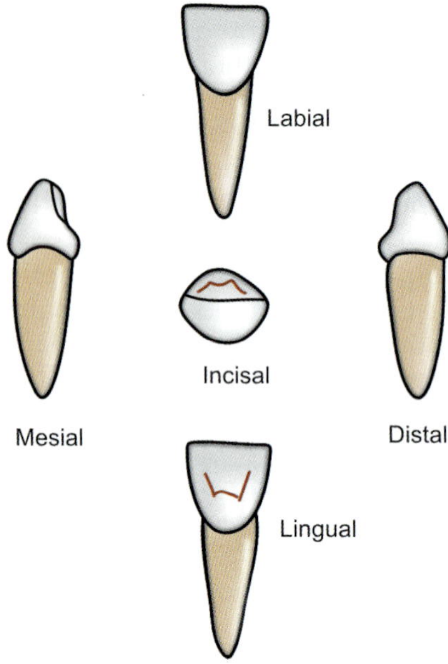

Fig. 2.5: Mandibular lateral incisor

- The primary mandibular lateral incisor is distinguished from the mandibular central incisor by the distoincisal angle, which is more rounded. In overall dimensions, the primary lateral incisor is somewhat longer but narrower than the primary central incisor.

Maxillary Canines (Fig. 2.6)

- They erupt at about 18 months of age.
- It is best described as being long and sharp.
- The crown is constricted at the cementoenamel junction.
- The marginal ridges on the primary canines are usually less distinct, but there is often a prominent cingulum.
- The long slender root is more than twice the crown length.
- Anatomy of the pulp: The pulp chamber follows the general contour of the tooth. The pulp horn is 3.2 mm from the cuspal tip.

Mandibular Canines (Fig. 2.7)

- The mandibular canines erupt at about 16 months of age.
- It is a long narrow tooth, much smaller than the primary maxillary canine.
- The distal marginal ridge is much lower than the mesial marginal ridge.
- The point of contact is very close to the cervical third of the tooth.
- The root is long and slender and is about twice the crown length.

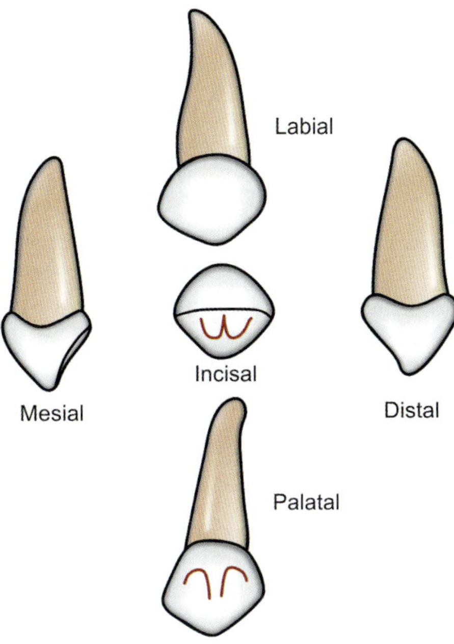

Fig. 2.6: Maxillary canine

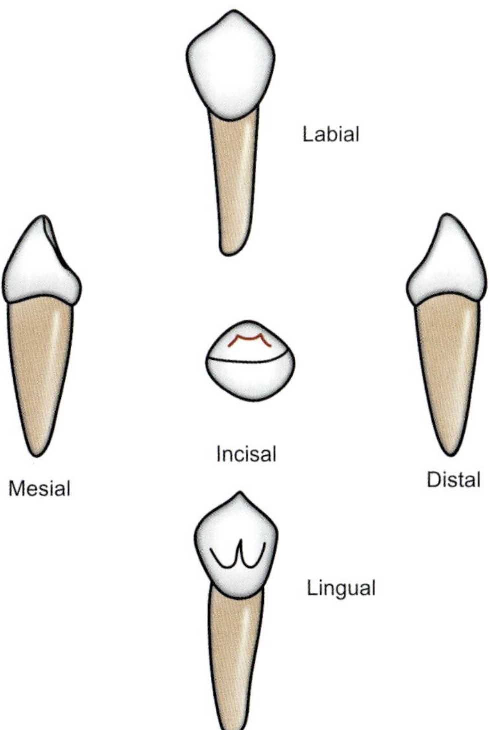

Fig. 2.7: Mandibular canine

- Anatomy of the pulp: The pulp chamber follows the general outline of the tooth form. The pulp is 3.0 mm from the cuspal tip.

Maxillary First Molars (Fig. 2.8)

- The primary maxillary first molars usually erupt by 16 months of age.
- The primary maxillary first molar resembles a molar and a premolar.
- The occlusal surface consists of three cusps, one each on the mesiobuccal and distobuccal surfaces and one on the lingual surface. This gives the tooth a square look.
- There are three slender roots, one beneath each cusp tip.
- A characteristic of all primary molars is that the furcation of the roots begins at the cementoenamel junction. This is not apparent in permanent molars. There is a very prominent buccal cervical ridge.
- Anatomy of the pulp: The pulp horns correspond to each cusp; the mesiobuccal pulp horn is the most prominent. The mesiobuccal pulp horn is 1.8 mm, the distobuccal pulp horn is 2.3 mm, and the palatal pulp horn is 2.0 mm from the cusp tip.

Mandibular First Molars (Fig. 2.9)

- This primary molar erupts by the 14-16th month of life.
- It has four cusps, two buccal and two lingual.
- The occlusal surface is narrow due to the convergence of the mesiobuccal and mesiolingual cusps.
- Transverse ridge is very prominent and divides the occlusal surface.

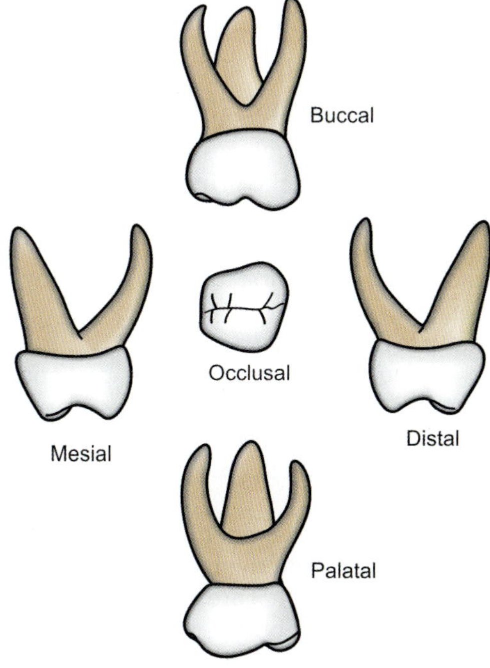

Fig. 2.8: Maxillary first molar

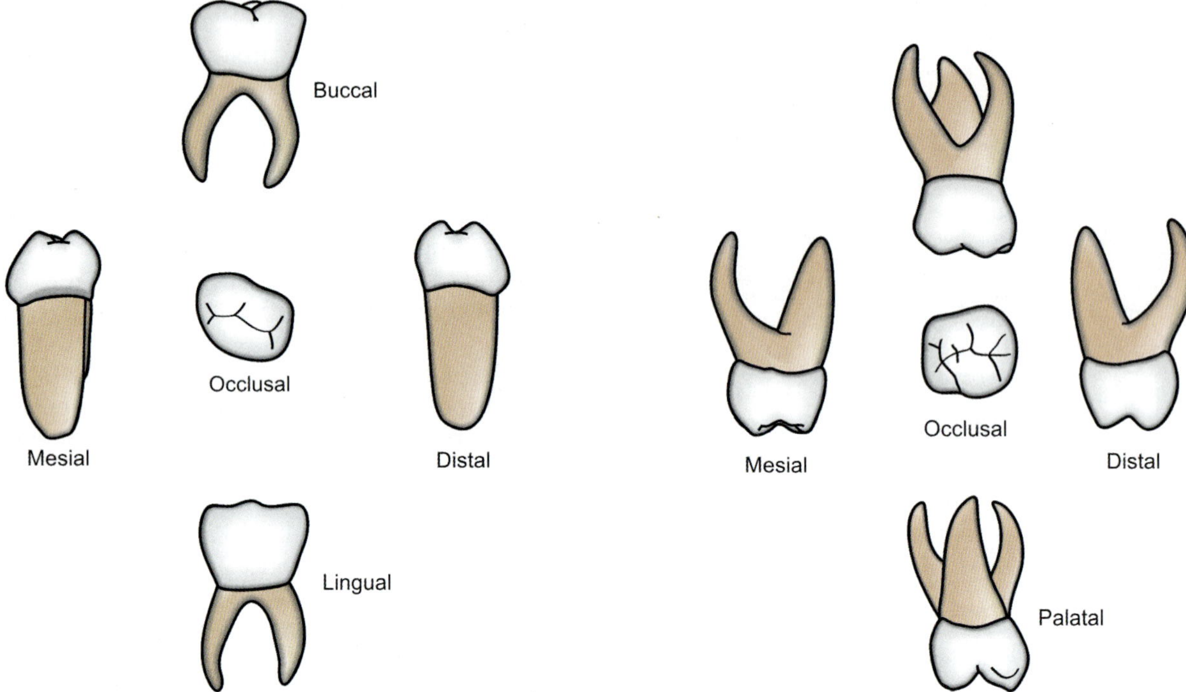

Fig. 2.9: Mandibular first molar

Fig. 2.10: Maxillary second molar

- The enamel of this tooth is uniformly thick.
- There are two broad but thin mesiodistal roots, one on the mesial aspect and one on the distal aspect.
- Anatomy of the pulp: There are four pulp horns with one pulp horn beneath each cusp. Both buccal and lingual mesial pulp horns are 2.1 mm from the DEJ while the distal pulp horns are 2.4 mm away from the DEJ.

Maxillary Second Molars (Fig. 2.10)

- The primary second molars are the last primary teeth to erupt, completing the primary dentition by 28-30 months of age.
- The primary maxillary second molar resembles the permanent maxillary first molar in appearance but is smaller.
- The tooth is rhomboidal.
- There are four cusps, two on the buccal and two on the lingual aspects.
- Often there is a fifth cusp or prominence, called as the tubercle of Carabelli on the palatal surface of the mesiopalatal cusp.
- A prominent transverse or oblique ridge connects the distolingual cusp with the mesiopalatal cusp.
- There are three roots that are curved to accommodate the developing tooth bud beneath.
- The enamel is usually 1.2 mm thick uniformly on the tooth.

- Anatomy of the pulp: There may be four or five pulp horns, which usually are most prominent beneath each cusp tip. The mesiobuccal pulp horn, as usual, is the largest and closest to the DEJ. The mesiobuccal pulp horn is usually 2.8 mm from the DEJ, while the distobuccal horn is 3.1 mm from the DEJ.

Mandibular Second Molars (Fig. 2.11)

- The primary mandibular second molar resembles a permanent mandibular first molar.
- There are five cusps, three on the buccal surface and two on the lingual.
- The enamel is uniformly 1.2 mm thick.
- There are two roots which are narrow mesiodistally but very broad buccolingually.
- The roots are somewhat curved to accommodate the developing tooth bud.
- Anatomy of the pulp: There are five pulp horns corresponding to the five cusp tips. The mesiobuccal pulp horn is the largest, extending 2.8 mm from the DEJ, while the distobuccal pulp horn is 3.1 mm from the dentinoenamel junction.

PRACTICAL APPLICATION OF UNDERSTANDING TOOTH MORPHOLOGY

Influence of primary tooth morphology for practical applications such as tooth preparations, stainless steel

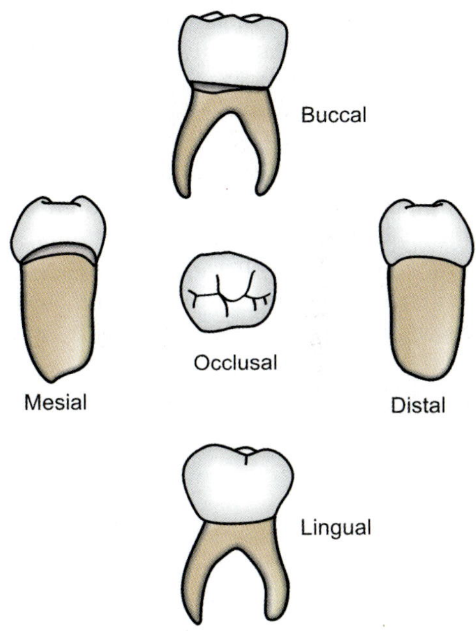

Fig. 2.11: Mandibular second molar

crown preparations, surgical procedures and pulp therapy are as follows:

1. Tooth preparations
   A. Modifications in the cavity depth and extension is required due to reduced thickness of enamel and dentin.
   B. Width of the occlusal cavity should be very much narrow in compliance with the narrow occlusal table.
   C. The interproximal contacts of primary teeth are broad and flat compared to those of permanent teeth. Use of a good wedge at the cervical part of the proximal box is necessary during material insertion and condensation into the proximal box.
   D. It is difficult to obtain an adequate gingival seat while preparing a Class II cavity due to the cervical constriction present in deciduous teeth. Trying to prepare a gingival seat in a deep cavity may lead to encroachment into pulp chamber.
2. Stainless steel crown preparations
   A. The prominent mesiobuccal cervical ridge of mandibular and maxillary first molars must be accommodated in the preparation of stainless steel crowns, which may otherwise result in a 'rocking' crown.
   B. The gingival contour of the cervical margin that varies from the buccal to lingual to proximal aspects should be replicated while fabricating the crown. The cervical border of the crown must flow parallel to this gingival contour.
   C. The cervical border of the crown must be placed below the cervical bulge of the tooth to obtain maximum retention.
3. Surgical procedures
   A. Conical roots of primary anterior teeth facilitate easy removal.
   B. Extraction of deciduous molar teeth must be made with great caution. The premolar tooth bud is located between the flared roots of primary molars, which may be avulsed during deciduous tooth extraction.
4. Pulp therapy
   Understanding of the anatomy of the pulp, the number and curvature of the root canals is important during pulp treatment procedures.

FURTHER READING

1. Ali Fayyad M, Jamani KD, Agrabawi J. Geometric and mathematical proportions and their relations to maxillary anterior teeth. J Contemp Dent Pract 2006;7(5):62-70.
2. Alwazzan KA. Variation in mesiodistal crown width and amount of tooth exposure between right and left maxillary anterior teeth. Egypt Dent J 1995;41(3):1283-6.
3. Bishara SE, Khadivi P, Jakobsen JR. Changes in tooth size-arch length relationships from the deciduous to the permanent dentition: a longitudinal study. Am J Orthod Dentofacial Orthop 1995;108(6):607-13.
4. Brown T, Margetts B, Townsend GC. Comparison of mesiodistal crown diameters of the deciduous and permanent teeth in Australian aboriginals. Aust Dent J 1980;25(1):28-33.
5. Dempsey PJ, Townsend GC. Genetic and environmental contributions to variation in human tooth size. Heredity 2001;86(Pt 6):685-93
6. Eger T, Muller HP, Helnecke A. Ultrasonic determination of gingival thickness. Subject variation and influence of tooth type and clinical features. J Clin Periodontol 1996; 23(9):839-45.
7. Gillen RJ, Schwartz RS, Hilton TJ, Evans DB. An analysis of selected normative tooth proportions. Int J Prosthodont 1994;7(5):410-7.
8. Heikkinen T, Alvesalo L, Tienari J. Deciduous tooth crown size and asymmetry in strabismic children. Orthod Craniofac Res 2002;5(4):195-204.
9. Kabban M, Fearne J, Jovanovski V, Zou L. Tooth size and morphology in twins. Int J Paediatr Dent 2001;11(5):333-9.
10. Kannapan JG, Swaminathan S. A study on a dental morphological variation. Tubercle of Carabelli. Indian J Dent Res 2001;12(3):145-9.
11. Kondo S, Wakatsuki E, Shun-Te H, Sheng-Yen C, Shibazaki Y, Arai M. Comparison of the crown dimensions between the maxillary second deciduous molar and the first permanent molar. Okajimas Folia Anat J 1996; 73(4):179-84.

12. Liu HH, Dung SZ, Yang YH. Crown diameters of the deciduous teeth of Taiwanese. Kaohsiung J Med Sci 2000;16(6):299-307.
13. Morrow LA, Robbins JW, Jones DL, Wilson NH. Clinical crown length changes from age 12-19 years: a longitudinal study. J Dent 2000;28(7):469-73.
14. Olsson M, Lindhe J, Marinello CP. On the relationship between crown forms and clinical features of the gingiva in adolescents. J Clin Periodontol 1993;20(8):570-7.
15. Olsson M, Lindhe J. Periodontal characteristics in individuals with varying form of the upper central incisors. J Clin Periodontol 1991;18(1):78-82.
16. Rhee SH, Nahm DS. Triangular-shaped incisor crowns and crowding. Am J Orthod Dentofacial Orthop 2000; 118(6):624-8.
17. Singh SP, Goyal A. Mesiodistal crown dimensions of the permanent dentition in North Indian children. J Indian Soc Pedod Prev Dent 2006;24(4):192-6.
18. Sterrett JD, Oliver T, Robinson F, Fortson W, Knaak B, Russell CM. Width/length ratios of normal clinical crowns of the maxillary anterior dentition in man. J Clin Periodontol 1999;26(3):153-7.
19. Tsai HH. Morphological characteristics of the deciduous teeth. J Clin Pediatr Dent 2001 Winter;25(2):95-101.
20. Tsai HH. Dental crowding in primary dentition and its relationship to arch and crown dimensions. J Dent Child (Chic.) 2003;70(2):164-9.
21. Yuen KK, So LL, Tang EL. Mesiodistal crown diameters of the primary and permanent teeth in southern Chinesea longitudinal study. Eur J Orthod 1997;19(6):721-31.
22. Yuen KK, Tang EL, So LL. Relations between the mesiodistal crown diameters of the primary and permanent teeth of Hong Kong Chinese. Arch Oral Biol 1996;41(1):1-7.

QUESTIONS

1. Enumerate the difference between the deciduous and permanent teeth. What is its clinical importance?
2. Explain with diagram the morphology of deciduous lower second molar.
3. Write the clinical application of understanding of tooth morphology.

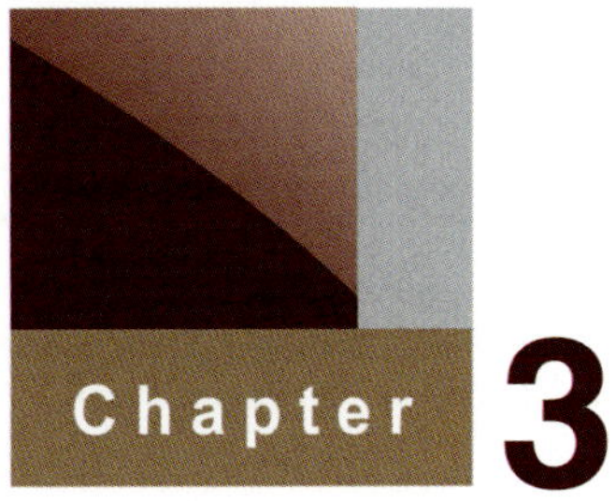

Chapter 3

Case History, Examination and Treatment Planning

INTRODUCTION

A thorough history, detailed examination and an accurate diagnosis, all of them are very essential for successful outcome of any treatment.

Children have different and distinct needs to be addressed at specific intervals, so the periodicities of professional oral health intervention and services are based on their individual needs and risk indicators. The first examination is recommended at the time of the eruption of the first tooth and no later than 12 months of age. Early detection and management of oral conditions can improve oral health and, in turn, the general health and well-being of the child.

Diagnosis and treatment planning thus includes assembling all the relevant facts obtained through history and examinations and to analyze each of them for determining the course of treatment.

NEED FOR PATIENT EVALUATION

1. To understand the difference between normal and abnormal.
2. In planning the treatment in a sequential order.
3. To determine the length of appointment.
4. To recognize any behavioral problems that may require treatment to be done under general anesthesia in a hospital setting.
5. To identify any medical problems that may require intervention or any modification in treatment.

Obtaining accurate data in a child is very difficult. The reasons may be any of the following:

1. Most of the times, it is the parent or the guardian who will be providing the required data about the child and not the child himself or herself.
2. It is impossible to observe everything a child does or says and make accurate records of what goes on.
3. Most children do not behave in the dental clinic the same way as they do at home or with their friends or teachers.
4. Data reported by parents and teachers may be inaccurate.
5. Information provided by parents or guardians is dependable on their emotional maturity.
6. Unless reports are made immediately after the observation, the parents may forget to mention minor yet important findings.
7. There may be a deliberate distortion by the observer to show the child or the parent in a favorable light.

The sequence of steps from case recording to implementation of the required plan are as follows:

1. **Vital statistics**
   a. Hospital registration number with date of first visit
   b. Name
   c. Age
   d. Sex
   e. Class and school
   f. Parents name and occupation
   g. Address and telephone number.
2. **Chief complaint**
3. **History**
   a. History of the chief complaint
   b. Medical history: Prenatal, natal, postnatal and present history
   c. Past dental history
   d. Family history
   e. Personal history: Oral hygiene, diet and oral habit history.
4. **Examination**
   - General examination
   - *Local examination*: Extraoral examination
     a. Shape of the head
     b. Shape of the face
     c. Facial profile
     d. Facial symmetry
     e. Facial divergence
     f. Facial height
     g. Temporomandibular joint
     h. Lymph nodes
     i. Eyes
     j. Nose
     k. Forehead
     l. Nasolabial angle
     m. Lips
     n. Mentolabial sulcus
     o. Chin.
   - *Local examination*: Intraoral examination
     a. Soft tissue examination
     b. Saliva
     c. Halitosis
     d. Hard tissue examination:
        - Teeth present
        - Hard tissue status
        - Occlusion: Molar, canine and incisal relationship
        - Curve of Spee
        - Mobility/depressibility of teeth
     e. Breathing pattern
     f. Swallowing pattern
     g. Physiologic spacing
     h. Midline

5. **Provisional diagnosis**
6. **Investigation**
7. **Final diagnosis**
8. **Treatment planning**
   a. Medical phase
   b. Systemic phase
   c. Preventive phase
   d. Corrective phase
   e. Maintenance and recall.

VITAL STATISTICS

Hospital Registration Number

It is recorded for the purpose of organized file keeping, billing and also legal purposes.

Date

Records patient's first visit which can be referred back to.

Name

Recording nick names are useful in pediatric practice. Children are at ease when they are referred to by the same names as they are referred at home.

Purpose of recording the patient's name is for:
- Identification
- To maintain records
- Communication
- To develop rapport with the patient.

Chronologic Age

It is one of the important details significant from the fact that a child is in a dynamic state of growth. Some of the reasons why recording age is important are:
- Behavior management techniques that have to be chosen are definitely age dependent.
- To relate the eruption and exfoliation sequence of teeth. It helps to compare the dental age of the patient with chronologic age and if needed to initiate any preventive or interceptive methods of treatment.
- To also compare the chronologic age with the skeletal and mental age.
- Understanding the period of growth spurts is important for treatment planning. Growth modifications by means of functional and orthodontic appliance elicit better response during the period of growth spurts.
- Certain diseases occur in certain age groups and it aids to diagnose a disease based on age factor.

Sex

- Certain diseases are specific to either of the sexes, such as hemophilia is common in males or juvenile periodontitis in females.

- Timing of eruption sequence also varies between males and female. Eruption is slightly earlier in females.
- Behavior management technique may vary depending on the sexes depending on the likes and dislikes of the child. Boys like toys such as cars and aeroplanes while girls like dolls. One can please a girl child by praising her dress or looks. A boy child would be more praised with regards to his activities than dress.
- Variation in timing of growth spurts is seen between girls and boys.

Class and School

- Helpful to correlate the patient's chronological age with mental age.
- Gives some indication regarding the socioeconomic background of the child.

Parent's Name and Occupation

- For communication
- Understanding the socioeconomic condition.

Address

- Communication
- Some areas are endemic to certain diseases or conditions. Example, if the patient is residing in the area with high water fluoride content, there is increased chance that he might be having dental or skeletal fluorosis.

CHIEF COMPLAINT

It is the reason which prompted the patient to seek dental treatment.

- Common reasons for seeking treatment includes pain, swelling and to improve esthetics or may be referred from other practitioner.
- While recording the chief complaint it must be made in the chronological order, that is what appeared first should be mentioned first.
  For example, if the patient complains of fever from yesterday, pain since four days and swelling began two days back. It should be recorded as follows:
  – Pain of 4 days duration
  – Swelling of 2 days duration
  – Fever of 1 day duration.

HISTORY

History of Chief Complaint

It includes extracting more information regarding the chief complaint that will be helpful in treatment planning.

For example, if the complaint is pain, the history to be obtained includes:

- *Location of pain:* It is required to identify the offending tooth or teeth.
- *Inception:* 'When did it start'? Pain that started few hours to days indicates that it is an acute condition, and similarly pain that is present for many days or months is most of the time related to a chronic condition.
- *Provoking factors or aggravating factors:* There may be some factors that initiate or increase the pain. For example, the pain that increases while lying down, is usually due to pulpal hyperemia or pain present only while eating may be due to deep caries (pressure through thin dentin to pulp) or reversible pulpitis. Spontaneous pain without any provoking factors indicates wide involvement of pulp and requires radical therapy such as pulpectomy.
- *Attenuating factors or relieving factors:* Understanding factors that reduce or stop the pain is also important. Pain that is relieved by removal of the stimuli indicates reversible pulpitis.
- *Duration:* Pain if present following a stimulus, for a short period or is transient in nature, indicates reversible pulpitis. Pain that begins on provocation and lingers on even after removal of stimulus indicates an irreversible pulpitis.
- *Intensity and quality:* Sharp, lacinating pain indicates acute condition and chronic condition is associated with dull, gnawing type of pain.
- *Radiation:* Pain can be radiated to other teeth or tissues. This makes it difficult to identify the diseased tooth or teeth. A tooth associated with chronic pain is most of the time radiated to the tooth in the opposite arch or the patient just cannot pinpoint the involved tooth. Pain due to only pulpal origin is also difficult to point.

> *Type of pain*—can be sharp, dull, continuous, intermittent, mild, severe, etc.
>
> *Pain in the pulp only*—is difficult to localize, as the pulp does not contain proprioceptive fibers unlike the pain of the periodontium.
>
> *Pain increased by lying down*—is due to increase in blood pressure to the head, which increases the pressure on the confined pulp.

Medical History

- Treatment must be postponed if the patient is suffering from acute illness such as mumps, chicken pox, etc.
- History of rhinitis, repeated cold, adenoidectomy, tonsillectomy should be carefully examined for

evidence of persisting nasal obstruction before undertaking orthodontic treatment with appliance such as oral screen, activator, etc.

- Patients with cardiac defects should be referred to a pediatrician. Antibiotic prophylaxis must be given prior to any treatment to minimize the risk of development of subacute bacterial endocarditis (SABE).
- During anticoagulant therapy, adjustment of anticoagulant dosage may be required.
- Communicable disease—precaution to avoid contacting the disease.
- Drug allergy or interactions
- History of psychological problems, if any must be obtained. This will help us during management of the child's behavior during the procedure.

Prenatal History

It includes history of the mother during her pregnancy period and includes about:

- Nutritional disorders
- *Drugs history*: Teratogens may cause abnormal development of the fetus and some drugs like tetracycline may cause discoloration of the teeth.
- *Diseases*: Viral infections are said to cause cleft lip or palate. German measles during first trimester may result in cleft lip and cleft palate.
- *Accidents/trauma*: Trauma may result in orofacial deformity, due to damage to the growth centers.
- Abnormal fetal position may result in abnormal pressure on some part of the face leading to facial asymmetry.

Natal History

It includes history of child at the time of birth.

- Injury to the temporomandibular joint at the time of birth such as may occur during forceps delivery can affect growth of the condyle and, in turn, the mandible.
- Cyanosis at birth may indicate congenital cardiac defect.
- Rh incompatibility that may lead to erythroblastosis fetalis.

Postnatal History

It includes history of the early infant period of the child.

- Includes history relating to the type and duration of feeding habits, nutritional disturbances.
- Trauma, childhood diseases
- Developmental milestones
- History of immunization.

Vaccination Schedule—Recommended by the Indian Academy of Pediatrics (2007)[1]	
Age	*Vaccines*
Birth	BCG
	OPV zero
	Hepatitis B1
6 weeks	DTPw1 / DTPa1
	OPV1,
	Hepatitis B2,
	Hib1
10 weeks	OPV-2 + IPV-2 / OPV-2
	DTPw-2 / DTPa-2
	Hib-2
14 weeks	OPV-3 + IPV-3 / OPV-3
	DTPw-3 / DTPa-3
	Hepatitis B-3
	Hib-3
9 months	Measles
15-18 months	OPV-4 + IPV-B1 / OPV-4
	DTPw booster-1 or DTPa booster-1
	Hib booster
	MMR-1
2 years	Typhoid
5 years	OPV-5
	DTPw booster-2 or DTPa booster-2
	MMR-2
10 years	Tdap
	HPV
Vaccines that can be given after discussion with parents	
More than 6 weeks	Pneumococcal conjugate
More than 6 weeks	Rotaviral vaccines
After 15 months	Varicella
After 18 months	Hepatitis A

Recent Medical History

It helps to alter or modify the treatment plan in accordance to the child's systemic condition. Please refer chapter on medically compromised children for further details. The history briefly includes:

- History of recent hospitalization or medication:
- Drug or any other allergy: Children normally tend to be more allergic to drugs, food items, etc. than adults and it suppresses as they grow.

When there is indication of an acute or chronic systemic disease or anomaly, dentist should consult the child's physician to learn the status of the condition, long range prognosis and the current drug therapy.

Dentist should be alert to identify potential communicable infections conditions that threaten the health of the patient and others as well. Then it is advisable to postpone non-emergency dental care.

Past Dental History

- Gives the attitude of the patient towards dentistry.
- History of previous bad experience needs careful handling.

Family History

- Provides some indication of the hereditarily influenced development of the patient.
- Attitude of the parents towards the oral hygiene, health and dentistry has to be assessed as it may be reflected in the behavior of children.
- Infectious diseases in the family such as tuberculosis should be carefully dealt with.

Personal History

Oral Habits History

- It includes recording the frequency, intensity, duration of the habits such as finger/thumb sucking, nail biting/lip biting, tongue thrusting, bruxism, mouth breathing, etc. Refer chapter on pernicious oral habits for details regarding examination for pernicious oral habits.

Oral Hygiene History

It includes history related to the maintenance of oral hygiene.
- Number of times and method of brushing.
- History regarding 'who' brushes the teeth is very important especially in children less than 5 years. Refer chapter on preventive dentistry for brushing techniques for children.
- Use of fluoridated of nonfluoridated dentrifices.
- *Brush:* Type of brush and how often it is changed.
- Other oral hygiene aids used like flossing, rinses, etc.
  For normal brushing techniques and preventive procedures refer chapter on Preventive Dentistry.

Diet History

- 24 hours recall history is routinely used. Ideal method would be to record a full week diet history including a weekend. Refer Chapter No. 11 for detailed diet history discussion.

EXAMINATION

General Examination

General Well-being of the Child

A brief survey of the entire body is made.

Height and Weight (Figs 3.1 and 3.2)

It is possible to determine whether an individual's growth is progressing normally or abnormally by comparing his/hers height and weight with the standard height and weight chart (Fig. 3.3).

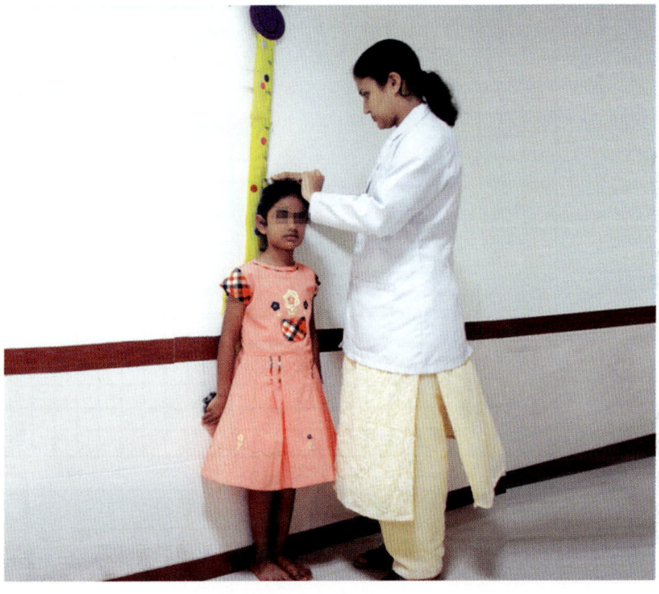

Fig. 3.1: Height can be measured using colorful measuring scale

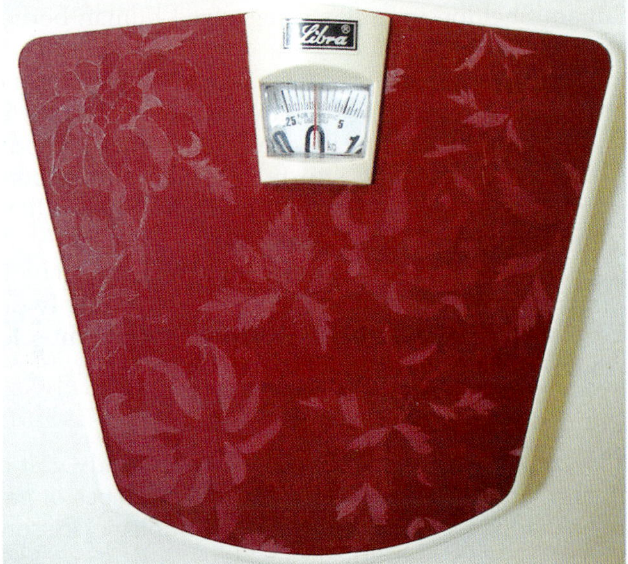

Fig. 3.2: Calibrated weighing machine should be used for measuring the weight of the child

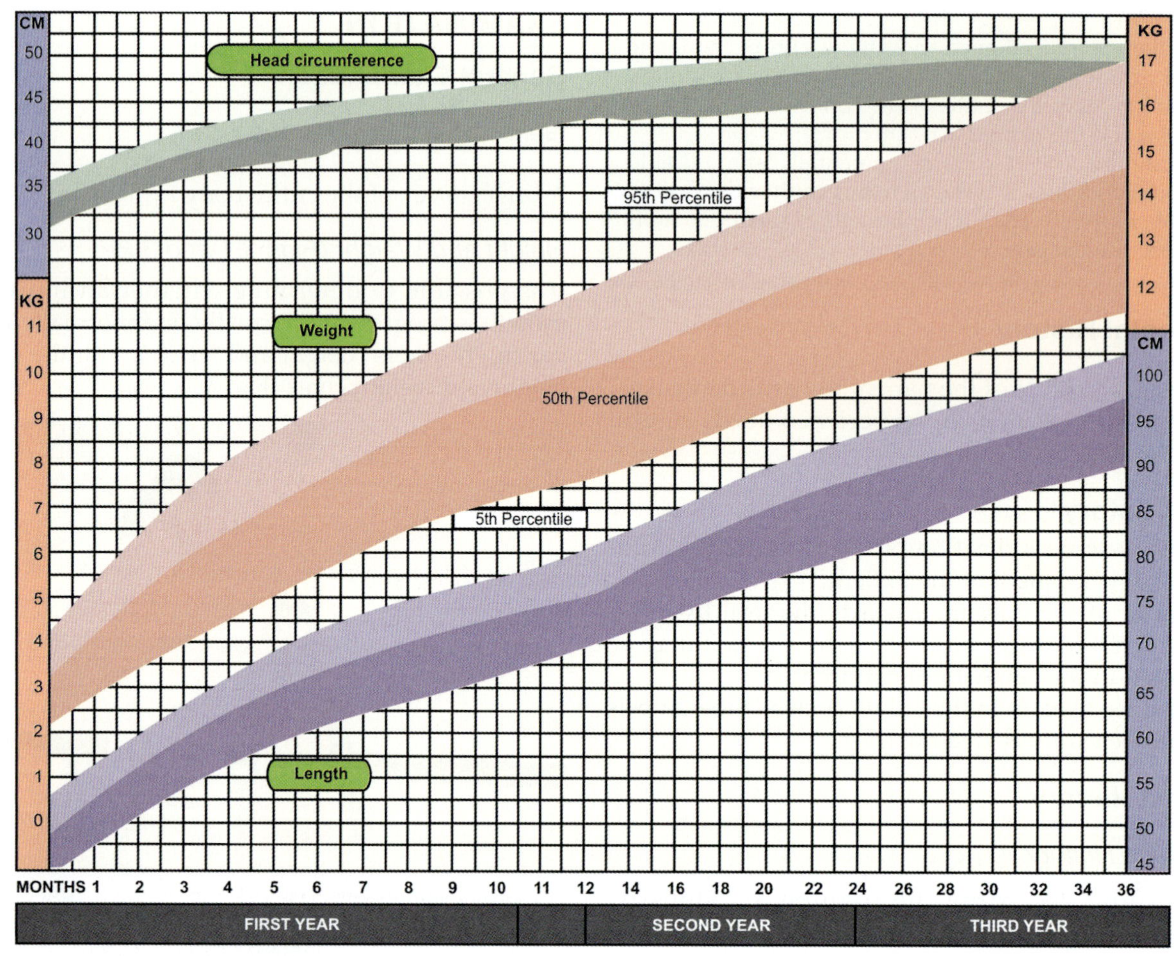

Fig. 3.3: Standard height and weight chart

Built

William Sheldon in 1940's categorized human bodies into three categories:
1. *Ectomorph:* Late maturer, tall, thin and fragile long and slender extremities with minimum subcutaneous fat and muscle. They have flat chest, lightly muscled body.
2. *Mesomorph:* Upright, sturdy, athletic. Muscle, bone and connective tissue predominate. They have a hard muscular body.
3. *Endomorph:* Early maturer, round shaped, usually stocky with abundant subcutaneous fat, highly developed digestive viscera, underdeveloped muscles with soft body.

Gait

Most common abnormal gait is weak, unsteady gait of lethargy and malaise in ill patients. Other types of gait are—waddling, equines, staggering, hemiplegic, scissors, ataxiac, stepped, shuffling or wobbly.

Speech

Speech disorders can be:
 i. Aphasia (loss of speech secondary to central nervous system damage).
 ii. Delayed speech (due to hearing loss, intellectual retardation, developmental retardation, poor environmental stimulation).
 iii. Stuttering or repetitive speech (where the child repeats some or most of the words and is due to psychological stress).
 iv. Cluttering is an unusual type of speech characterized by repetition of words or phrases, false starts, changes in context in the middle of the sentence and general verbal confusion.

Local Examination

Patients Frankfort Horizontal (FH) plane should be parallel to the floor during examination (Fig. 3.4).

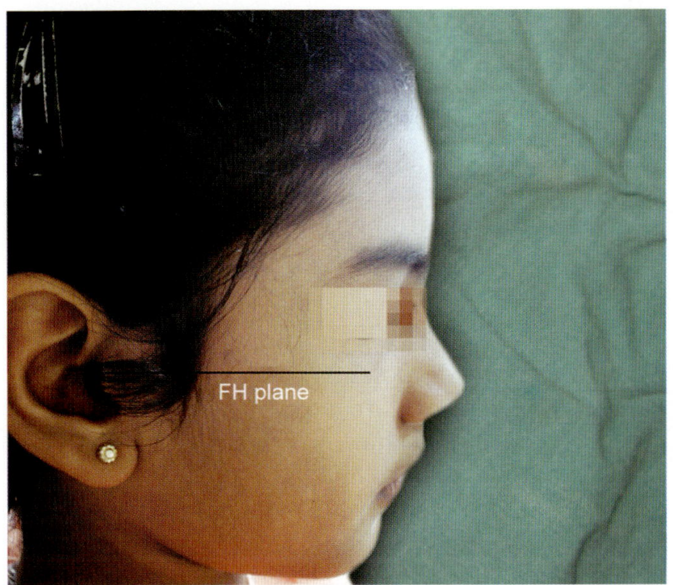

Fig. 3.4: Frankfort horizontal plane

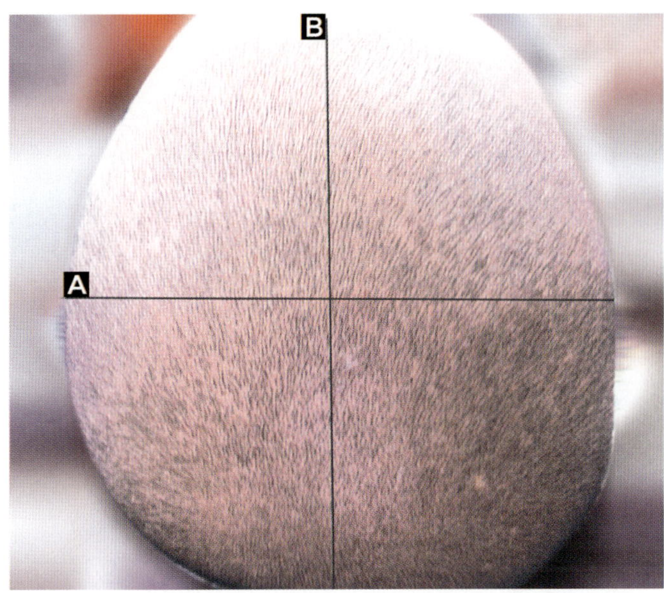

Fig. 3.5: Measuring the shapes of the head: (A) Transverse dimension; (B) Anteroposterior dimension

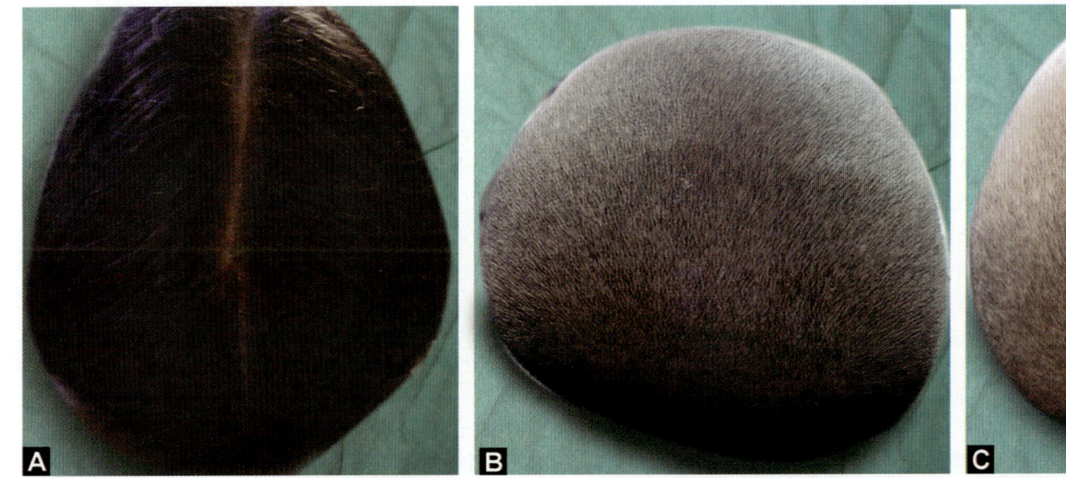

Figs 3.6A to C: Different shapes of head: (A) Dolichocephaly; (B) Mesocephaly; (C) Brachycephaly

Extraoral Examination

Shape of the Head (Fig. 3.5)

Cephalic index (CI) =

$$\frac{\text{Maximum skull width (transverse) dimension}}{\text{Maximum skull length (Anteroposterior dimension)}}$$

Shape of the head can be classified as (Figs 3.6A to C):
- *Mesocephalic:* Average, cephalic index (CI) is 76.0 – 80.9
- *Dolichocephalic:* Long and narrow, CI is < 75.9
- *Brachycephalic:* Broad and short, CI is 81.0 – 85.4
- *Hyperbrachycephalic:* CI is > 85.5.

Shape of the Face (Fig. 3.7)

Morphologic facial index,

$$\text{MFI} = \frac{\text{Morphologic facial height (point N to Gn)}}{\text{Bizygomatic width (ZY to ZY)}}$$

Shape of the face can be classified as (Figs 3.8A to C):
- *Dolichoprosopic or leptoprosopic:* High facial skeleton, long and narrow – Oval, MFI is 88.0 – 92.9

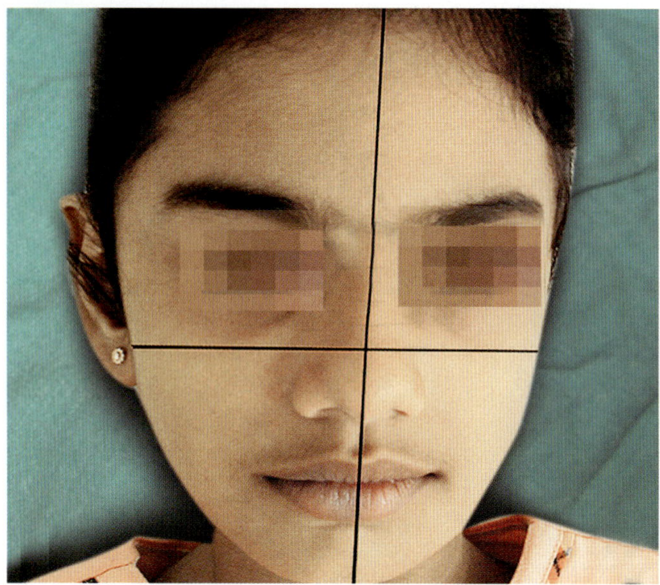

Fig. 3.7: Recording the shapes of the face

- *Euryprosopic:* Low facial skeleton, broad and short – round, MFI is 79.0 – 83.9.
- *Mesoprosopic:* Average – Square, MFI is 84.0 – 87.9.

Facial Profile (Fig. 3.9)

Nasion, point A and the pogonion are considered. Facial profile can be shown (Figs 3.10A to C):

- *Straight:* When all the 3 points are in the same vertical plane, seen in Class I malocclusion.
- *Convex:* If point A is ahead or pogonion is behind, seen in Cl II div 1 malocclusion.
- *Concave:* If point A is behind or pogonion is front, seen in Cl III malocclusion.

Facial Symmetry

It is better visualized from above the head, the operator standing behind the patient as shown in Figure 3.11. Gross asymmetry can be due to:
- Abscess due dental infections
- Parotid enlargement
- Hemifacial hypertrophy/atrophy
- First arch syndrome
- Unilateral condylar hyperplasia
- Unilateral ankylosis of TMJ.

Facial Divergence (Fig. 3.12)

Facial angle (FA) is used, which is formed by NA-Pog soft tissue line and FH line.
It can be of three types:
- *Orthognathic:* FA is approximately 90°
- *Posteriorly divergent:* Low FA
- *Anteriorly divergent:* High FA

Facial Height (Fig. 3.13)

Upper facial height
- From the bridge of the nose to the lower border of the nose or NA to ANS—45% of the total facial height.

Lower facial height
- From the lower border of the nose to the lower border of the chin (ANS to Me)—55% of the total facial height.

Lower facial height	
Increased	*Lowered*
1. Skeletal open bite	1. Growing children
2. Long face syndrome	2. Skeletal deep bite
	3. Cl II div 2

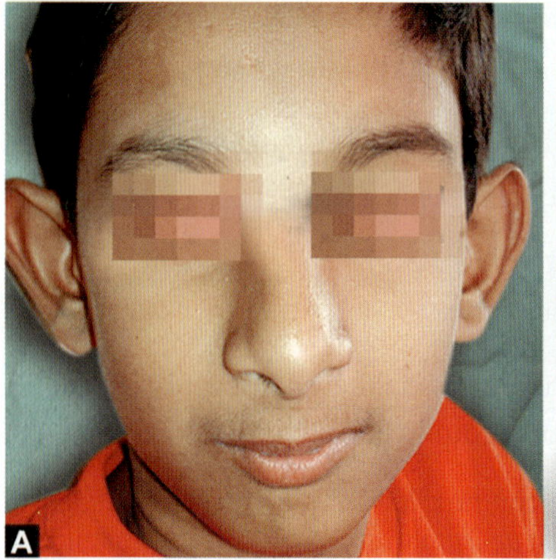
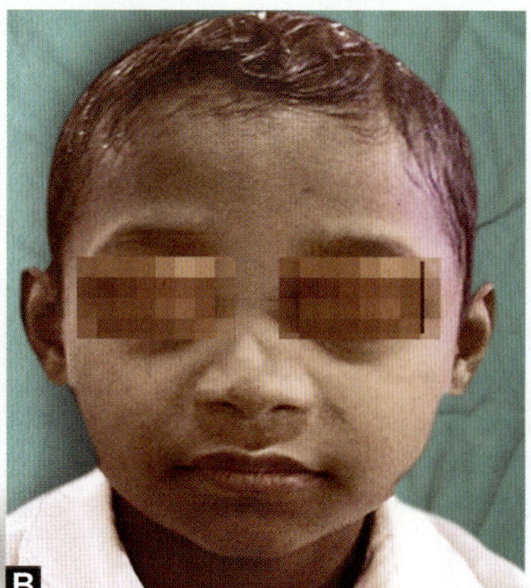
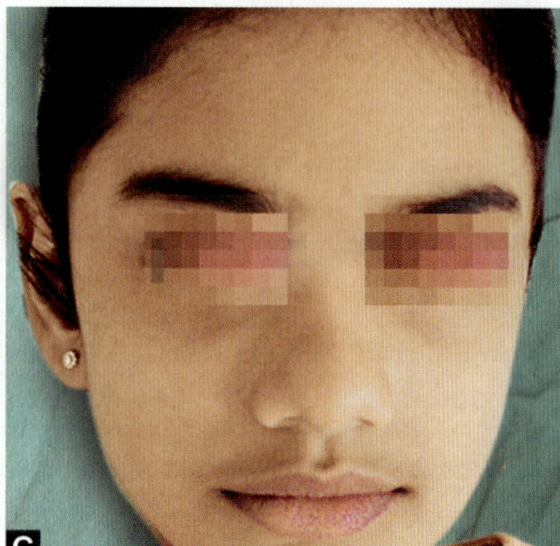

Figs 3.8A to C: Different shapes of the face: (A) Dolichoprosopic or leptoprosopic; (B) Euryprosopic; (C) Mesoprosopic

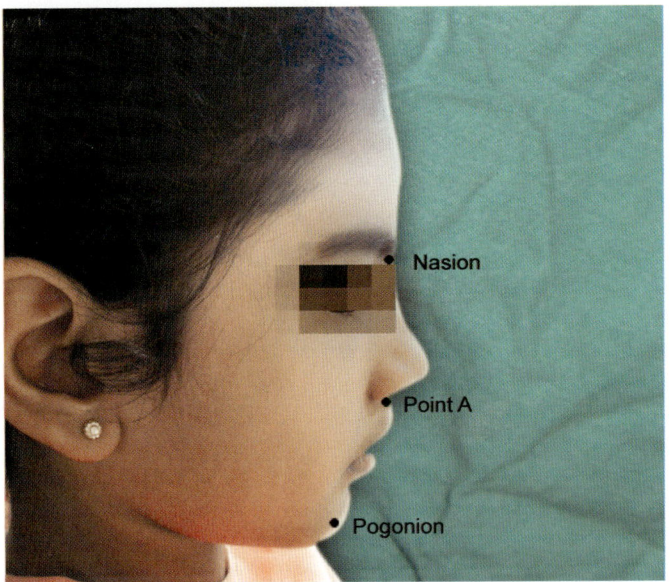

Fig. 3.9: Landmarks used for recording the profile of the face

Temporomandibular Joint

Temporomandibular joint (TMJ) is palpated by standing in front of the patient. This helps to visualize the movement of the mandible during the opening and closure of the jaw and thus note any discrepancies. The head of each mandibular condyle can be palpated by placing the index finger in front of the tragus and the posterior border of the condyle can be palpated by placing the index finger in the external acoustic meatus.

Examination of TMJ (Figs 3.14 to 3.16)

- It reveals pain on pressure and synchrony of action of left and right condyle.
- Discrepancies of TMJ such as muscular imbalances, anatomic deviations, swellings or redness over joint region, trismus and spasm of muscles can be noted.
- Palpation of muscles of mastication is also very important. Lateral pterygoid and masseteric pain is also encountered associated with TMJ problems.

Path of Closure: Altered

- Occlusal prematurities
- Lingually or palatally erupting incisor
- Cl II div 1—habitual forward positioning
- Cl III—forward displacement
- Backward path of closure or posterior displacement
- Lateral path of closure in unilateral crossbite cases

Clicking may be initial, intermediate, terminal and reciprocal.
- Initial clicking: Sign of retruded condyle in relation to disk.
- Intermediate clicking: Unevenness of the condylar surfaces and of the articular disk which slides over one another during the movements.
- Terminal clicking: Most common and is due to the condyle being moved too far anteriorly in relation to the disk on maximum jaw opening.
- Reciprocal clicking: Occurs during opening and closing and expresses an incoordination between displacement of the condyle and disk. Clicking of the joint is rare in children.

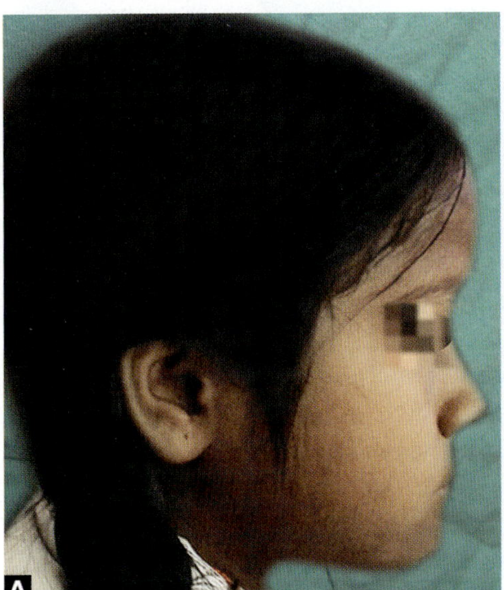
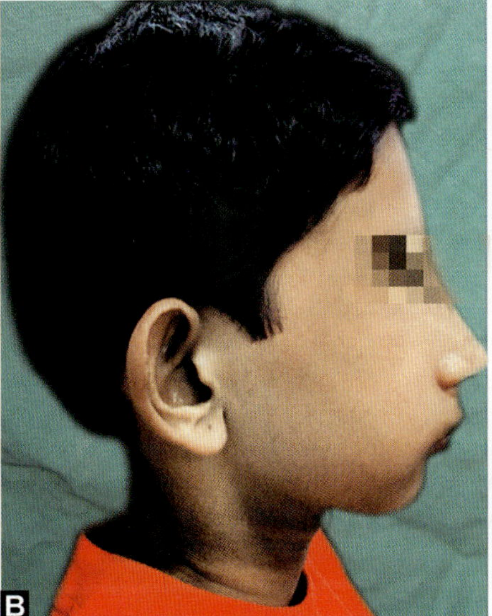
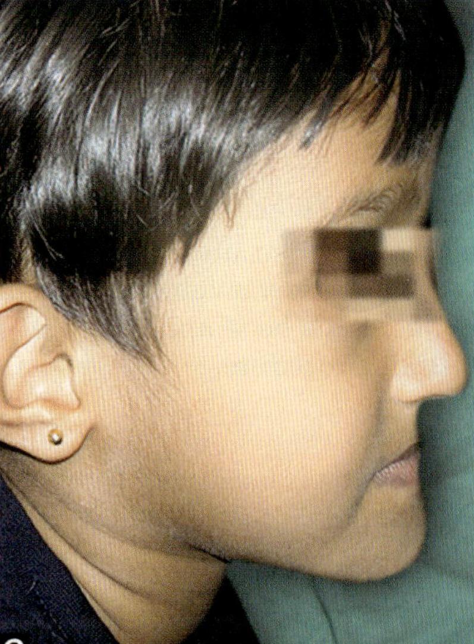

Figs 3.10A to C: (A) Straight; (B) Convex; (C) Concave profile of the face

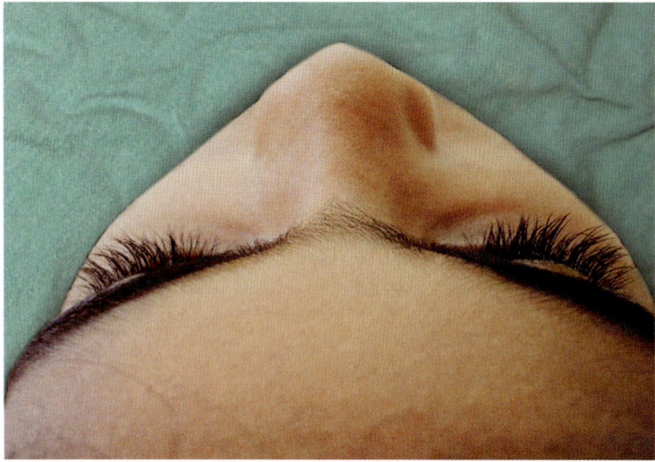

Fig. 3.11: It is easy to differentiate the change in facial symmetry when visualized from this view

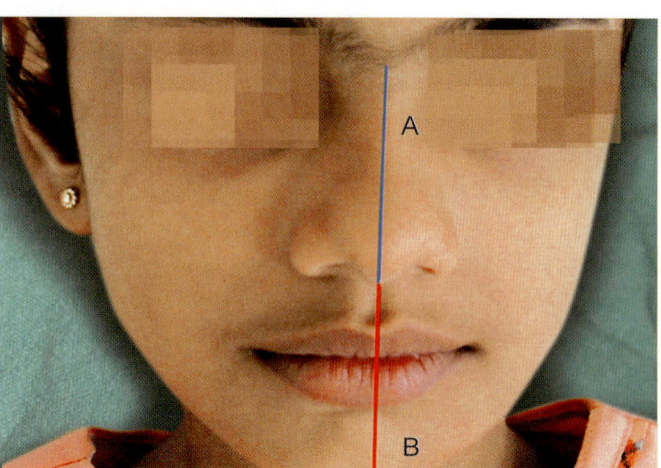

Fig. 3.13: Facial height (A) Upper facial height (Blue line); (B) Lower facial height (Red line)

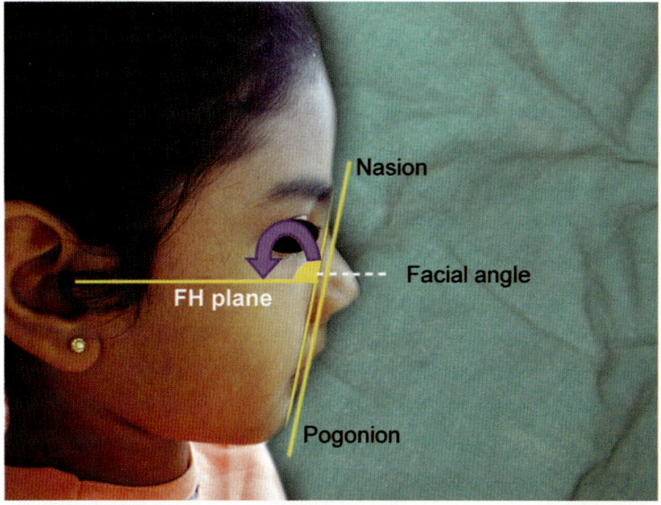

Fig. 3.12: Facial angle formed by NA-Pog soft tissue line and FH line

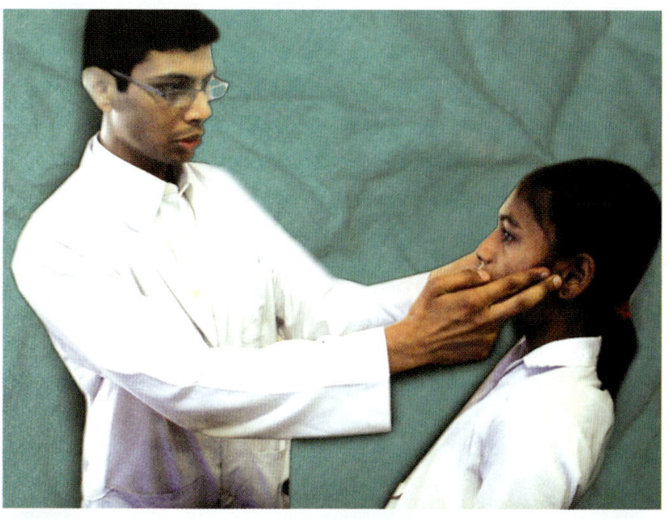

Fig. 3.14: Operator should stand in front of the patient to observe the path of closure of mandible

Lymph Nodes (Figs 3.17A and B)

Submandibular and submental lymph nodes are the ones commonly involved during dental infections. Other nodes in the head and neck area should be checked as routine procedure.

Eyes

Inflammation associated with maxillary teeth may extend to the orbital region causing swelling of the eyelids and conjunctivitis. Eyes also serve as indicators for anemia, jaundice, etc.

Nose

- Contour (nasal bridge) can be—straight, convex, crooked.
- *Size*: Height should be about 1/3rd of total facial height. Microrhinic is associated with high root of the nose, short nasal bridge and an elevated tip. Large nasal profile is associated with deep root of the nose, long nasal bridge and a protruding lip.
- Ratio between the horizontal length with the height of the nose is 2:1.
- *Nostrils:* Width is approximately 70% of the length of the nose.
- Certain infectious diseases leave their marks on nose, e.g. saddle nose in congenital syphilis.
- Identifying deviated nasal septum is important in mouth breathers.

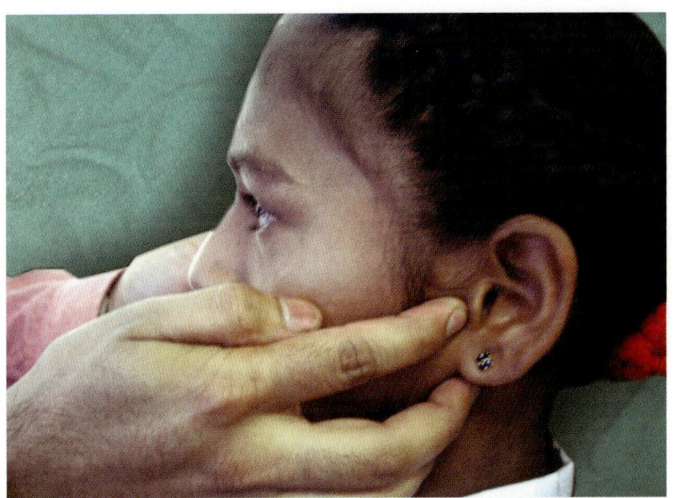

Fig. 3.15: Index finger is placed in front of the tragus to palpate the anterior border of the condlye

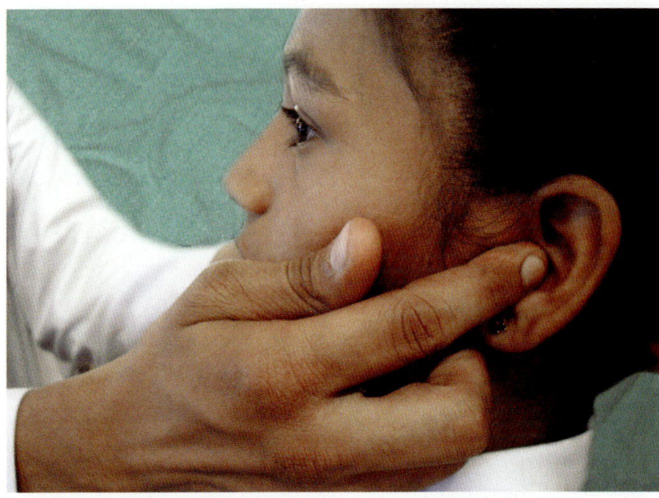

Fig. 3.16: Index finger is placed in the external acoustic meatus to palpate the posterior border of the condlye

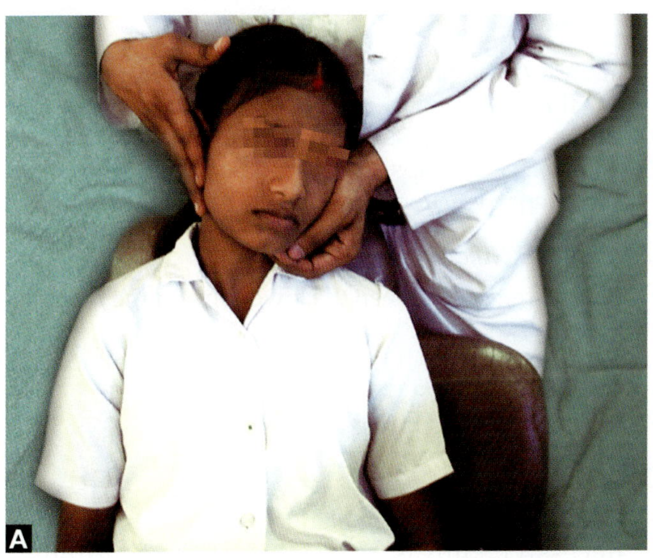

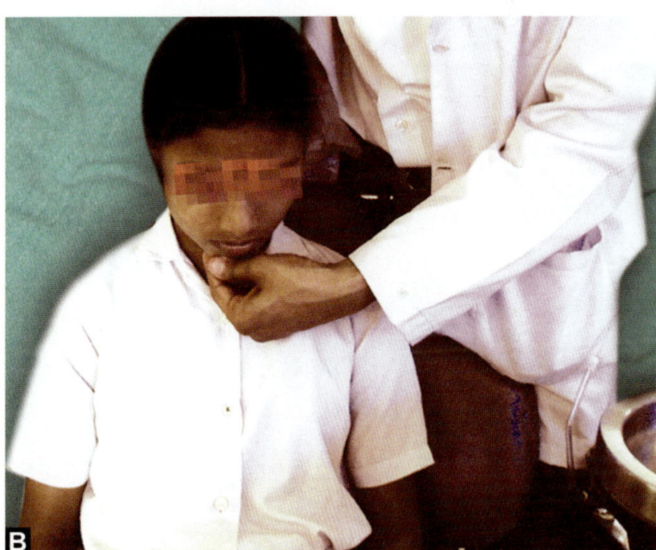

Figs 3.17A and B: Examination of the lymph nodes: (A) Submandibular lymph nodes; (B) Submental lymph nodes

Forehead

- Profile of face is influenced by the shape of the forehead and nose.
- Harmonious facial morphology = height of the forehead should be 1/3rd of the entire face height that is it must be as long as the middle and lower third.
- Height of the forehead (Upper 1/3rd of the face) = distance of hairline to the glabella (middle 1/3rd is from glabella to subnasal and lower 1/3rd from subnasal to menton).
- Contour can be flat, protruding or oblique. Steep forehead is usually associated with prognathic dental bases than with flat forehead.

Nasolabial Angle (Fig. 3.18)

- It is the angle formed between lower border of nose to the upper lip and is 90-110°.
- Decreased in cases of proclined maxilla, tense upper lip, prognathic upper teeth.
- Increased in retrusive maxilla, retruded upper teeth.

Lips

- *Normally competent:* Touch each other lightly or with 0-1 mm of gap (Fig. 3.19). When the lips do not approximate each other at rest they are termed as incompetent (Fig. 3.20).

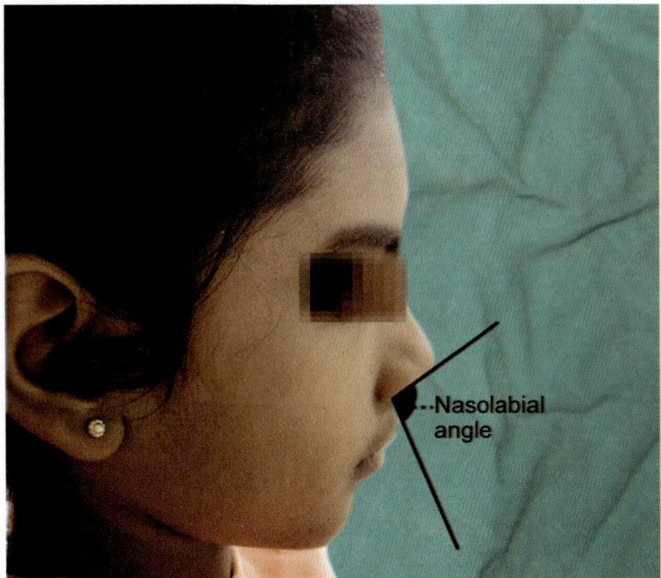

Fig. 3.18: Nasolabial angle

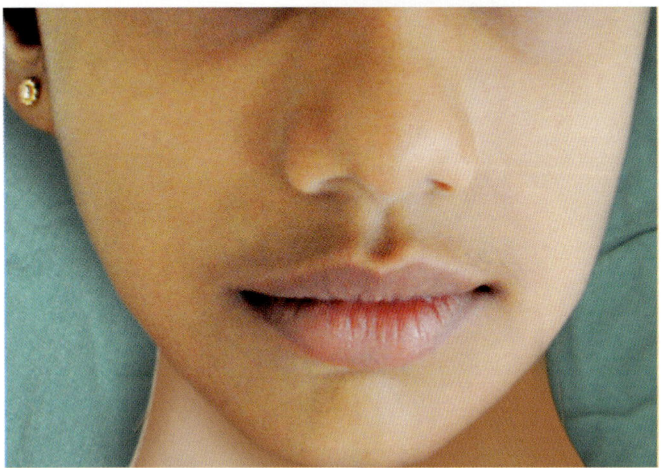

Fig. 3.19: Normal competent lips

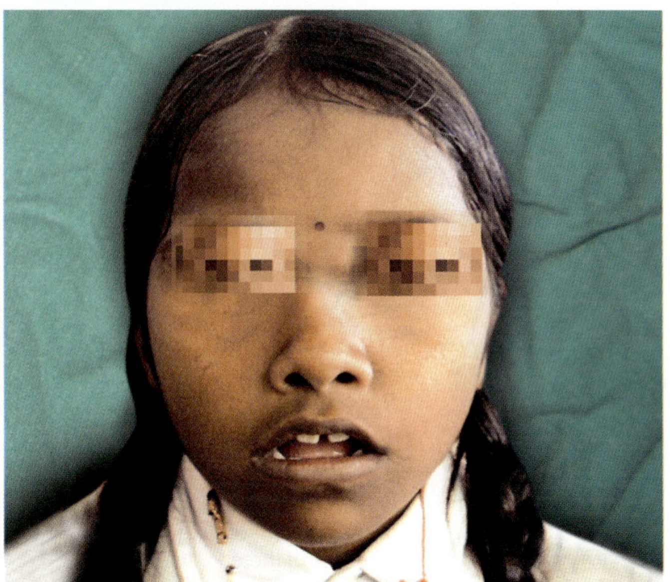

Fig. 3.20: Incompetent lips

- *Length:* Upper lip covers the entire labial surface of upper anterior teeth except the incisal third or incisal 2-3 mm.
- *Tonicity and color:* Normal is pink and firm, hypo-active lip is lighter in color and is flaccid.
- Hypotonic lip is flaccid.
- Lip protrusion is influenced by the thickness of the soft tissue, tone of the muscles, position of the anterior teeth and configuration of underlying bony structures.
- Lip steps (profile) are of three types (Figs 3.21A to C).
  i. *Positive lip step:* Protruded lower lip associated with Cl III relation.
  ii. *Normal lip relation* has a mild negative lip, with upper lip mildly protruded compared to the lower lip.
  iii. *Marked negative lip step:* Protruded upper lip, Cl II relation.
- Ulcers, vesicles, fissures, crusts and abrasions are frequently seen on lips and should be noted. Nutritional and allergic reactions may also cause changes in lips.

Mentolabial Sulcus (Fig. 3.22)

- It is the region between the lower lip and the mentalis muscle.
- Normal: Seen in Cl I occlusion.
- Deep: Cl II div 1.
- Shallow: Seen in bimaxillary protrusion.

Chin (Fig. 3.23)

- Chin prominence is related to mandibular position. Recessive chin is associated with mandibular retrognathism or Cl II molar relation. Prominent or prognathic chin is associated with mandibular prognathism or Cl III molar relation. Normally positioned chin is associated with straight profile or Cl I molar relation.
  Normal: Seen in Cl I occlusion
- Increased height of the chin alters the position of the lower lip and interferes with the lip closure.

Intraoral—Soft Tissue Examination

Soft tissue should be examined for 3C's, change in the color, contour and consistency.

Change in Color

It may be a change to red (inflammation), blue (hematoma, bruise) or white (electric or thermal burns, candida infection).

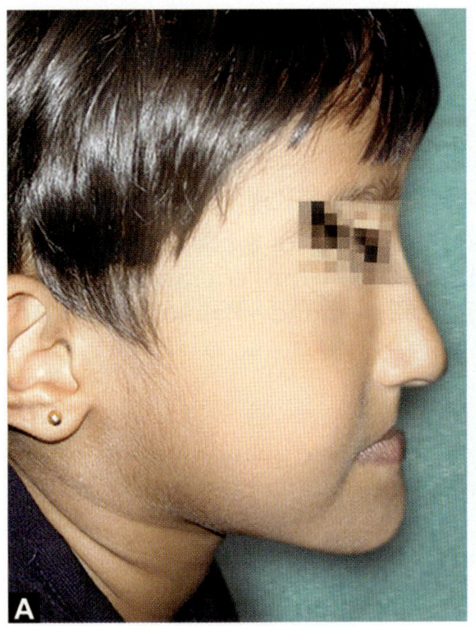 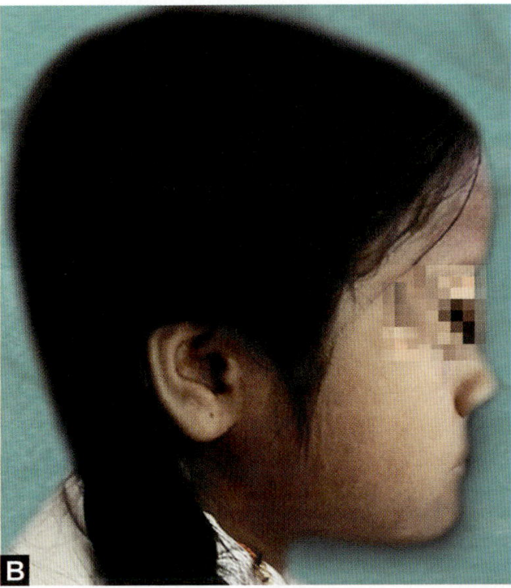 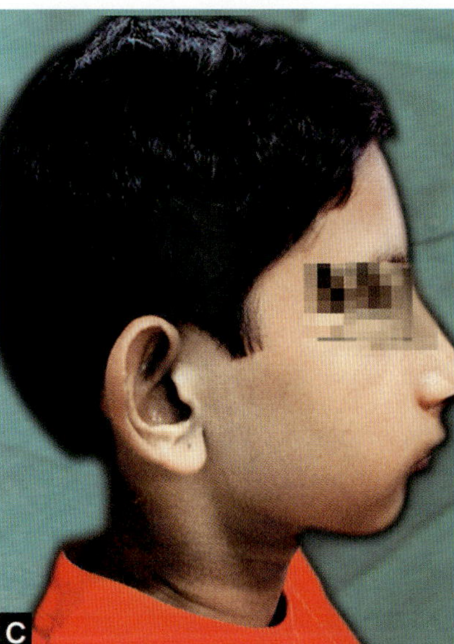

Figs 3.21A to C: Lip profile: (A) Positive lip step; (B) Normal lip step; (C) Negetive lip step

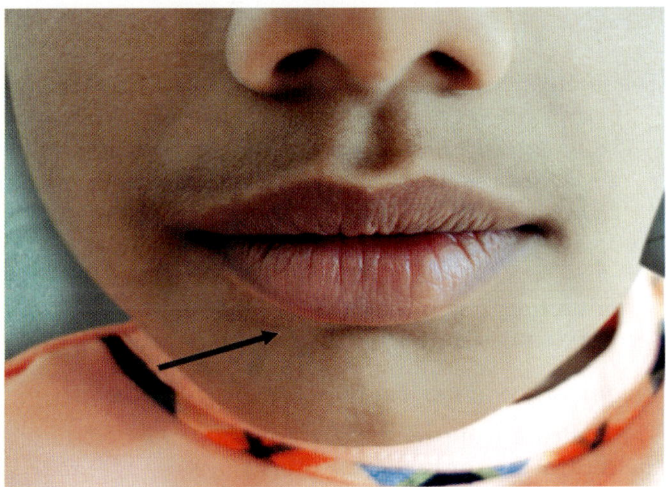

Fig. 3.22: Mentolabial sulcus

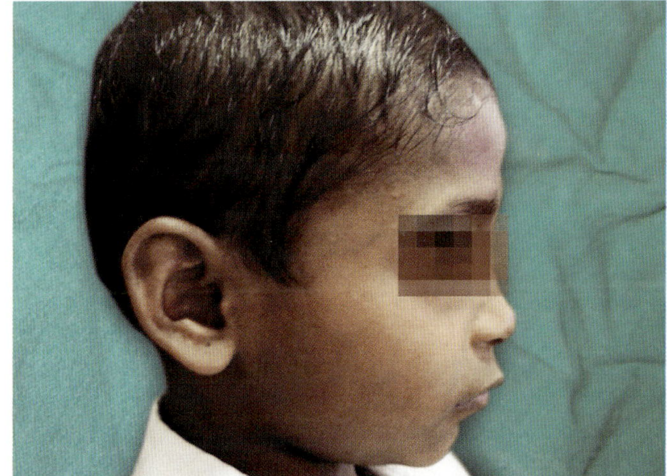

Fig. 3.23: Chin examination

Change in Contour

It may be due to either a swelling (abscess, papilloma) or ulcer (aphthous, traumatic).

Change in Consistency

It may be soft (inflammation), firm (mucocele) or hard (bony exostosis).

Gingiva (Figs 3.24 and 3.25)

- High maxillary labial frenal attachment may be responsible for abnormal spacing between the central incisors (Fig. 3.26).
- Redness and swelling of gingiva may be seen associated with gingivitis (Fig. 3.27).

- Draining fistula on the attached gingiva accompanied by a tooth that is tender, painful and mobile are usually diagnostic of abscessed teeth.

Tongue

- The size, shape, color and movement of the tongue should be noted.
- Dryness of tongue—indicates dehydration.
- Tongue is coated in febrile state.
- Abnormal lingual frenum can result in 'tongue tie' or ankyloglossia (Fig. 3.28).

Saliva

- May be thin, normal or viscous.

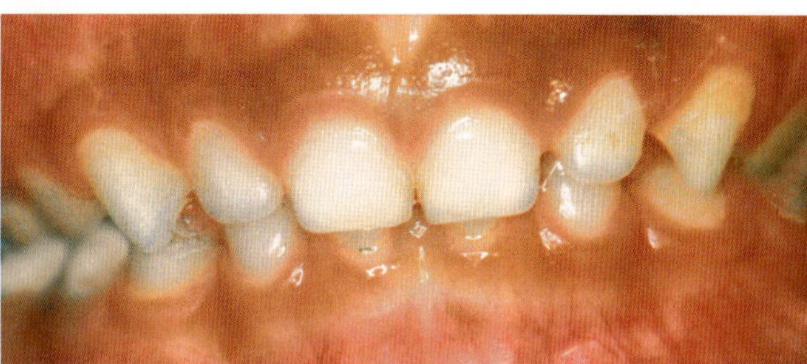

Fig. 3.24: Normal healthy gingiva

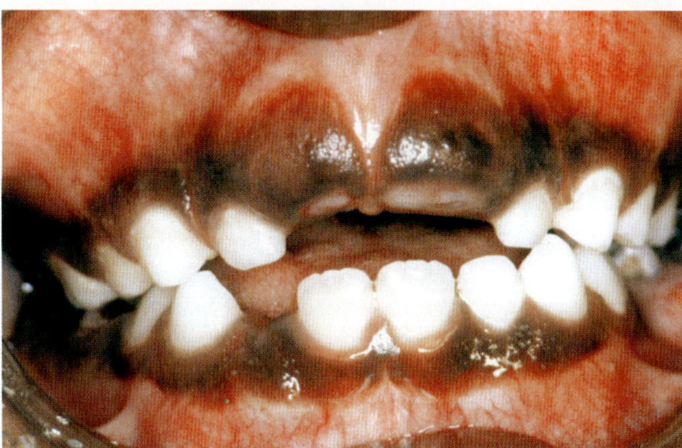

Fig. 3.25: Normal healthy gingiva with melanin pigmentation

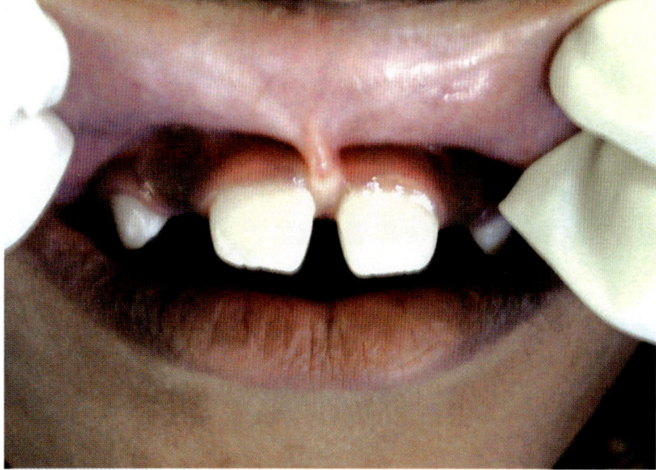

Fig. 3.26: High frenum attachment causing midline diastema

- Altered secretions are seen in systemic conditions such as mumps, Sjogren's syndrome, etc.

Halitosis

- May be due to poor oral hygiene, blood in mouth, dehydration, sinusitis, infection of adenoid tissue, disturbances of alimentary tract, etc.

Intraoral—Hard Tissue Examination

Basic instruments used for examination include a mouth mirror, explorer, straight probe, tweezer and a spoon excavator (Fig. 3.29).

(a) Teeth Present (Fig. 3.30)

There are different systems used for tooth numbering, of which the one recommended by the Federation Dentaire Internationale (FDI) and Zsigmondy-Palmer system are commonly used.

FDI System

The dental arches are divided into quandrants, the upper and lower, right and left. Each quadrant is denoted by a number as:

Permanent Dentition	1	2
	4	3
Deciduous Dentition	5	6
	8	7

The teeth are numbered as follows:

Permanent teeth
18,17,16,15,14,13,12,11,21,22,23,24,25,26,27,28
48,47,46,45,44,43,42,41,31,32,33,34,35,36,37,38
Deciduous teeth
55,54,53,52,51,61,62,63,64,65
85,84,83,82,81,71,72,73,74,75

Thus the first number denotes the quadrant and second denotes the tooth.

Zsigmondy-Palmer Tooth Numbering System

The teeth are grouped in quandrants and numbered from the central incisor to the last molar.

Deciduous Dentition	E D C B A	A B C D E
	E D C B A	A B C D E
Permanent Dentition	8 7 6 5 4 3 2 1	1 2 3 4 5 6 7 8
	8 7 6 5 4 3 2 1	1 2 3 4 5 6 7 8

For example, an upper right permanent first molar is denoted as ⎽6⎸ or ⎽6⎸

(b) Hard Tissue Status

i. *Decayed teeth* (Fig. 3.31): The teeth should be cleaned thoroughly before attempting to check for decay. Refer for siagnosis of caries.

ii. *Discoloration* (Figs 3.32 and 3.33): Difference should be made regarding discoloration which may be due

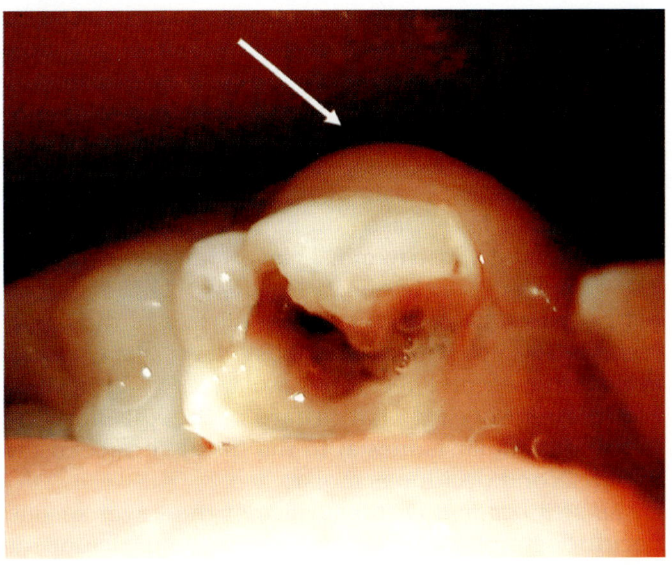

Fig. 3.27: Swelling associated with a nonvital tooth changing the contour of the gingiva

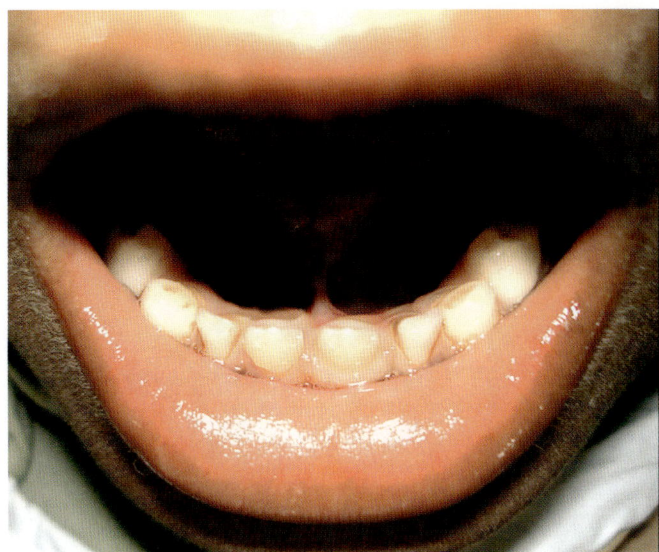

Fig. 3.28: Tongue tie or ankyloglossia

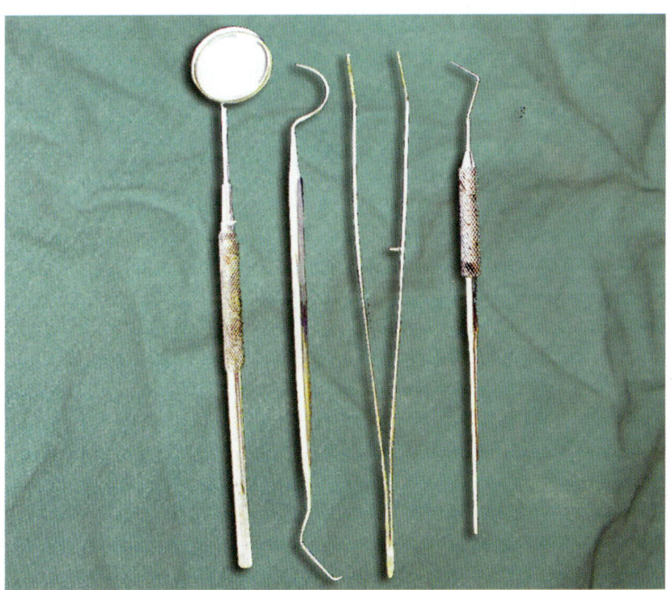

Fig. 3.29: Instruments that are required for examination

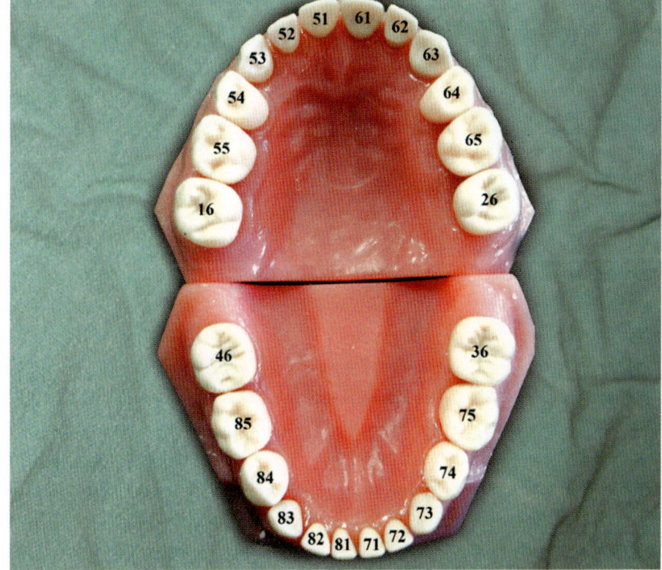

Fig. 3.30: Teeth denoted by FDI system of tooth numbering

to extrinsic or an intrinsic reason. Food stains or tobacco stains cause discoloration on the surface of the tooth. The cause for discoloration in a nonvital tooth is due to intrinsic reasons. Other reasons that cause intrinsic change in the color are enamel hypoplasia, fluorosis, etc.

iii. Other abnormal findings (Figs 3.34 and 3.35): Such as rotated teeth, mobile tooth, root stumps, etc. should be noted.

(c) Occlusion

Molar relationship

(i) Permanent teeth: Classified based on Angle's[2] classification (Figs 3.36A to C).

Cl I molar relation: Mesiobuccal cusp of the upper first permanent molar occludes with the mesiobuccal groove of the lower first permanent molar.

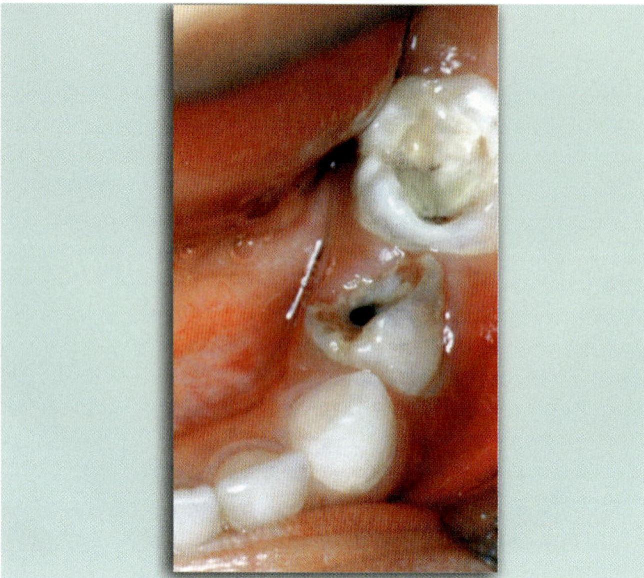

Fig. 3.31: Decayed teeth

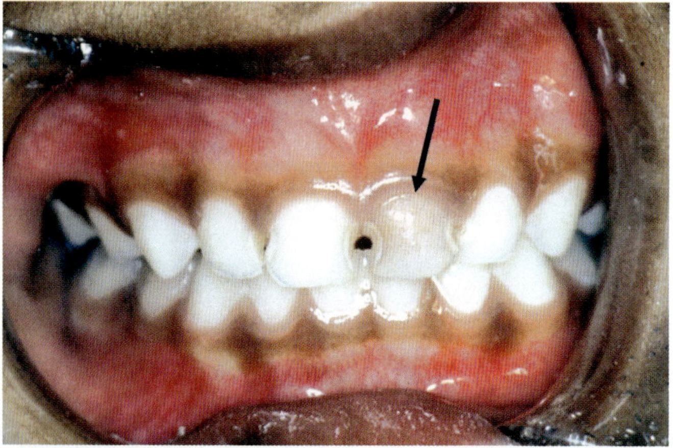

Fig. 3.32: Discolored nonvital tooth

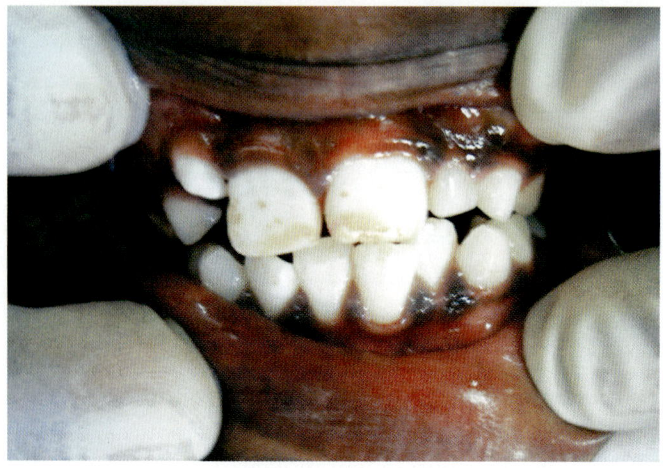

Fig. 3.33: Discoloration due to enamel hypoplasia

Cl II molar relation: Distobuccal cusp of the upper first permanent molar occludes with the mesiobuccal groove of the lower first permanent molar.

Cl III molar relation: Mesiobuccal cusp of the upper first permanent molar occludes in between the lower first and second permanent molar.

(ii) *Deciduous teeth:* Based on Baume's[3] terminal plane relationship into flush terminal plane, mesial step terminal plane and distal step terminal plane (Figs 3.37 A to C).

Flush terminal plane relation: Distal surface of the upper second deciduous molar is in line with the distal surface of the lower second deciduous molar.

Mesial step relation: Distal surface of the lower second deciduous molar is mesial to the distal surface of the upper second deciduous molar.

Distal step relation: Distal surface of the lower second deciduous molar is distal to the distal surface of the upper second deciduous molar.

Please refer the chapter on development of occlusion for the importance of these relations in relation to the permanent molar occlusion.

Canine relationship: It can be class I, II or III (Fig. 3.38).

Cl I relation: Distal slope of the lower canine occludes with the mesial slope of the upper canine.

Cl II relation: Mesial slope of the lower canine occludes with the mesial slope of the upper canine.

Cl III relation: Lower canine is placed more mesially than Cl I relation almost extending between the lateral and central incisor.

Incisal relationship (Figs 3.39A to C): The upper and lower incisors can be related in both horizontal and vertical planes.

(i) Overjet

- Horizontal overlapping of upper and lower teeth.

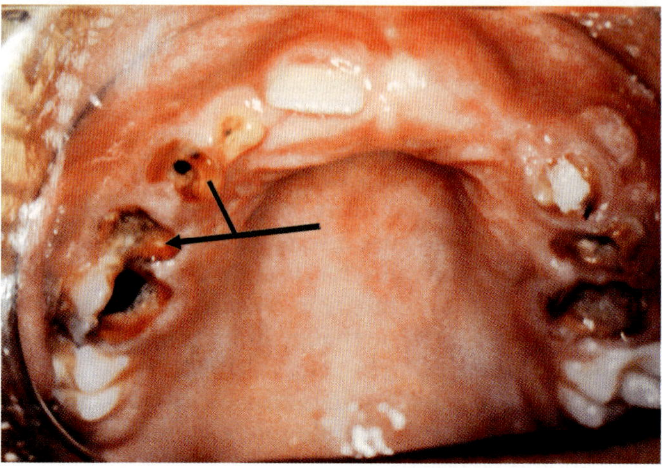

Fig. 3.34: Root stumps

- It is measured from labial surface of lower anterior to incisal edges of upper anterior teeth, when in centric occlusion.
- Normal is 2-3 mm.

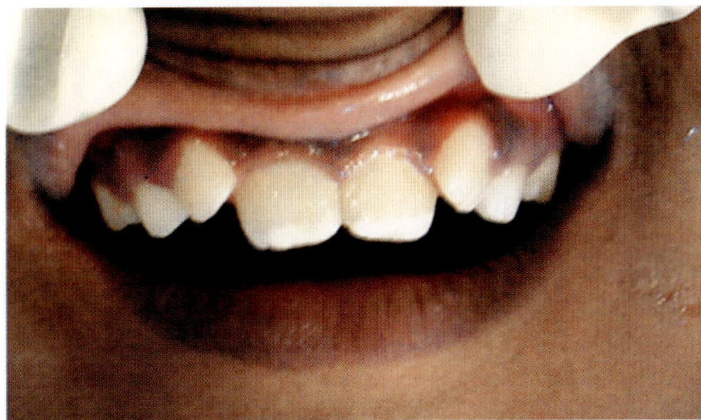

Fig. 3.35: Malocclusion

(ii) Overbite

- Vertical overlapping of the incisors
- It is measured from the incisal edge of the lower incisors to the point of extension of the upper incisor on the labial surface of the lower incisors when in centric occlusion.
- Normal is 2-3 mm.
- Deep bite is when overbite >2-3 mm.
- When lower incisors contact the palatal mucosa, it is termed as complete deep bite.
- Closed bite is observed in Cl II div 2 where the upper anterior teeth overlaps lower anterior completely.
- Open bite is described when there is no contact between the upper and the lower anterior teeth.
- True deep overbite is due to infraocclusion of molars with large freeway space.
- Pseudo deep overbite is due to overeruption of incisors with small freeway space.

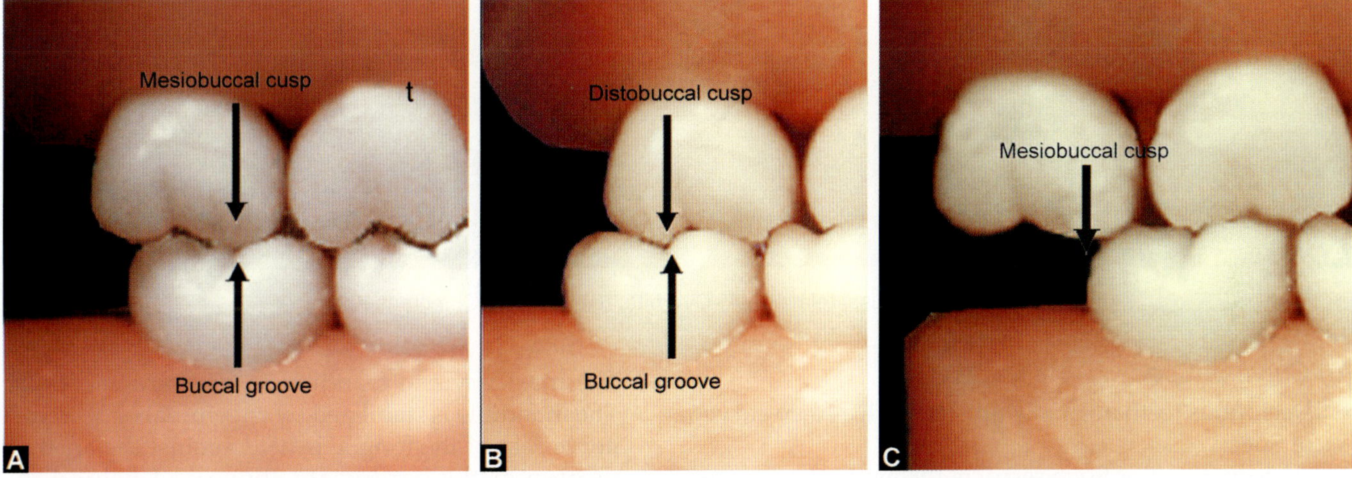

Figs 3.36A to C: Angle's permanent molar relation: (A) Class I; (B) Class II; (C) Class III

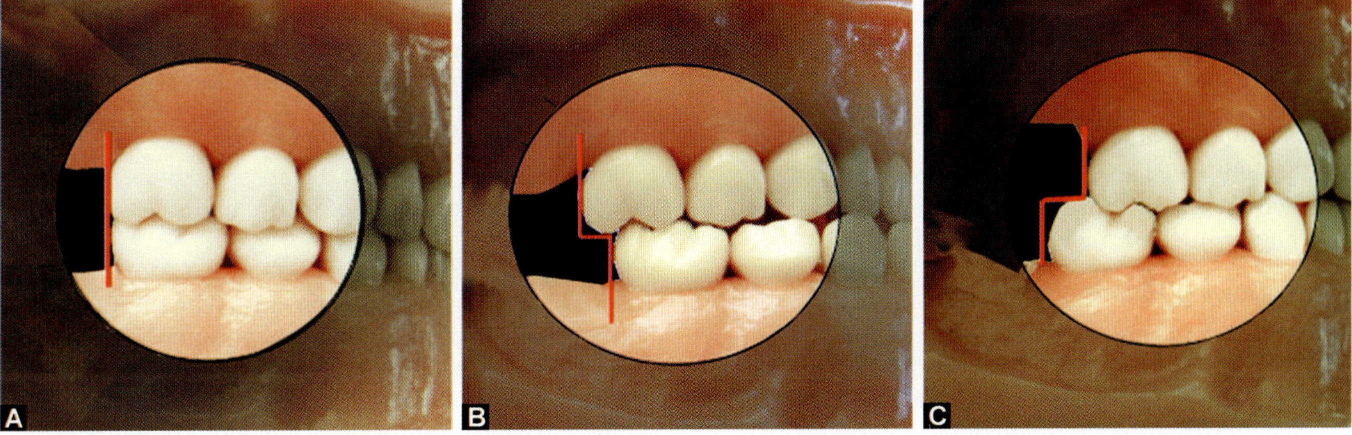

Figs 3.37A to C: Deciduous molar relation: (A) Flush terminal plane relation; (B) Mesial step relation; (C) Distal step relation

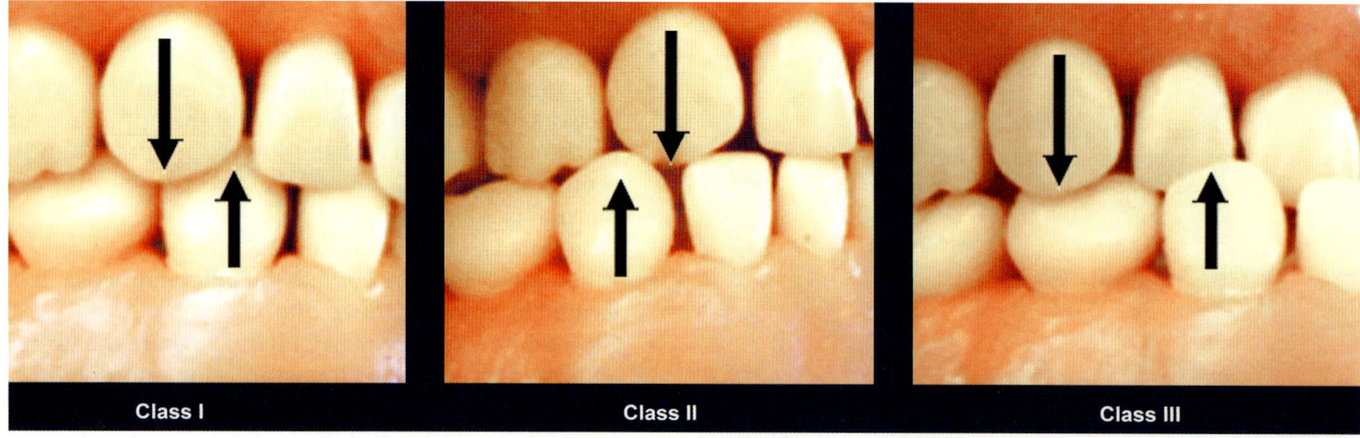

Fig. 3.38: Canine relations

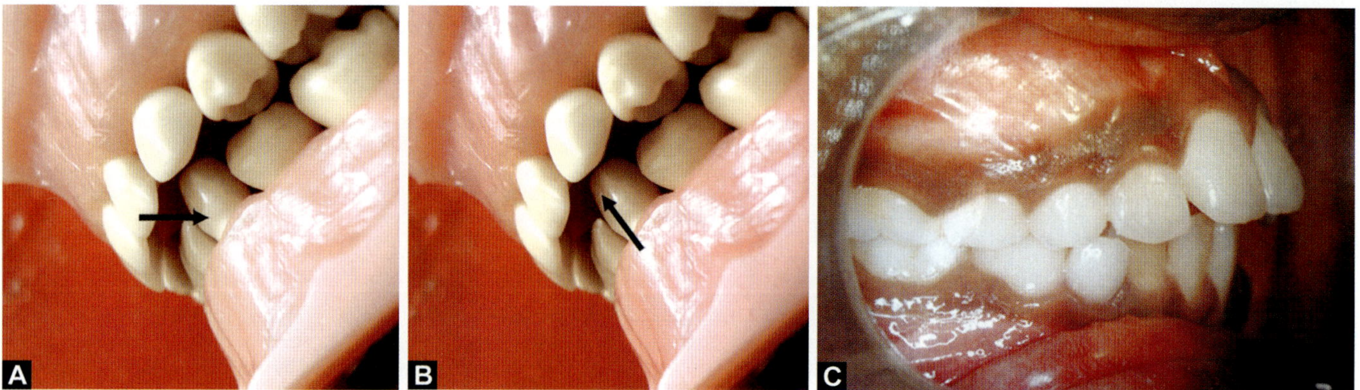

Figs 3.39A to C: Incisal relation: (A) Overbite; (B) Overjet; (C) Increased overjet

(d) Curve of Spee

- Deciduous teeth normally present with a steep curve of Spee.
- A steep curve of Spee restricts the amount of space available for the upper teeth and is often combined with crowding.
- A flat curve allows a good occlusion.
- A reverse curve of Spee creates excessive space in the upper jaw.

(e) Breathing Pattern

- It can be nasal, oral or combination
- Methods to diagnose abnormal breathing is given in chapter titled Pernicious Oral Habits.

(f) Swallowing Pattern

Normal patterns are:
- *Normal infantile pattern:* Seen before the eruption of the buccal teeth in the primary dentition. Mandible is stabilized by contraction of facial muscles.
- *Normal mature pattern:* Attained by 18 months of age.

The maxillary and mandibular teeth are in contact. The mandible is stabilized by trigeminal or V cranial nerve. Tip of the tongue is held against the anterior portion of the hardpalate above and behind the incisors with minimal contraction of the lip. The middle portion of the tongue touches the middle of the hardpalate and the posterior portion forms 45° with the posterior pharyngeal wall.

- *Abnormal patterns:* It is discussed in Chapter 6.

(g) Physiologic Spacing (Fig. 3.40)

It can be present or absent. Its absence gives some idea regarding the probability of future malocclusion.

(h) Dental Midline

The midline of the dentition coincides with the interincisal line between the upper and the lower central incisors. The upper interincisor line also coincides with the center of the philtrum or the midpalatine raphe. The patient is asked to occlude in centric occlusion. An imaginary line is drawn extending from between the upper central incisors and

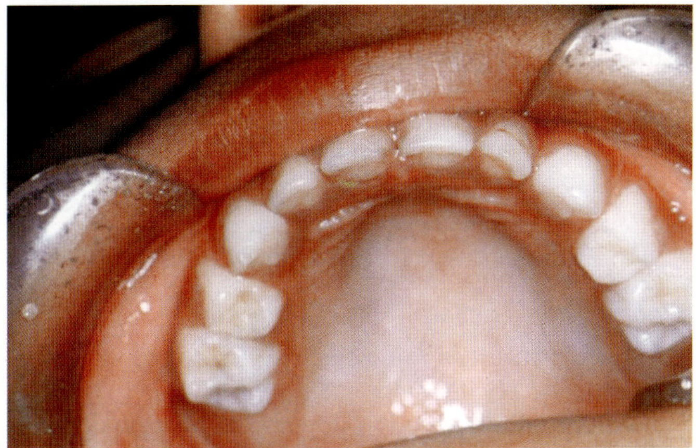

Fig. 3.40: Normal spacing present in deciduous dentition

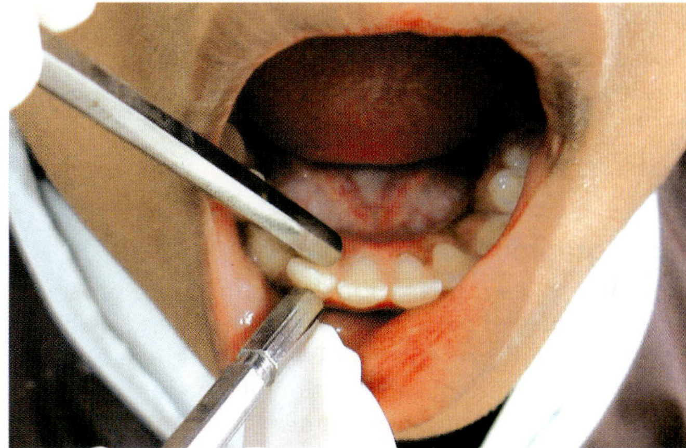

Fig. 3.42: Position of the instruments while checking the mobility of the tooth

passing down between the lower central incisors. This line should be in straight line and coincide with philtrum or mid palatine raphe. Any deviation (Fig. 3.41) must be noted and the etiology assessed.

Midline shift usually occurs due to supernumerary tooth (where the midline shifts towards opposite side) premature loss of tooth or teeth, proximal caries, missing tooth or teeth (where the midline shifts towards the same side).

(i) Mobility/Depressibility of Teeth

Mobility is checked using two blunt instruments such as the handle of the mouth mirror as shown in Figure 3.42. Mobility is the labiolingual movement of the tooth whereas depressibility is the movement of the tooth in an apical direction. Based on the amount of tooth movement it can be graded as:

- *First degree*—barely visible
- *Second degree*—1 mm or less
- *Third degree*—>1 mm or vertical

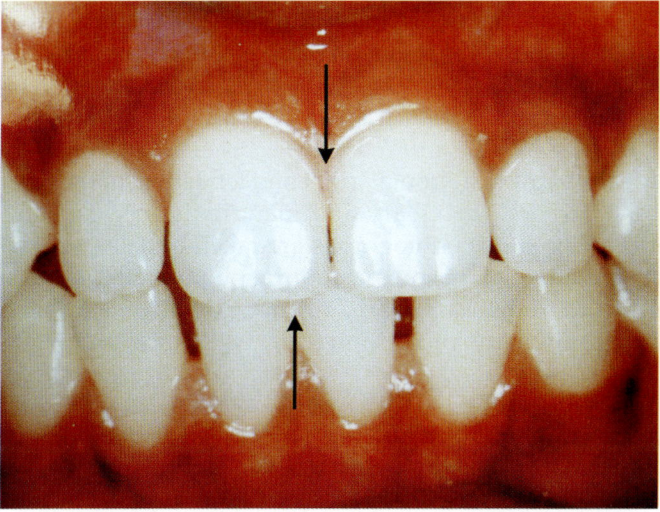

Fig. 3.41: Note the deviation in the dental midline

May be due to the purulent exudate in periapical region, advanced periodontal disease, horizontal root fracture in middle or coronal 1/3rd or chronic bruxism.

PROVISIONAL DIAGNOSIS

Diagnosis is the art of identifying a disease from its signs and symptoms followed by thoughtful interpretation of the data.

Provisional diagnosis is a general diagnosis based on clinical impression without any laboratory investigation.

INVESTIGATION

Percussion

- Reveals the status of the periodontium and not of pulp.
- During inflammation in the periodontal space the tooth is pushed corronally due to the exudate that gets accumulated. There is also pressure that is built due to continuous formation of exudate in a confined periodontal space. When the tooth is tapped the tooth is pushed back into the socket which stimulates the nerve ending present in the periodontal space causing pain. Thus pain on percussion means that the tissues in the periodontal space are inflamed.
- Children should be explained the steps involved during the test. They must be explained the difference between the sensation that is felt during tapping of a normal tooth and the actual pain. Normally children mistake the feel of tapping for pain.
- First a normal tooth must be percussed followed by the affected tooth. This helps in comparing the sensation felt by the child.
- Percussion should be done first lightly with index finger followed by the handle of the mouth mirror.

- Tapping on each cusp may, at times, reveal the presence of crown fracture.

Positive response to percussion may be due to:

- Teeth undergoing orthodontic movement
- Recent high restoration
- An apical or lateral periodontal abscess.

Radiographic Examination

- IOPA gives information regarding—the presence or absence of permanent teeth, shape and position of the teeth present, relative state of development of teeth, extent of calcification of developing tooth, path of eruption of permanent teeth, morphology and inclination of the root of permanent tooth, etc.
- Crown, roots, root canal, lamina dura, bony architecture and other anatomic landmarks should be examined for carious destruction, depth of restoration, internal resorption, incomplete apices, etc.
- If the canal appears to change quickly from dark to light it indicates bifurcated or trifurcated root canal.
- If the outline of the root is unclear or deviates, an extra root should be suspected.
- A great deal of bone destruction might have occurred before radiographic signs are evident. Loss of cancellous bone is undetectable until at least 66% of the mineral content of the cortical bone in the direct path of the X-ray beam has been lost. Hence a periapical lesion is usually larger than its radiographic image.
- Vertical fractures are difficult to identify.
- Horizontal fractures may be confused with bone trabeculae. This may be differentiated by noting that the lines of bone trabeculae extend beyond the border of the root, but a root fracture often causes a thickening of the PDL.
- Please refer the Chapter on Radiology for further information of different types of radiographs and their indications.

Pulp Testing

This is not routinely used in children as their pain perception varies due to incomplete roots which are either resorbing or developing. Objective of this test is to elicit a pulpal response for a particular stimuli. The stimuli can be thermal or electric.

Thermal

Heat or cold stimuli can be used. Preferred temperature for heat test is 65.5°C. Gutta-percha stick, hot water, or heated instrument tip can be used as the source of heat. Ethyl alcohol, ice sticks or carbon dioxide can be used as the source for applying cold stimuli.

Response to Vitality Testing

It may be nil, moderate transient, painful transient or painful lingering and each indicating the status of the pulp as follows:

- Nil = nonvital pulp or false –ve
- Moderate transient = normal
- Painful transient = reversible pulpitis
- Painful lingering = irreversible pulpitis

Electric Pulp Testing

- This test utilizes mild electric current to stimulate nerve and elicit a response.
- It is contraindicated in patients with pacemakers.
- False positive reading is observed with extensive vital restorations, anxiety, moist gangrenous pulp, and failure to isolate the tooth.
- False negative reading is observed with thick insulating base, recently traumatized tooth, incomplete root formation, excessive calcification, partial necrosis and patients taking sedatives.
- The main disadvantage of electric pulp tester is that it merely suggests whether the tooth is vital or not and does not provide information on the health, integrity or vascular supply of pulp.

Study Models and Model Analysis

- Model analysis is done to detect arch size and tooth size discrepancies.
- Study models should be neat and well detailed. Alveolar process should also be recorded.
- The top surface of upper model and lower surface of the lower base should be parallel when models are in occlusion.
- Midline of the palate is at right angles to the rear surface of the model.
- The base of the cast must be 25% of the total height of the cast and the remaining 75% is the anatomic details of the cast.

Photographs

Ideally extra oral (frontal, right and left lateral of the face) and intraoral (maxillary and mandibular occlusal and frontal occlusal) photographs are taken initially prior to any treatment. This pre procedural photographs serve as a record for later comparison. They also aid to study the facial symmetry, profile and facial type of the patient.

Cephalometric Study[4,5] (Fig. 3.43)

Use of Cephalometrics

- Study of growth and development
- Case diagnosis
- Treatment planning

- Dictating the prognosis
- Studying the craniofacial abnormalities
- Prediction of growth

Cephalometric analysis

Skeletal

- SNA: To know the anteroposterior position of the maxilla in relation to the anterior cranial base.
  - Normal—82°
  - Increased—prognathic maxilla
  - Decreased—retrognathic maxilla
- SNB: Anteroposterior positioning of mandible to anterior cranial base.
  - Normal—80°
- ANB: Maxillomandibular relation or skeletal base relationship
  - CL I—2-4°
  - CL II—> 4°
  - CL III—<2°
- Facial angle: Anteroposterior position of mandible in relation to FH plane
  - (Facial plane to FH plane)
  - Normal—76°
  - Increased—prognathic mandible
  - Decreased—retrognathic mandible
- FMA: Frankfurt mandibular plane angle (FH plane to mandibular plane), gives the idea of mandibular growth pattern.
  - Average—25°
  - Increased—high angle case (vertical growth pattern)
  - Decreased—low angle case (horizontal growth pattern)
- Y axis to FH plane (growth axis)
  - Indicates the type of growth which the mandible is likely to undergo.
  - Normal—66°
  - Increased—vertical growth pattern
  - Decreased—horizontal or forward growth pattern

Dental

Assessment of upper incisors

- Upper incisors to NA plane in degree (22°) and in mm (4 mm).
  - Increased—proclined
  - Decreased—retroclined

Assessment of lower incisors

- Lower incisor NB plane in degree (25°) and in mm (4 mm).
  - Increased—proclined
  - Decreased—retroclined

Interincisal angle: Formed by the long axis of upper and lower incisors.
  - Normal—131°

Supplemental Diagnostic Aids

- *Occlusal radiographic view*: Used for location of impacted canine or mid palatal suture area

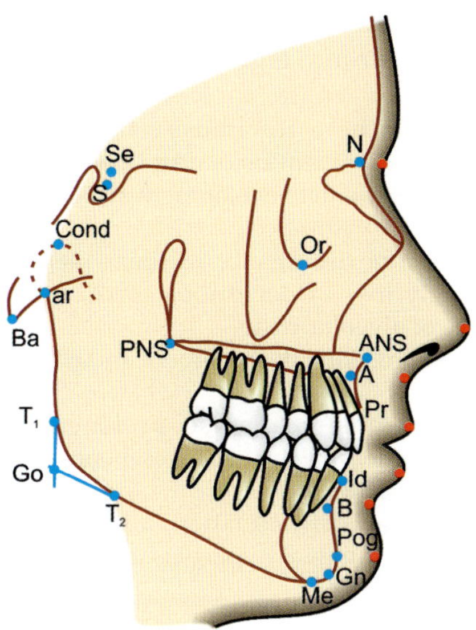

Fig. 3.43: Cephalometric points: N—Nasion; S—Sella; Se—Mid point of the entrance to sella; Cond—Condylion; Ar—Articulare; Ba—Basion; T_1—Most posterior point on ramus in the region of the angle of mandible; T_2—Most inferior and posterior point on the body of the mandible; Go—Gonion; Me – Menton; Gn—Gnathion; Pog—Pogonion; B—Point B; Id—Infradentale; Pr—Prosthion; A—Point A; ANS—Anterior nasal spine; PNS—Posterior nasal spine; Or—Orbitale

- Tube shift technique
- PA view
- *EMG*: To conform the clinical diagnosis of muscle function, e.g. Cl II div 1 is associated with hyperactive mentalis = 85-90 MV.
- *BMR*: In hypothyroidism there is delayed eruption which may cause malocclusion and is associated with reduced BMR.
- *Diagnostic set up*: Teeth are removed and resembled replaced in position simulating the post-treatment position.
- *Hand wrist radiograph:*
  - Estimates the skeletal age.
  - Carpal bones, epiphysis, phalanges, metacarpals provide a clue to bone growth in the body as a whole
  - Ossification occurs in these bones after birth and before maturity
  - Inspection of carpal radiographs to assess the growth by evaluating the following—shape of the carpal bones, degree of ossification of the skeleton, time and order of appearance of carpals.

  The stages of mineralization of the carpal bones are determined. Then the development of metacarpal bones and phalanges are evaluated. Standard tables and analysis of Bjork are useful which divide the maturation process of bones of the hand between the 9th to 17th year into eight developmental stages.

> *Dental age:* Can be estimated by the stage of tooth development, mineralization or eruption on a radiograph.
> - Acceleration in dental development and eruption timing can be:
>   *True*—endocrine disturbances, diabetes mellitus, etc.
>   *False*—early loss of deciduous teeth, inflammatory processes of alveolar bone
> - Retardation in dental development and eruption timing can be:
>   *True*—severe organic disease, prolonged periods of deficiency, endocrine disturbances, bone disease, environmental influence, etc.
>   *False*—post-traumatic situation, alveolar bone hyperplasia, fibrous gingival hyperplasia, etc.

FINAL DIAGNOSIS

It is a more confirmed diagnosis analyzing all the available data including the results of investigation.

TREATMENT PLANNING

Treatment planning is the orderly or sequentially arrangement of the various treatment needs of the patient to provide maximum benefit to the patient as a whole.

Advantages of Treatment Planning

1. Re-diagnosis at every visit is avoided.
2. Serial appointments can be given on the first day as the patient's treatment needs are already planned in a sequencial order.
3. Instruments can be prepared well in advance before the patient's arrival for the treatment.
4. Total fee estimation can be done.

Treatment plan must be discussed with the parents and permission taken before performing any treatment on the child. Information relating to the following must be given:
- Dental need of their child including the treatment as well as the preventive measures.
- Amount of time required to perform the treatment.
- Total cost.

Sometimes it may be difficult to perform any treatment in the normal out-patient clinical setup and may require hospitalization such condition includes very young child < 2 years with rampant caries, where cooperation may be difficult to achieve.
- Child with concurrent medical problem such as cystic fibrosis, chronic heart disease, kidney disease, etc.
- Child with congenital or developmental handicapping condition such as mental, emotional or physical.

Planning the treatment can be made based on five different phases
a. Emergency phase
b. Medical/referral phase
c. Systemic phase
d. Preventive phase
e. Corrective phase
f. Maintenance and recall

Emergency Phase

All the problems that require immediate actions, such as relieving the child from pain, attending to a trauma, etc. should be done in this stage.

Medical/Referral Phase

In this phase patients with positive medical history are referred to pediatrician for evaluation and consent. It may also be required to modify the dosage or change a particular drug as per the requirement of the treatment.

Systemic Phase

Any medication given to modify dental treatment is included in this phase, such as premedication for behavior management or antibiotic prophylaxis to a child with congenital cardiac defect.

Preventive Phase

This phase is the first phase of treatment. It is aimed at providing preventive therapy to prevent or minimize dental disease. It includes:
  i. Oral prophylaxis and fluoride treatment
  ii. Pit and fissure sealant application
  iii. Oral hygiene counseling
  iv. Diet counseling
  v. Orthodontic consultation

Corrective Phase

It includes providing treatment or management of the disease process.
  i. Extractions
  ii. Restorations
  iii. Minor surgical procedures
  iv. Space maintainers
  v. Minor orthodontic corrections
  vi. Prosthetic rehabilitation

Maintenance and Recall

Patients are recalled at regular intervals following the completion of the required treatment. This is done as a preventive measure for early detection of disease and also for biannual topical fluoride application. Patients at high risk are maintained at 2-3 months recall and low risk at 6 months recall.

Modification

Treatment planning may be modified during the procedure based on:
1. Estimation of cooperation from the patient and parents.
2. Assessment of the condition of the teeth and the oral hygiene.
3. Whether extraction is needed or not.
4. Nature of tooth movement and type of appliance required.

Guideline and Recommendations based on Age for the Periodicity of Examination and Dental Services (AAPD Recommendation, 2009)[6]

6 to 12 Months

1. Complete the clinical oral examination with adjunctive diagnostic tools (e.g. radiographs as determined by child's history, clinical findings, and susceptibility to oral disease) to assess oral growth and development, pathology, and/or injuries; provide diagnosis.
2. Provide oral hygiene counseling for parents, including the implications of the oral health of the caregiver.
3. Remove supragingival and subgingival stains or deposits as indicated.
4. Assess the child's systemic and topical fluoride status (including type of infant formula used, if any, and exposure to fluoridated toothpaste) and provide counseling regarding fluoride. Prescribe systemic fluoride supplements, if indicated, following assessment of total fluoride intake from drinking water, diet, and oral hygiene products.
5. Assess appropriateness of feeding practices, including bottle and breastfeeding, and provide counseling as indicated.
6. Provide dietary counseling related to oral health.
7. Provide age-appropriate injury prevention counseling for orofacial trauma.
8. Provide counseling for non-nutritive oral habits (e.g. digit, pacifiers).
9. Provide required treatment and/or appropriate referral for any oral diseases or injuries.
10. Provide anticipatory guidance.
11. Consult with the child's physician as needed.
12. Complete a caries risk assessment.
13. Determine the interval for periodic reevaluation.

12 to 24 Months

1. Repeat 6 to 12 month procedures every 6 months or as indicated by individual patient's risk status/susceptibility to disease.
2. Assess appropriateness of feeding practices—including bottle, breastfeeding, and no-spill training cups and provide counseling as indicated.
3. Review patient's fluoride status—including any child care arrangements which may impact systemic fluoride intake and provide parental counseling.
4. Provide topical fluoride treatments every 6 months or as indicated by the individual patient's needs.

2 to 6 Years

1. Repeat 12 to 24 month procedures every 6 months or as indicated by individual patient's risk status/susceptibility to disease. Provide age-appropriate oral hygiene instructions.
2. Scale and clean the teeth every 6 months or as indicated by individual patient's needs.
3. Provide pit and fissure sealants for caries—susceptible primary molars and permanent molars, premolars, and anterior teeth.
4. Provide counseling and services (e.g mouthguards) as needed for orofacial trauma prevention.
5. Provide assessment/treatment or referral of developing malocclusion as indicated by individual patient's needs.
6. Provide required treatment and/or appropriate referral for any oral diseases, habits, or injuries as indicated.
7. Assess speech and language development and provide appropriate referral as indicated.

6 to 12 Years

1. Repeat 2 to 6 year procedures every 6 months or as indicated by individual patient's risk status/susceptibility to disease.
2. Provide substance abuse counseling (e.g. smoking, smoke-less tobacco).
3. Provide counseling on intraoral/perioral piercing.

12 Years and Older

1. Repeat 6 to 12 year procedures every 6 months or as indicated by individual patient's risk status/susceptibility to disease.
2. During late adolescence, assess the presence, position, and development of third molars, giving consideration to removal when there is a high probability of disease or pathology and/or the risks associated with early removal are less than the risks of later removal.

3. At an age determined by patient, parent and pediatric dentist, refer the patient to a general dentist for continuing oral care.

Informed Consent

The informed consent process is a detailed process of informing the patient or the custodial parent or, in the case of minors, legal guardian regarding the diagnosis and treatment required and the associated problems that might be encountered. They should also be told about alternate treatment plan if any. It also allows them to make educated decision and participate and retain autonomy over the health care received. Informed consent also may decrease the practitioner's liability from claims associated with miscommunication. A written form should be used with the required information and signed by the child's guardians. Consent forms should be procedure specific, with multiple forms likely to be used. It is also important to discuss the behavior management technique that will be used and prior written consent taken for the same.

Items appearing on a consent form should include:
1. Name and date of birth of patient;
2. Name, relationship to patient, and legal basis for adult to consent on behalf of minor.
3. Description of specific treatment in simple term.
4. Alternatives to treatment.
5. Potential adverse sequelae specific to the procedure.
6. An area for the patient or parent/guardian to indicate all questions have been answered.
7. Signature lines for the dentist, parent or legal guardian, and a witness.

REFERENCES

1. IAP Guidebook On Immunization, Indian Academy Of Pediatrics, 2007.
2. Angle EH. Treatment of malocclusion of teeth 7th Ed. Philadelphia, SS White manufacturing Co. 1907.
3. Baume LJ. Physiologic tooth migration and its significance for the development of occlusion II. The biogenesis of accessional dentition. J Dent Res 1950;29:331.
4. Broadbent BH. A new X-ray technique and its application to orthodontia, Angle Orthod 1931;1:45.
5. Graber TM. Cephalometric Techniques: types of analysis, interpretation and longitudinal observations Pediatric Dentistry, scientific foundation and clinical practice, Stewart RE, Barber TK, Troutman KC, Wei SHY, 1982; 288-302.
6. AAPD Recommendation, 2009.

FURTHER READING

1. American Dental Association. Principles of Ethics and Code of Professional Conduct. Available at: "http://www.ada.org/prof/prac/law/code/index.asp". Accessed April 12, 2008.
2. Andria LM, Leite LP, Dunlap AM, Cooper EC, King LB. Mandibular first molar relation to variable lower face skeletal components. Angle Orthod 2007;77(1):21-8.
3. Auvenshine RC. Temporomandibular disorders: associated features. Dent Clin North Am 2007;51(1):105-27, vi. Review.
4. Bishara SE, Jakobsen JR, Vorhies B, Bayati P. Changes in dentofacial structures in untreated Class II division 1 and normal subjects: a longitudinal study. Angle Orthod 1997;67(1):55-66.
5. Bishara SE, Jakobsen JR. Longitudinal changes in three normal facial types. Am J Orthod. 1985;88(6):466-502.
6. Broadbent JM. TMJ in your practice. Funct Orthod. 2006 Summer-Fall;23(2):38-45.
7. Graff-Radford SB. Temporomandibular disorders and other causes of facial pain. Curr Pain Headache Rep 2007;11(1):75-81. Review.
8. Haynes S. Prevalence of upper lip posture and incisor overjet. Community Dent Oral Epidemiol 1977;5(2):87-90.
9. Karlsen AT, Krogstad O. Morphology and growth in convex profile facial patterns: a longitudinal study. Angle Orthod 1999;69(4):334-44.
10. Karlsen AT. Longitudinal changes in Class I subjects with moderate mandibular skeletal protrusion. Angle Orthod 1998;68(5):431-8.
11. Keski-Nisula K, Keski-Nisula L, Makela P, Maki-Torkko T, Varrela J. Dentofacial features of children with distal occlusions, large overjets, and deepbites in the early mixed dentition. Am J Orthod Dentofacial Orthop 2006;130(3):292-9.
12. Matoula S, Pancherz H. Skeletofacial morphology of attractive and nonattractive faces. Angle Orthod 2006; 76(2):204-10.
13. McIntyre GT, Millett DT. Lip shape and position in Class II division 2 malocclusion. Angle Orthod 2006;76(5):739-44.
14. Turkkahraman H, Gokalp H. Facial profile preferences among various layers of Turkish population. Angle Orthod 2004;74(5):640-7
15. Wiese M, Hintze H, Svensson P, Wenzel A. Comparison of diagnostic accuracy of film and digital tomograms for assessment of morphological changes in the TMJ. Dentomaxillofac Radiol 2007;36(1):12-7.
16. Zaitseva V, Son'kin V. Statistical and physiological distinction of constitution types. J Physiol Anthropol Appl Human Sci 2005;24(4):327-31.
17. Zhang X, Hans MG, Graham G, Kirchner HL, Redline S. Correlations between cephalometric and facial photographic measurements of craniofacial form. Am J Orthod Dentofacial Orthop 2007;131(1):67-71.

QUESTIONS

1. What is vital statistics?
2. Explain chief complaint and the history related to it.
3. Give the vaccination schedule recommended for children.
4. What is the importance of past dental, family and personal history?
5. What is the relevance of oral habits and oral hygiene history?
6. Explain the FDI and Zsigmondy-Palmer tooth numbering system.
7. Write in detail the deciduous and permanent molar relationship.
8. Explain the canine and incisor relationship.
9. Curve of Spee and deciduous dentition.
10. Write the different types of swallowing patterns.
11. Physiologic spacing.
12. What are the reasons of dental midline shift?
13. What is the difference between provisional and final diagnosis.
14. Enumerate different investigation procedures.
15. What is the role of percussion and pulp testing in examination?
16. Use of cephalometrics in investigation.
17. Enumerate supplemental diagnostic aids.
18. Explain dental age.
19. What are the advantages of treatment planning?
20. What are the different phases of treatment planning?
21. What is informed consent?

Growth and Development

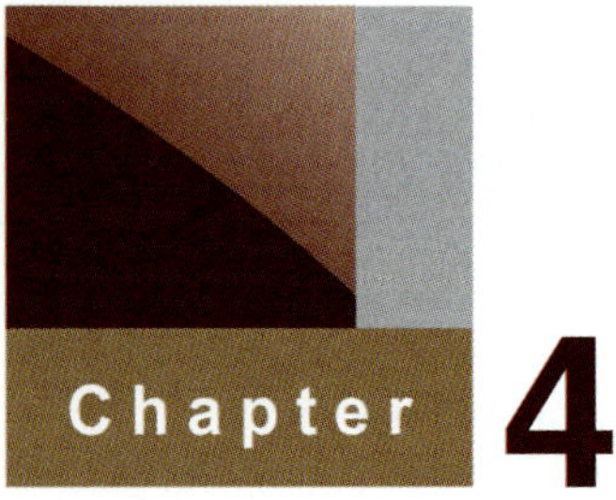

CRANIOFACIAL GROWTH

DEFINITION OF GROWTH AND DEVELOPMENT

Growth is defined as an increase in mass, which means that it is a process that leads to an increase in the physical size of a cell, tissue organ or organism as a whole.

Development is defined as progress towards maturity. It is the naturally occurring unidirectional changes in life. Growth and development go hand in hand and hence most of the time are dealt together.

FACTORS INFLUENCING GROWTH

1. Genetic factors
2. Maternal factors
3. Environmental factors

Genetic Factors

Size at birth relates to about
- 18% to genome of the fetus
- 20% to the maternal genome
- 32% to the maternal environmental factors
- 30% to unknown factors

After birth, growth rate is primarily related to its own genetic make up. Thus neonates who are small for gestational age but have the genetic capacity to catch up to the normal range generally show accelerated growth within the first 6 months of postnatal life. Size at birth correlates best with the size of the mother.

Maternal Factors

1. *Role of uterine constraints or the size of the uterus:* The fetus increases in size and fills the entire uterine cavity as it grows. During the last months the uterine constraints may limit the growth of the fetus.
2. *Role of placenta:* Placenta grows by increasing the cells until 35 weeks of gestation. Later the growth is due to increase in cell size. By 38–40 weeks of gestation the placenta reaches its full growth and later shows signs of deterioration or regression. So a post-mature infant may be under weighed.
3. *Socioeconomic factors:* Lower the socioeconomic status the smaller is the size of the child.
4. *Maternal health:* Rubella, Rh incompatibility or other ill-health affecting the mother will directly affect the development of the fetus.
5. *Tobacco:* Smoking is most damaging as it affects the fetal heart rate and alters the chemical content of the fetal blood.
6. *Emotions:* Fetal activity and heart rate increases in mild maternal stress. Severe and prolonged maternal stress lead to 'blood borne anxieties' which affect the postnatal as well as prenatal development.
7. *Nutrition:* Fetus is able to obtain adequate nutrition for prenatal growth, even at the expense of depleting the mother. It, therefore, requires severe malnourishment in mother to have its effect on the child. Alcohol, if sparing used has no effect. If used frequently and heavily it is likely to damage the child's physical and mental development.
8. *Endocrine factors:* Endocrine disturbances in mother will directly influence the fetal growth. Example, maternal diabetes causes excessive fetal growth and thus an overweight baby.
9. *Other maternal factors adversely affecting fetal growth:* Toxemia, hypertension, renal and cardiac diseases, use of exogenous agents such as ethanol, nicotine, hydantoin, warfarin, etc.

Environmental Factors

1. Postnatal growth and development of a child depends on both the genetic and environmental factors.
2. Environmental factors that influence growth and development are socioeconomic factors, smoking, emotions, nutrition, endocrine factors and general health.

NORMAL HUMAN GROWTH

The time from conception to birth is described in three phases:
1. Period of ovum
2. Period of embryo
3. Period of fetus

1. Period of ovum (Conception—10 days)
   - This period is from fertilization to implantation (up to 10–14 days).
   - Rapid internal development is seen.
   - Implantation in the uterine wall occurs after about 10 days of fertilization.
2. Period of embryo—2–8 weeks
   - Accessory apparatus like placenta, umbilical cord and amniotic sac develop during this period.
   - External and internal features start to develop and function.
   - Sex can be identified.
   - Growth in the head region is proportionally much greater than the rest of the body.
   - By the end of this period the embryo measures 1½ to 2" in length.
3. Period of fetus—8–40 weeks
   - Growth continues
   - Nerve cells that are present since the third week, increase rapidly in number during the second, third and fourth months.
   - Internal organs assume nearly adult positions by fifth lunar month.

> The development of face begins during the 4th week of intrauterine life. It is seen as consisting of one frontonasal process, two maxillary processes and two mandibular processes.

Relation of maxilla to mandible during growth:

Embryonic stage—mandibular process is larger
Fetal stage—maxilla is more developed
By 11 weeks—mandible grows rapidly and equals maxilla
By 13-20th week—lag in mandibular growth
At birth—mandible seems to be retrognathic to maxilla

Intrauterine life is characterized by very rapid growth, with peak growth velocity at about the 4th month. The growth rate decreases during the last 5 months. Following birth, growth rate continues to decrease. This is the period when the infant makes adjustments for the maternal factors that influence birth length and weight.

Scammon's Growth Curve

It represents the differential growth of the body tissues. The lymphoid tissues, genital tissues and neural tissues grow at different rates and are different from the general growth of the other tissues of the body and represented in a graph as in Figure 4.1.

Lymphoid tissues grow during childhood. The growth of the neural tissues is complete at a early stage of life at about 7 years, whereas the growth of genital tissues begins only at puberty. The growth of the body in general comprising of skeletal system, muscles and the visceras grow and develop throughout from birth with periods of low and rapid growth throughout and represented as an 'S' curve in the graph.

Features Seen at Birth (Fig. 4.2)

- Tiny mouth and small chin
- Small face, eyes appear big
- Forehead and top of the head are big
- Bones that compose the cranium are not fused
- Broad and flat face
- Underdeveloped mandible
- Cranium is nearest to adult size

By 1 year, the infant is growing near the projected growth rate and by 2 years, the growth rate is dependent on the genetic make up of the child itself. From 2–3 years growth is slow and steady till puberty.

Growth of cranial vault is complete before that of maxilla. And maxillary growth is complete before mandibular growth.

3–6 Years

- Cartilage in the skeletal system is getting replaced by bone and all the bones become more calcified and harder.
- Face becomes larger, wider, longer and more detailed.
- It will become evident to some degree which children have natural athletic ability and which do not.
- Soft tissue prominence of nose and mandible continue to increase.
- Lowering of palatal vault is seen, due to sutural growth and apposition on the oral side of the palate and resorption on the nasal side.

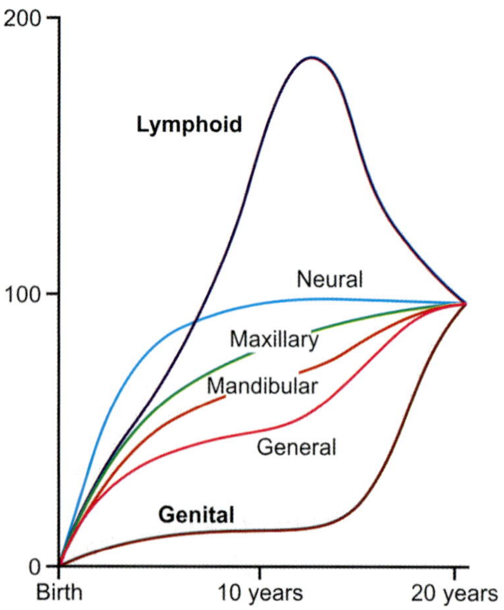

Fig. 4.1: Scammon's growth curve

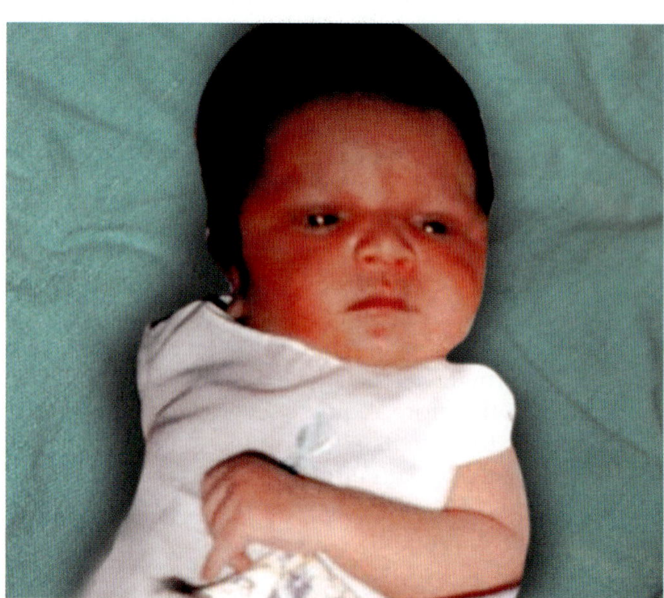

Fig. 4.2: Newborn baby

- Transverse growth of the face comes to an end much earlier than other dimensions.

6–12 Years

Most remarkable proportional change in the body during these years results from the lengthening of the child's limbs. Boys are generally slightly taller and heavier than girls until around 10 years. From 10–15 years girls become slightly taller and heavier than boys for a brief period. Neural and cranial growth are found to be almost entering completion.

>12 Years (Adolescence)

It is usually associated with puberty, which is the landmark in physical development when an individual becomes capable of sexual reproduction. It is paralleled by the development of genital tissue and secondary sexual characteristics. There is an increase in the mass of muscles, redistribution of body fat and increase in the rate of skeletal growth. A growth spurt is associated with this time of life.

GROWTH SPURTS

Growth does not occur uniformly throughout the life. Certain periods of life exhibit faster or more growth compared to other periods. Such bouts of sudden accelerated growth are termed as growth spurts.
Periods of growth spurts are:
a. Just before birth
b. One year after birth
c. Mixed dentition period—boys at 8–11 years and girls at 7–9 years.
d. Adolescent period—boys at 14–16 years and girls at 11–13 years.

Clinical Importance

Orthodontic appliances such as myofunctional appliances are usually prescribed during these growth spurt periods, taking advantage of the active growth. Orthopedic surgeries such as done for the correction of bimaxillary protrusion are done preferably after cessation of the growth, otherwise it may result in relapse and failure.

> Influence of Hormones on Growth:
> *Increase in growth rate*—growth hormone, thyroxin, insulin
> *Decrease in growth rate*—corticosteroids
> *Increase in skeletal ossification*—parathormone, vit D, calcitonin
> *Increase in skeletal maturation and pubertal growth*— thyroxin, gonadotropins, adrenal steroids

MEASURES OF GROWTH

Standard normal growth measures can be studied based on either cross-sectional data or longitudinal data. Cross-sectional data compare the height of a child at a given time with the heights of other children in general population. Longitudinal study includes collection and comparing a single child over a period of time.

Growth Assessment Parameters

The parameters used to assess growth are:
1. Chronologic age
2. Biologic age
   - Morphologic age/height and weight age
   - Skeletal age
   - Dental age
   - Sexual age
3. Behavioral age
4. Facial age
5. Mental age

Chronologic Age

Chronologic age is calculated from the child's date of birth. This, by itself is, not an accurate indicator of stage of development, nor is it a good predictor of growth potential.

Height and weight age

A standard growth curve (Fig. 4.3) is used to assess and characterize a child's height, compared to that of children of the same chronologic age. The child's own growth curve can be expressed by constructing a growth velocity curve, plotting height increments per year for each chronologic age. Weight standard curves have been constructed, although the abnormal variation in weight in otherwise normal children limits the usefulness of these curves as a sole indicator of development.

Skeletal age

The areas of ossification are recognizable on a radiograph and can be compared to the normal sequence of developmental changes that occur from birth to adulthood.

A characteristic pattern of progression of ossification of epiphyseal centers can be identified. Each endochondral bone begins with a primary center of ossification, which changes in shape, size and contour until fusion occurs. Any of the skeletal growth centers may be used, but the hand and wrist have been commonly used as the area may be easily radiographed with minimal radiation exposure to the rest of the body. The union of the epiphyses with their diaphyses occurs in a specific order, which in females is advanced by 3–4

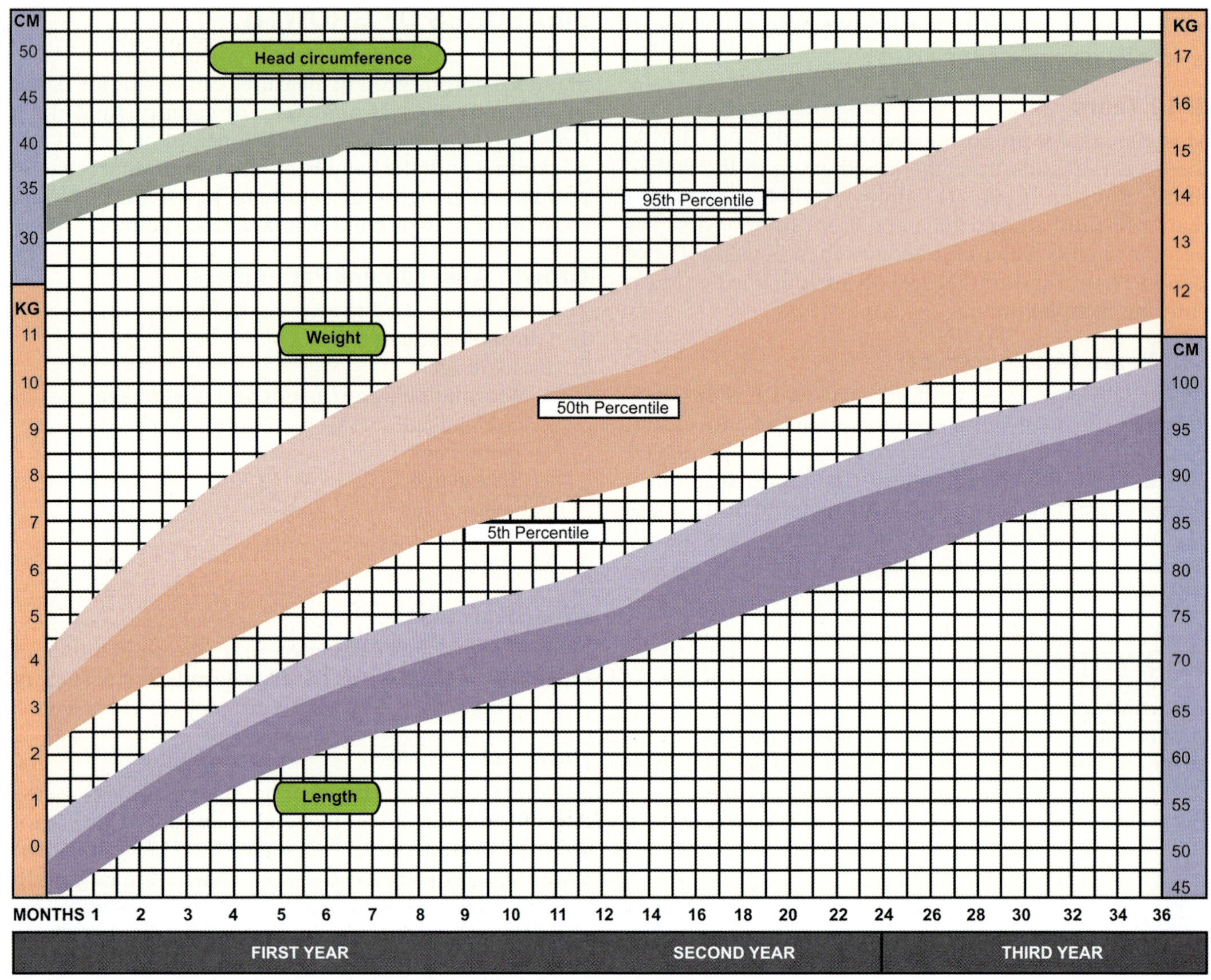

Fig. 4.3: Standard growth curve chart

years compared to that in males. Between the ages of 12.5 and 14 years the most active transformation of the epiphyseal cartilages occurs concurrently with peak height velocity.

Skeletal age was found to be more highly correlated with menarcheal age than with height and weight. Menarche usually occurred soon after the fusion of the epiphysis of the distal phalanges with their shafts.

Dental age

Dental age indicator involves recognizing the teeth clinically present in the oral cavity in comparison to dental eruption charts. It also involves scoring based on the amount of calcification, according to the amount of crown and root formation or based on the different stages of tooth development. Dental age can be very well calculated using Nolla's (Fig. 4.4) or Demirjian's method (Figs 4.5A to H).

1. Absence of crypt
2. Initial calcification
3. 1/3rd of the crown completed
4. 2/3rd of the crown completed
5. Crown almost completed
6. Crown completed
7. 1/3rd of root completed
8. 2/3rd of root completed
9. Root almost completed
10. Apical end of root development completed.

Sexual age

Tanner outlined stages of secondary sexual characteristics and their relation to the pubertal growth spurt in

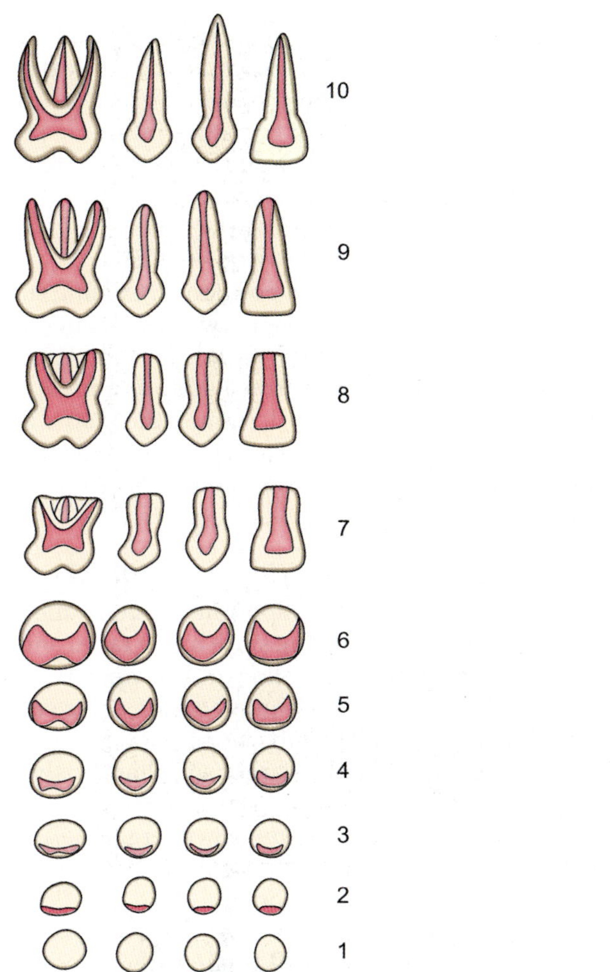

Fig. 4.4: Stages of development of teeth based on Nolla's method

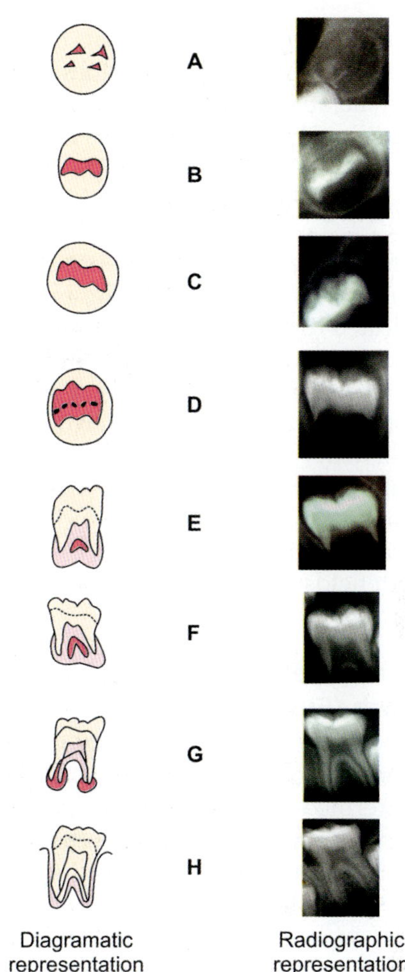

Diagramatic representation   Radiographic representation

Figs 4.5A to H: Stages of tooth development used for calculating the dental age as per Demirjian's method. (A) Beginning of calcification seen at the superior level of the crypt in the form of inverted cone; (B) Fusion of the calcified points to form the occlusal outline; (C) Enamel formation is complete at the occlusal surface. Its extension and convergence towards the cervical region is seen; (D) Crown formation is complete down to the cementoenamel junction; (E) Initial formation of the root is seen; (F) Bifurcation appears to give roots a more distinct outline; (G) Walls of the root canal are parallel. Apical ends of the roots are open; (H) Apical ends of the roots are closed

height categorizing them into five stages. Stage one is prepubertal and stage five is a mature adult.

Behavioral Age

It is based on the behavior of the patient, which can be social or activity based.

Facial Age

It is an anthropometric measurements and development of a facial growth velocity curve using measurements from serial cephalometric radiographs similar to the standard height curves.

Mental Age

Mental age is based on the IQ or understanding ability of the child. Any explanation given to children regarding the instruments or procedure should be done in accord with the mental age of the child.

PRACTICAL SIGNIFICANCE OF PREDICTING DEVELOPMENT

1. *Mature size:* It is possible to predict at a fairly early age what the child's adult physique will be.
2. *Educational planning:* Plans regarding education can be made based on the child's early intellectual aptitude.
3. *Preparation for next stage:* At every stage of development, the child can be prepared for the next stage.

4. *Vocational planning:* Early physical, intellectual and personality development gives clues as to what the child may be able to do vocationally in adulthood. These clues can be used by parents and teachers.

MECHANISMS OF GROWTH

Growth of facial skeleton is not a simple mechanism. There are no symmetrical enlargements but is associated with complicated differential growth mechanism.

The mechanisms important for bone growth in craniofacial regions are:
- A. Endosteal and periosteal bone growth
- B. Cortical drift
- C. Relocation and remodeling
- D. V' principle
- E. Surface principle
- F. Growth fields
- G. Displacement

Endosteal and Periosteal Bone Growth (Fig. 4.6)

When there is growth of a particular bone by the deposition of bone on the inner or endosteal surface of the bone it is termed as endosteal bone growth. Similarly periosteal bone growth is seen when bone deposition occurs on the outside or in the periosteum. Both types of growths are seen in facial and cranial bones.

Cortical Drift

All bone structures have one growth principle in common, termed as 'drift' by Enlow. The cortical plate drifts in the direction of growth by selective deposition on the outer side and resorption on the inner side. The

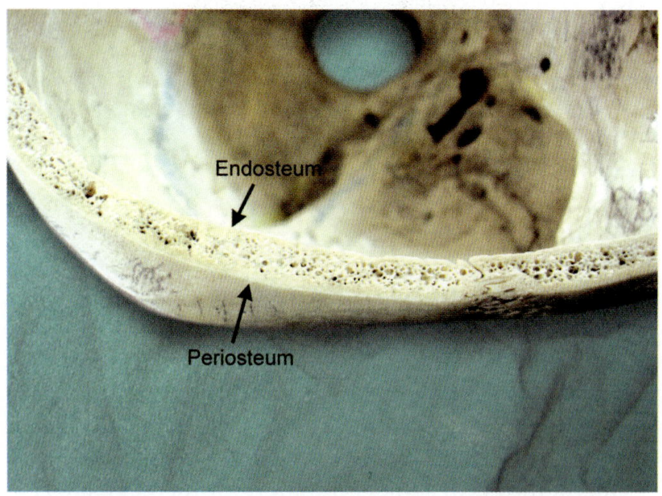

Fig. 4.6: Endosteum and periosteum of the skull bone

rate of deposition and resorption is almost similar thus maintaining the thickness of the cortical plate. The teeth follow the drift of the alveolar bone while the jaws are growing and thus maintaining their position within the surrounding bony structures despite the bone displacement.

Relocation and Remodeling

Due to new bone deposition on existing surface, all other parts of the structure undergo shifts in relative position, a movement which is termed as 'relocation'. As a result of this process, further adaptive bone remodeling is necessary in order to adjust the shape and size of the bone to the new relationship. Remodeling is based on relocation and is a secondary result of the displacement process.

Expanding 'V' Principle (Fig. 4.7)

This principle is important to study the facial skeleton growth mechanism, since many facial and cranial bones have a 'V' configuration or 'V' shaped regions. Such areas grow by bone resorption on the outer surface of the 'V' and deposition on the inner surface. The 'V' moves away from its tip and enlarges simultaneously. Thus increase in size and growth movements are a unified process resulting in enlargement in overall size, movement of the entire 'V' structure towards its own wide end leading to continuous relocation.

Surface Principle (Fig. 4.8)

According to this, bone sides which face the direction of growth are subject to deposition and those opposite to it undergo resorption. The direction of growth is not the same for all the areas of the bone as each region of a structure has its own specific growth pattern.

Growth Fields

Bone growth is controlled by so-called growth fields. They are distributed in a characteristic pattern across the surface of a given bone and have either depository or resorptive activity. Growth fields have a pace making function, which is controlled by soft tissues. The soft tissues act as functional matrix to control bone growth whereas the bone itself only reports, via a feed-back mechanism which is connected to the connective tissues, when the shape, size and biomechanical aspects coincide with the functional requirement.

Displacement (Figs 4.9A and B)

Apart from direct bone growth due to deposition and resorption, the process of displacement, that is the translatory movement of the whole bone caused by the

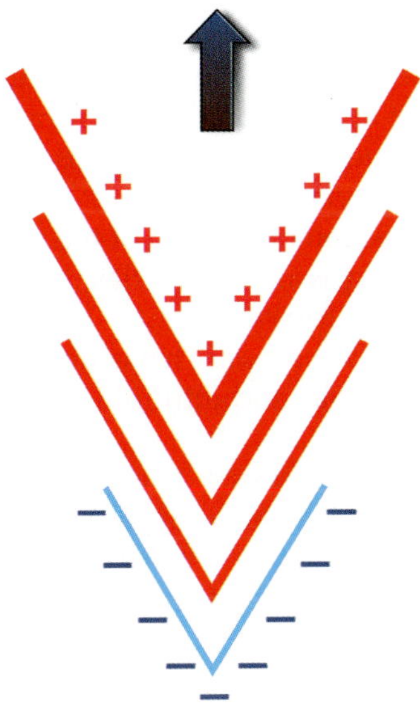

Fig. 4.7: Expanding 'V' principle of growth

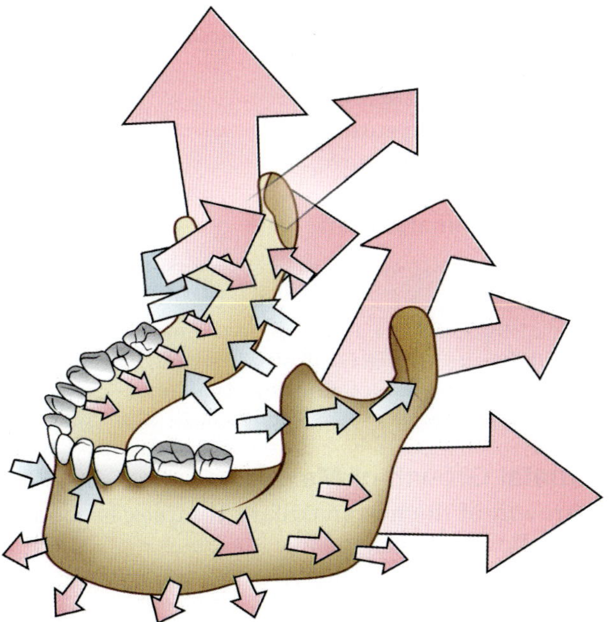

Fig. 4.8: Surface principle of growth

surrounding physical forces, is the second characteristic mechanism of skull growth. The entire bone is carried away from its articular interfaces with adjacent bones.

Displacement in conjunction with bone's own growth is termed 'primary displacement' by Enlow. The degree of displacement exactly equals the amount of new bone deposition, although the direction of displacement is always opposite to that of bone deposition. Bone displacement due to the enlargement of bones and soft tissues which are nearby or not immediately adjacent is termed 'secondary displacement.'

Functional Matrix Theory

Osteogenesis is mostly influenced by local functional demands. For example, an increase in the size of the brain influences the increase in size of the cranium.

Each component of the bone consists of two parts, the functional matrix and the skeletal unit. Functional matrix includes functioning spaces and the soft tissue components required for a specific function. The functional matrix carries out a given function, whereas the skeletal units such as bone and cartilage protect and support the functional matrix and are adaptable.

There are two types of functional matrices, the periosteal matrix and the capsular matrix. Periosteal matrix is best represented by muscle attachment. Capsular matrices are divided into three types—the neurocranial, orbital and orofacial.

The capsular and periosteal matrices have a completely different effect on the growth processes. Capsular matrix exerts a direct influence on the macroskeletal units and functional cranial components. It is responsible for changes in the three dimensional position of the skeletal unit. Periosteal matrix exerts direct influence on the microskeletal unit and the functional cranial components or perichondral or endochondral growth processes. Thus the periosteal matrix changes the shape and size of the corresponding microskeletal unit.

POSTNATAL GROWTH

Cranium

The growth processes occurring at the cranial base, maxilla and the mandible are all related to each other at various sutures and the temporomandibular joint.

The cranial base grows postnatally by complex interaction between the following three growth processes:
A. Extensive cortical drift and remodeling
B. Elongation at synchondroses
C. Sutural growth

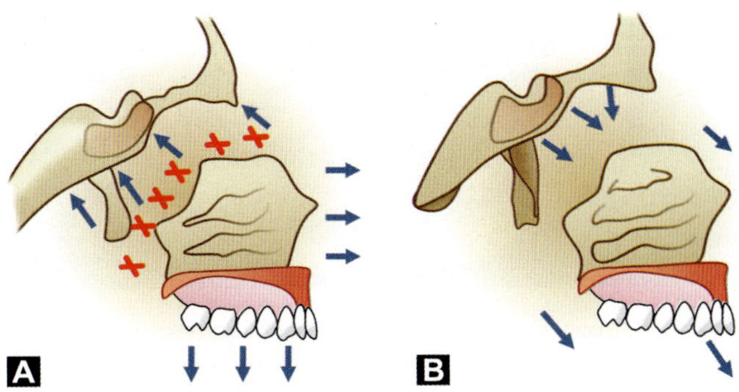

Figs 4.9A and B: Displacement

Cortical Drift and Remodeling

Remodeling is a process where bone deposition and resorption occur that bring about change in size, shape and relationship of the bone.

The elevated ridges and bony partitions in the cranial base show bone deposition.

The predominant part of the floor shows bone resorption, which helps in increasing the intracranial space to accommodate the growing brain.

The cranial base is perforated by the passage of a number of blood vessels and nerves communicating with the brain. The foramina that allow the passage of these nerves and blood vessels undergo drifting by bone deposition and resorption so as to constantly maintain their proper relationship with the growing brain.

Elongation at the Synchondroses

Most of the bones of the cranial base are formed by a cartilaginous process. Later the cartilage is replaced by bone. However, small parts of cartilage may remain at the junction of various bones. These areas are called synchondroses. They are important growth sites of the cranial base. The important synchondroses found in the cranial base are (Fig. 4.10):

A. Spheno-occipital synchondrosis
B. Sphenoethmoid synchondrosis
C. Intersphenoid synchondrosis
D. Interoccipital synchondrosis

Spheno-occipital synchondrosis: It is a cartilaginous junction between the sphenoid and the occipital bones. The spheno-occipital synchondrosis is the principal growth cartilage of the cranial base during childhood and is active up to the age of 12–15 years. The sphenoid and the occipital segments then become fused in the midline by the age of 20 years.

Since the direction of growth of the spheno-occipital synchondrosis is upwards, it carries the anterior part of the cranium bodily forwards.

Sphenoethmoid synchondrosis: This is a cartilaginous band between the sphenoid and ethmoid bones. It ossifies at later years of age.

Intersphenoidal synchondrosis: It is a cartilaginous band between the 2 parts of the sphenoid bone. It ossifies at birth.

Intraoccipital synchondrosis: This ossifies by 3–5 years of age.

Sutural Growth

The cranial base has a number of bones that are joined to one another by means of sutures. Some of the sutures that are present and influence the growth of the cranium are (Fig. 4.11):

1. Sphenofrontal suture
2. Frontotemporal suture
3. Sphenoethmoid suture
4. Frontoethmoid suture
5. Frontozygomatic suture

> **Timing of cranial base growth**
>
> A. By birth, 55-60% of adult size is attained.
> B. By 4-7 years, 94% of adult size is attained.
> C. By 8-13 years, 98% of adult size is attained.

Postnatal Growth of Maxilla

The growth of the nasomaxillary complex is produced by the following mechanisms:

A. Displacement
B. Growth at sutures
C. Surface remodeling

Displacement

Maxilla is attached to the cranial base by means of a number of sutures. Thus the growth of the cranial base has a direct bearing on the nasomaxillary growth.

Nasomaxillary complex grows in a downward and forward direction as the cranial base grows. This is referred to as secondary displacement, as the actual enlargement of these parts is not directly involved. The passive displacement of the maxilla is an important growth mechanism during the primary dentition years but becomes less important as growth of cranial base slows.

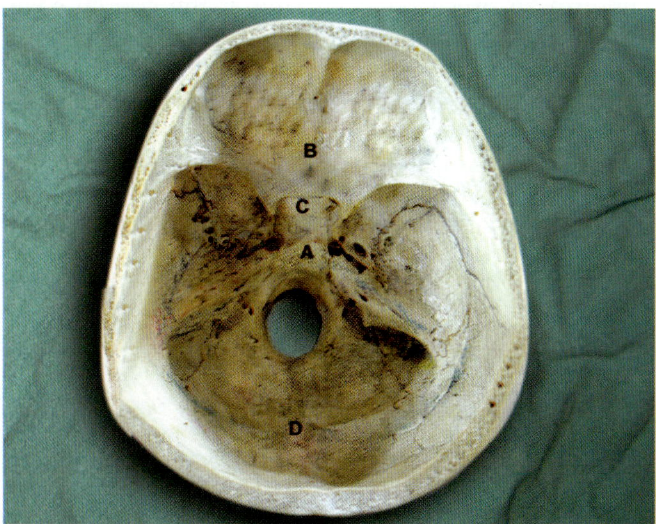

Fig. 4.10: Positions of the important synchondroses of the cranial base: (A) Spheno-occipital synchondrosis; (B) Sphenoethmoid synchondrosis; (C) Intersphenoid synchondrosis; (D) Interoccipital synchondrosis

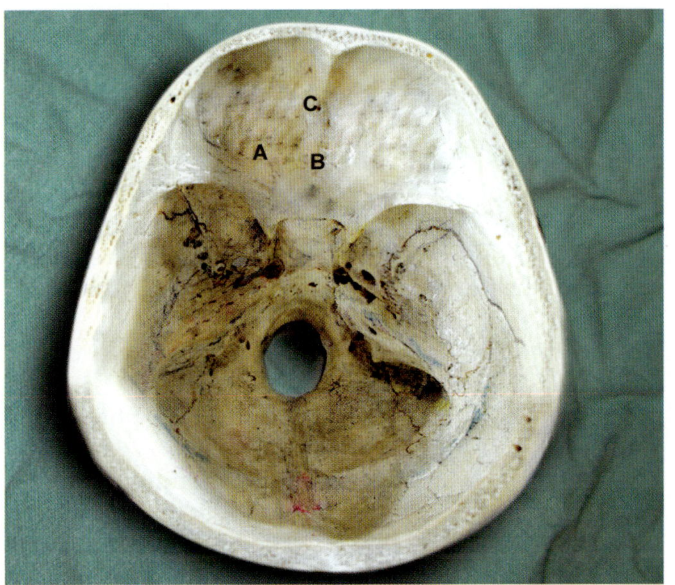

Fig. 4.11: Important sutures at the cranial base: (A) Sphenofrontal suture; (B) Sphenoethmoid suture; (C) Frontoethmoid suture

Primary type of displacement is also seen in a forward direction. This occurs by growth of the maxillary tuberosity in a posterior direction resulting in the whole maxilla being carried anteriorly. The amount of this forward displacement equals the amount of posterior lengthening.

Growth at Sutures

The maxilla is connected to the cranium and cranial base by a number of sutures. These sutures include (Fig. 4.12):
1. Frontonasal suture
2. Frontomaxillary suture
3. Zygomaticotemporal suture
4. Zygomaticomaxillary suture
5. Pterygopalatine suture

These sutures are all oblique and more or less parallel to each other, which allows the downward and forward repositioning of the maxilla as growth occurs at these sutures. As growth of the surrounding soft tissue occurs, the maxilla is carried downwards and forward. This leads to opening up of space at the sutural attachments. New bone is now formed on either side of the suture. Thus the overall size of the bones on either side increases.

Surface Remodeling

In addition to the growth occurring at the sutures, massive remodeling by bone deposition and resorption occurs to bring about:
1. Increase in size
2. Change in shape of bone
3. Change in functional relationship

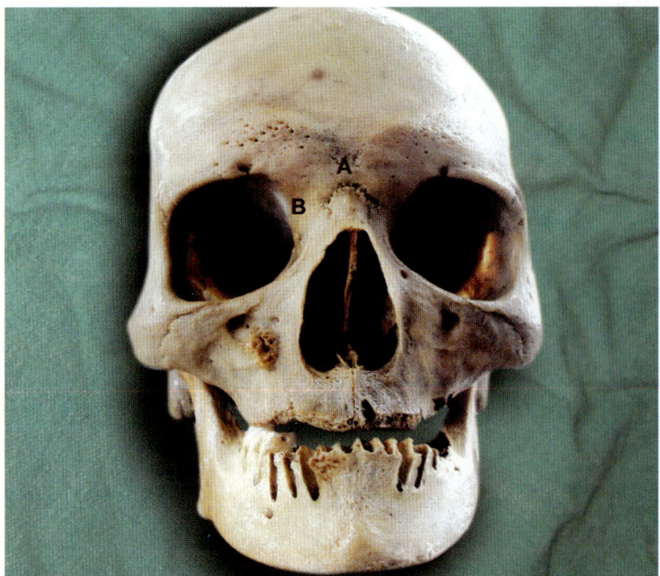

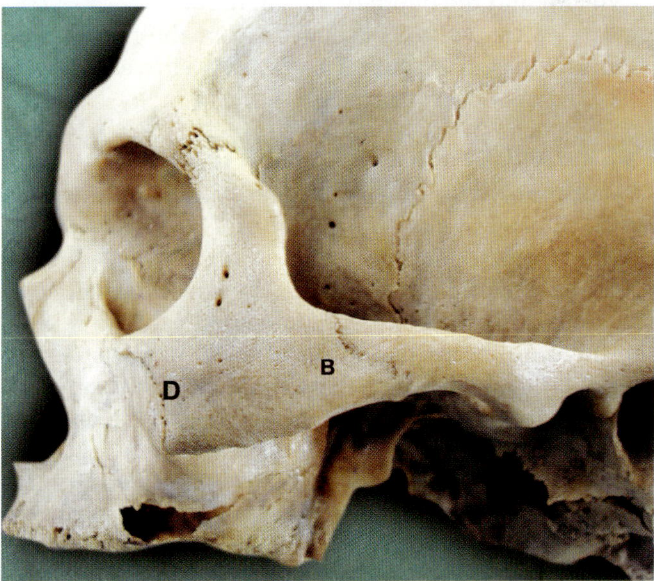

Fig. 4.12: Important sutures through which maxilla is connected to the cranial base: (A) Frontonasal suture; (B) Frontomaxillary suture; (C) Zygomaticotemporal suture; (D) Zygomaticomaxillary suture

It is characterized by:
- Resorption occurs on the lateral surface and deposition on the medial rim of the orbit.
- Bone deposition occurs along the posterior margin of the maxillary tuberosity. This causes lengthening of the dental arch and enlargement of the anteroposterior dimension of the entire maxillary body. This helps to accommodate the erupting molars.
- Bone resorption occurs on the lateral wall of the nose leading to an increase in size of the nasal cavity.

- Bone resorption is seen on the floor of the nasal cavity and there is bone deposition on the palatal side. Thus a net downward shift occurs leading to increase in maxillary height.
- Resorption on the anterior surface and deposition on the posterior surface of the zygomatic bone results in the movement of the bone in a posterior direction.
- The face enlarges in width by bone formation on the lateral surface of the zygomatic arch and resorption on its medial surface.
- The anterior nasal spine prominence increases due to bone deposition. In addition there is resorption from the periosteal surface of labial cortex. As a compensatory mechanism, bone deposition occurs on the endosteal surface of the labial cortex and periosteal surface of the lingual cortex.
- As the teeth start erupting, bone deposition occurs at the alveolar margins. This increases the maxillary height and the depth of the palate.
- The entire wall of the sinus except the mesial wall undergoes resorption. This results in increase in size of the maxillary antrum.

Postnatal Growth of Mandible (Fig. 4.13)

Developmentally and functionally the mandible is made of several skeletal subunits. The basal bone or the body of the mandible forms one unit, to which is attached the alveolar process, the coronoid process, the condylar process, the angular process, the ramus, the lingual tuberosity and the chin. Thus the study of postnatal growth of the mandible is made easier and more meaningful when each of the developmental and functional parts are considered separately.

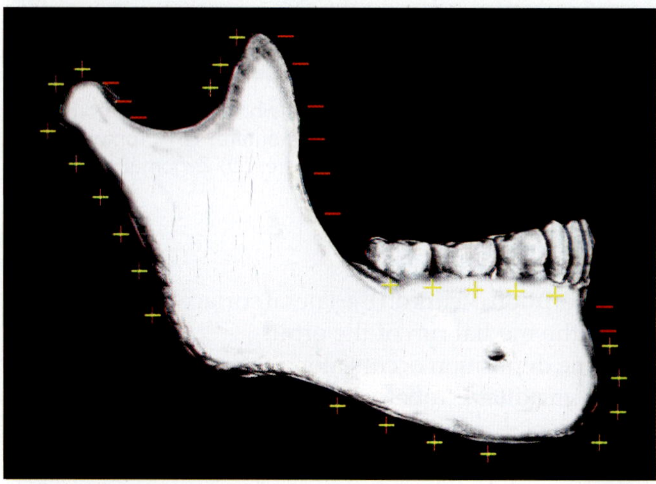

Fig. 4.13: Areas of bone deposition (+) and resorption (–) in mandible

The right and the left halves of the mandible fuse by one year after birth. Chin prominence increases as the child grows along with lengthening of the body of the mandible.

The ramus moves progressively posteriorly by a combination of deposition and resorption. Resorption occurs on the anterior part of the ramus, while bone deposition occurs on the posterior region. This results in a 'drift' of the ramus in a posterior direction, which aids to:

- Accommodate the increasing mass of masticatory muscles inserted into it.
- Accommodate the enlarged width of the pharyngeal space.
- Facilitate the lengthening of the mandibular body, which in turn accommodates the erupting molars.

This results in the conversion of former ramus bone into the posterior part of the body of mandible. In this manner the body of the mandible also lengthens. Thus the additional space made available by means of resorption of the anterior border of the ramus is made use of to accommodate the erupting permanent molars.

Resorption also takes place on the posteroinferior aspect of the angle of mandible while deposition occurs on the anterosuperior aspect on the lingual aspect. On the buccal side, resorption occurs on the anterosuperior part and deposition occurs on the posterosuperior aspect. This result in flaring out of the angle of the mandible as age advances.

The lingual tuberosity moves posteriorly by deposition on its posteriorly facing surface. The prominence of the tuberosity is increased by the presence of a large resorption field just below it. This resorption field produces a sizable depression, the lingual fossa and deposition on the medial surface of the tuberosity itself accentuates the prominence of the lingual tuberosity.

Alveolar process develops in response to the presence of tooth buds. As the teeth erupt the alveolar process develops and increases in height by bone deposition at the margins. The alveolar bone adds to the height and thickness of the body of the mandible and is particularly manifested as a ledge extending lingual to the ramus to accommodate the 3rd molars. In case of absence of teeth, the alveolar bone fails to develop and it resorbs in the event of tooth extraction.

At birth the chin is usually under-developed. As age advances the growth of chin becomes significant and is influenced by sexual and specific genetic factors. Usually males have prominent chins compared to females. The mental protuberance forms by the deposition of bone during childhood.

The growth of the coronoid process follows the enlarging 'V' principle. Viewing the longitudinal section of the coronoid process from the posterior aspect, it can be seen that deposition occurs on the lingual (medial) surfaces of the left and right coronoid process. There is also associated increase in the height of the coronoid process.

Viewing it from the occlusal aspect, the deposition on the lingual of the coronoid process brings about a posterior growth movement in the 'V' pattern.

The mandibular condyle forms an important growth site. The head of the condyle is covered by a thin layer of cartilage called the condylar cartilage. The role of the condyle in the growth of mandible has remained a controversy, there are two schools of thought regarding the role of the condyle.

A. It was earlier believed that growth occurs at the surface of the condylar cartilage by means of bone deposition. Thus the condyle grows towards the cranial base. As the condyle pushes against the cranial base, the entire mandible gets displaced forwards and downwards.

B. It is now believed that the growth of soft tissues including the muscles and connective tissues carries the mandible forwards away from the cranial base (carry away phenomenon). Bone growth follows secondarily at the condyle to maintain constant contact with the cranial base.

Growth and development of the face is a combination of the growth of the entire cranium, the maxilla and the mandible. If there is hindrance in this growth in any one of the complexes it can result in serious deformity in the entire facial skeleton. Common example is the early synostosis of the cranial sutures results in syndromes such as Crouzon's or the Aperts Syndrome characterized by severe changes in the cranium as well in the orbit, nose, maxilla and mandible.

FURTHER READING

1. Arat M, Koklu A, Ozdiler E, Rubenduz M, Erdogan B. Craniofacial growth and skeletal maturation: a mixed longitudinal study. Eur J Orthod 2001;23(4):355-61.
2. Avery JK. Prenatal Growth. In: Moyers RE (Ed). Handbook of Orthodontics. 4th Ed. Year Book Medical Publishers, Inc. Chicago 1988.
3. Bishara SE, Jakobsen JR. Longitudinal changes in three normal facial types. Am J Orthod 1985;88(6):466-502.
4. Björk A, Skieller V. Postnatal growth and development of the maxillary complex. In: Mc Namara JA (Ed). Factors affecting the growth of the midface, craniofacial growth series. AnnArbor, Mich Centre for Human Growth and Development, University of Michigan 1976;61-99.
5. Broadbent BH Sr, Broadbent BH Jr, Golden WH. Bolten standards of dentofacial developmental growth. St Louis CV Mosby Co 1975.
6. Demirjian A, Goldstein H, Tanner JM. A new system of dental age assessment. Hum Biol 1973;45:211-27.
7. Dogan S, Oncag G, Akin Y. Craniofacial development in children with unilateral cleft lip and palate. Br J Oral Maxillofac Surg 2006;44(1):28-33. Epub 2005 Nov 18.
8. Enlow DH. Handbook of facial growth, 2nd Ed. Philadelphia, WB Saunders Co 1982.
9. Enlow DH. Principles of bone remodeling. Springfield Ill Charles C Thomas 1963.
10. Enlow DH. The human face New York. Hoeber Medical Division, Harper and Row, 1968 (Moyers RE, Enlow DH. Growth of the craniofacial skeleton in Moyer RE, Handbook of Orthodontics 4th Ed. Year Book Medical Publishers, Inc. Chicago 1988.
11. Eteson DJ. Determination of developmental age. Pediatric Dentistry, Scientific foundation and clinical practice. Stewart RE, Barber TK, Troutman KC, Wei SHY, 1982;11-31.
12. Funatsu M, Sato K, Mitani H. Effects of growth hormone on craniofacial growth. Angle Orthod 2006;76(6):970-7.
13. Gomes AS, Lima EM. Mandibular growth during adolescence. Angle Orthod 2006;76(5):786-90.
14. Hesby RM, Marshall SD, Dawson DV, Southard KA, Casko JS, Franciscus RG, Southard TE. Transverse skeletal and dentoalveolar changes during growth. Am J Orthod Dentofacial Orthop 2006;130(6):721-31.
15. Kasai K, Moro T, Kanazawa E, Iwasawa T. Relationship between cranial base and maxillofacial morphology. Eur J Orthod 1995;17(5):403-10.
16. Krogman WM. Biological timing and dentofacial complex. J Dent Child 1968;35:176,328,377.
17. Langman J. Medical Embryology, 4th Ed. Baltimore, Williams and Wilkins Co 1988;268-306.
18. Lux CJ, Conradt C, Burden D, Komposch G. Transverse development of the craniofacial skeleton and dentition between 7 and 15 years of age—a longitudinal postero-anterior cephalometric study. Eur J Orthod 2004;26(1):31-42.
19. Lux CJ, Conradt C, Burden D, Komposch G. Three-dimensional analysis of maxillary and mandibular growth increments. Cleft Palate Craniofac J 2004;41(3): 304-14.
20. Moore RN. Postnatal development in Stewart RE, Barber TK, Troutman KC, Wei SHY. Pediatric Dentistry, Scientific foundations and clinical practice. The CV Mosby Company 1982.
21. Moss ML, Salentijn L. The primary role of functional matrices in facial growth. Am Jn Orthod 1969;55:566-77.
22. Moss ML. The differential roles of periosteal and capsular functional matrices in orofacial growth. Europ Jn Orthod 2007;29:96-101.
23. Moyers RE. Handbook of Orthodontics, 4th Ed. Year Book Medical Publishers, Inc. Chicago 1988.
24. Nanda RS, Ghosh J. Longitudinal growth changes in the sagittal relationship of maxilla and mandible. Am J Orthod Dentofacial Orthop 1995;107(1):79-90.

25. Nolla CM. The development of the permanent teeth. J Dent Child 1960;27:254-66.
26. Proffit WR, Fields HW. Contemporary orthodontics 3rd Ed Mosby Co 2000.
27. Rakosi T, Jonas I, Graber TM. Orthodontic -diagnosis. Edited by Rateitschak KH, Wold HF. Thieme Pub, 1993.
28. Riesmeijer AM, Prahl-Andersen B, Mascarenhas AK, Joo BH, Vig KW. A comparison of craniofacial Class I and Class II growth patterns. Am J Orthod Dentofacial Orthop 2004;125(4):463-71.
29. Root AW. Failure to thrive and problems of growth. In Textbook of Pediatric Dentistry Braham RL, Morris ME. 2nd Ed. CBS Publishers and Distributors, New Delhi 1990.
30. Scammon RE. The measurements of Man by Harris JA, Jackson CM, Paterson DG and Scammon RE. Minneapolis, University of Minnesota Press p193.
31. Snodell SF, Nanda RS, Currier GF. A longitudinal cephalometric study of transverse and vertical craniofacial growth. Am J Orthod Dentofacial Orthop 1993;104(5): 471-83.
32. Tanner JM, Whitehouse RH, Marshall WA, et al. Assessment of skeletal maturity and prediction of adult height (TW 2 method), New York, Academic Press Inc. 1975.

QUESTIONS

1. Define growth and development.
2. Enumerate the factors influencing growth and discuss each of them in detail.
3. Describe Scammon's growth curve.
4. What are growth spurts? What are the different periods of growth spurts?
5. Discuss the different growth assessment parameters.
6. What is dental age. Discuss Demirjian's method.
7. Enumerate the different mechanisms of growth. Explain each of them.
8. Explain in detail functional matrix theory.
9. Describe the postnatal growth of mandible.
10. Describe the postnatal growth of maxilla.

PSYCHOLOGICAL GROWTH

INTRODUCTION

Psychology is a combination of scientific analysis and clinical application of behavior. Behavior of each individual varies depending on the age, mood and environment. Behavior is the action of what the person thinks, understands, analyses and persues. It is an observation that can be seen, recorded and studied. Understanding psychology will help dentist to detect any deviations in normal behavior that might interfere with treatment process. Psychology thus comprises of systematized knowledge that is gathered through carefully measuring and observing events and summarized to form theories.

Understanding psychology will help dentist to detect any deviations in normal behavior that might interfere with treatment process.

DEFINITION

Psychology

Psychology can be defined as "the science dealing with human nature and behavior. It also includes understanding of the pattern of mental processes characteristic of an individual". Psychology thus is scientific study of behavior and mental process. It comprises of systematized knowledge that is gathered through carefully measuring and observing events and summarized to form theories.

Behavior

Behavior is defined as any change observed in the functioning of the organism. It is the action of what the person thinks, understands, analyses and presumes. It is an observation that can be seen, recorded and studied and is the result of interaction between the innate instincts and those which are learned. While in animals, majority of behaviors are instinctive, in humans majority of behaviors are learned. The older the individual, the more complex the behavioral pattern and more prominent the overlay of the learned behavior.

The term development is used to describe a series of changes that are progressive occurring as a result of maturation and experience, and implies qualitative change. This progressive maturation helps a person to adapt to the environment.

Developmental Psychology

Developmental psychology is a branch of psychology concerned with physical, cognitive and social change throughout the life span. It is study of how individuals grow and change throughout life.

Child Psychology

Child psychology is the study of child's behavior including physical, cognitive, motor, linguistic, perceptual, social and emotional characteristics from birth through adolescence.

Psychologic growth and development generally proceed in a relatively predictable, logical and sequential order. An understanding of the developmental tasks and behaviors common to specific age groups will equip the dentist with the knowledge of the particular needs or fears of children and adolescents. It will also enable the dentist to detect deviations in these patterns which may interfere with the treatment process.

Importance of psychological development of the child in pediatric dentistry:
- To understand the behavior of the child
- To understand the emotional makeup of the child
- To establish effective communication
- To deliver dental service in a meaningful and effective manner
- To develop a treatment planning
- For patient and parent education.

VALUES OF KNOWING THAT CHILDREN DEVELOP DIFFERENTLY

Different Expectations

All children of the same age cannot be expected to behave in the same way. A child who comes from a culturally deprived environment cannot be expected to learn or read as early as a child whose parents put high value on education and encouraged the child to be interested in reading.

Basis of Individuality

The child, who is different from members of the group, provided the difference is not so great so as to be conspicuous, will be interesting to other children and will be able to contribute something different to the group activities.

Child Rearing must be Individualized

One child may respond favorably to authoritarian control because it gives a feeling of security while another child will respond with antagonism and resentment.

Prediction is Difficult

Even when it is known how the average person reacts in a given situation, it is never possible to predict how a specific person will react. One person for example may find a joke 'hilariously funny', while another person may find it 'boring and stupid'.

MAJOR DEVELOPMENTAL PERIODS IN THE DEVELOPMENT OF A CHILD TO A FULL MATURED ADULT

Prenatal Period (Conception to Birth)

It is strongly agreed that the development of psychology does not begin only after birth, but is also influenced deeply by the conditions before birth. This period is very important for some of the following reasons:
- The hereditary characteristics that form the found-ation for the later development are formed at this stage.
- Unfavorable conditions during development may stunt the development potential to the extent of extreme deviation.
- Proportionally greater growth and development occurs during this stage than at any postnatal period.
- This period is very sensitive to physical and chemical hazards.

Newborn (Birth to 10–14 Days)

This is the period of the newborn or the neonate. During this time, the infant must adjust to a totally new environment outside the mother's body. Growth is temporarily at a standstill.

Conditions Influencing Adjustment to Postnatal Life
- *Prenatal development:* Prenatal environment plays a major role in the development of the fetus.
- *Experiences associated with birth:* Difficulty during birth may have adverse effect on the postnatal adjustments.
- *Length of gestation period:* A postmature infant adjusts more quickly and successfully to the postnatal environment than the infant born at full term. Similarly, a prematurely born baby usually experiences complications in adjusting to the postnatal environment.
- *Parental attitudes:* Positive parental attitude will help the newborn adjust quickly to postnatal environment.
- *Postnatal care:* The amount of stimulation, attention and the degree of confidence the infant will receive influences the postnatal adjustment to life.

Characteristics of an Infant
- *Activities:* These can be divided into mass activity and specific activity. Mass activity indicated involvement of the entire body whereas specific activity involving limited area such as reflex response to touch. These activities gradually increase. Long labor or heavily sedated mother during child birth may cause the infant to be relatively inactive for few days following birth. Infants delivered by cesarean section are the least active of all.
- *Vocalization:* Two kinds of sounds a child produces, one is crying and the other is explosive sounds. Crying begins at birth. Shortly after birth the cry changes in pitch and intensity. The explosive sounds are in simpler terms called as 'coos' or 'gurgles'.
- *Learning:* Conditioned reflex in infants is not development exception being regarding feeding.
- *Emotions:* The emotions in a child is concentrated around being satisfied or not with relation to hunger, temperature or feeling secure. They are very sensitive to parental depression and lack of stimulation.
- *Vision:* Newly borns have a shorter field of vision to about one-half that of an adult. Color vision is either absent or minimal.
- *Hearing:* It is the least developed sense at birth. Hearing improves within the first three or four days of birth.
- *Taste perception:* Infants have a keen sense of taste.
- *Skin sensitivity:* Sensitivity to touch, pressure and temperature are well-developed. The infant is more sensitive to cold than heat.

Babyhood (2 Weeks to 2 Years)
At first, babies are completely helpless. Gradually, they learn to control their muscles so that they can become increasingly self-reliant. This change is accompanied by a growing resentment against being babied and a growing desire to be independent.

Characteristics of the Period
- *True foundation age:* During this period many behavior patterns, attitudes and emotional expressions are being established.

- *Age of rapid growth and change:* Rapid change due to growth also means varied activities tending to become more independent. Individuality improves and socialization begins. Development of concepts such as that of space, weight, time, beauty, etc. begins.
- *Beginning of creativity:* As they become more independent they tend to explore. Creativity is seen in routine activities such as play and communication.
- *Sense organ:* Eye muscles are well developed and coordinated. Hearing develops rapidly.
- *Early skills:* Babies go a long way from initially learning to hold the bottle of milk in two hands to feeding themselves with spoon. They also learn to dress with assistance. They learn to scribble with a pencil or crayon and even cut paper with a scissor.
- *Speech development:* The ability to comprehend the meaning of what others are trying to communicate to them and the ability to communicate using words, gestures and expression develop.
- *Emotions:* Anger, fear, curiosity, joy and affection are some of the emotions that a baby exhibits. Babies are fearful sudden stimulus, loud noise, strange persons, dark room, etc.

Childhood (2 Years to 11 Years)

This is divided into:

A. *Early childhood (2-6 years):* Preschool or 'pregang age'. The child seeks to gain control over the environment and starts to learn to make social adjustments.
B. *Late childhood (6-11 years):* It is the period of sexual maturity and beginning of adolescence. The major development is socialization. This is the elementary school age or the 'gang age.'

Characteristics of the Period

- *Skills:* The skills learnt in babyhood improves significantly. Leg skills improve such as running, galloping, climbing, etc.
- *Speech:* Vocalization and comprehension improves markedly. Children try to communicate by gestures, speech and expressions. They form three to four word sentences by age of two years and six to eight word sentences by three to four years.
- *Emotions:* Conflicts during play are common and are the reason for anger among children. They express anger through temper tantrums, crying stamping, etc. They develop fear through scary stories, movies, etc. Jealously develop especially when their parent's attention is diverted to other children.
- *Concept development:* Concepts such as of life and death, bodily functions, numbers, time, social awareness, etc. develop.

Puberty/Adolescence (11 Years to 16 Years)

The word puberty is derived from the Latin word Pubertas, which means "age of manhood." It refers to the process of physical changes by which a child's body becomes an adult body capable of reproduction. Growth accelerates in the first half of puberty and reaches completion by the end.

Characteristics of Puberty

- *Is an overlapping period:* It denotes the closing years of childhood and the beginning years of adolescence.
- Lasts for two to four years. Children who pass through puberty in two years or less are regarded as "rapid maturers", while those who require three to four years to complete the transformation into adults are regarded as "slow maturers".
- *Puberty is divided into three stages:* Prepubescent stage (the secondary sex characteristics begin to appear but the reproductive organs are not yet fully developed), pubescent stage (the time when the criteria of sexual maturity appear—the menarche in girls and the first nocturnal emissions in boys) and postpubescent stage (the secondary sex characteristics become well developed and the sex organs begin to function in a mature manner).
- *Puberty is a time of rapid growth and change:* Puberty is also characterized by rapid growth and marked changes in body proportions, and is termed as "adolescent growth spurt" or the "puberty growth spurt". This growth spurt lasts for a year or two before children become sexually mature and continue for six months to a year afterward. Thus the entire period of rapid growth lasts for almost three years. The other periods of life that have rapid growth are the prenatal period and the first half of the first year of life.
- *Effects on physical well-being*
  - Increased fatigue, listlessness, and other unfavorable symptoms.
  - Digestive disturbances are frequent, and appetite is finicky. The prepubescent child is upset by glandular changes and changes in the size and position of the internal organs.
  - Anemia is common at this period, not because of marked changes in blood chemistry, but because of erratic eating habits, which in turn, increase the already present tendency to be tired and listless.
- *Desire for isolation*
  - Children usually withdraw from peer and family activities and instead quarrel with them.
  - They spend much time in day-dreaming.
  - They also refuse to communicate with others.

- *Boredom*
  - Pubescent children are bored with the play they formerly enjoyed, with schoolwork, with social activities, and with life in general.
- *Incoordination*
  - Rapid and uneven growth affects habitual patterns of coordination, and the pubescent child is clumsy and awkward for a time. As growth slows down, coordination gradually improves.
- *Social antagonism*
  - The pubescent child is often uncooperative, disagreeable, and antagonistic.
- *Heightened emotionality*
  - They are very moody, sulky, with temper outbursts, and a tendency to cry at the slightest provocation.
- *Loss of self-confidence*
  - The pubescent child, lacks in self-confidence and is afraid of failure although was formerly very self-assured.

The term adolescence is derived from the Latin word 'Adolescere' meaning to grow to maturity. It encompasses mental, emotional and social maturity. Adolescence is the period of psychological and social transition between childhood and adulthood.

Characteristics of Adolescence

- 'Childish' behavior diminishes.
- Confusion of role exists as an adolescent is neither a child nor an adult.
- Period of 'storm and stress'. It is a period of heightened emotional tension during physical and glandular changes.
- Increased peer-group influence. This is seen in behavior, likings, way of dressing, etc.
- Gangism begins. Friends are formed based on similarity in values and interests.
- They tend to be more social and like to attend parties, play games, travel, etc.

> John Bowlby stated (Attachment theory) that the interaction between a child and its caregiver is very important during the systematic progression from childhood to adulthood. Problems in this relation would lead to a child to be insecure who finds it difficult to adjust and develop relationships.

THEORIES OF PSYCHOLOGICAL DEVELOPMENT

The theories of psychological development can be studied as follows:

I. Psychodynamic theories and behavior learning theories.

Psychodynamic Theories

In general, psychodynamics, is the study of the interrelationship of various parts of the mind, personality, or psyche as they relate to mental, emotional, or motivational forces especially at the subconscious and unconscious level.

1. Psychoanalytical theory by Sigmund Freud, 1905
2. Hierarchy of needs by Abraham Maslow, 1954
3. Psychosocial theory by Erik Erikson, 1963

Behavior Learning Theories

Learning is a permanent change in behavior that occurs as result of practice or experience. Every behavior of a person such as way of dressing, eating, thinking, attitude towards other people, etc. is influenced by past learning. Understanding learning patterns will help during behavior management process. Some of the principles used in understanding behavior learning are:

1. Classic conditioning by Ivan Pavlov, 1927
2. Operant conditioning theory by BF Skinner, 1938
3. Cognitive theory by Jean Piaget, 1952
4. Social learning theory by Albert Bandura, 1963

II. Another classification given in literature is:
  1. Psychodynamic theories, e.g. psychoanalytical theory, psychosocial theory
  2. Behavior learning theories, e.g. classic conditioning, operant conditioning theory, social learning theory
  3. Cognitive theories, e.g. Piaget's cognitive development theory
  4. Humanistic theories, e.g. hierarchy of needs.

III. Stage theories and nonstage theories:

Stage theories: Each stage represents a distinct, coherent structural mode of feeling and are hierarchically organized based on age. e.g. Piaget's cognitive theory, Sigmund Frued's psychoanalytical theory.

Nonstage theories: Psychological development is regarded as a continuous sequence of development, not governed by age. e.g. behavior learning theories.

PSYCHODYNAMIC THEORIES

Psychoanalytical Theory (Sigmund Freud, 1905)

Psychodynamics is the systematized study and theory of the psychological forces that underlie human behavior, emphasizing the interplay between unconscious and conscious motivation. The original concept of "psychodynamics" was developed by Sigmund Freud. Freud's theory has 2 primary ideas: One, the adult behavior is exclusively determined by the childhood experiences. Two, the story of personality development is the story of how to handle antisocial impulses in socially acceptable ways.

Psychic triad: The building blocks of personality according to psychoanalytic theory are three systems or forces. They are:

a. Id
b. Ego
c. Superego

The mental life of a person is defined by his activity and interaction. Id, ego, and superego are functions of the mind rather than parts of the brain and do not necessarily correspond one-to-one with actual somatic structures of the kind dealt with by neuroscience.

Id

The Id comprises the part of the personality structure that contains the basic drives. It is present since birth, impulse ridden and strives for immediate pleasure or gratification. Thus Id is governed by pleasure principle. It represents unregulated instinctual drives and energies striving to meet bodily needs and desires and is present since birth. Examples are hunger, thirst, sexual drive, aggression, etc. These drives are necessary for the survival of the species. It also includes motivational and emotional impulses. The Id wants its wishes immediately and directly fulfilled regardless of the circumstances. The newborn is all "Id", wanting food right away when hungry, urinating without consideration of time and place, and so forth. Ego and superego usually temper Id as the individual grows up in the society.

Freud divided the Id's drives and instincts into two categories: Life and death instincts. Life instincts (Eros) are those that are crucial to pleasurable survival, such as eating and copulation. Death instincts (Thanatos), are our unconscious wish to die, as death puts an end to the everyday struggles for happiness and survival. Freud noticed the death instinct in our desire for peace and attempts to escape reality through fiction, media, and drugs. It also indirectly represents itself through aggression.

Superego

It is similar to social conscience. It is derived from familial and cultural restrictions placed upon the growing child. The superego thus contains all of the moral lessons the person has learned in their life, initially from parents and later from friends and others. It represents the regulations imposed on the individual by society and culture. Superego formation continues during school age and is present through the entire life.

It has two divisions.

a. *Conscience:* Discourages the expression of behavior seemed undesirable by parents and elders. It develops primarily under scorn or threats of punishment. When the parent says to the child who has been dishonest in a particular situation: "You are bad"; the next time child enters the same situation, he says to himself the same words. In this way, the child controls his behavior much as parents would control it. It is responsible for sense of guilt.

b. *Ego Ideal:* Arises largely through encouragement, praise and rewards given to the child, when she has strived and achieved certain goals the parents desired, e.g. child may be praised for hardwork in school or taking music lessons. Ego ideal also develops as the child identifies with older persons such as parents, teachers, sports hero, etc. and tries to imitate them.

The superego works in contradiction to the Id. The superego strives to act in a socially appropriate manner, whereas the Id just wants instant self-gratification. The superego controls our sense of right and wrong and guilt. It helps us fit into society by getting us to act in socially acceptable ways. Freud's theory implies that the superego is a symbolic internalization of the moral and cultural regulations. If Id is stronger and superimposes upon superego, restrictions set by superego would be weak and ineffective, leading to the possibility of unsocialized behavior.

Ego

As the growing infant learns to react to the outer environment, the expression of Id becomes modified. There emerges a new dimension called ego, which is the executive of problem solving dimension of the personality, now operating in the service of Id. The ego assists the Id in achieving its ends, taking into account the conditions of the external environment. Ego acts according to the reality principle; i.e. it seeks to please the Id's drive in realistic ways that will benefit in the long-term rather than bringing grief. The child discovers that sucking clothes does not satisfy hunger and wet diapers are uncomfortable. He seeks to alter these conditions by calling out to the mother.

Thus with increase in age, psychological processes such as perceiving, learning, remembering and reasoning develop which alter the ego. The child gradually refrains from acting solely according to biological principles. The ego comprises that organized part of the personality structure that includes defensive, perceptual, intellectual-cognitive, and executive func-tions and becomes more organized as individual matures. By adolescence, ego processes are well emerged. The ego separates what is real. It helps us to organize our thoughts and make sense of them and the world around us. The ego is the part of the mind that contains the consciousness. Ego acts as a mediator between Id and super ego. Ego tries to bring together the wishes of the Id, and the moral attitudes of the superego. The ego can and might postpone the requirements or needs of Id keeping in mind the reality and deciding on what may be the best course of action to attain goals of the Id and superego.

When the ego is personified, it is like a slave to three harsh masters: the Id, the superego, and the external world. It has to do its best to suit all three, thus is constantly feeling hemmed by the danger of causing discontent on two other sides. It is said, however, that the ego seems to be more loyal to the Id, preferring to gloss over the finer details of reality to minimize conflicts while pretending to have a regard for reality. But the superego is constantly watching everyone of the ego's moves and punishes it with feelings of guilt, anxiety, and inferiority. To overcome this ego employs defense mechanisms. They lessen the tension by covering up our impulses that are threatening.

Example: If a person sees the food displayed on the shelf of a bakery and wants to take it from the shelf and eat it to satisfy his hunger. This is Id. Superego stops him from doing this, because it is not socially and culturally right to take the food from the shelf of the bakery. Now to satisfy Id under the norms of superego, ego convinces him to go to the counter, pay the money and take the desired food.

Defense Mechanisms

These are unconscious responses that the ego of an individual makes in an attempt to cope with and reduce anxiety that arises due to conflict between Id and superego. Due to these, the individual is able to ward off crisis which might otherwise overwhelm him; which is a positive function. They also serve a negative function wherein it leads to self-deception and prevents the individual from realistically coping with life.

There are ten types of defense mechanisms which are commonly employed. They are:

1. *Projection:* Individual projects personal feelings of inadequacy onto someone else in order to feel more comfortable, e.g. the individual who has failed to perform a task, but blames the machine for the failure.
2. *Denial:* Permits the person to disown the existence of a threatening and unwelcome reality, e.g. patient who denies existence of a tooth with abscess due to fear regarding dental treatment.
3. *Repression:* Process of unconscious forgetting which allows for the suppression of painful experiences into the subconscious mind. This often emerges later in the form of Freudian slips by unconscious motivation.
4. *Rationalization:* Development of logical excuse to explain behavior because the real motive is unacceptable. Something we cannot get becomes something we did not want any way. This often helps to bolster our self-esteem, but if over used can prevent the individual from confronting the situation, e.g. a parent, who is anxious about child's dental treatment, postpones the treatment saying 'there is no pain anyway.'
5. *Intellectualization:* Related to rationalization and also involves reasoning. The intensity of the anxiety is reduced by retreat into detached, unemotional, abstract language. Temporarily separating emotional and cognitive components helps the individual to deal with the parts of an experience when it is too much to handle, e.g. an adolescent may describe his new experiences with sex and independence in an abstract and impersonal plane.
6. *Sublimation:* Redirection of socially unacceptable drives into socially approved channels to allow the discharge of instinctive impulses in an unacceptable form. Seen in individuals who have a healthy and mature ego, e.g. an unmarried girl who wants children, raises animals or plants instead.
7. *Reaction formation:* Development of a behavior opposite to that dictated by unconscious impulses so that a socially acceptable trait is inappropriately exaggerated. If an individual too strident in the crusades against child abuse, it is likely that he is unconsciously harboring the opposite feelings. The unwanted motives are controlled under a disguise.
8. *Identification:* Assumption of the quality of someone else to vent frustration or create fantasy, e.g. an adolescent imitating a sports star whom he idolizes.
9. *Regression-age-inappropriate response:* Behavioral relapse to a more infantile manner as a result of confrontation with anxiety producing situation. For example: Faced with prospect of going to school for the first time, the child may resort to baby talk or start sucking his thumb.
10. *Displacement:* The motive remains unaltered but the person substitutes the original goal object for a different one, e.g. when a newborn baby is the center of attention, the older child may become

jealous; prevented from harming the baby, the child breaks a doll.

Freud's Notion of Unconscious Process

This explains the irrational behavior exhibited by individuals. Freud proposed three levels of consciousness or awareness: the conscious, the preconscious and the unconscious.

Conscious level: At this level we are aware of certain things around us and of certain thoughts.

Preconscious level: At this level are memories or thoughts that are easily available with a moment's reflection, e.g. what we had for breakfast, our date of birth, etc.

Unconscious level: It contains memories, thoughts and motives which we cannot easily recall. We repress or banish from consciousness, ideas, memories and feelings or motives that are disturbing or unacceptable to us. We do not choose to repress an idea or impulse, it happens unconsciously, triggered by the anxiety or pain of the experience.

All of id is unconscious, the ego and superego are present at all three levels of consciousness.

From the schematic representation it is evident that id forms the major part of the psychic structure. It also represents that a large part of the personality remains unconscious.

This unconscious part of the personality is responsible for dreams and verbal accidents which are now called as Fruedian slips (e.g. a reporter having a problem with his marriage writes "cold wife" instead of "cold wave"). They are disguised manifestation of id motives. Too much repression into the unconscious results in neurosis.

The theory of psychoanalysis says that the human personality is significantly influenced by two basic forces, sex and aggression which constantly seek expression in the individual. These impulses are part our inborn nature. Denial of their expression, as often required by the society does not result in their disappearance, but they are expressed in disguised form and this process is called as unconscious motivation. It takes place in three steps: conflict, repression and symbolic behavior.

Psychosexual Stages

Psychoanalytic theory emphasizes on childhood influences. The earliest years are the formative ones, setting the stage for adult personality. As the child matures, it experiences satisfactions as well as problems in the context of his own body. The libido is directed to different areas of the body: mouth, anus and genitals which are called erogenous zones as their stimulation results in pleasure to the individual. These body areas become foci of interest at different growth stages and hence they are called psychosexual stages, meaning that psychological development is related to successive sexual interests.

Libido was Freud's word for psychic and sexual energy. How libido is expressed depends on the stage of development. If it is over satisfied or unsatisfied, fixation takes place. Fixation is the failure of normal psychological development where the child shows continued attachment to an old stage even after moving to a new one. Behavior patterns or problems from the fixated stage persist, often into adulthood.

Oral Stage: 0–1 Year

This occurs from birth to about 1 year, and the libido is focused on the mouth. The primary zone of pleasure is the oral region and infants obtain gratification by stimulation of oral areas. The child's concern is to obtain food. If food requirements are regularly satisfied during this period by breast or bottle feeding, the child develops a sense of trust and optimistic outlook. If these needs are not met, feelings of uncertainty and pessimism are likely outcomes. These feelings persist in the adult personality.

Result of oral stage disturbance

According to Freud, disturbance of the oral stage may result in a permanent fixation on the oral channel for gratification. It may result in adult behaviors pertaining to oral cavity such as smoking, overeating, thumb-sucking, and pencil chewing. Typical resulting personality traits include impatience, passivity, greedi-ness, dependence and a preoccupation with giving and taking.

Anal Stage: 1–3 Years

The child experiences pleasure from the elimination of feces. According to Freud, this brings them into conflict with their parents. Random elimination (as demanded by the Id) incurs parental displeasure. Withholding elimination (as requested by the parents) is denying the demands of the Id. This results in conflict and may have important implications for behaviors later in life. Here individuals have their first encounter with rules and regulations, as they learn toilet training. For the first time Id must be brought in control of emerging ego. This encounter with rules and regulations will dictate the later behavior with rules and regulations. When done successfully, it provides a sense of independence and autonomy.

Result of anal stage disturbance

If the demands were too harsh or lenient, they are likely to have later consequences. Too little gratification in this stage results in an 'anal' or obsessive character who has a wish to make a terrible mess and therefore must build defences against this, such as orderliness, rigidity, and hatred of waste. They are also obstinate, stingy, punctual and possessive. Too much gratification will result in opposite behaviors like untidiness, hot temper and destructiveness.

Phallic Stage: 3–6 Years

The focus of gratification in this stage is on the genitals. Children take an increasing interest in their own genitals, and show a curiosity about other people's bodies. There is an increasing awareness of sex roles and emerging interest in the parent of the opposite sex. Freud called this Oedipus complex in boys and Electra complex in girls. Both the names are derived from early Greek drama in which offspring sought relations with the parent of opposite sex, regarding the like-sexed parent as a rival. Freud implies that the major conflict faced during this stage is the Oedipal/Electra conflict. Resolution occurs by identification where the boy imitates the behavior patterns of the father and the girl child that of the mother. Resolution of this conflict should result in the attachment to the parents. The superego strength (of conscious and ego ideal) of a person in later life depends largely on the events in the phallic stage.

> **Oedepus Complex:**
> It is the tendency of young boy child being attached more to the mother than the father.
> **Electra Complex:**
> It is the tendency of the young girl child developing an attraction towards father.

Result of phallic stage disturbance

According to Freud, the conflicts may result in homosexuality, authority problems, and rejection of appropriate gender roles if not resolved.

Latency Stage: 7–12 Years

This lasts from about the age of 7 until puberty, and is a period of consolidation. Previous libido drives become passive and increased importance is placed on peer development and character formation. Repressed sexual drives during this stage may be redirected into other activities, such as the formation of friendships, or hobbies. Personality identification begins and tries to socialize. A temporary truce is called between Id and ego and the superego becomes more firmly internalized.

Genital Stage : >12 Years

This stage begins with puberty and is characterized by appearance of mature heterosexual interests. Competitiveness with the parent of the same sex recurs. However, these feelings are repressed and the target of sexual arousal is projected to outside the tiny circle of self and family. There is reopening of struggle to gain mastery and control over the impulses of Id and super ego. There are fluctuating extremes in the emotional behavior due to variation in hormonal imbalances. If earlier conflicts have been adequately resolved, the individual settles into task of establishing mature relationship with other people.

Result of Genital Stage Disturbance

The individual cannot reach maturity, cannot shift the focus from his own body, his own parents and their immediate needs to larger responsibilities involving others.

Psychosocial Theory (Erik Erikson, 1963)

Erik Erikson has modified Freud's theory and postulates that society responds to the child's basic needs or developmental tasks. He combines both internal psychological factors and external social factors to explain psychological development throughout the life of an individual.

Erikson's stages of psychosocial development explain eight stages through which a healthily developing human should pass from infancy to late adulthood. The first five are during childhood and adolescence. In each stage the person confronts, and hopefully masters, new challenges. In each stage the individuals are influenced by the psychosocial environment to develop more or less toward one extreme of the conflicting personality qualities dominant at that stage. Each stage builds on the successful completion of earlier stages. The challenges of stages not successfully completed may be expected to reappear as problems in the future. Erikson states that each of these processes occurs throughout the lifetime in one form or another, and he emphasizes these "phases" only because it is at these times that the conflicts become most prominent.

1. Trust vs Mistrust (Infants, 0 to 1 Year)

- Psychosocial crisis: Trust vs mistrust
- Virtue: Hope
- Significant social relationship: Mother

The first stage centers on the infant's basic needs being met by the parents. The infant depends on the parents, especially the mother, for food, sustenance, and comfort. The early interdependency of mother and child is described as a symbiotic relationship. The child's relative understanding of world and society comes from the parents and their interaction with the child. If the parents expose the child to warmth, regularity, and dependable affection, the infant's view of the world will be one of trust—that others are dependable and reliable. If the parents fail to provide a secure environment and to meet the child's basic need, are neglectful or even abusive, a sense of mistrust results—that the world is in an undependable, unpredictable, and possibly dangerous place. Stranger anxiety or separation anxiety seen in this period but is soon mastered by the initiation of the hide and seek game. This allows the toddler to get a firm image of the mother. If separation anxiety is not overcome, fear of abandonment persists.

The tight bond between the child and parent at this stage is reflected in the form of separation anxiety, when the child is separated from the parent. Hence it is preferable to do the treatment with the parent present in the operatory, preferably with child being held by one of the parents. A child who has not developed a sense of trust is likely to become a frightened and uncooperative patient in later ages who has difficulty in establishing rapport and trust with the dentist and staff.

2. Autonomy vs Shame and Doubt (Toddlers, 2 to 3 Years)

- Psychosocial crisis: Autonomy vs shame and doubt
- Main question: "Can I do things myself or must I always rely on others?"
- Virtue: Will
- Significant social relationship: Parents

The child is moving away from the symbiotic relationship of the mother and tries to assert independence. The child learns to delay immediate gratification based on reality principle such as by achieving bowel and bladder control. As the child gains control over eliminative functions and motor abilities, they begin to explore their surroundings. However, the sense of judgment is not yet developed. What the child wants is not necessarily what the adult wants as they are concerned about the child's health, safety as well as others' rights. The child tries to assert control by temper tantrums and saying "no" to everything. Hence this period is often referred to the period of "terrible twos". These behaviors represent the child's effort to achieve autonomy and control when faced with restrictions of the outside world.

The parents should provide a strong base of security from which the child can venture out to assert their will. The parent's patience and encouragement helps foster autonomy in the child. The parent's decision on how much freedom should be allowed is important. If the parent is highly permissive, the infant encounters difficulties it cannot handle, may become overwhelmed, doubting itself and not developing a sense of independence. Highly restrictive parents, also, are more likely to instill the child with a sense of doubt as the child feels shameful of being capable of so little.

As they gain increased muscular coordination and mobility, toddlers become capable of satisfying some of their own needs. They begin to feed themselves, wash and dress themselves, and use the bathroom. If caregivers encourage self-sufficient behavior, toddlers develop a sense of autonomy—a sense of being able to handle many problems on their own. But if caregivers demand too much too soon, refuse to let children perform tasks of which they are capable, or ridicule early attempts at self-sufficiency; children may instead develop shame and doubt about their ability to handle problems.

This stage is decisive in producing personality characteristics of love as opposed to hate, cooperation as opposed to selfishness, freedom of expression as opposed to self-consciousness.

To obtain cooperation of the child in this stage, is to have the child think that whatever the dentist wants was his or her own choice, not required by the dentist. For a 2-year-old child seeking autonomy, it is all right to open your mouth if you want to, unacceptable if someone tells you to do so. One way to achieve this, is to offer reasonable choices whenever possible, for example, letting the patient choose the color of the drape. The dentist should keep in mind that the child at this stage varies between being a little devil, who says no to every wish of parents or the dentist and retreats to the parents like a little angel in moments of dependence. As a result, complex dental treatment of children at this stage is quite challenging and usually carried out under sedation or general anesthesia.

3. Initiative vs Guilt (Preschool, 4 to 6 Years)

- Psychosocial crisis: Initiative vs guilt
- Main question: "Am I good or am I bad?"
- Virtue: Purpose
- Significant social relationship: Family

The child is learning to master the world around him, learning basic skills and principles like things fall down, not up; round things roll. He learns how to zip and tie, count and speak with ease. At this stage, the child wants to begin and complete his own actions for a purpose. The initiative is shown by physical activity, extreme curiosity and questioning, aggressive talking. Through playful fantasy, child becomes a teacher, doctor, hairdresser or any other character that captures his imagination. At this stage, child is inherently teachable.

The child's willingness to try new things is facilitated or inhibited by the response of the parents. If the parent recognizes child's initiative and channels the activity into manageable tasks, so that the child succeeds, it influences future initiative. As part of the initiative, the child eagerly models the behavior of whom he respects. The opposite of initiative is guilt that occurs due to goals that are contemplated but not attained, from acts initiated but not completed, from acts of rebuke by the person whom the child respects.

If parents and preschool teachers encourage and support children's efforts, while also helping them make realistic and appropriate choices, children develop initiative—independence in planning and undertaking activities. But if, instead, adults discourage the pursuit of independent activities or dismiss them as silly and bothersome, children develop guilt about their needs and desires. The child's ability to initiate new ideas depends on how well he is able to express his new thoughts and do new things without feeling guilty about expressing a bad idea or failing to achieve what was expected.

A successful first visit to dentist can produce a sense of accomplishment. An exploratory visit with mother present and a short treatment time can help to give a child a sense of accomplishment. The child is very curious about dental office and asks questions about things there. A prolonged first visit, with elaborate treatment procedures with which the child was not able to cope up, results in guilt that accompanies failure.

4. Industry vs Inferiority (Childhood, 7 to 12 Years)

* Psychosocial crisis: Industry vs inferiority
* Main question: "Am I successful or worthless?"
* Virtue: Competence
* Significant social relationship: School, neighborhood

At this stage, the child works to acquire academic and social skills. This will allow him to compete with others in an environment where recognition is given to those who produce. The child also learns the rules of the world. Children at this age are becoming more aware of themselves as individual. They work hard at "being responsible, being good and doing it right." They are now more reasonable to share and cooperate. They also get to form moral values, recognize cultural and individual differences and are able to manage most of their personal needs and grooming with minimal assistance. At this stage, children might express their independence by being disobedient, using back talk and being rebellious.

Erikson viewed the elementary school years as critical for the development of self-confidence. Ideally, elementary school provides many opportunities for children to achieve the recognition of teachers, parents and peers by producing things—drawing pictures, solving addition problems, writing sentences, and so on. If children are encouraged to make and do things and are then praised for their accomplishments, they begin to demonstrate industry by being diligent, persevering tasks until completed and putting work before pleasure. If children are instead ridiculed or punished for their efforts or if they find they are incapable of meeting their teachers' and parents' expectations, they develop feelings of inferiority about their capabilities. The child can either develop a feeling of competence or inability by being shaped by the interplay of inherited and environmental factors.

A key to behavioral guidance of children of this age group is to set attainable intermediate goals, clearly outlining how to achieve this including the rules of the dental office, and rewarding once it is achieved.

5. Identity vs Role Confusion (Adolescents, 13 to 19 Years)

* Psychosocial crisis: Identity vs role confusion
* Main question: "Who am I and where am I going?"
* Ego quality: Fidelity
* Significant social relationship: Peers, society

It is the stage of psychosocial development in which a unique personal identity is acquired. Adolescent is a time of radical change: the great body changes accompanying puberty, the ability of the mind to search one's own intentions and the intentions of others, the suddenly sharpened awareness of the roles society has offered for later life. The adolescent is newly concerned with how they appear to others. In later stages of adolescence, the child develops a sense of sexual identity.

There is a feeling of belonging to larger group and realization that one can exist outside family. The influence of the peer group is predominant and members of the peer group become role models. At the same time, some separation from the peer group is necessary to establish one's own identity and value. Values and tastes of the parents and authority are likely to be rejected.

As they make the transition from childhood to adulthood, adolescents ponder the roles they will play in the adult world. Initially, they are apt to experience some role confusion—mixed ideas and feelings about the specific ways in which they will fit into society and may experiment with a variety of behaviors and activities (e.g. tinkering with cars, babysitting for neighbors, affiliating with certain political or religious groups). Often, this leads to conflict with adults over religious and political orientations. Another area where teenagers are deciding for themselves is their career choice, and often parents want to have a decisive say in that role. Eventually, most adolescents achieve a sense of identity regarding who they are and where their lives are headed.

Identity crisis: Occurs when goal identification and self-identity is not achieved. Adolescents are confronted by the need to re-establish for themselves and to do this in the face of an often potentially hostile world. This is often challenging since commitments are being asked for before particular identity roles have formed. At this point, one is in a state of 'identity confusion', i.e. reluctance to commit, but society normally makes allowances for youth to "find themselves," and this state is called 'the moratorium': when a person can freely experiment and explore—what may emerge is a firm sense of identity, an emotional and deep awareness of who he or she is.

Each stage that came before and that follows has its own 'crisis', but even more so at this stage, for this marks the transition from childhood to adulthood. This emerging sense of self will be established by 'forging' past experiences with anticipations of the future. In relation to the eight life stages as a whole, the fifth stage corresponds to the crossroads. In many individuals this stage can extend into their twenties or even later.

At this stage it is important to motivate the adolescent for the required dental treatment. A treatment procedure can be successfully carried out only if the patient wants it and just according to the wishes of the parent. An internal motivation, where in the individual has a desire to correct the disease or the defect which he has perceived, will determine the success of the treatment. Acceptance among peer group is another important factor to be considered while treating for esthetic and orthodontic problems.

Hierarchy of Needs (Abraham Maslow, 1954)

Maslow's theory of hierarchy of needs is a humanistic theory in psychology, which focuses on personality as self. The theory focuses on the individual's subjective perception of self, the world and the self within the world and is an example of humanistic theory. According to these theories, both self-image and executive functions by the individual give the notion of self. People's attitude about themselves, their perceived traits, abilities and weaknesses contribute to self-image. A self-process where the individual thinks, remembers, perceives, plans and manages are termed as executive functions.

Maslow believed that human beings have higher and transcendent nature. Hence unlike Freud, who studied emotionally disturbed people and drew his conclusions, he studied models of people who have fulfilled their potentialities. He identified a hierarchy of basic human needs that motivate individual behavior. Human beings are motivated by unsatisfied needs, and that certain lower needs need to be satisfied before higher needs can be addressed. Only when these basic needs are met an individual can achieve his full potential and attain self-respect, self-fulfillment, self-worth, self-determination.

The basic needs were classified based on hierarchy as:
Level 1 (Physiologic needs): Include basic needs for survival such as hunger, thirst, clothing, etc. Human beings direct energy sources in first fulfilling these necessities.

Level 2 (Security): This need for shelter and employ-ment. This ensures protection, stability, pain avoidance. Safety needs are mostly psychological in nature. A secure home and family is required for sense of security. A child from a family where parents have a marital discord will have less sense of security.

Level 3 (Social): This need to be loved and have a sense of belonging. The individual needs have a sense of affection, acceptance and inclusion when being with parents, peers or in other social groups.

Level 4 (Esteem): Competency and skill needs; to feel wanted. This depends on the competency and success of the individual at school or at work. Acknowledgment and appreciation received after an achievement also enhances self-esteem which in turn instills a sense of independence.

Level 5 (Self-actualization): Realization of self: realiz-ation of one's potential and does what he is best suited or intended to do. Thus a musician must make music; an artist must paint and so on. Maslow considered that only a small group of individuals achieve this level. This should not be confused attaining with fame and fortune. Self-actualization by the individuals enhances the culture of the society.

Lower levels of needs have to be fulfilled for the functioning of higher level of needs. The higher the level of fulfillment, it is more likely the individual accepts and adjusts to new situations (Fig. 4.14).

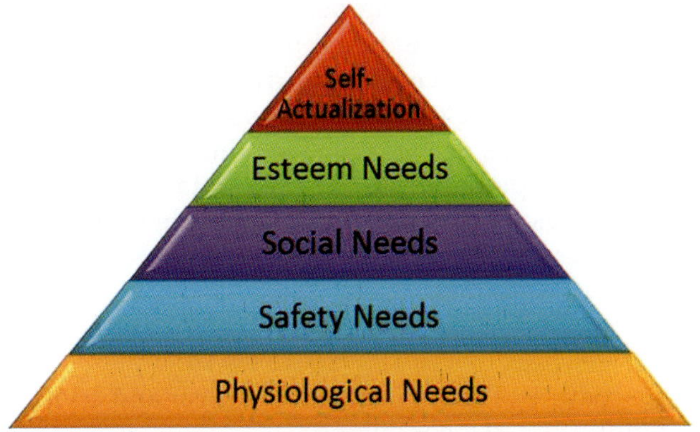

Fig. 4.14: Maslow's hierarchy of needs chart

Behavior Learning Theories

Classic Conditioning (Ivan Pavlov, 1927) (Pavlovian or respondent conditioning, Pavlovian reinforcement)

Classical conditioning is a form of associative learning that was first demonstrated by Ivan Pavlov.

The typical procedure for inducing classical conditioning involves presentation of a neutral stimulus along with a stimulus of some significance. Presentation of the significant stimulus necessarily evokes an innate, often reflexive, response. Pavlov called these the unconditioned stimulus (US) and unconditioned response (UR), respectively. The neutral stimulus could be any event that does not result in an overt behavioral response from the organism under investigation. Pavlov referred to this as a conditioned stimulus (CS). If the CS and the US are repeatedly paired, eventually the two stimuli become associated and the organism begins to produce a behavioral response to the CS. Pavlov called this the conditioned response (CR).

Pavlov's classic experiment involved presentation of food to a hungry dog, along with another stimulus, ringing of the bell. The sight and smell of the food (US) elicits salivation by a reflex mechanism (UR). When the bell was rung each time the food was presented (CS), in a relatively short period of time, the auditory stimulus of the ringing bell itself resulted in salivation (CR). Thus classical conditioning operates by a simple process of association of one stimulus with another. This mode of behavior learning is also sometimes referred to as *learning by association.*

Many of our subjective feelings such as violent emotions fear or anxiety in a particular situation is a conditioned response. A face, a scene or a voice may be a conditioned stimulus for the emotional response. When there is stimulus generalization, it may be difficult to trace back the conditioned beginnings and thus the origin of the emotional response cannot be traced.

Classical conditioning occurs readily in a young child very often in the dental office. A child who has an earlier experience of pain during injection in a pediatrician's clinic will learn to associate the pain with the surroundings of the clinic including the white coat worn by the pediatrician. In the dental clinic, if the surroundings are similar including the white coat of the dentist, the child associates this conditioned stimulus with pain of injection.

First Visit

White coat + Pain of injection → Fear and crying
(Neutral   (Unconditioned
stimulus)   stimulus)   (Response)

Second Visit

Sight of white coat → Fear and crying
(Conditioned stimulus)

Stimulus reinforcement: Association between conditioned and unconditioned stimulus is strengthened every time they occur together. Every time the child is taken to a hospital and something painful is done, the association between pain and the general atmosphere of the clinic becomes stronger. The child concludes that only bad things happen at such a place and shows crying behavior as soon as he enters the hospital.

Stimulus extinction: If this association between the conditioned and unconditioned stimuli is not reinforced, or if conditioned stimulus is presented without the unconditioned stimulus a number of times, extinction of the conditioned behavior occurs. While reinforcement requires only occasional pairing, extinction takes a longer time. If the conditioned association of pain in doctor's office is strong, it takes many visits without pain experience to extinguish crying behavior as soon as the child enters the hospital.

The extinction does not completely erase conditioning. Upon reconditioning (presentation of unconditioned stimulus with conditioned stimulus) spontaneous recovery occurs more rapidly than the original is conditioning.

Stimulus generalization or stimulus substitution: Conditioned responses occur to stimuli that have never been paired with a specific stimulus if the stimulus is similar to the conditioned stimulus. Pavlov noticed that the dog began salivating when the bell was replaced by a buzzer or similar sound producing machine. Development of phobia in children to a specific environment or action may be due to stimulus generalization most of the time. Thus painful experiences in the physician's office may be generalized to dental office.

Stimulus discrimination or differential conditioning: Conditioned response to stimuli that have never been paired with a specific stimulus does not occur if the stimuli are perceived by the individual as dissimilar to the conditioned stimulus. If the dentist's office appearance is different from that of the clinician or if the first visit is not painful, child learns to discriminate from the experience in physician's office.

Application of classical conditioning: Used in systematic desensitization which is a measure used to overcome extreme fear or phobias. The first step is to teach person to relax and then presented with various grades of fear producing stimuli. At each step, the person is taught to relax. Thus relaxation is associated with the fear producing stimuli. For example: For an adolescent who is afraid of needles, first the child is asked to relax, and needle shown by the dentist from a distance. Next by varying the time for which it is seen and the distance of the syringe, each time the stimulus being stronger and the patient learning to relax, the fear of the needle will be overcome. The patient will finally relax during the actual administration of the local anesthetic.

Other feelings and emotions for a particular type of situation are also developed by classical conditioning.

Operant Conditioning Theory (BF Skinner, 1938) (Instrumental Conditioning; Stimulus-Response Theory)

Operant conditioning is the use of consequences to modify the occurrence and form of behavior. Operant conditioning is distinguished from classical conditioning in that operant conditioning deals with the modification of "voluntary behavior" or operant behavior. The theory highlights the role of individual's conscious determination as opposed to unconscious determination of behavior as in classical conditioning theory. Operant behavior "operates" on the environment and is maintained by its consequences. Whereas behaviors conditioned via classical conditioning procedure are not maintained by consequences. In classical conditioning a stimulus leads to a response whereas in the operant conditioning, the response becomes the further stimulus.

The basic principle of operant conditioning is that the consequence of a behavior is in itself a stimulus that can affect future behavior. This means that the consequence determines the probability of that response occurring again in a similar situation. If the consequence of a certain response is pleasant or desirable, the response is more likely to repeat in future. If a particular response produces unpleasant consequence, it is less likely to repeat in future.

The main dependent variable is the rate of response that is developed over a period of time. New operant responses can be developed and shaped by reinforcing close approximations of the desired response.

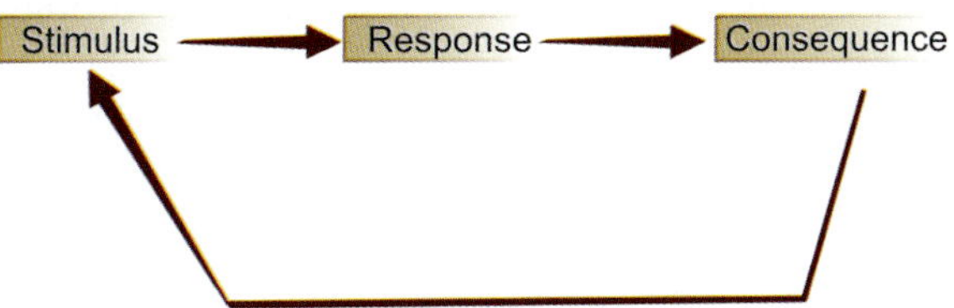

Four basic types of operant conditioning—based on the nature of the sequence.

Reinforcement: The consequence increases the likelihood of behavior in future. It can be verbal or material.

a. *Positive reinforcement:* Pleasant consequence follows a response and the behavior that led to this consequence is more likely to repeat in future.

For example, following a cooperative behavior in the dental clinic, the child is given a toy as a reward for good behavior. The child is likely to behave well in future dental visits.

Reward can be material, social or activity.

Primary reinforcers: Which satisfy the physiological needs such as hunger, thirst, etc.

Secondary reinforcers: Which satisfy needs other than physiological ones, e.g. praising, showing affection enhances the desire to achieve. These are often referred to as conditioned reinforcers when they are paired with the primary reinforcer. Conditioned reinforcers have a large role to play in dental situations as parents often use them to shape the behavior of the child.

b. *Negative reinforcement:* Involves the withdrawal of an unpleasant stimulus after a response. The word 'negative' refers to the response that leads to removal of the undesirable stimulus.

It is important to reinforce only desired behavior, e.g. if a child is apprehensive about the treatment procedure but copes and behaves well during the procedure, understands that the procedure time is shortened due to the good behavior, then the procedure is negatively reinforced.

c. *Omission:* Also called as time-out or omission training, involves removal of a pleasant stimulus after a particular response, e.g. if a child shows temper tantrums during treatment and his mother is sent out of the operatory as a consequence of this behavior.

d. *Punishment:* Unpleasant stimulus is presented after a response. This results in decrease in behavior that prompted punishment, e.g. the dentist speaks in a raised voice to the child when child fails to obey the dentist's commands.

For punishment to be effective, even if it is mild, it should be consistent and paired with positive reinforcement when undesired behavior is suppressed and the desired behavior is obtained. Punishment should be sparingly used in the dental clinic as it often results in fear and anger. It can even lead to classically conditioned fear response. However, mild forms of punishment like voice control can be used in a child with temper tantrums. In voice control, dentist speaks in a firm and loud voice to gain the attention of the child and conveys the message that the behavior is unacceptable. To avoid fear response, the child should be rewarded immediately upon improvement in behavior.

In general, positive and negative reinforcements are the most suitable types of operant conditioning. This is because they increase the likelihood of a particular behavior recurring rather than attempting to suppress a behavior as in case of omission and punishment.

The smaller the interval between response and reinforcement, the faster is the conditioning. In other words, all the four types of operant conditioning must be contingent upon response for them to be effective.

Extinction is the lack of any consequence following a behavior. When a behavior is inconsequential, producing neither favorable nor unfavorable consequences, it will occur with less frequency. When a previously reinforced behavior is no longer reinforced with either positive or negative reinforcement, it leads to a decline in the response. After a time period, if reinforcement is presented again after the desired response, spontaneous recovery can occur. Stimulus generalization and stimulus discrimination occur in operant conditioning also.

The key feature of this form of learning is that some action or behavior of the learner is instrumental in bringing about a change in the environment that makes the action more or less likely to occur again in the future. Thus the response is contingent with the behavior and in turn the future behavior. An individual learns to produce a voluntary response where the outcome results in bringing about the reoccurrence of the stimulus. The response to a stimulus which produces a satisfactory outcome will be repeated whereas those which met disagreeable results will tend to diminish. This theory thus explains development or continuation of new behavior as a result of reinforcement.

If the desired response is not obtained in a given situation, by reinforcing each approximation to the desired behavior, the desired behavior is obtained. This is learning by approximation or behavior shaping. Initially a continuous reinforcement is given, where every positive step towards the desired response is reinforced. Once the basic desired response is established, to increase the frequency of the desired response, later intermittent reinforcement is used. This makes the individual work harder for reinforcement.

Reciprocal conditioning: Operant conditioning involves mutual reinforcement. The response of one member supports the response of other. Thus when the individual operates in his environment, the environment operates on the individual as well.

Applications: Contingency management which uses all four operations.
- Aversive conditioning is a form of punishment.
- Behavior shaping

Two-factor theory of conditioning: Emotions are learned through classical conditioning and the responses for coping with emotions are acquired through operant conditioning. Complex behavior is thus a combination of classical and operant conditioning wherein each form of conditioning makes different contributions to the total learning situation.

Cognitive Theory (Jean Piaget, 1952)

Also called as Piaget's theory of cognitive development, it is a comprehensive theory about the nature and development of human intelligence first developed by Jean Piaget. It is a developmental stage theory which deals with the nature of knowledge itself and how humans come gradually to acquire it, construct it, and use it.

The term *cognition* means knowing or under-standing. *Cognitive development* refers to mental development and includes a wide range of human mental abilities like intelligence, mental processes such as perceiving, recognizing, recalling, interpreting information and reasoning. Cognitive process involves selection of the information, making alterations in the selected information by association with the items already known, elaboration of the information in thought, storage of information in memory and when needed, retrieval of the information. Thus cognition is a form of learning wherein there is change in the behavior of the organism due to experience.

Cognitive structure: Two components
Schema: Relatively simple mental structure present from birth. They are the mental representation of objects which can be modified on seeing new objects, which in turn results in recognition of the object.
Operations: Arise much later in life, more complex and reversible. They are flexible mental actions which can be combined with one another to solve problems. At first, they are concrete but become more abstract or hypothetical and carried out with increased reasoning with age.

Cognition occurs by three processes: They operate in different ways at different age levels.
Assimilation: Incorporation of new knowledge through the use of existing schemes.
Accommodation: Modification of child's existing sch-emes to incorporate new knowledge.

Ability of accommodation is related to mental development and the chronologic age of the individual.
Equilibration: The tendency of the developing individual to stay 'in balance' intellectually by filling in gaps in knowledge and by restructuring beliefs when they fail to test against reality.

Piaget claims that the thinking of children is not just a simpler version of the thinking of adults. It is qualitatively different. The understanding of the reality slowly changes with maturation and experience. The sequence of these changes can be divided into four periods or stages, according to chronologic age.

According to the theory, intelligence is the basic mechanism of ensuring equilibrium in the relations between the person and the environment. This is achieved through the actions of the developing person on the world. At any moment in development, the environment is assimilated in the schemes of action that are already available and these schemes are transformed or accommodated to the peculiarities of the objects of the environment, if they are not completely appropriate.

Thus, the development of intelligence is a continuous process of assimilations and accommodations that lead to increasing expansion of the field of application of schemes, increasing coordination between them, and increasing abstraction.

Jean Piaget emphasizes that childhood development proceeds from an egocentric position through a predictable step like consistent expansion by incorporation of learned experiences. This theory tries to explain the development based on the influence of behavior on thought processes.

Periods of cognitive growth is grouped into 4 major periods. Development into the next stage is possible if previous stages have been mastered.
1. Sensorimotor period
2. Preoperational period
3. Period of concrete operations
4. Period of formal operations.

Sensorimotor Period: Birth to 24 Months

It is period of sensory input and motor output. Infants construct an understanding of the world by coordinating sensory experiences (such as seeing and hearing) with physical, motoric actions. Infants gain knowledge of the world from the physical actions they perform on it. They are concerned not with thinking about things but rather experiencing them. Thus the infant merely senses things and acts upon them and hence the name sensorimotor period. These senses become gradually organized by coordinating and storing information gained from various sensory organs. The sensory modalities are integrated and the infant becomes able to look towards an object, make a sound or reach toward an object he desires. The infant is egocentric but begins the task of decentration where he gradually differentiates himself from the world around him.

Social influence plays a major role in the development of the object permanence. The child becomes upset when the mother or caretaker is absent and goes in search of her as she is object of the most concern to the child. Separation anxiety begins at the age of 6 months as the child develops the sense of object permanence and the visual ability to recognize strangers.

Preoperational Period: 18 Months to 7 Years

It is a transitional period from the sensorimotor period to the concrete operations. The hallmark of the preoperational stage is sparse and logically inadequate mental operations. During this stage, the child learns to use and to represent objects by images, words, and drawings. The child, however, is still not able to perform operations; tasks that the child can do mentally rather than physically.

The important characteristics are:

Language development: The child's representational ability has become more sophisticated and uses language to communicate ideas to others. The capacity develops to form mental symbols representing things and events not present and children use words to symbolize these absent objects. However, they go by the external appearance of the object and do not consider other aspects such as its function. The identity concept is more primitive. Thus "a coat" is the one which he wears and the one worn by daddy should have a different name. At this age, language is understood in its literal sense and meaning of idioms, sarcastic or ironic statements are not understood. The child understands only concrete things (opposite of abstract). Concepts that cannot be seen, heard, smelt, tasted or felt such as time, health are not grasped by the child.

Symbolic play: The child is able to have a mental representation of objects that are not present and engages in pretend play. This is possible due to representational thought—the ability to form mental symbols to represent objects or events that are not present.

Trial and error: The child understands himself and his surrounding environment by becoming a little explorer, seizing opportunities for picking and dropping, poking and rubbing, twisting and pulling, shaking and breaking. The child attains his normal intellectual growth due to these explorations. Thus the cognitive growth is mainly influenced by the intellectual stimulation he gets from his surrounding environment.

Reasoning: They are capable of transductive reasoning—from particular to particular. They can understand cause—effect relationship but is limited to a particular event or object. They are not capable of inductive reasoning (from particular to general) or deductive reasoning (from general to particular). As result a volley of questions may be asked to the adult such as "How" and "Why".

Egocentrism: The child is unaware of other perspectives except his own view point. Thus defined, it does not mean selfishness, but instead refers to intellectual limitation. It may be of two types: perceptual and cognitive.

Perceptual egocentrism: Preschoolers do not realize that other people see things from a view point different from theirs; e.g: a young girl playing hide and seek, shuts her eyes and says " Ha,Ha, you can't see me!"

Cognitive egocentrism: Children find it difficult that other people do not know their thoughts. In communicating with others children often forget themselves in the role of listener and to adapt their message to that person.

Thus, it will be useless to point out how proud his parents will be if he cooperated for the dental treatment as the child can't see the parent's point of view. Instead if the dentist shows the decayed discolored teeth and says "your teeth will be better if these germs are out of them" it is accepted by the child.

Animism: Is the belief that inanimate objects are capable of actions and have lifelike qualities. For example, a child who gets hit by the edge of the door while running says that the door has gone mad and hit him badly. Essentially everything is seen as being alive by the child, so stories that have inanimate objects with life are acceptable. Animism can be used to dentist's advantage by giving life-like names and qualities to equipments, e.g. the handpiece is the "Whistling Willie" who is happy and sings while he polishes the child's teeth.

Centration: Child focuses on single striking feature of an object or event. The child is impressed with how things appear, rather than how they were made. This is illustrated by Piaget's conservation experiment, the aim of which is to determine whether the child can recognize that altering a substance's appearance does not change its basic properties. In Piaget's most famous task, a child is presented with two identical beakers containing the same amount of liquid. The child usually notes that the beakers have the same amount of liquid. When one of the beakers is poured into a taller and thinner container, a preschool child says that the two beakers now contain a different amount of liquid. The child simply focuses on the height and width of the container compared to the general concept. Piaget believes that if a child fails the conservation-of-liquid task, it is a sign that they are at the preoperational stage of cognitive development. The child also fails to show conservation of number, matter, length, volume, and area as well. Children at this stage are unaware of conservation.

The dental staff should use immediate sensations rather than abstract reasoning in discussing oral hygiene methods and prevention of dental caries at this stage. A preoperational child will have trouble understanding "Brushing and flossing remove food particles, which in turn prevents bacteria from forming acids, which cause dental decay." Instead "Brushing makes your teeth feel clean and smooth" will be understood better by the child.

During this period marked inconsistencies appear in the child's thinking. The child often acknowledges understanding something with true sincerity, only to be betrayed by completely opposite actions shortly thereafter.

The period is subdivided into two stages:

Preconceptual substage (2-4 years): Where there is rapid development of language and begins to engage in symbolic play.

Perceptual or intuitive substage (4-7 years): Charact-erized by increased reasoning but fails the test of conservation. Confuses reality with fantasy and cannot think of reversibility.

Period of Concrete Operations: 7–11 Years

The stage is characterized by the appropriate use of logic and reasoning by the school child. Important processes during this stage are:

Conservation: Understanding that quantity, length or number of items is unrelated to the arrangement or appearance of the object or items. The child can successfully pass through the conservation experiments.

Decentering: Where the child takes into account multiple aspects of a problem to solve it. For example, the child will no longer perceive an exceptionally wide but short cup to contain less than a normally-wide, taller cup.

Elimination of egocentrism: Develops the ability to view things from another's perspective. Animism declines.

Seriation: The ability to sort objects in an order according to size, shape, or any other characteristic. For example, if given different-shaded objects they may make a color gradient.

Transitivity: The ability to recognize logical relation-ships among elements in a serial order, and perform 'transitive inferences' (for example, if A is taller than B, and B is taller than C, then A must be taller than C).

Classification: The ability to name and identify sets of objects according to appearance, size and consistency. The child can compare and classify.

Reversibility: The child understands that numbers or objects can be changed, then returned to their original state. For this reason, a child will be able to rapidly determine that if 4 + 4 equals t, t − 4 will equal 4, the original quantity.

During this period intelligence is demonstrated through logical and systematic manipulation of symbols related to concrete objects and the child undergoes enormous surge in intellectual development guided by academic rigor. However, the child is not capable of abstract reasoning and thinking.

During dental treatment, instructions should be based on concrete objects. " Brush your teeth in up and down strokes for front teeth; back and forth strokes for back teeth, twice a day" may be less understood than saying and demonstrating " This a model of your teeth. The brush should be held in this way for front teeth and moved in up and down direction, in this manner."

Period of Formal Operations: 11–18 Years

In this stage, individuals move beyond concrete experiences and begin to think abstractly, reason logically and draw conclusions from the information available, as well as apply all these processes to hypothetical situations.

During this stage the young adult is able to understand such things as love, "shades of gray", logical proofs and values. The young adult begins to entertain possibilities for the future and is fascinated with what they can be. The adolescent's thought process is similar to adults and can understand concepts like health, disease and prevention. Hence he should be treated like an adult.

Adolescents are changing cognitively also by the way they think about social matters. They begin to imagine their world in a serious way, as an ideal one and thus differ from adult way of thinking. They often compare their real world with the ideal one; often rebel and change their lifestyles. He often moves away from conventional standards of morality towards construction of his own moral principles.

Adolescent egocentrism governs the way that adolescents think about social matters. It is a new form of expression of egocentrism wherein the adolescent considers what others are thinking about, others are thinking the same thing as him. Because young adults are experiencing tremendous biologic changes due to growth and sexual development they are more concerned about bodies, actions and feelings.

Adolescent egocentrism can be dissected into two types of social thinking:
  a. Imaginary audience involves attention getting behavior and heightened self-consciousness. This makes them susceptible to peer influence.
  b. Personal fable: Adolescents sense of personal uniqueness and invincibility which makes them think "because I am unique, I am not subject to consequences other will experience".

The egocentrism can affect the acceptability of dental treatment. A treatment which results in improved esthetics is easily accepted as the adolescent thinks that he will be better accepted by peers. On the other hand, an orthodontic removable appliance may not be accepted as he fears ridicule by his peers. Encouraging the reluctant teenager to try it and then judge the peer response is likely to make him wear the appliance. A typical adolescent also feels that health problems concern somebody else and neglects his own health concerns.

Social Learning Theory (Albert Bandura, 1963)

People learn through observing others' behavior, attitudes, and outcomes of those behaviors. One forms an idea of how new behaviors are performed, and on later occasions this coded information serves as a guide for action. Social learning theory explains human behavior in terms of continuous reciprocal interaction between cognitive, behavioral, and environmental influences.

Learning by observation is also called modeling. The person observed, who provides information about the behavior by performing the behavior for the observer is called model. The individual learns by observing and thinking and is facilitated by reinforcement. Learning is done by observing someone else; hence it is called social learning.

Modeling is governed by inter-related sub-processes: Two distinct stages:
1. Acquisition of the behavior
2. Performance of the behavior.

Acquisition of Behavior
Attentional process

A child can observe many behaviors and thereby acquires potential to perform them, without immediately demonstrating or performing the behavior. The model should be observed closely and the modeled behavior should not be too complex for them to comprehend. Whether the child can actually performs an acquired behavior depends on several factors:

The characteristics of the model: Model should be liked and respected. For this reason usually parent or older sibling serves as a model to the child. For an adolescent, peers in the older age group serve as models.

Expected consequence of the behavior: If a child observes an older sibling refuses to obey his father's command; sees punishment follows refusal, he is less likely to defy his father on future occasion. An anticipated reinforcement will strengthen attention.

If the younger child observes the older sibling getting rewarded for his good behavior during dental treatment, he is likely to behave the same way when his turn for treatment comes. Because the parent is an important role model for the young child, the mother's attitude towards dental treatment is likely to influence the child's approach. Thus an anxious mother results in anxious child in the dental clinic.

Retention process

Observer must be able to reproduce the behavior of the model when the model is no longer present. The response pattern must be memorized and coded in a symbolic form. Mental and physical rehearsal of the modeled activities will increase their retention. Thus learning requires cognitive development where all the operations with regard to a particular sequence need to be understood, e.g. a 6-year-old child will model action only and will not understand the motivation or consequences of the action. A 10-year-old child will also understand the motivation and consequence of the action.

Performance of the Behavior

Motoric reproduction process

Amount of reproduction occurs based on level of skills and physical capabilities the child has attained. These skills must be coordinated and refined through self-corrective adjustments based on the performance feedback.

Reinforcement/Motivational process

Positive incentives are provided. Includes motives such as a past (i.e. traditional behaviorism), promised (imagined incentives) and vicarious (seeing and recalling the reinforced model) reinforcements.

From early infancy the child strives to have his basic needs met in order to reduce tension and to create a satisfied pleasure feeling. The infant quickly learns in a reflexive manner that certain behaviors on his part elicit responses from his parents. If these responses are pleasing and rewarding to the child, the initial behavior will be repeated over and over and will eventually become part of his behavior and personality. This approval or disapproval of the mother acts as a powerful reinforcer of certain behavior in the child and permits the mother to shape and modify the child's behavior toward socially acceptable behavior.

In dentistry, observational learning may be either positive or negative. The child may be made to imitate either a live model or audiovisual model in order to elicit cooperative behavior. The parent's prior experience with dental health professionals will greatly influence their child's attitudes. Children may overhear their parents discussing their dental experiences or may see their parents suffering before, during, or after a dental appointment.

FURTHER READING

1. Baghdadi ZD. Principles and application of learning theory in child patient management. Quintessence Int 2001;32(2):135-41.
2. Bjorklund DF, Pellegrini AD. Child development and evolutionary psychology. Child Dev 2000;71(6):1687-708.
3. Bonetti D, Pitts NB, Eccles M, Grimshaw J, Johnston M, Steen N, Glidewell L, Thomas R, Maclennan G, Clarkson JE, Walker A. Applying psychological theory to evidence-based clinical practice: identifying factors predictive of taking intra-oral radiographs. Soc Sci Med 2006;63(7):1889-99. Epub 2006 Jul 14.
4. Davis-Sharts J. An empirical test of Maslow's theory of need hierarchy using hologeistic comparison by statistical sampling. ANS Adv Nurs Sci 1986;9(1):58-72.
5. Delamater AR, Oakeshott S. Learning about multiple attributes of reward in Pavlovian conditioning. Ann N Y Acad Sci 2007;7.
6. Delitala G. Incorporating Piaget's theories into behavior management techniques for the child dental patient. Gen Dent 2000;48(1):74-6. Review.
7. Do C. Applying social learning theory to children with dental anxiety. J Contemp Dent Pract 2004;15;5(1):126-35. Review.
8. Fernald LD, Fernald PS. Munn's Introduction to Psychology. 5th ed. AITBS Publishers and distributors (Regd.) Delhi, 2003pp 69-73, 178-92, 398-423, 433-4.
9. Hoare P. Essentials of child psychiatry. Churchill Livingstone, Edinburgh 1st ed. 1993;5-26.
10. Horner AJ. On the limits of psychoanalytic theory: a cautionary perspective. J Am Acad Psychoanal Dyn Psychiatry 2006 Winter;34(4):693-707.
11. Landry SH, Smith KE, Swank PR, Miller-Loncar CL. Early maternal and child influences on children's later independent cognitive and social functioning. Child Dev 2000;71(2):358-75.
12. Malerstein AJ, Ahern MM. Piaget's stages of cognitive development and adult character structure. Am J Psychother 1979;33(1):107-18.
13. Mathewson RJ, Primosch RE, Robertson D. Fundamentals of Pediatric Dentistry. Quintessence Publishing Co., Inc. Chicago, 2nd ed, 1987;139-42.
14. Mathewson RJ. Fundamentals of Dentistry in Children 1st ed. 1982;21-43.
15. Mayer SJ. The early evolution of Jean Piaget's clinical method. Hist Psychol 2005;8(4):362-82.
17. McIver FT, Profitt WR. Social and behavioral development in Contemporary Orthodontics. Profitt WR, Fields HW, Sarver DM. (Editors); 4th ed. Mosby Inc, Elsevier, New Delhi 2007;58-70.
18. McMillan S. Behavior of children and adolescents. In Pediatric dentistry: Scientific Foundations and Clinical Practice. Stewart RE, Barber TK, Troutma KC, Wei SHY. Editors. CVMosby Company 1982;150-6.

19. Meissner WW. Freud's methodology. J Am Psychoanal Assoc 1971;19(2):265-309.
20. Morgan CT, King RA, Weiz JR, Scholper JS. Introduction to Psychology. 1st ed. New Delhi: Tata McGraw Hill Publishing Company Limited 1993;137-79:409-509.
21. Muthu MS, Sivakumar N. Pediatric dentistry: Principles and Practice. 1st ed. Noida: Reed Elsevier India Pvt. Limited 2009;35-50.
22. Pinkham JR. Personality development. Managing behavior of the cooperative preschool child. Dent Clin North Am 1995;39(4):771-87. Review.
23. Sarles RM. Psychologic growth and development in Pediatric Dental Medicine. Forrester DJ, Wagner ML, Fleming J (editors) 1981. Lea and Febiger, Philadelphia 27-37.
24. Vassalli G. The birth of psychoanalysis from the spirit of technique. Int J Psychoanal 2001;82(Pt1):3-25.

QUESTIONS

1. Define psychology, behavior and child psychology.
2. Explain the importance of psychological development of the child in pediatric dentistry.
3. Enumerate the theories of psychological development.
4. What is psychic triad?
5. Explain different stages of development based on Freud's theory?
6. Write in detail the psychosocial theory by Erik Erikson?
7. What are the developmental changes seen in an adolescent?
8. Explain the importance of understanding classic conditioning theory for dental practice.
9. What are the periods of cognitive growth according to Jean Piaget?
10. Explain the characteristics of the childhood period.

EMOTIONAL AND SOCIAL DEVELOPMENT

INTRODUCTION

Emotions are an outcome of intellectual ability, ability to understand and imagination. They play an important role in life and affect the personal and social adjustments. Emotions serve as a form of communication, leave their mark on facial expressions, form the essence of everyday experiences and contribute to personality development. At birth, emotions are simple and undifferentiated. With age, emotional responses are more differentiated and less diffuse or random.

CONDITIONS RESPONSIBLE FOR EMOTIONAL MATURATION

1. **Role of maturation:** Refers to intellectual development and growth of imagination and understanding with age. The growth of endocrine glands by puberty also influences the emotional states.
2. **Role of learning:** Five kinds of learning contribute to the development of emotional patterns during childhood.
   a. **Trial and error learning:** Based on the satisfaction obtained after the expression of emotions.
   b. **Learning by imitation:** Emotions are learnt by observation.
   c. **Learning by identification:** By copying the emotional reaction of a person whom the child admires.
   d. **Conditioning:** Learning by association. This occurs increasingly up to early childhood.
   e. **Training:** Learning under guidance. Children are taught the approved way of responding when a particular emotion is aroused. Through training children are stimulated to respond to stimuli that gives rise to pleasant emotions and discouraged from emotionally responding to stimuli that give rise to unpleasant emotions.

Both maturation and learning influence development of emotions, but learning is more important as it is more controllable. Because these two factors affect emotional development, emotions of young children differ markedly as compared to adults.

STAGES OF EMOTIONAL AND SOCIAL DEVELOPMENT

Infancy

Refers to the first two weeks of life and suggests extreme helplessness and dependency on parents or caregivers. Factors affecting infant's emotional and personality development are:
1. Disturbed prenatal environment such as prolonged stress suffered by the mother.
2. Parental attitudes especially maternal attitudes after birth: A mother who is relaxed and able to provide a good postnatal care confidently, will enhance infant's emotional and social adjustment later in life. A warm, intimate and continuous relationship with mother or caretaker is necessary during this period. Attachment towards the mother is more than that with father.
3. Hereditary traits: For a healthy development, the parental attitudes should be in harmony with hereditary traits.

Babyhood

Refers to the first two years of life following the brief two-week period of infancy. In the second year of life the baby is often referred to as toddler, who has achieved enough body control to relatively independent. Babyhood is often referred to as foundation age, as attitudes, emotional expression and behavior patterns established during this period persist for lifetime. Although they are modified with age, the first two years set the pattern for personal and social adjustments.

There are two distinctive characteristics:
1. The intensity of emotional response is too great for the stimuli that give rise to them, especially anger and fear. They are brief in duration and easily give way to other emotions when distracted.
2. Emotions are easily conditioned, e.g. pain of injection during inoculation at the earlier visit can be reluctant to enter the doctor's clinic.

Common Emotional Patterns

Anger: Arises when the babies are not let to do what they want to do. Response is in the form of kicking, screaming and waving the arms. A toddler may also jump up and down, throw himself on the floor or hold his breath.

Fear: Arises due to loud noises, strange persons, objects, situations, dark rooms, high places, animals or any sudden unexpected stimulus. The baby's response is of withdrawal from the stimulus along with whimpering or crying, sometimes holding the breath. Shyness, a form of fear where the individual shrinks from contact with strangers is seen by first year of life. This exhibited in the form of crying, turning the head away from stranger and clinging to a familiar person for protection.

Curiosity: Anything new can stimulate child's curiosity. As the fear wanes, curiosity develops which is seen in facial expression—facial muscles become tense, mouth is slightly opened, with protruding tongue. This is followed by grasping of the object, shaking, banging or sucking the object.

Joy: It is stimulated mostly due to physical well-being, being played with, tickled, watching or listening to others. It is expressed as a smile or laugh along with movement of arms and legs. When the joy is intensified, cooing or gurgling or shouting with glee along with intensified arm and leg movements are seen. The sight of a human face or a high pithched sound of a voice can bring about smile.

Affection: It is shown towards who take care of baby's bodily needs and shows affection. A toddler may also show affection towards his toys or family pet. Affection is expressed by hugging, patting or kissing the loved object.

Happiness: Generally babies are happier in the first year of life than second year. The intimate relationship of the caregivers with the baby due to its dependency keeps the baby except during times of teething or when baby is sick. During the second year of life as the dependency decreases, temper tantrums are shown by the babies when they are not allowed to do what they want to do. Also the adults usually try to instil a sense of discipline and morality by spanking, harsh words and angry facial expressions which the baby resents. However, rewarding the baby by approval and affection given by the parents during play and other activities of the baby increases happiness.

However, all these responses are modified by conditioning or past experiences. For example, a baby cared only by family members is likely to be more fearful of strangers than a baby who is exposed to outsiders. Response of the elders can also modify the future manifestation of emotions, e.g: if a child is punished for banging objects, the curiosity towards newer objects may just be expressed by just looking or touching it.

A dominance of pleasant emotions like curiosity and joy is dependent on the environment in which the child has grown up and is an indicator of social adjustments in new situations.

Social Development

Early social experiences leave their mark on the personality, which remains throughout life. Positive attitudes towards self are found in a person whose early social experiences are favorable. Social experiences during babyhood lay the foundation for behavior in adolescence and adulthood. Child who cries excessively as a baby tends to be aggressive and shows more attention getting behavior. Social experiences during this period are mainly from situations at home. Thus the parental or caregiver's response or attitude towards baby's emotional response plays an important role in social development. The parent plays the role of disciplinarian by telling the child what not to do. Parental warmth makes the child eager to maintain parent's approval and understand parent's reasons for prohibition. Consistency overtime and between parents is also important to learn discipline.

At six weeks, the baby acknowledges the caregivers with a social smile. By fifth month babies like to be picked by anyone who approaches them. They cannot differentiate strangers from known people. However, they recognize and react differently to smiling and angry faces. At sixth or seventh month, babies can differentiate between "friends" and stranger. By eight or nine months baby attempts to imitate speech and gestures of others. A one-year old baby reacts to the warning "no-no". This changes to stubborn resistance to requests and demand from adults which is manifested as physical withdrawal or angry outbursts by sixteen months. At eighteen to twenty four months, a more socially acceptable behavior is observed. The baby cooperates during a number of routine activities such as being fed, bathed and dressed. The baby also shows more interest in play materials, shows interest in sharing it with other babies, marking the beginning of establishment of new social relationships. However there is little cooperation, the play pattern is mostly "parallel play" where they play their own way without regard to what others are doing. Play is the foundation of creativity and problem solving. It also gives scope for the child to learn by exploring its environment. It removes boredom, keeps the child amused thereby preventing the detrimental effects of crying behavior. This ability to keep himself amused instils a sense of self-sufficiency, self-confidence and cooperation, which help the child to cope with problems in life as he grows older. During this period children often develop attachment to a particular toy during this period, which reduces anxiety and enhances adjustment to the new situation.

Childhood

Begins when the relative dependency of babyhood is over, at approximately two years and extends to the time when the child is sexually mature. Childhood is divided into two separate periods:

Early childhood: Extends from 2-5 years

Late childhood: Extends from 6 years to the time the child becomes sexually mature.

The transition from early childhood to late childhood is marked by change in the psychological make as the child begins formal schooling.

Early childhood: This is often referred to as preschool age, as children are considered not old enough both physically and mentally to cope with formal schooling. It is considered as a time for preparation for formal schooling.

Emotions are intense during this period and characterized by temper tantrums, intense fears and unreasonable outbursts of jealousy. This can be traced partly to the fatigue due to strenuous and prolonged play, too little eating and taking too short a nap. But mostly it is because, children during this period feel that they are capable of doing more than their parents permit them to do and revolt against the restrictions. They also become angry when they find that they are incapable of doing what they think they can do successfully. If parents set unrealistically high standards, they experience more emotional tension.

Common Emotional Patterns

Anger: Due to conflicts over play things or thwarting of wishes. Child resorts to loud crying or screaming, stamping, kicking, jumping up and down.

Fear: Fear is acquired by both conditioning and imitation. Stories, pictures, television programs and movies with frightening elements instils a sense of fear. The child's fear is expressed by running away, hiding and crying. As the child grows older, overt fear responses like crying decrease due to social pressure. They learn to avoid situations that are frightening. Some children may show extreme shyness leading to generalized timidity which affects the social relationships.

Jealousy: It is seen when the parental attention shifts towards a younger sibling. In a bid to gain attention, they often revert to infantile behavior such as bed wetting, pretending to be ill or being naughty and indulging in mischiefs. They also become envious of abilities and material possessions of the other child. They often verbalize the wishes to have what other child has.

Grief: Loss of anything they love such as pet or toy can cause grief which is expressed by crying or losing interest in normal activities such as eating.

Joy: A sense of physical well-being, slight calami-ties such as watching someone falling on the ground, sudden unexpected noises, playing pranks on others, accomplishing difficult tasks can bring joy. It is expressed by clapping, laughing, jumping up and down or hugging the object or person that has made them happy.

Curiosity: Arises about anything new they see or hear and also about their own bodies and bodies of others. This results in asking a volley of questions to the adults or sometimes child explores things himself.

Affection: Express love towards people who care for them, pets or play things by hugging, patting or kissing. As the child grows older the affection is also expressed verbally. Adults especially teachers, who show interest in children and willingness to help them quickly win their affection.

Happiness: Depends mainly on the environment at home than outside home. Acceptance by others, Achievements and Affection are the three As that lead to happiness.

Factors Influencing Emotions

Age: The intensity of emotions varies with age. For example, as the children grow older they are no longer afraid of many fear causing stimuli. Feelings of jealousy increase with age and temper tantrums are at their peak between two to four years.

Sex: Temper tantrums tend to be more in boys while fear, jealousy, affection are more in girls.

Family size: Children from larger families are likely to envious other's material possessions. First born children display more jealousy and more violent behavior than their siblings.

Child rearing practices and the environment at home: It has a major influence on emotional behavior in early childhood. Children of more authoritarian parents are more likely to show angry outbursts. If the aspirations of parents are unrealistically high, children are doomed to failure. This leaves an indelible mark on the self concept of the child. Presence of siblings often results in competition and comparison at home and if done in a unhealthy way, can lead to negative feelings and low self-esteem.

Social development: The preschool age is also referred to as the pregang age because this is the age at which child begins to interact and socialize with other peers. The social attitudes and patterns of social life are established during this period. A pleasurable social contact with other children reinforces him to make more social contacts and spend more time talking and playing with his peers. In the beginning, the pattern of playing is limited to parallel play which soon changes to associative play in which children engage in similar activities with other children towards the end of early childhood. Child may also remain an onlooker where he watches other children playing during which he learns how others make social contacts. These activities are rudiments of team play seen in late childhood. The following are some of the behavior patterns seen in early childhood:

1. Imitation of the attitude and behavior of the person whom they admire.
2. By third year, cooperative play begins and children learn that sharing toys wins social acceptance. Thus selfish and egocentric behavior is gradually replaced by generosity as they come across their peers and new social situations. This depends on how many contacts children have with people outside their home.
3. Social contact results in feelings of sympathy and empathy towards others.
4. Desire to excel and outdo others is apparent by fourth year.
5. Peer approval becomes more important than adult approval.
6. Resistance to adult authority is seen. Physical resistance is gradually replaced by verbal resistance or pretending not to hear the requests. This negativism in its extremes results in aggressive behavior initially in the form of physical destructiveness which is replaced with name calling or blaming others as the child grows older.
7. Until four years of age, boys and girls play together harmoniously. After this segregation in play activities between boys and girls is seen mainly due to social perception.
8. Attachment behavior with parents is gradually shifted to people outside home such as teachers, friends, etc. Children usually have an attachment object such as a toy or blanket or pet. Children who feel lonely may have imaginary playmates who have qualities similar to real playmate, and play as they want them to play.
9. Toys play an important role in play activities where the toys are involved in imaginary role playing or make believe games. Variety in play activities due to guidance by adults enhances their creativity.
10. Books on fairy tales, rhymes cartoons in television fascinate the child.
11. Children have a great interest in self and love to talk about their toys, clothes, etc.

Late Childhood

The beginning of late childhood is marked entry of the child into formal schooling and hence school environment will have great influence in attitudes and behavior of the child. It is elementary school age, where the child is expected to acquire the rudiments of knowledge which are considered essential for successful adjustment to adult life. It is critical period in the achievement drive wherein the children are rated as being achievers, under-achievers and over-achievers.

Emotional patterns: The common emotional patterns are similar to those of early childhood. However, they differ from early childhood in two ways:

1. The kind of situations that give rise to them:
   Older children are far more likely to become angry when a derogatory comment is made than younger children understanding level of older ones is better. Curiosity arises only in situations or about things which are markedly different from known ones. Periods of heightened emotionality may be seen due to illness, being tired, when the child enters a new school, change in family situation such as parental divorce. However, late childhood is considered as a period of relative emotional calm because due to improved skills, children are able to accomplish tasks which they could not when they were younger. During this period children also learn to provide an outlet for pent up emotional energy.

   A child who is more popular or seen as an achiever will express his emotions in a more socially acceptable way than a child who is less popular or non-achiever as he is less anxious. Happiness is linked to performance at school, relationship with family members and peers. Thwarting of desires, constant fault finding, teasing or making unfavorable comparisons with other children will lead to anger.

2. The form of emotional expression:
   Older children discover that expression of emotions especially unpleasant emotions are unacceptable socially especially among their peers. Thus they learn that temper outbursts are babyish, withdrawal reactions to fear is cowardly and hurting others in jealousy is poor sportsmanship. Fear and shyness is usually seen in the form of blushing, stuttering, talking as little as possible and nervous mannerisms such as pulling the clothing. Thus there is a strong incentive to learn to control the outward expression of their emotions. However, at home, the emotional expression may be similar to early childhood due which parents often complain that "he is not acting his age". The method of expressing emotions varies markedly with gender. Girls often show temper outbursts or dissolve

into tears whereas boys express their anxieties by being sulky. Boys are more likely to express anger and curiosity while girls are more likely to express fears, worries and feelings of affection. This gender variation in expression of emotions is mostly due to social perceptions. Pent up emotional energy is cleared either by crying in private, laughing and playing with other children or by discussing with their friends. This helps them to cope with emotional stress. As the child grows older, the latter ways are used rather than crying as they find it to be socially unacceptable.

Social behavior: It is characterized by peer activities where they are not satisfied to play at home alone or with siblings or family members. They want to be with their peers and feel dissatisfied and lonely when they are not with them. Late childhood is often referred to as the gang age as they are not satisfied with having one or two friends but are a part of a group and have increasingly strong desire to be accepted to be a member of the gang. They engage in play activities with their group, usually behave and dress in a similar way to get a sense of belonging to the gang. The members of the gang usually belong to the same sex. Gang belonging improvises socialization as being a part to gang children learn many things such as socially acceptable behavior, compete with others, conform to group standards and cooperate, be loyal to the group, learn to be a good sport, learn to play various games and sports. It also gives them a sense of independence and motivates them to take up responsibilities. However, friction with adults in the family increases as they spend less time at home or fail to carry out home work. Also children may not accept or be hostile towards peers who do not belong to the gang. Children who are not accepted by the gang spend time in solitary activities like reading, watching television, etc.

Influence of the Family

Children's work in school and attitude towards school is greatly influenced by that of family members. A good family environment encourages better social adjustments. Democratic child training methods lead to a better social life than authoritarian and permissive child training methods. They also have a major influence on the self-concept. Children often compare the qualities of their parents with that of their peers.

Adolescence

It lasts from the time of puberty till eighteen years. It is the period where the individual undergoes mental, emotional and physical maturity. The period is divided into early and late adolescence, the dividing line is placed at seventeen years.

Adolescence is the period where the individual attains puberty which occurs between 11–14 years. During this period there is rapid growth in the body. The individual attains secondary sexual characteristics and sexual maturation. The adolescent needs to adjust to changes in the body growth and may often show clumsy or nervous behavior. The antagonism to the opposite sex in late childhood changes to attraction which results in mental conflicts. Adolescents also try to achieve emotional independence.

Emotional patterns: Most adolescents go through a period of emotional 'storm and stress' due to new social expectations. This turmoil of adolescence is due to surging drive to adulthood with its privileges and reponsibilities and a regressive pull backward towards security and comfort of childhood. Emotions are often intense, uncontrolled and seemingly irrational but stabilize with each passing year of adolescence. Moodiness, sulkiness, temper outbursts and tendency to cry at the slightest provocation is seen during the period of onset of puberty. Worry, anxiety and irritability are heightened during this period. Depression, irritability and negative moods are more marked in girls during the early menstrual periods. Adolescents may also show loss of self-confidence and fear of failure when the individuals are not prepared well by their parents to face the changes that take place during puberty. Emotional patterns seen in late childhood are seen in adolescents as well, but the situations and reaction may differ. Being treated like a child and being treated unfairly provokes anger. Temper tantrums give way to sulking, refusing to speak or loudly criticizing the person who angered them. Envy towards others with more material possessions is seen. Towards end of adolescence, emotional maturity occurs. They show willingness to disclose their problems, attitudes and feelings and this depends on how secure they feel about social relationships. They also learn to clear the pent up emotional energy more by laughing or by involving in strenuous activities rather than crying.

Social development: When puberty changes begin, the following behavior patterns are seen:
1. Withdrawal from peer and family activities
2. Spend much time in day dreaming about how misunderstood and mistreated they are.
3. Bored with play, school work and social activities which they formerly enjoyed.

To achieve the goal of adult behavior patterns, the adolescents learn to make new adjustments eventually. They spend most of their time outside home with the members of the peer group. Thus peers have greater influence on adolescent attitudes, speech, interests, appearance and behavior than the family. Instead of hanging on in large groups, they are seen in groups of three or four friends which are close, personal friendships. Friend are viewed as ones who are dependable, trusted and someone to talk to. However instability, quarrel are quite common when their expectations are not met, due to their inexperience in judging people and themselves and then they may move on to new set of friends. As adolescence progresses, peer group influences begin to wane and establishing one's identity gains priority. They are now able to judge the members of the opposite sex as well as members of their own sex better and make necessary social adjustments.

The traits of an adolescent which lead to acceptance by peer group are:
1. Cheerful and confident personality
2. Appearance and attire conforms to that of peers
3. Reputation of being a good sport or one who is fun to be with
4. Personality traits such as extroversion, truthfulness, sincerity, unselfishness which lead to good social adjustments
5. Being resourceful, responsible and cooperative

The opposite characteristics may lead to alienation by peers.

During this period the personal interests are in terms of clothes they wear, their appearance, acceptance by the peer group, educational achievements and having a sense of independence. If adults in the family do not understand the new cultural values of the peer group, friction usually results. Parents may also become impatient about failure to assume responsibilities. Adolescents also resent the punitive and critical attitudes of the parents when adolescents neglect their school work. The greatest rebellion occurs in homes where one parent has greater authority. In contrast, egalitarian marriage relationships between parents along with democratic way of upbringing results in better adjustments between parents and adolescents.

Emotional Dominance

The emotions that become dominant affect children's personalities and in turn their social adjustments. The dominant emotions determine the child's temperament. The dominant emotion is determined by the environment in which they grow up.

A predominance of pleasant emotions is essential for normal development. These emotions lead to feeling of security which help children approach problems with self-confidence and react to minor obstacles with emotional tension. They are readily accepted by others and successful in whatever they do.

Conditions contributing to emotional dominance:
1. **Health:** Good health encourages dominance of unpleasant emotions.
2. **Home environment:** If the relationship between the adults is good and the temperament of adults is such that unpleasant emotions such as jealousy, animosity is kept to minimum, dominance of pleasant emotions occurs in children also.
3. **Child training:** Authoritarian child training where punitive methods are used encourages unpleasant emotions, while democratic or permissive child training leads to expression of pleasant emotions. Over protective parents who think of danger in everything encourage dominance of fear in children. If parents have high aspirations which the child is not able to fulfill, he/she will have a sense of guilt. Repeated experiences can make unpleasant emotions dominant in their lives. Even an authoritarian atmosphere at school may contribute to dominance of unpleasant emotions.
4. **Relationship with peers:** If well accepted by the peer group, there is dominance of pleasant emotions.

Emotional tolerance, which is the ability to control unpleasant emotions helps in making good personal and social adjustments. Emotional tolerance develops if parents follow democratic child training method. Lack of emotional control leads to periods of heightened emotionality during anxiety provoking situations such as dental treatment or ill health.

FURTHER READING

1. Balswick JO, Macrides C. Parental stimulus for adolescent rebellion. Adolescence 1975;10:253-66.
2. Bischof NA. A system approach toward the functional connections of attachment and fear. Child Development 1975;46:801-17.
3. Denzin NK. Play, Games and Interaction. Sociological quarterly 1975;6:458-78.
4. Eckerman CO, Whately JL. Infant's reaction to unfamiliar adults varying in novelty. Developmental Psychology 1975;11:562-6.
5. Elizabeth B Hurlock. Child development. New Delhi: Tata McGraw Hill Publishing Company Limited, 1997, 6th ed. 191-253.
6. Elizabeth B Hurlock. Developmental psychology: A life span approach. Tata McGraw Hill Publishing Company Limited, 1981 5th ed. 52-259.
7. Joseph TP. Adolescents from the view of the members of an informal adolescent group. Genetic Psychology Monographs 1969;79:3-88.
8. Laura E Berk. Child development. Prentice Hall India Private Limited 3rd ed. 1994;389-413.

9. Maw WH, Maw EW. Social adjustment and curiosity of fifth grade children. Journal of Psychology 1975;90:137-45.
10. Ross HS. The influence of novelty and complexity on exploratory behaviour in 12 month-old-infants. Journal of experimental child psychology 1974;17:436-51.
11. Rutter M, Graham MP, Chadwick OFD, Yule W. Adolescent turmoil: Fact or fiction. Journal of child psychology and psychiatry and allied disciplines 1976; 17:35-6.
12. Sarles RM. Psychologic growth and development in Pediatric Dental Medicine. Forrester DJ, Wagner ML, Fleming J. editors. Lea and Febiger, Philadelphia 1981;27-37.
13. Stonag LW. Implication of infant behavior and environment for adult personalities. Annals of the New York Academy of Sciences 1966;132:782-6.
14. Waldrop MF, Halverson CF. Intensive and extensive peer behaviour: Longitudinal and cross sectional analysis. Child Development 1974;45:19-26.

QUESTIONS

1. Explain the principles of motor development.
2. Explain different stages in motor development.
3. What is learning motor skill?
4. Define speech and language.
5. What are the stages of speech and language development?
6. What are the four prespeech forms of communication?
7. Factors affecting speech and language development.
8. Explain the stages of emotional and social development.

SPEECH AND LANGUAGE DEVELOPMENT

INTRODUCTION

Speech is a tool for communication. To be able to communicate with others, all individuals must be capable of two distinct functions—comprehend what others are trying to communicate and react appropriately by speaking. Communication can be in any form of language: Written, spoken, gesticulative, musical or artistic of which spoken language is easily understood.

DEFINITION

Speech: Implies vocal and verbal expression of language appropriate to the environment of speaker and listener.
Language: This is a system of communication among human beings, who comprehend and use symbols possessing arbitrary conventional meanings.

STAGES OF SPEECH AND LANGUAGE DEVELOPMENT

Understanding the speech and language development pattern in children is essential as communication is an important tool in behavior management and communication with the child should be age appropriate.

Infant

The vocalization of the newborn infant can be divided into two categories: Crying and explosive sounds out of which crying predominates. The infant cry is the first mode of communication the individual has with the outside world. Because of the variations in the cry of the infant it is possible to tell what the infant wants. Bodily activity that accompanies crying is a signal that infant needs attention. It is thus a form of language.

In addition to crying, the infant makes explosive sounds which are commonly referred to as 'coos' or 'gurgles'. They are uttered without meaning or intent and occur purely by chance when vocal muscles contract. These are gradually strengthened into babbling which later develops into speech.

Babyhood

The foundation communication through speech is laid during babyhood.
Comprehension: The ability to understand is greater than the ability to speak during this period. The speaker's facial expression, tone of voice and gestures help babies understand what is being said to them. Pleasure, anger and fear can be comprehended as early as third month of life. Until babies are eighteen month old words should be combined with gestures such as pointing to the object for better understanding. The level of understanding depends on the baby's own intellectual abilities and also on how it is stimulated and encouraged by the family members.

Learning to speak: As babies are not mature enough to speak like adults, it is substituted by prespeech communication forms.

Four prespeech forms of communication appear in developmental pattern of learning to talk:

1. **Crying:** It is the most frequently used form in early months of life. The cry of the newborn gradually becomes differentiated, so that by third to fourth week of life it is possible to tell what the cry signifies by its tone, intensity and accompanying bodily movements. For example, hunger cries are loud and interrupted by sucking movements. Pain is expressed by shrill loud cries, interrupted by groaning and whimpering. Cries from colic are accompanied by a peculiar, high pitched scream, with alternate and forceful flexion and extension of the legs.

2. **Babbling:** The explosive sounds seen in infancy gradually develop into babbling. Over a period of time some will form the basis of real speech. It begins in the second or third month of life, reaches its peak in eighth month and then gives way to real speech. It completely disappears by the time babyhood comes to an end.

3. **Gestures:** Babies use gestures as a substitute to speech. They often combine them with words to imply sentences. By outstretching the arms and smiling, babies communicate the idea that they want to be picked up. When they push away plates saying 'no' they are trying to say that they do not want food.

4. **Emotional expressions:** It is the most effective form of prespeech communication. Babies use facial expressions to communicate their emotional state to others. When the babies are happy, they relax their bodies, wave their arms and legs, smile and make cooing sounds as a form of laughter. Babies also find it easier to understand what others are trying to communicate through facial expressions. An angry

face of the mother is quickly understood than the words " I am angry".

The tasks involved in learning to speak are:

Pronunciation: It is learnt partly by trial and error and partly by imitating adult speech. Consonants are learnt later than vowels and dipthongs. By eighteen months, the baby's speech becomes more comprehensible to adults.

Vocabulary building: Names of people and objects are learnt first, followed by verbs such as 'give', 'take' and then few adjectives and adverbs such as 'nice', 'naughty'. Vocabulary increases with age. Often they may just imitate words what others say, without knowing the meaning they imply.

Sentences: Baby's first sentences appear by twelve to eighteen months. A single word (holophrase) is used as a sentence, e.g: "Where daddy?"

Early Childhood

Most of the prespeech communications are abandoned. Young children no longer babble, their crying is greatly reduced. They use gestures mainly as supplements to speech rather than as substitute. However, use of emotional expression is still predominant.

During early childhood there is a strong motivation to learn to speak, as it gives a sense of independence and also enhances social interaction with peers in preschool. Through the medium of speech children can communicate their likes and dislikes.

Comprehension during this period is greatly dependent on the listening skills. Listening to radio or television during this period is said to improve listening skills. In addition, speaking slowly but clearly, using distinct but simple words is important.

Speaking skills: Rapid strides are made in terms of pronunciation, vocabulary and forming sentences. The time spent by parents in speaking to children enhances their speaking abilities. Three to four word sentences are formed by three years of age. These sentences are often lacking in conjunctions and prepositions. By the end of early childhood six to eight word sentences are formed by children. Child also learns about numbers and colors. However, consonants such as s, z, d, g, st, str etc. are still not pronounced correctly by many children. The content of speech is usually egocentric. They like to talk about their families, their interests and material possessions. Some children may talk incessantly (chatter box) while others are non-talkers (silent Sams). Factors contributing to non-talking trait are low intelligence, authoritarian parents, and bilingual homes. Usually girls are more talkative at this age than boys.

Late Childhood

Speech is seen as an essential tool for acceptance in a group. Simpler forms of communication such as crying and gesturing are socially unacceptable. They understand the importance of comprehension to maintain communication with the peer group. They have improved concentration due to training at school. Improvement in speech occurs due to parents, teachers at school who encourage conversation, correct mispronunciation and teach the meanings of new words. Reading habits developed by children, listening to radio or watching television also improves listening and speaking skills. By the time the child is in 6th grade, most children know 50,000 words which cover a wide range, related to color, money, numbers, etiquette, time, etc. Children also catch up correct pronunciation after hearing the words once or twice. The length and complexity of sentences increase with age. They may ask questions regarding word or a phrase which they do not understand. The content of speech shifts from egocentric to a more socialized form. They commonly boast about their superior skills and achievements rather than material possessions. The content of speech may vary based on intellectual and socialization skills. The chatter box stage is replaced by more controlled selection of speech. As childhood draws to close, children talk increasingly less.

Adolescence

Speech at this age depends on the training they have received at school regarding vocabulary, pronunciation and forming sentences. It is also influenced by the personality type and breadth of their experience. They talk to adults in lengthier sentences as compared to peers, where even phrases may be used. Conversation with peers is centered on variety of topics such as families, pets, clothes, trips, movies, television programs, sports and tabooed subjects such as sex and sex organs. Children feel more comfortable to discuss these topics with their contemporaries. Children who talk more have more self-confidence and likely to be more popular among peers.

Factors affecting speech and language development are:
1. Severe hearing loss or deafness
2. Neurologic disorders
3. Prolonged severe illness
4. Intelligence level
5. Low socioeconomic status
6. Sex: Boys catch up later than girls
7. Home environment: Parental language stimulation, language skills and attitude towards language use

8. Family size: Only child develops language faster than a family with number of siblings
9. Bilingualism: If two or more languages are spoken at home
10. Genetic influences.

FURTHER READING

1. Cole RM, Cole JE. Development and disorders of speech and language in Pediatric Dental Medicine. Forrester DJ, Wagner ML, Fleming J (editors). Lea and Febiger, Philadelphia 1981;81-7.
2. Elizabeth B Hurlock. Child development. Tata McGraw Hill Publishing Company Limited, 6th ed. 1997;161-86.
3. Elizabeth B Hurlock. Developmental psychology: A life span approach. Tata McGraw Hill Publishing Company Limited, 5th ed. 1981;52-259.
4. Vaughn GR, Hithcock HP, Akin J. Communicative disorders in children in Clinical Pedodontics. Finn SB editor, 4th ed. WB Saunders Company, USA. 1995; 590-5.

MOTOR DEVELOPMENT

INTRODUCTION

Motor development is the development of control over bodily movements through the coordinated activity of nerve centers, nerves and muscles.

PRINCIPLES OF MOTOR DEVELOPMENT

1. Motor development depends on neural and muscular maturation: Lower nerve centers located in spinal chord are better developed at birth than higher nerve centers located in brain. Thus reflexes are better developed at birth.
   Mass activity present at birth develops into a pattern of voluntary activities. This corresponds to the development of cerebellum which controls the balance in early years and reaches its mature size by 5 years. The cerebrum which controls the skilled movements also matures by 5 years. However, the striated muscles which control voluntary movements develop at a slower rate throughout childhood years. Voluntary coordinated action is impossible before they are sufficiently mature.
2. Motor development follows the laws of developmental direction and hence a predictable pattern.
   The cephaplocaudal (head–to–foot) sequence of development is shown by the fact that early in babyhood, there is greater movement in the head region than the rest of the body. As the neuromuscular mechanisms mature, there is better controlled movement in the trunk and later in the leg region. Motor development also proceeds in the proximodistal direction. In reaching for an object, the baby uses shoulders and elbows before wrists and fingers. The predictable pattern is evident in the change from mass to specific activities.
3. Learning skills cannot occur until the child is maturationally ready: Trying to teach the child skilled movements before the nervous system and muscles are well developed is a wasted effort. This is also true of the process the child may initiate.
4. Indivdual differences in motor development is due to the following factors:
   a. Genetic constitution of the body and intelligence.
   b. Favorable prenatal conditions result rapid postnatal motor development.
   c. Good health and nutrition in early postnatal life.
   d. Stimulation, encouragement and opportunities to move all parts of the body speed up motor development. Overprotectiveness by parents stifles motor development.
   e. Prematurity, physical handicaps such as blindness can delay motor development.

STAGES OF MOTOR DEVELOPMENT

At birth: Reflexes; mass activity
First 4-5 years after birth: Control of gross movements such as walking, running, jumping and so on.
After 5 years of age: Control of finer coordination which involves smaller muscle groups such as grasping, throwing, catching balls, writing, using tools.

Sequence of Motor Development

- Social smiles: 3 months
- Holding the the head up in prone position: 1 month
  - In sitting position: 4 months
- Turning: From side to back: 2 months
  - From back to side: 4 months
  - Complete: 6 months
- Sitting: Pulls to sitting position: 4 months
  - With support: 5 months
  - Without support: 9 months
- Bowel control: 2 years
- Bladder control: 2-4 years
- Hitching (backward movement in crawling position): 6 months
- Crawling (prone body pulled by arm and leg kicks): 7 months
- Creeping on hands and knees: 9 months
- Standing with support: 8 months
  - Without support: 11 months
- Walking with support: 11 months
  - Without support: 12-14 months
- Grasp: Reach and grasp: 4 months
  - Picking up objects using fingers: 8 months

LEARNING MOTOR SKILLS

Motor skills are fine coordinations in which smaller muscles play a major role. They can be broadly divided into:

1. *Self-help skills:* Self-feeding, dressing, grooming, bathing.

2. *Social help skills:* Helping with work at home, school or peer group.
3. *Play skills:* Ball play, roller skating, manipulating toys.
4. *School skills:* Writing, drawing, painting, dancing, clay modelling.

Childhood is the ideal age for learning motor skills because the bodies are more pliable; they have fewer previously learned skills which conflict with new ones; and children are more adventuresome. Essential factors for learning motor skills are:

a. Readiness to learn
b. Opportunity to learn
c. Opportunities for practice
d. Good model who can be imitated
e. Guidance to imitate the model correctly
f. Motivation to keep the interest from lagging
g. Each skill is learnt individually, e.g. holding a spoon during self-feeding is different from holding a crayon
h. Skills should be learnt one at a time.

Methods of Learning Motor Skills

1. *Trial and error learning:* Having no guidance and no model, child tries different act at random. This results in skills below child's capacities.
2. *Imitation:* Child observes the model (parent or older child) and tries to reproduce the behavior of the model. Though faster than trial and error method, is limited by faults in the model.
3. *Training:* Learning under guidance and supervision where the model demonstrates the skill and sees that the child imitates correctly.

Society has a major role in the development of motor skills. Motor skills give a sense of independence, help in socialization, instill self-confidence and also ensure good physical health. Delayed motor development or unrealistic expectations about motor skills can have negative effects on personality development and social adjustments. It can affect the self-esteem of the child, leading to emotional and behavioral problems. It may result in feelings of inferiority, a sense of dependency, resentment toward adults, difficulty in social adjustments, jealousy towards other children and timidity. They may show lack of initiative because they are afraid, they may not perform successfully.

FURTHER READING

1. Elizabeth B Hurlock. Developmental psychology: A life span approach. Tata McGraw Hill Publishing Company Limited, 5th ed. 1981;52-259.
2. Elizabeth B Hurlock. Child development. Tata McGraw Hill Publishing Company Limited, 6th ed. 1997;161-86.
3. Laura E Berk. Child development. Prentice Hall India Private Limited 3rd ed. 1994;389-413.

DEVELOPMENT AND ERUPTION OF TEETH

INTRODUCTION

The development and subsequent eruption of the teeth is a complex procedure that occurs simultaneously with the growth and development of the entire facial complex. The development of teeth starts at about 5-6 intrauterine week, in the primitive oral cavity also called as stomodeum which is lined with low squamous cells that form the oral ectoderm. The cells that underlie the oral ectoderm are neural crest or ectomesenchymal in origin.

Initially at this stage neither the upper nor the lower jaws show separate lip or gum region. The separation lips and cheeks from the gums are closely related with the development of the teeth. As the primordial of the teeth appears and develop, the cells of the oral epithelium thickens in the region of the lip, cheek, vestibule of the mouth and the site of the origin of dental lamina to form the primary epithelial band which gives rise to vestibular lamina and dental lamina. Vestibular lamina forms the vestibule.

The dental lamina is a band of epithelium that invades the underlying ectomesenchyme along each of the dental arches. The dental lamina serves as a primordium for the ectodermal portion of the teeth. The total activity of dental lamina extends over a period of at least 5 years, except in the third molar region where its activity is prolonged. As the teeth develop they loose their connection with the dental lamina and break up by mesemchymal invasion. Remnants of dental lamina persist as epithelial pearls or islands within the jaw and in the gingiva.

The development of teeth can be studied by dividing it into different stages based on the shape they acquire during development or based on physiologic changes they undergo as follows:

DEVELOPMENT OF TEETH

Teeth development can be divided based on the shape and physiologic changes as follows:

Based on Change of Shape

1. Bud stage
2. Cap stage
3. Bell stage
4. Advanced bell stage

Based on Physiologic Changes

1. Initiation
2. Proliferation
3. Morpho and histodifferentiation
4. Apposition

Bud Stage/Initiation

The first epithelial invasion into the mesenchyme of the jaw to form a tooth occurs that resembles a bud and is called as enamel organ (Fig. 4.15). Different teeth are initiated at different and definite time. Enamel organ forms the enamel of the tooth. Lack of initiation results in the absence of tooth development leading to congenitally missing tooth and conversely abnormal initiation may lead to supernumerary teeth as well.

The initiation processes occur along each jaw which marks the beginning of development of deciduous teeth. The timing will differ for anterior teeth and the posterior teeth. Anterior teeth develop earlier than the posterior teeth.

As the formation of the enamel organ continuous the ectomesenchymal cells below this increase in number and appear denser than the surrounding mesenchyme to form the dental papilla. The dental papilla and the enamel organ are surrounded by dental sac. The tooth bud at this stage lies close to the oral epithelium.

Cap Stage/Proliferation

As the growth continues regular changes in the size and proportion of the growing tooth germ is seen leading to the formation of a cap shaped enamel organ, characterized by a shallow invagination on the deep surface of the bud (Fig. 4.16). The enamel organ at this stage consists of 3 layers, enamel knot and enamel cord. The three layers are the outer enamel epithelium, inner enamel epithelium and stellate reticulum.

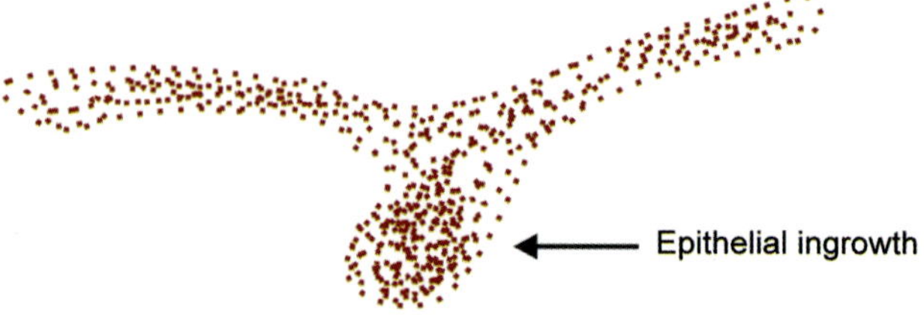

Fig. 4.15: Bud stage of tooth development: Condensation of the ectomesenchyme leading to bud shaped epithelial ingrowth

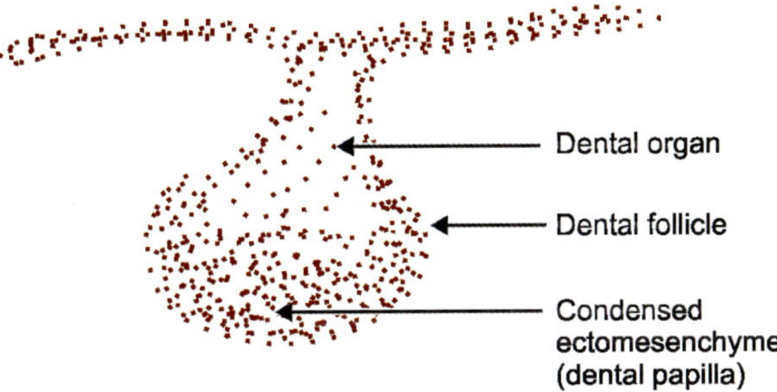

Fig. 4.16: Cap stage of tooth development: The dental organ assumes the shape of a cap and overlies the dental papilla

i. *Outer enamel epithelium:* Cuboidal cells covering the convexity
ii. *Inner enamel epithelium:* Tall columnar cells in the concavity.
iii. *Stellate reticulum:* These are polygonal cells in the center between the outer and the inner enamel epithelium. They tend to separate as intercellular fluid is produced and assume a branched reticular form. This layer acts as a cushion which supports and protects the delicate enamel forming cells.
iv. *Enamel knot:* Densely packed cells in the center of the enamel organ.
v. *Enamel cord:* Vertical extension of the enamel knot extending to the outer enamel epithelium.

The dental papilla shows active budding of capillaries. The pheripheral cells adjacent to inner enamel epithelium enlarge and later differentiate into odontoblasts.

Bell Stage/Morphological and Histological Differentiation

In this stage, cells undergo definite morphologic as well as functional changes and acquire appositional growth potential. This phase reaches its highest development in the bell stage just before the beginning of enamel and dentin formation (Fig. 4.17).

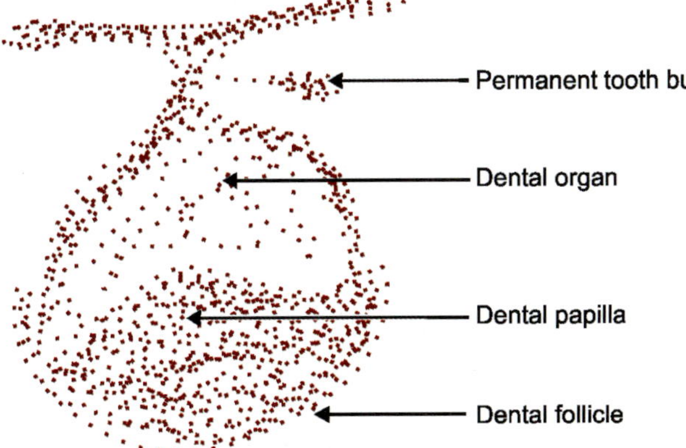

Fig. 4.17: Bell stage of tooth development: The undersurface of the dental organ deepens, giving it a bell shape

At this stage the enamel organ consists of four layers, they are:
   i. Inner enamel epithelium, made of single layer of tall columnar cells called as ameloblasts.
   ii. Stratum intermedium, consisting of squamous cells. This layer is essential for enamel formation along with inner enamel epithelium cells.
   iii. Stellate reticulum are starshaped and secrete glycosaminoglycans.
   iv. Outer enamel epithelium, the cells flatten to a low cuboidal form.

The pheripheral cells of the dental papilla differentiate into odontoblasts that form the dentin.

The dental sac initially shows a circular arrangement of its fibers resembling a capsular structure and later as the root development continues differentiates into periodontal fibers.

At the last stages of bell stage, the cervical portion of the enamel organ gives rise to the epithelial root sheath of Hertwig. The inner and outer enamel epithelium meet each other at the rim of the enamel organ-junctional zone known as cervical loop.

> The cells forming ameloblasts are tall columnar, 4-5 μm in diameter and 40 μm high. These cells are attached to each other by functional complexes and to stratum intermedium by desmosomes. The nucleus is centrally located, cytoplasm contains free ribosomes, few endoplasmic reticulum, mitochondria, Golgi complex and increased glycogen content.

Advanced Bell Stage/Apposition

In this stage, there is deposition of the matrix of the dental hard tissues in a layer like pattern and is additive (Fig. 4.18).

ROOT FORMATION

- Begins after enamel and dentin formation has reached the future cementoenamel junction.
- The outer and inner enamel epithelium blend at the future cementoenamel junction into a horizontal plane to form the epithelial diaphragm. This narrows the wide cervical opening of the tooth germ.
- Hertwig's epithelial root sheath moulds the shape of the root and initiates radicular dentin formation.
- Hertwig's epithelial root sheath cells loose their structural continuity and close relation to the surface of the root, when the first layer of dentin has been laid down.

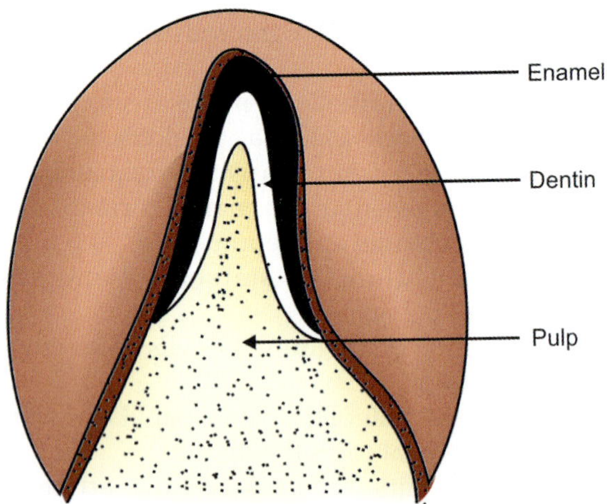

Fig. 4.18: Advanced bell stage of tooth development: Dental lamina is disintergrating. The crown pattern of the tooth is established by folding of the inner dental epithelium

- At the last stages, the wide apical foramen is reduced first to the width of the diaphragmatic opening itself and later is further narrowed by apposition of dentin and cementum to the apex of the root. Differential growth of the epithelial diaphragm in multirooted teeth causes the division of the root trunk into 2 or 3 roots.

> During the development, if the cells of the epithelial root sheath remain adherent to the dentin surface, they may differentiate into fully functioning ameloblasts and produce enamel called as enamel pearls.

> **Early development and calcification of primary teeth**
>
> First macroscopic indication of morphologic development—11-12 ½ IU week
> Incisors begin to develop morphologic characteristics—13-14 IU week
> Canines begin to develop morphologic characteristics—14-16 IU week
> Initial calcification of incisors—16 IU week
> Initial calcification of canines—17 IU week
> First evidence of calcification of first molar—15 ½ IU week
> First evidence of calcification of second molar—18-19 IU week.

Permanent Dentition

The permanent tooth develops from the dental lamina as the result of the proliferative activity within the dental lamina at a point where it joins the dental organ of deciduous tooth germ. This leads to the formation of another epithelial cap and associated ectomesenchymal response on the lingual aspect of the deciduous tooth germ.

The entire deciduous dentition is initiated between 5th-8th intrauterine week. The successional permanent teeth are initiated between 20th intrauterine week to 10th post natal month. The permanent first molar is initiated at the 20th intrauterine week and the second permanent molar at the 5th year of life.

> Time scale of human tooth development:
> Dental lamina formation—42-48 IU day
>   Duration   ↓   8-10 Days
> Bud stage of deciduous incisors, canine and molars—55-56 IU day
> Duration   ↓   43 Days
> Bell stage of deciduous teeth—14th week
> Duration   ↓   28 Days
> Dentin and functional ameloblasts seen in deciduous teeth—18th week

Chronology of Human Dentition

Kronfelld in 1935 first described the chronology of human dentition (Both deciduous and permanent). Lunt later in 1974 modified the earlier version (only for deciduous dentition) and the same is being followed till date.

TOOTH ERUPTION

The process of eruption involves the movement or change of position of the tooth from the deeper portion of the jaws into the oral cavity until it achieves occlusal contact with adjacent and opposing teeth. A tooth begins its movement once its crown formation is completed (It takes about 5 years from crown completion to complete eruption of an individual tooth).[6] Tooth emergence is also associated with the formation of root. It is said that a tooth erupts into the oral cavity, approximately ¾ of the root is formed and reaches the occlusion before the complete formation.

Various Factors Influence the Timing of Eruption

1. Genetic factor
2. Sex
3. Socioeconomic conditions
4. Birth weight
5. Systemic disorders
6. Hormones and vitamins
7. Local causes

Dentition	Jaw	Tooth	First evidence of calcification	Crown completion	Eruption	Root completion
Deciduous	Upper	Central Incisor	13–16 weeks IU	4 months	10 (8–12) months	1 ½ years
		Lateral Incisor	14–16 ½ weeks IU	5 months	11 (9–13) months	2 years
		Canine	15–18 weeks IU	9 months	19 (16–22) months	3 ¼ years
		First Molar	14 ½–17 weeks IU	6 months	16 (13–19) months	2 ½ years
		Second Molar	16–23 ½ weeks IU	10–12 months	29 (25–33) months	3 years
	Lower	Central Incisor	13–16 weeks IU	4 months	8 (6–10) months	1 ½ years
		Lateral Incisor	14–16 ½ weeks IU	4 ¼ months	13 (10–16) months	1 ½ years
		Canine	16–18 weeks IU	9 months	20 (17–23) months	3 ¼ years
		First Molar	14 ½–17 weeks IU	6 months	16 (14–18) months	2 ¼ years
		Second Molar	17–19 ½ weeks IU	10–12 months	27 (23–31) months	3 years
Permanent	Upper	Central Incisor	3–4 months	4–5 years	7–8 years	10 years
		Lateral Incisor	10 months	4–5 years	8–9 years	11 years
		Canine	4–5 months	6–7 years	11–12 years	13–15 years
		First Premolar	1 ½–1 ¾ Years	5–6 years	10–11 years	12–13 years
		Second Premolar	2–2 ½ Years	6–7 years	10–12 years	12–14 years
		First Molar	At birth	2 ½–3 years	6–7 years	9–10 years
		Second Molar	2 ½–3 years	7–8 years	12–13 years	14–16 years
		Third Molar	7–9 years	12–16 years	17–21 years	18–25 years
	Lower	Central Incisor	3–4 months	4–5 years	6–7 years	9 years
		Lateral Incisor	3–4 months	4–5 years	7–8 years	10 years
		Canine	4–5 months	6–7 years	9–10 years	12–14 years
		First Premolar	1 ¾–2 years	5–6 years	10–12 years	12–13 years
		Second Premolar	2 ¼–2 ½ years	6–7 years	11–12 years	13–14 years
		First Molar	At birth	2 ½–3 years	6–7 years	9–10 years
		Second Molar	2 ½–3 years	7–8 years	11–13 years	14–15 years
		Third Molar	8–10 years	12–16 years	17–21 years	18–25 years

Genetic Factor

Genes play a definite role in tooth eruption and have been estimated to be about 78%.

Sex

It is observed that the teeth of girls erupt slightly earlier than those of boys. The average amount of tooth development for girls is about 3% ahead that of boys. The difference may vary from 2 months [first molar] to 10 months (maxillary canine). Intially during the formation stage, there was no sex difference up to the stage of calcification, and the difference begins only from the crown completion stage.

Socioeconomic Condition

Socioeconomic levels are known to affect eruption. Retarded eruption of anterior teeth and accelerated emergences of the posterior dentition has been linked to low socioeconomic status in all racial groups.

Birth Weight

Low birth weight has been associated with delayed emergence of permanent teeth and conversely early eruption has been associated with increased birth weight.

Systemic Disorders

Precocious eruption is rare and is observed less commonly than retarded eruption.

Delay in permanent tooth eruption is associated with Down's syndrome, cleidocranial dysostosis, hypothyroidism, hypopituitarism and hemifacial atrophy.

Precocious eruption is seen in precocious puberty, hyperthyroidism, hemifacial hypertrophy, Sturge-Weber syndrome and hyperpituitarism.

Hormones and Vitamins

Thyroid, pituitary [growth hormone], and parathyroid hormones are essential for normal eruption of teeth.

Vitamins like vitamin B complex, A, C and D aid either directly or indirectly for tooth eruption.

Local Causes

Ankylosis of primary teeth delays the eruption of permanent tooth.

Dental caries and periapical infection of primary teeth, resulted in early eruption of the corresponding permanent tooth.

Very early extraction of a primary molar delays gingival eruption of the successor.

> Time required for a tooth to reach occlusion after piercing the gingival tissue varies from 3–30 months.
> Root completion is complete approximately 1½ years for deciduous teeth and 3 years for permanent teeth after eruption.

Sequence of Eruption

The mandibular I permanent molars are often the first permanent teeth to erupt. The most favorable sequence of eruption of permanent teeth in the mandible is first molar, central incisor, lateral incisor, canine, first premolar, second premolar and second molar.

In maxilla the sequence is as follows, the first molar, central incisor, lateral incisor, first premolar, second premolar, canine and second molar.

This sequence of eruption is important to maintain arch length adequacy. For example, if the premolars erupt first there is a tendency for them to tip mesially due to extra space (mesiodistal width of premolars is less than the mesiodistal width of the deciduous molars) and thus causing loss of arch length.

> All mammalians have gomphosis type of tooth attachment to the jaws but the eruption process or mechanism differs. There are three basic mechanisms of tooth eruption in mammalians.
> 1. *Continuously growing tooth:* There is no separation between anatomical crown and root. Continuous growth of the tooth at the apex and continuous eruption occur throughout the life of the animal. Clinical crown is constantly replaced by a root covered with enamel in progressive stages of development. With the loss of tooth substance due to occlusal attrition more tooth substance is extruded from the socket to maintain clinical crown, e.g. rodent incisor teeth.
> 2. *Continuously extruding tooth:* There is a definite crown and anatomical root. The tooth begins erupting by partially emerging from the investing tissue, revealing only a fraction of the large enamel surface. The enamel
>
> *Contd...*

Contd...

> beneath the gingiva is covered with cementum enabling supraalveolar fibers to be attached to the tooth. As the tooth wears off, more of the anatomical crown extrudes and the epithelial attachment migrate apically, but since no new tooth structure is being formed, the continuous tooth eruption results in a gradual loosening and final exfoliation of the tooth, e.g. lower incisors of sheep and cattle.
> 3. *Continuously erupting teeth:* Mild amount of tooth extrusion occurs throughout with resultant addition of alveolar bone at the base of the socket, e.g. human teeth.
>
> Rate of eruption of human teeth—140 μm/day during the most rapid period, i.e. during the time of gingival emergence and 5 μm/day as the teeth reaches occlusal plane.
>
> In a radiographic study, it was found that the interval between crown completion and beginning of eruption until the tooth is in full occlusion is approximately 5 years for permanent teeth.

ERUPTION PATTERN

The eruptive movements of tooth can be divided as:
1. Pre-eruptive tooth movements
2. Eruptive movements
3. Posteruptive tooth movements

Pre-eruptive Movements

These are the movements made within the bone before the tooth begins to erupt.

Development of the tooth and jaws occurs simultaneously. As the jaw grows the developing teeth are carried along in their direction of growth. Thus the deciduous molar tooth germ moves or is carried in a backward direction, the anterior tooth germ in a forward direction.

Pre-eruptive movements are combination of two factors:
A. Total bodily movement
B. Growth in which one part of the tooth germ remains fixed while the rest continues to grow leading to change in the center of the tooth germ. This explains how the deciduous incisors maintain their position relative to the oral mucosa as the jaws increase in height.

Eruptive Movements

Eruption normally starts when the root formation begins. The periodontal ligament develops only after root formation has been initiated and once established, it is remodeled to permit continued eruptive tooth movement, which is achieved by the fibroblasts.

As the eruptive movements begin the enamel of the crown is still covered by a layer of ameloblasts and remnants of enamel organ together called as reduced enamel epithelium. The bone covering the erupting teeth is soon resorbed and the crown passes through the connective tissue of the mucosa, which is broken down in advance of erupting tooth. This reduced enamel epithelium and oral epithelium fuse and form a solid knot of epithelial cells over the crown of the tooth. The central cells of this mass of epithelium degenerate, forming an epithelial canal through which crown of the tooth erupts. During eruption the cells of the reduced enamel epithelium lose their nutritive supply and degenerate, thus exposing enamel.

When the erupting tooth appears in oral cavity, it is subjected to environmental factors that help determine its final position in the dental arch.

Theories of Mechanism of Tooth Eruption

Many theories have been proposed to explain the mechanism of eruption but it seems that eruption is a multifactorial process.

Possible mechanisms currently favored although not mutually exclusive, are:

A. Papillary constriction theory
B. Bony remodeling
C. Epithelial path theory
D. Cushioned hammock theory
E. Root formation
F. Hydrostatic pressure
G. Selective deposition and resorption of bone around the tooth
H. Periodontal ligament—traction.

Papillary constriction theory

Dental papilla constricts because of decrease in the volume of the pulp cavity by continuous dentin formation and this generates a propulsive force.

Bony remodelling

Forces acting during eruption are similar to that seen in cranial bone sutures. The sutural connective tissue grows as a result of tension created by the growing brain. The bones thus move apart. The space thus created is transformed into bone keeping the sutural width more or less the same. Similarly, the connective tissue of dental follicle and periodontal ligament proliferate and the tooth and crypt are pushed away from each other. The crypt cannot move, but the tooth moves away and this space is filled by growing root and bone apposition.

Eruption is due to the differential growth between tooth and bone.

Epithelial path theory

Hair, nail and salivary gland are end product of the epithelial down growth. They return to the surface by the path, down which the original epithelium grew. Enamel is also an epithelial structure and so returns back to the surface.

Cushioned hammock theory

This theory states that root grows and pushes against the cushion hammock ligament which passes from one side of the socket wall to the opposite. Recent works have shown that this Hammock ligament does not extend across the socket, but only separates the pulp from the follicle.

Root formation

According to this theory, as the root grows apically there is a force generated in an opposite direction that propels the tooth occlusally. This theory is not accepted as the force generated is not adequate to push the tooth into occlusion.

Hydrostatic pressure

It is known that teeth move in their socket in synchrony with the arterial pulse, and this was said to be responsible for movement of tooth during eruption. But it is difficult to link such observations to eruptive tooth movements and does not have adequate experimental support.

Selective deposition and resorption of bone around the tooth

The inherent growth pattern of the jaws moves the teeth by selective deposition and resorption of bone in the immediate neighborhood of tooth. But whether they are completely responsible for eruption of tooth is clearly not understood.

Periodontal ligament traction

If the normal architecture of the periodontal ligament is disturbed experimentally by interfering with collagen synthesis, eruptive tooth movement is either slowed or stopped. The contractility of fibroblasts in the periodontal ligament is said to exert comparatively large and sustained tractional forces that is useful to push the tooth in occlusal direction as occurs during eruption.

Posteruptive Movements

- They are the movements made by the tooth after it has reached its functional position in the occlusal plane. Posteruptive tooth movements help in readjustment of the tooth in the socket. This is achieved by the formation of new bone at the alveolar crest and on the socket floor to keep pace with the increasing height of the jaws. Such movements can be in axial, mesial or distal directions.

- Axial movement is the movement in occlusal direction the tooth makes to compensate for occlusal wear.
- Mesial or proximal drift involves a combination of two separate forces resulting from occlusal contact of teeth and contraction of the trans-septal ligaments between them.

Clinical and radiographic changes associated with tooth eruption (Figs 4.19 to 4.23) again discussed later in the book.

Problems during Eruption of Teeth

Difficult Eruption/Teething

In most children, the eruption of primary teeth is preceded by increased salivation and the child would want to put the hand and fingers into the mouth. Some children become restless and fretful, exhibit increase in the amount of finger sucking or rubbing of the gum, drooling and loss of appetite during the time of eruption of the primary teeth. It is coincidentally associated with diarrhea, fever and even convulsions and is not directly attributed to eruption. All these features may be due to mouthing of contaminated toys or teethers which the children use to rub the gums.

Local conditions observed during teeth eruption are gum inflammation, ulcer in mouth, cheek flush and cheek rash. Inflammation of the gingival tissues before complete emergence of the crown may cause a temporary painful condition that subsides within a few days.

Symptoms often associated with teething are:
- Irritability (most prevalent)
- Restlessness
- Drooling
- Disturbed sleep
- Decreased food consumption
- Increased fluid intake
- Diarrhea
- Fever, and rash.

Management

Treatment for teething is symptomatic and palliative. If the child is having extreme difficulty, the application of a nonirritating topical anesthetic gel may bring temporary relief. The parent can apply the anesthetic gel to the affected tissue over the erupting tooth 3 or 4 times a day. The child can be given vegetables such as carrot

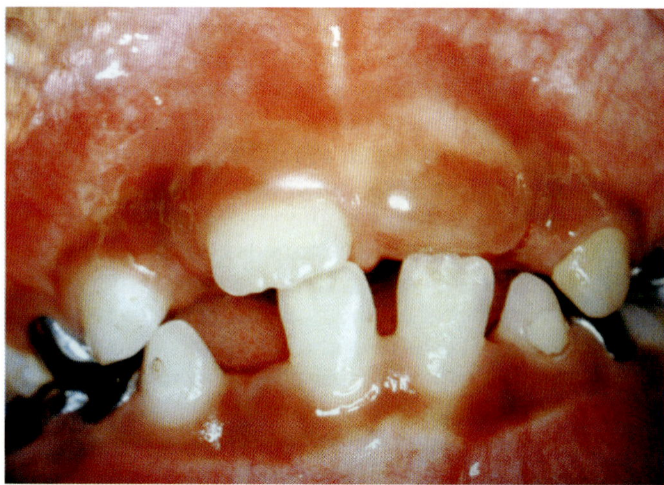

Fig. 4.19: Pre-eruptive swelling seen on the ridge just before tooth eruption

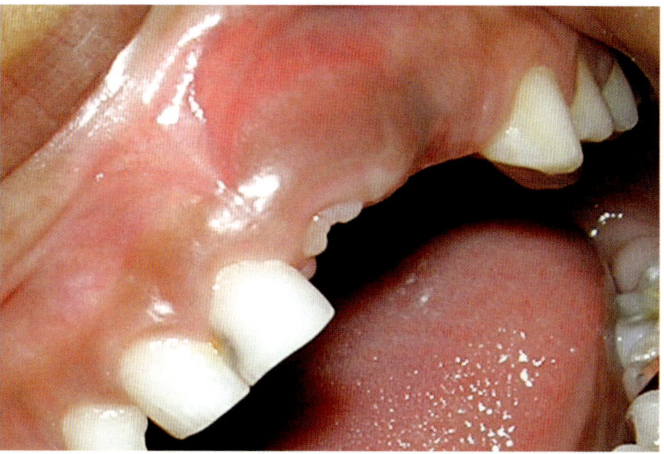

Fig. 4.20: Tooth seen erupting through the gingiva

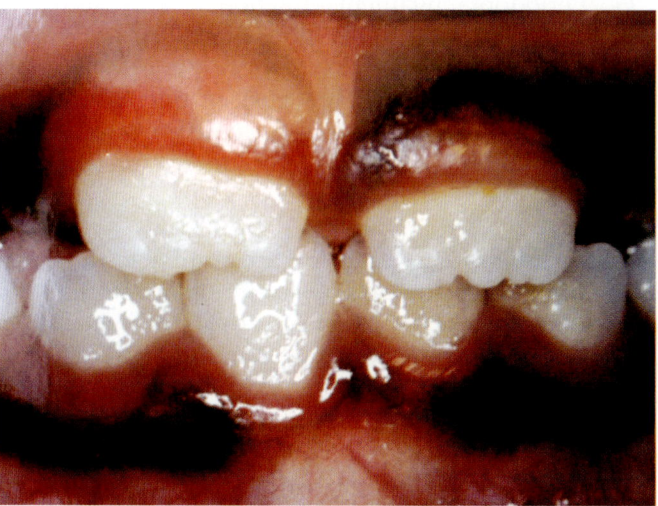

Fig. 4.21: Teeth in the process of eruption

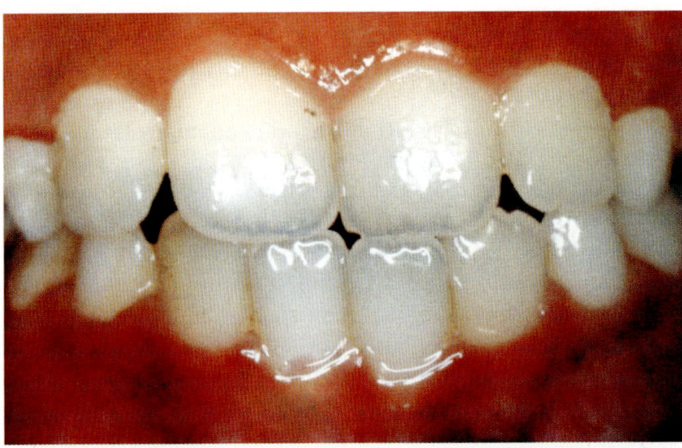

Fig. 4.22: Fully erupted permanent incisors

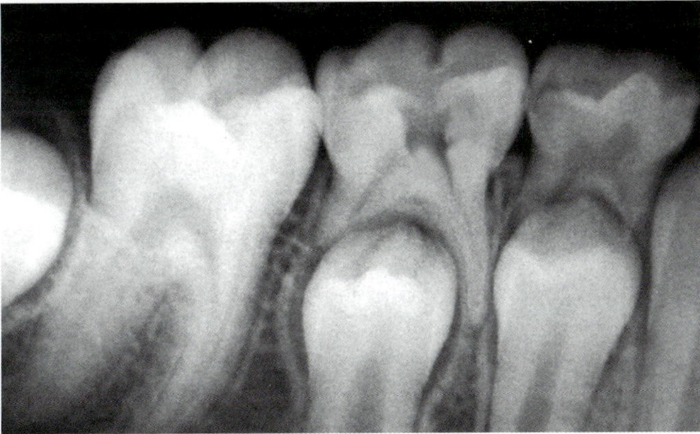

Fig. 4.23: Note the pattern of physiologic root resorption of lower first and second deciduous molars seen during the eruption of the premolars

that are hard and chewable to bite onto it. This may give some relief to the child. Commercially available sterile and clean teethers can also be used. Reassuring the parents is helpful. Fever, if present, should be treated with acetaminophen. If the fever is persistent, the child should be referred to a pediatrician. Use of a chewable object and topical anesthetics will help relieve local irritation.

Eruption Hematoma/Eruption Cyst

It appears as bluish purple, elevated area of tissue, which develops a few weeks before the eruption of a primary or permanent tooth. This blood filled cyst is most frequently seen in primary second molar or permanent first molar region. Within a few days the tooth breaks through the tissue and the hematoma subsides. Since it is self-correcting, treatment is usually unnecessary.

Eruption Sequestrum

Sequestrum is a tiny spicule of nonviable bone overlying the crown of an erupting permanent molar. They have little or no clinical significance, as they usually sequestrate spontaneously.

Natal and Neonatal Teeth

- Natal teeth are those that are present at birth and neonatal are those that erupt within the first 30 days of birth.
- Natal teeth may resemble normal primary teeth. In about 85% of the cases they are prematurely erupted deciduous incisors. Otherwise they may appear poorly developed, small, conical shaped, yellowish brown opaque, and have hypoplastic enamel and dentin, poor texture, and small root.
- The mandibular incisor region is the most prevalent location.
- The condition is probably attributed to superficial positioning during the formation of the involved tooth germ.
- Natal and neonatal teeth that lack root structure, will usually exfoliate prematurely during infancy, presenting a potential hazard for aspiration.
- Natal and neonatal teeth seem to have familial predilection (in about 15%).
  They may be sometimes associated with three syndromes:
  A. Chondroectodermal dysplasia or Ellis Van Creveld syndrome
  B. Hallermann-Streiff syndrome
  C. Pachyonychia congenita syndrome
- Natal teeth appear more frequently than neonatal teeth in a ratio of 3:1.
- A sharp incisal edge of the natal or neonatal teeth may lacerate the tongue and cause difficulty while breastfeeding. Although there seems to be a risk that the teeth may be aspirated, there is no recorded document. In such cases it may be extracted or otherwise left without extraction. Where possible, extraction should be avoided until after the tenth postnatal day to avoid hemorrhage, due to possibility of vitamin K deficiency present.
- Riga-Fede disease: It is characterized by the formation of an ulcer on the ventral surface of the tongue caused by the natal or neonatal teeth rubbing against the teeth. It is also called a Fede's disease or Riga-Fede syndrome.

Epstein Pears, Bohn's Nodules and Dental Lamina Cysts

They are inclusion cysts and are of three types:
A. Epstein pearls—formed along the median palatine raphe. They are considered remnants of epithelial tissue trapped along the raphe as the fetus grows.

B. Bohn's nodules—formed along the buccal and lingual aspects of the dental ridge and on the palate away from the raphe. They are considered remnants of mucous gland tissue and histologically are different from Epstein pearls.

C. Dental lamina cysts—they are found on the crest of maxillary and mandibular ridges. They originated from remnants of the dental lamina.

Ankylosis (Submerged Tooth)

It is the aberration of tooth eruption in which the continuity of the periodontal ligament has been compromised and the tooth is fused to the underlying bone.

The tooth appears submerged and does not occlude with the opposing tooth, as the ankylosed tooth is in the state of static retention whereas in the adjacent areas eruption and alveolar growth continues.

There are high chances for the occurrence of many ankylosed teeth when a patient is diagnosed to have one or two ankylosed tooth in oral cavity.

Mandibular primary molars are the teeth most often observed to be ankylosed. Ankylosis of anterior primary tooth usually follows any kind of trauma. Familial occurrences (non-sex linked) have been noted.

Diagnosis of an ankylosed tooth can be made based on the following points:

- No contact with opposing molar
- Not mobile inspite of advanced root resorption
- Comparing the sound by taping the involved and adjacent tooth. Ankylosed tooth exhibits solid sound, but a normal tooth has a cushioned sound
- Break in the continuity of periodontal membrane.

Management of Ankylosed Tooth

A. Surgical removal, if the permanent successor is present.

B. If permanent teeth are missing, functional occlusion is established with stainless steel crowns on the affected tooth.

Understanding tooth development and eruption will guide a practitioner to diagnose or differentiate normal from an abnormal. Constant evaluation or observation of the development of teeth and occlusion can be included under preventive dentistry program thus intervening any developing malocclusion at its early stage.

Delayed Eruption

- Seen in Down Syndrome, cleidocranial dysplasia, hypothyroidism, hypopituitarism or achondroplastic dwarfism. Other conditions associated with delayed eruption are fibromatosis gingivae, Albright hereditary osteodystrophy, chondroectodermal dysplasia, Gard-ner syndrome, hypophosphatemia, etc.

FURTHER READING

1. Alexander SA, et al. Multiple ankylosed teeth, J Pedodo 1980;4:354-9.
2. Bodenhoff J, Gorlin RJ. Natal ad neonatal teeth: Folklore and fact, Pediatrics 1963;32:1087-93.
3. Brown ID. Some further observations on submerging deciduous molars. Br J Orthod 1981;8(2):99-107.
4. Burdi AR, Moyers RE. Development of the dentition and occlusion in Moyers RE. Handbook of Orthodontics 4th Ed. Year Book Medical Publishers, Inc. Chicago 1988.
5. Davit-Beal T, Chisaka H, Delgado S, Sire JY. Amphibian teeth: current knowledge, unanswered questions, and some directions for future research. Biol Rev Camb Philos Soc 2007;82(1):49-81.
6. Demirjian A, Levesque GY. Sexual difference in dental development and prediction of emergence. J Dent Res 1980;59:1110-22.
7. Ferreira AN, Silveira L, Genovese WJ, de Araujo VC, Frigo L, de Mesquita RA, Guedes E. Effect of GaAIAs laser on reactional dentinogenesis induction in human teeth. Photomed Laser Surg 2006;24(3):358-65.
8. Fromm A. Epstein's Pearls, Bohn's Nodules and inclusion cysts of the oral cavity. J Detn Child 1967;34:275-87.
9. Gron AMP. Prediction of tooth emergency. J Dent Res 1962;41:573-85.
10. Hu B, Nadiri A, Kuchler-Bopp S, Perrin-Schmitt F, Peters H, Lesot H. Tissue engineering of tooth crown, root, and periodontium Tissue Eng 2006;12(8):2069-75.
11. Illingworth RS. Teething, Dev Med Child Neurol 1969; 11:376-7.
12. Lunt RC, Law DB. A review of the chronology of calcification of deciduous teeth. J Am Dent Assoc 1974; 89:599-606.
13. Maciejewska I, Spodnik JH, Domaradzka-Pytel B, Sidor-Kaczmarek J, Bereznowski Z. Fluoride alters type I collagen expression in the early stages of odontogenesis. Folia Morphol (Warsz) 2006;65(4):359-66.
14. Mc Donald RE, Avery DR, Dean JA. Eruption of the teeth: Local, systemic and congenital factors that influence the process. Dentistry for the child and adolescent 9th Edition, Elsevier Mosby 2011;150-76.
15. Miyaji H, Sugaya T, Kato K, Kawamura N, Tsuji H, Kawanami M. Dentin resorption and cementum-like tissue formation by bone morphogenetic protein application. J Periodontal Res 2006;41(4):311-5.
16. Opydo-Szymaczek J, Borysewicz-Lewicka M. Variations in concentration of fluoride in blood plasma of pregnant women and their possible consequences for amelogenesis in a fetus. Homo 2006;57(4):295-307. Epub 2006 Jul 14.
17. Orban BJ. Oral Histology and Embryology. St. Louis CV Mosby 1976.
18. Orban BJ. Growth and movement of the tooth germs and teeth. Am Dent Assoc J 1928;15:1004.
19. Remmers D, Bokkerink JP, Katsaros C. Microdontia after chemotherapy in a child treated for neuroblastoma. Orthod Craniofac Res 2006;9(4):206-10.
20. Sartaj R, Sharpe P. Biological tooth replacement. J Anat 2006;209(4):503-9.

21. Seppala M, Zoupa M, Onyekwelu O, Cobourne MT. Tooth development: 1. Generating teeth in the embryo. Dent Update 2006;33(10):582-4, 586-8, 590-1.

22. Tencate AR. Oral Histology 3rd Ed St. Louis Mosby, 1989.

23. Thesleff I. The genetic basis of tooth development and dental defects. Am J Med Genet A 2006;140(23):2530-5. Review.

24. Ye L, Le TQ, Zhu L, Butcher K, Schneider RA, Li W, Besten PK. Amelogenins in human developing and mature dental pulp. J Dent Res 2006;85(9):814-8.

25. Zhu J, King D. Natal and neonatal teeth. J Dent Child 1995;62:123-8.

QUESTIONS

1. Describe the stages of tooth development based on the shape.
2. Describe the mechanism of root formation.
3. Discuss in detail the chronology of human dentition.
4. What are the factors influencing tooth eruption?
5. Explain the sequence of eruption of deciduous and permanent dentition.
6. Describe the eruption of tooth.
7. What are the problems encountered during eruption of teeth?

DEVELOPMENT OF OCCLUSION

At birth, the alveolar ridges are plain firm tissue with no teeth on them. As the child grows steady changes are seen both on and within the ridge. The alveolar ridge grows and enlarges while the teeth develop to attain their final shape and size within the jaws. As per the predetermined time individual teeth erupt and aligne and come into a full fledged occlusion with each other.

The study of this development of occlusion can be divided into the following developmental periods (Fig. 4.24):

1. *Pre-dental/dentate period:* This is the period after birth during which the neonate does not have any teeth. It usually lasts for 6 months after birth. The characteristic feature is the alveolar ridge that are called as gum pads.
2. *The deciduous dentition period:* The initiation of primary tooth buds occurs during the first six weeks of intrauterine life. The primary teeth begin to erupt at the age of about 6 months. The eruption of all primary teeth is completed by 2-2½ years of age when the second deciduous molars come into occlusion.
3. *The mixed dentition period:* The mixed dentition period begins at approximately 6 years of age with the eruption of the first permanent molars. During the mixed dentition period, the deciduous teeth along with some permanent teeth are present in the oral cavity.
4. *The permanent dentition period:* This period is characterized by the presence of all permanent teeth.

PREDENTAL/DENTATE PERIOD

Gum Pads

Features of Gumpads (Figs 4.25 and 4.26)

- The alveolar processes at the time of birth are known as gum pads. The gum pads are pink, firm and are covered by a dense layer of fibrous periosteum.
- They are horse-shoe shaped and develop in two parts, the labiobuccal portion and the lingual portion. The labiobuccal portion develops before the lingual

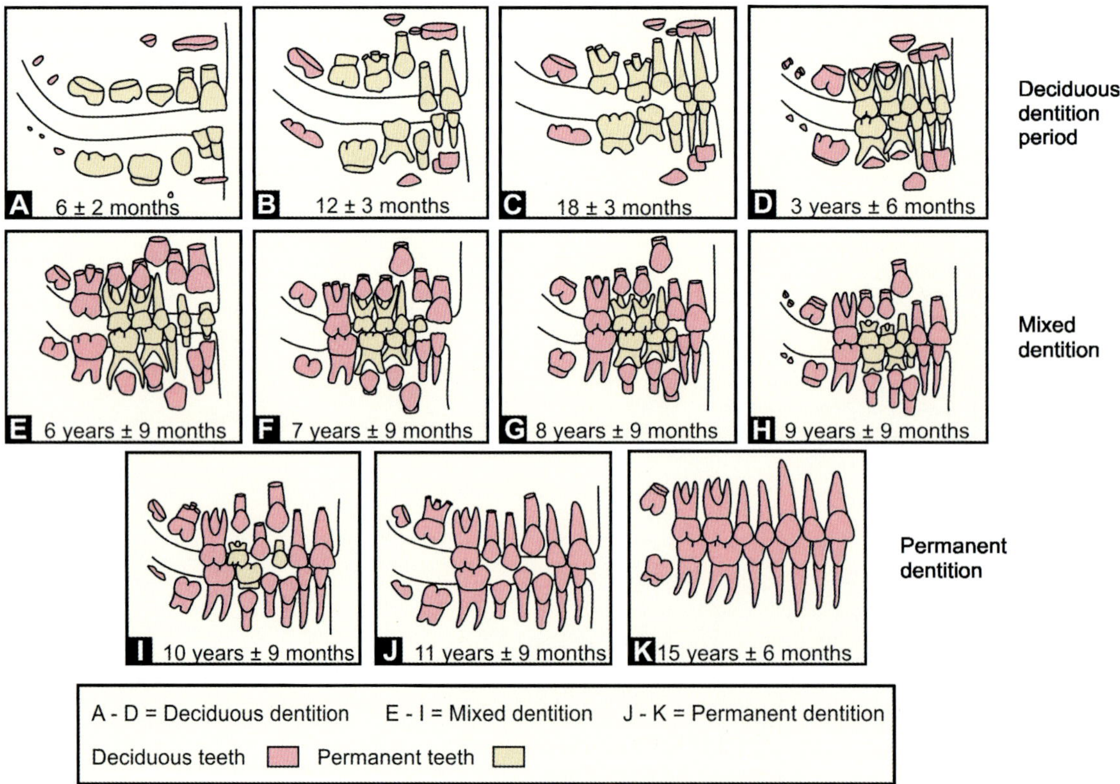

Fig. 4.24: Various developmental stages of teeth

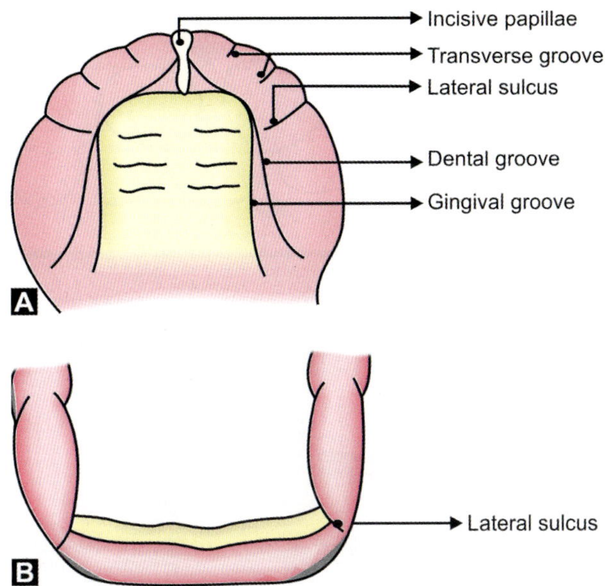

Figs 4.25A and B: (A) Upper gum pad; (B) Lower gum pad

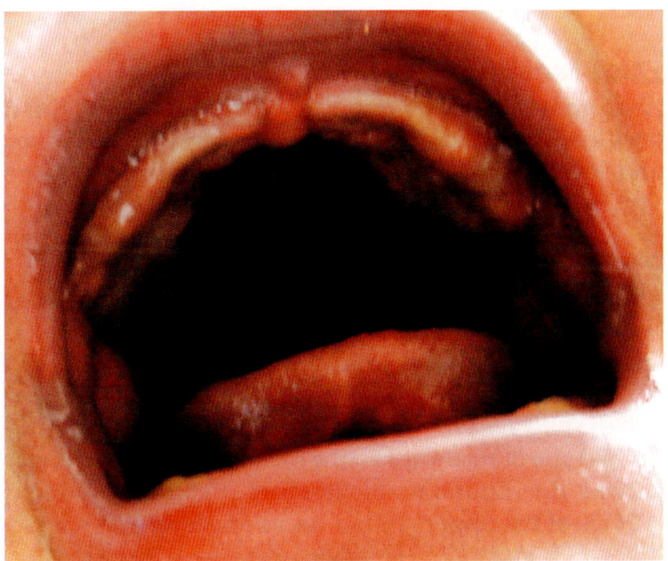

Fig. 4.26: Upper gum pad in a newborn child

portion. The two portions of the gum pads are separated from each other by a groove called the dental groove.

- The gum pads are divided into ten segments by ten grooves called transverse grooves. Each of these segments consists of one developing deciduous tooth sac.
- The transverse groove between the canine and first deciduous molar segment is called the lateral sulcus. The lateral sulci are useful in judging the interarch

relationship at a very early stage. The lateral sulcus of the mandibular arch is normally more distal to that of the maxillary arch.

- The gingival groove separates the gum pad from the palate and floor of the mouth in upper and lower arch separately.
- The upper and lower gum pads are almost similar to each other. The upper gum pad is both wider as well as longer than the mandibular gum pad. Thus when the upper and lower gum pads are approximated, there is a complete overjet all around. This space is occupied by the tongue resulting in tongue thrust (infantile tongue thrust). Contact occurs between the upper and lower gum pads in the first molar region (Fig. 4.27). The upper lateral sulcus is positioned much anteriorly to the lower lateral sulcus.

DECIDUOUS DENTITION PERIOD

Eruption Age and Sequence of Deciduous Dentition

The mandibular central incisors are the first teeth to erupt into the oral cavity. They erupt at around 6-7 months of age. A variation of 3 months from the mean age has been accepted as normal.

The sequence of eruption of the deciduous dentition is:

Central Incisor – Lateral Incisor – First Molar – Canine - Second Molar.

The primary dentition is usually established by 2½ years of age following the eruption of the second deciduous molars. Between 3-6 years of age, the dental arch is relatively stable and very few changes occur.

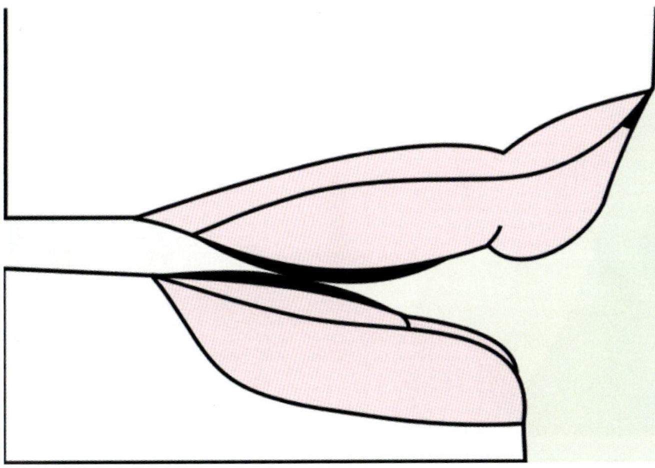

Fig. 4.27: Gum pads in occlusion

Features of Deciduous Dentition Period

1. Spacing in deciduous dentition
2. Terminal plane relation of the deciduous molars
3. Deep bite
4. The dental arches are wide U shaped
5. Flat curve of Spee
6. Shallow cuspal interdigitation
7. Incisors are more vertically placed

Spacing in Deciduous Dentition (Fig. 4.28)

Spacing normally exists between the deciduous teeth. These spaces are called physiological spaces or developmental spaces. The presence of spaces in the primary dentition is important for the normal development of the permanent dentition and absence of spaces in the primary dentition is an indication that crowding of teeth may occur when the larger permanent teeth erupt.

Spacing seen mesial to the maxillary canines and distal to the mandibular canines are wider than in other areas. These physiological spaces are called Primate spaces or Simian spaces or Anthropoid spaces as they are seen commonly in primates (Figs 4.29A and B). These spaces help in placement of the canine cusps of the opposing arch.

Terminal Plane Relation of the Deciduous Molars (Figs 4.30A to C)

The mesiodistal relation between the distal surfaces of the upper and lower second deciduous molars is called the terminal plane. They can be of three types as given by Baume:

A: Flush Terminal Plane (37%)
B: Mesial Step Terminal Plane (49%)
C: Distal Step Terminal Plane (14%)

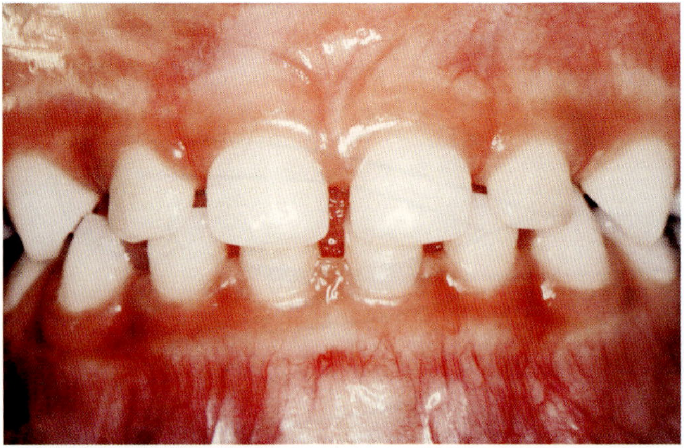

Fig. 4.28: Generalized spacing seen in deciduous dentition

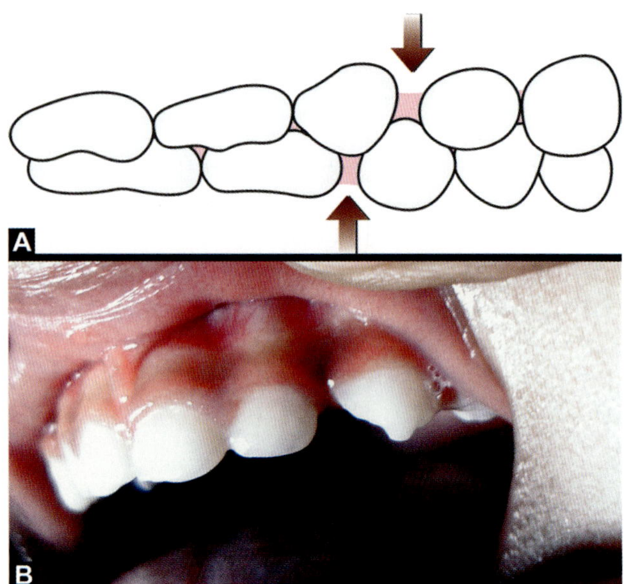

Figs 4.29A and B: Primate space: (A) Diagrammatic representation of the primate space; (B) Primate space in a 2-year-old child seen between deciduous upper lateral incisor and canine

Flush Terminal Plane

A normal feature of deciduous dentition is a flush terminal plane where the distal surfaces of the upper and lower second deciduous molars are in the same vertical plane.

Mesial Step Terminal Plane

In this type of relationship the distal surface of the lower second deciduous molar is more mesial to the distal surface of the upper second deciduous molar.

Distal Step Terminal Plane

In this type of relationship the distal surface of the lower second deciduous molar is more distal to the distal surface of the upper second deciduous molar.

Deep Bite (Fig. 4.31)

A deep bite may occur in the initial stages of development. The deep bite is accentuated by the fact that the deciduous incisors are more upright than their successors. The lower incisal edges often contact the cingulum area of the maxillary incisors. This deep bite is later reduced due to the following factors:

A. Eruption of permanent posterior teeth.
B. Attrition of incisors.
C. Forward and downward movement of the mandible due to growth.

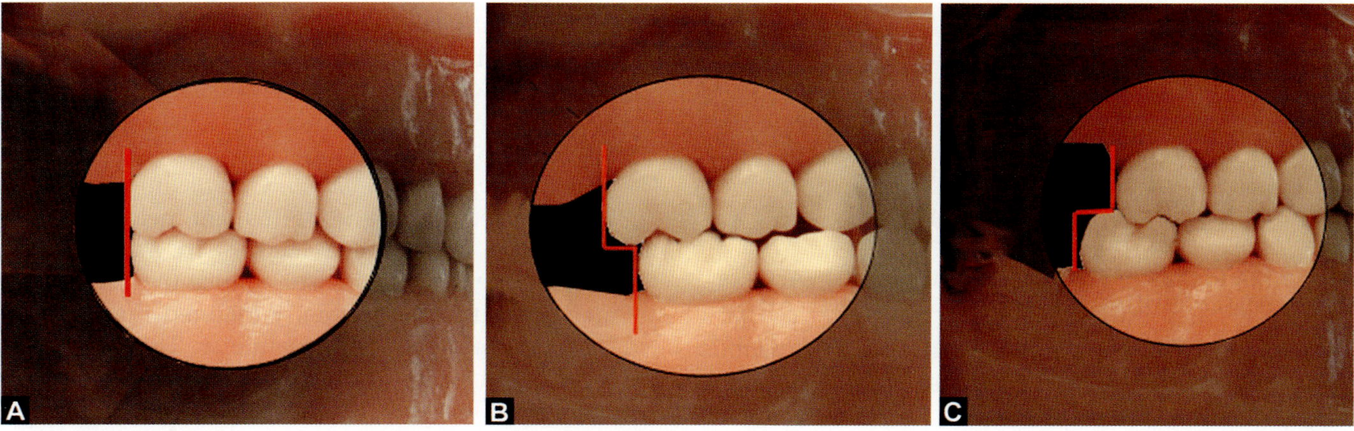

Figs 4.30A to C: Terminal plane relation of deciduous molars: (A) Flush terminal plane (37%); (B) Mesial step terminal plane (49%); (C) Distal step terminal plane (14%)

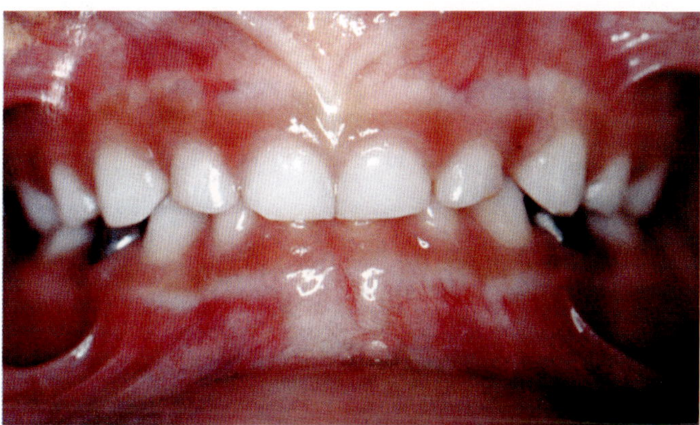

Fig. 4.31: Deep bite seen in deciduous dentition

MIXED DENTITION PERIOD

The mixed dentition period can be divided into three phases:
1. First transitional period
2. Inter transitional period
3. Second transitional period

First Transitional Period

The first transitional period is characterized by the emergence of the first permanent molars and the exchange of the deciduous incisors with the permanent incisors.

Eruption and Attainment of Occlusion of the First Permanent Molars (Figs 4.32A to C)

The mandibular first molar is the first permanent tooth to erupt at around 6 years of age. The location and relationship of the first permanent molar depends much upon the distal surface relationship between the upper and lower second deciduous molars. The first permanent molars are guided into the dental arch by the distal surface of the second deciduous molars. The deciduous molar relation determines the permanent molar relation as the later erupts into occlusion.

The shift in lower molar from the initial relation to final occlusion can occur in two ways. They are designated as the early and the late mesial shift. The forward movement of the first permanent molar utilizing the primate space is termed as early mesial shift. When the deciduous second molars exfoliate the permanent first molars drift mesially utilizing the leeway space. This occurs in the late mixed dentition period and is called late mesial shift.

Occlusion of First Permanent Molar when Deciduous Molars are in Flush Terminal Plane Relation

The erupting first permanent molars may also be in a flush or end on relationship. For the transition of such an end on molar relation to a class I molar relation, the lower molar has to move forward by about 3 – 5 min relative to the upper molar. This occurs by utilization of the primate space (Early mesial shift) and by differential forward growth of the mandible.

Early shift occurs during the early mixed dentition period. The eruptive force of the first permanent molar is sufficient to push the deciduous first and the second molars forward in the arch to erupt in class I molar relationship.

Many children lack the primate space and in this situation the erupting permanent molars are unable to move forward to establish Class I relationship. In these cases, when the deciduous second molars exfoliate, the permanent first molars drift mesially utilizing the leeway space. This occurs in the late mixed dentition period and is called late mesial shift.

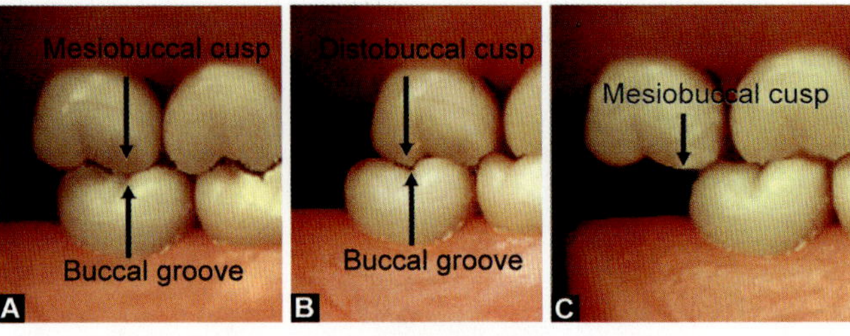

Figs 4.32A to C: Occlusion of first permanent molar: (A) Class I relation; (B) Class II relation; (C) Class III relation

Occlusion of First Permanent Molar when Deciduous Molars are in Mesial Step Terminal Plane Relation

In this type of relationship the distal surface of the lower second deciduous molar is more mesial than that of the upper. Thus the permanent molars erupt directly into Angle's class I occlusion. This type of mesial step terminal plane most commonly occurs due to early forward growth of the mandible. If the differential growth of the mandible in a forward direction persists, it can lead to an Angle's Class III molar relation. If the forward mandibular growth is minimal, it can establish a class I molar relationship.

Occlusion of First Permanent Molar when Deciduous Molars are in Distal Step Terminal Plane Relation

This is characterized by the distal surface of the lower second deciduous molar being more distal to that of the upper. Thus the erupting permanent molars may be in Angle's class II occlusion. Later the relation may shift to class I if the forward mandibular growth is extensive.

Exchange of Incisors

During the first transitional period the deciduous incisors are replaced by the permanent incisors. The mandibular central incisors are usually the first to erupt. The permanent incisors are considerably larger than the deciduous teeth they replace. This difference between the amount of space needed for the accommodation of the incisors and the amount of space available for this is called incisal liability. The incisal liability is roughly about 7 mm in the maxillary arch and about 5 mm in the mandibular arch.

Incisal Liability is Overcome by the following Factors

A. *Utilization of physiologic spaces seen in primary dentition:* The physiologic or the developmental spaces that exist in the primary dentition are utilized to partly account for the incisal liability. The permanent incisors are much more easily accommodated in normal alignment in cases exhibiting adequate interdental spaces than in an arch that has no space.

B. *Increase in inter-canine width:* An increase in inter-canine width of both the maxillary as well as the mandibular arches allows the much larger permanent incisors to be accommodated in the arch previously occupied by the deciduous incisors.

C. *Change in incisor inclination:* One of the differences between deciduous and permanent incisors is their inclination. The primary incisors are more upright than the permanent incisors. Since the permanent incisors erupt more labially inclined they tend to increase the dental arch perimeter. This is another factor that helps in accommodating the larger permanent incisors.

Inter-transitional Period

This is a relatively quite phase and no active tooth eruption is seen.

In this period the maxillary and mandibular arches consist of deciduous and permanent teeth. Between the permanent incisors and the first permanent molars are the deciduous molars and canines. This phase during the mixed dentition period is relatively stable and no change occurs.

Second Transitional Period

The second transitional period is characterized by the replacement and alignment of the deciduous molars and canines by the premolars and permanent cuspids respectively.

The features of second transitional period are:
1. Leeway space of Nance
2. Ugly duckling stage.

Leeway Space of Nance (Fig. 4.33)

The combined mesiodistal width of the permanent canines and premolars is usually less than that of the deciduous canines and molars. The surplus space is called Leeway space of Nance. The amount of leeway space is greater in the mandibular arch than in the maxillary arch. It is about 1.8 mm (0.9 mm on each side of the arch) in the maxillary arch and about 3.4 mm (1.7 mm on each side of the arch) in the mandibular arch. This excess space available after the exchange of the deciduous molars and canines is utilized for mesial drift of the mandibular molars to establish class I molar relation.

Ugly Duckling Stage (Broadbent Phenomenon) (Figs 4.34A and B)

It is a transient or self-correcting malocclusion seen in the maxillary incisor region between 8-9 years of age, seen during the eruption of the permanent canines. As

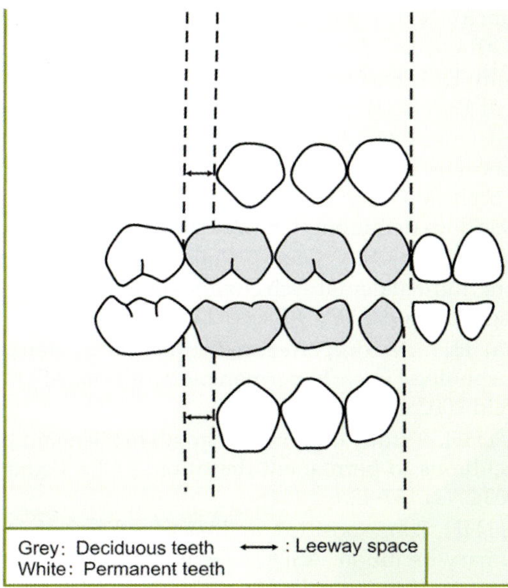

Fig. 4.33: Leeway space of Nance

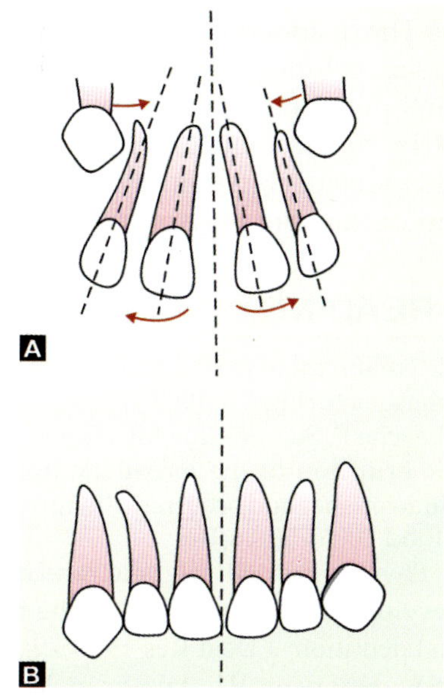

Figs 4.34A and B: Broadbent phenomenon

the developing permanent canines erupt, they displace the roots of the lateral incisors mesially. This results in transmitting of the force onto the roots of the central incisors which also get displaced mesially. A resultant distal divergence of the crowns of the incisors occurs leading to creation of diastema in the incisor region.

Broadbent named this as the ugly duckling stage as children tend to look ugly during this phase of development. Parents are often apprehensive during this stage and consult the dentist. This condition usually corrects by itself when canines erupt as the pressure is transferred from the roots to the crown of the incisors.

PERMANENT DENTITION PERIOD

The permanent dentition is complete with the eruption and alignment of the maxillary canines which is the last tooth to erupt into the oral cavity excepting the third molars.

The permanent molar relation is classified into three types, as given by Angle:

Angle's Class I: The mesiobuccal cusp of the maxillary first permanent molar occludes with the buccal groove of the mandibular first permanent molar.

Self-correcting Aromalies/Transient Malocclusion and their Correction

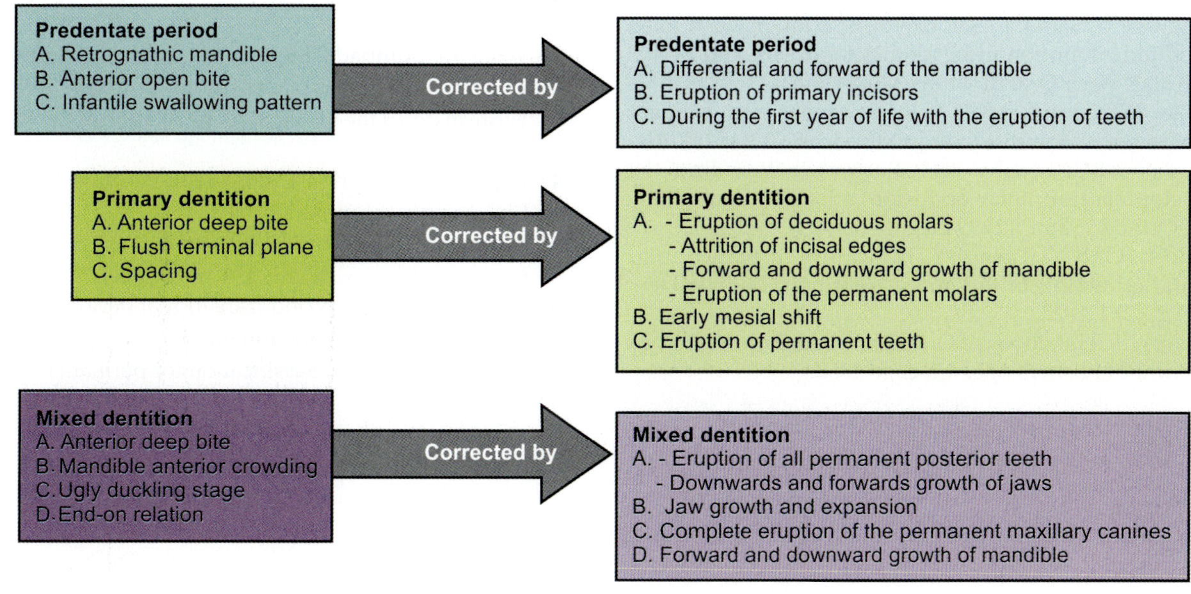

Angle's Class II: The distobuccal cusp of the maxillary first permanent molar occludes with the buccal groove of the mandibular first permanent molar.

Angle's Class III: The mesiobuccal cusp of the maxillary first permanent molar occludes in between the lower first and the second permanent molars.

FURTHER READING

1. Angle EH. Treatment of malocclusion of teeth 7th Edn. S S White Manufacturing Co. 1907.
2. Barberia-Leache E, Suarez-Clua MC, Saavedra-Ontiveros D. Ectopic eruption of the maxillary first permanent molar: characteristics and occurrence in growing children. Angle Orthod 2005;75(4):610-5.
3. Baume LJ. Physiologic tooth migration and its significance for the development of occlusion II. The biogenesis of accessional dentition. J Dent Res 1950;29:331.
4. Bishara SE, Hoppens BJ, Jakobsen JR, Kohout FJ. Changes in the molar relationship between the deciduous and permanent dentitions: a longitudinal study. Am J Orthod Dentofacial Orthop 1988;93(1):19-28.
5. Bishara SE, Jakobsen JR, Treder JE, Stasi MJ. Changes in the maxillary and mandibular tooth size-arch length relationship from early adolescence to early adulthood. A longitudinal study. Am J Orthod Dentofacial Orthop 1989;95(1):46-59.
6. Bishara SE, Jakobsen JR. Individual variation in tooth-size/ arch-length changes from the primary to permanent dentitions. World J Orthod 2006 Summer;7(2):145-53.
7. Bishara SE, Khadivi P, Jakobsen JR. Changes in tooth size-arch length relationships from the deciduous to the permanent dentition: a longitudinal study. Am J Orthod Dentofacial Orthop 1995;108(6):607-13.
8. Clinch L. Variations in the mutual relationship of the upper and lower gum pads in the newborn child. Trans Br Soc Study Orthod 1932;91-107.
9. El-Nofely A, Sadek L, Soliman N. Spacing in the human deciduous dentition in relation to tooth size and dental arch size. Arch Oral Biol 1989;34(6):437-41.
10. Foster TD, Grundy MC. Occlusal changes from primary to permanent dentitions. Br J Orthod 1986;13(4):187-93.
11. Leighton BC, Feasby WH. Factors influencing the development of molar occlusion: a longitudinal study. Br J Orthod 1988;15(2):99-103. Review.
12. Melo L, Ono Y, Takagi Y. Indicators of mandibular dental crowding in the mixed dentition. Pediatr Dent 2001;23(2):118-22.
13. Moyers RE. Handbook of Ordodontics 4th Edn. Year Book Medical Publishers, Inc. Chicago 1988.
14. Nance HN. The limitations of orthodontic treatment. Am J. Orthod 1947;33:177, 253.
15. Ranly DM. Early orofacial development. J Clin Pediatr Dent 1998;22(4):267-75. Review.
16. Rodrigues CH, Mori M, Rodrigues AA, Nascimento EJ, Goncalves FM, Santana KC. Distribution of different types of occlusal contacts at maximal intercuspal position in deciduous dentition. J Clin Pediatr Dent 2003;27(4):339-46.
17. Slaj M, Jezina MA, Lauc T, Rajic-Mestrovic S, Miksic M. Longitudinal dental arch changes in the mixed dentition. Angle Orthod 2003;73(5):509-14.
18. Tsai HH. A computerized analysis of dental arch morphology in early permanent dentition. ASDC J Dent Child 2002;69(3):259-65, 234.
19. Tsai HH. A study of growth changes in the mandible from deciduous to permanent dentition. J Clin Pediatr Dent 2003;27(2):137-42.
20. Tsai HH. Tooth-position, arch-size, and arch-shape in the primary dentition. ASDC J Dent Child 2001;68(1):17-22, 10.
21. Warren JJ, Bishara SE, Yonezu T. Tooth size-arch length relationships in the deciduous dentition: a comparison between contemporary and historical samples. Am J Orthod Dentofacial Orthop 2003;123(6):614-9.
22. West CM. The development of the gums and their relationship to the deciduous teeth in the human fetus. Contrib Embryol 1925;16:25.
23. White TC, Gardiner HJ, Leighton BC. Orthodontics for dental students, 3rd Ed. Mac Millan India Ltd. 1996.
24. White TC, Gardiner HJ, Leighton BC. Orthodontics for dental students, 3rd Ed. Mac Millan India Ltd. 1996.
25. Zuccati G, Ghobadlu J, Nieri M, Clauser C. Factors associated with the duration of forced eruption of impacted maxillary canines: a retrospective study. Am J Orthod Dentofacial Orthop 2006;130(3):349-56.

QUESTIONS

1. What are gumpads. Explain the features of gumpads?
2. Explain the features of deciduous dentition period.
3. Write in detail the terminal plane relation of the deciduous molars.
4. Explain the eruption and attainment of occlusion of the first permanent molars.
5. What is incisal liability and explain the methods of its overcome?
6. What is first and second transitional period?
7. What is broadbent phenomenon?
8. Explain the Angles classification for permanent dentition.

Behavior Guidance in Dental Practice

INTRODUCTION

One of the most important aspects of treating a child patient is the management of the behavior. Without the child's cooperation, dental treatment becomes difficult if not impossible. Most of the children enter the dental clinic with some kind of fear and anxiety which is usually transferred to them from parents, relatives, friends or it may be just an imagination.

The process of modifying a child's behavior was termed 'Behavior Management'. But this was modified by American Academy of Pediatric Dentistry (AAPD) as 'Behavior Guidance'. The main aim of this concept was to improve communication and partner with the child and the parent towards a positive attitude and providing good oral health.[1]

DEFINITION[2,3]

Behavior pedodontics: Defined as a 'discipline which focuses upon the psychological, social and learning problems of children and adolescents as they relate to the dental situations'.

Behavior: 'As any change in the functioning of an organism.'

Behavior guidance: Means by which the dental health team effectively and efficiently performs treatment for a child and at the same, installs a positive dental attitude.

Behavior shaping: It is that procedure which very slowly develops behavior by reinforcing successive approximations of the desired behavior until the desired behavior comes to be. It is sometimes called as 'Stimulus-response theory.'

Fear: Physiopsychological response to a realistic threat or danger to one's existence.

Anxiety: Fear of the unknown

Phobia: 'Pathological fear, attached to a certain stimulus learned in his career'. It is deep seated and is provoked by any stimulus which resembles the original episode.

EMOTIONAL DEVELOPMENT

Characteristics of Commonly Seen Emotions in a Child[3,4]

Distress or Cry

Cry during childhood is a primary emotion expressed due to hunger, dislike to specific environment, etc. School going children are under social pressure and hence cry for reasons such as trauma, etc. Young adults do not express emotions with loud cry, but may cry in private without exhibition.

Different types of cry are:

a. **Obstinate cry:** It is characterized by loud high pitched cry. It may be associated with kicking and biting.

b. **Frightened cry:** It is characterized by deep sobbing and tears rolling down. The child is willing to cooperate but the cry is due to the fear of the unknown.

c. **Hurt cry:** It is a low volume cry with small whimpers in between. The child may hold his breath and tightens his body in anticipation of pain.

d. **Compensatory cry:** It is a slow monotonous sound made without any tears or sobbing. Such children usually cooperate with the treatment.

ANGER

A child may be upset for reasons relating to dentistry, home or even school. These emotions may be expressed as anger. Physical expression of anger may vary from throwing objects, attacks, kicking, running violently or even shouting loudly.

FEAR

According to Sidney Finn, fear is a primary emotion for survival against danger, which is acquired soon after birth. Most of the time parents instill the fear of dentistry in their children as a means of punishment. Fear should be channeled in the correct direction such as those that causes harm to the child's existence or well being. Children should be taught that dental office is not a place to fear, and the parents should never employ dentistry as threat.

Types of Fear

Objective Fear

They are produced by direct physical stimulation. They are the responses to stimuli that are felt, seen, heard, smelt or tasted and are not liked or accepted.

Objective fear of dentistry usually is the result of previous improper dental handling. They fear white uniforms and smell of certain drugs and chemicals in hospital. It is the responsibility of the dentist to change the fear by tender loving care and gaining confidence.

Subjective Fear

Most of the children would not have visited a dental clinic before, but are afraid of the dental procedures. These are based on the feelings and attitudes that have been suggested to the child by others about dentistry without the child having had the experience personally. Parents may tell the child about an unpleasant or pain producing situation undergone by them and this fear may be retained in the child's mind.

Subjective fear are of 2 types: Suggestive and imaginative.

Suggestive fear: It may be acquired by observing or imitating fear and then the child develops a fear for the same object as real and genuine. Child's anxiety is closely correlated with parental anxiety. Children frequently identify themselves with parents. If the parent is sad the child feels sad and if the parent displays fear the child is fearful.

Imaginative fear: A mother who fears going to the dentist may transmit this unconsciously to her child who is observing her. Such kind of fear may be displayed by the parent and acquired by the child without either being aware of it and are deep seated and difficult to eradicate. Even a clenching of the child's hand in the dental office in an unconscious gesture can create suspicion and fear in the child.

A fearful child matures to become a fearful parent and a fearful parent produces a fearful child leading to a viscous cycle.

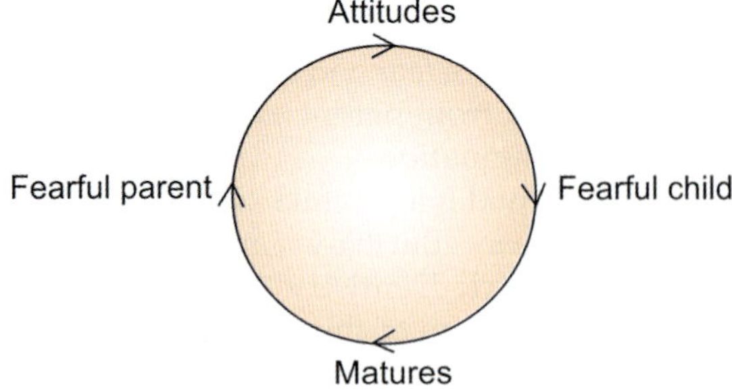

Nature and Value of Fear

The emotional stimulus is released or discharged by way of the automatic nervous system through hypothalamus, which is modified by cortical interference, so that man can control his emotions. In young children who cannot rationalize, behavior is produced which is difficult to control. As a child's mental age increases these responses can be controlled more and more by the cortex through higher psychic functions.

Fear is of great value, when it is given the right direction. Fear helps people to be prepared against danger. It should be channeled in the direction of real danger and in this way, it will act as a protective mechanism against real danger. Since dentistry or dental procedures are not threat, dentistry should never be used as a threat to children.

Anxiety

It is same as fear but without the known reasons or fear of the unknown.

Phobia

It is an extreme irrational fear, defined as a persistent, excessive, unreasonable fear of a specific object, activity or situation that results in a compelling desire to avoid the dreaded object.

ADAPTIVE CHANGES SEEN IN CHILDREN AT DIFFERENT STAGES OF DEVELOPMENT[3,5]

The expression and intensity of child's fear varies with emotions, illness and age. The sleepy child shows more fear and irritation than the widely awake child, because he has a lower tolerance to discomfort. A physically healthy child will respond more actively than the child who is weak and medically handicapped. A mentally alert child will respond more intelligently and rapidly than the mentally retarded individual.

Birth to 1 Year

This is the beginning of adaptation with the caregiver and environment. If there is any trouble in this, it may lead to problems in adaptation and interaction. Cognitive development begins with sensorimotor changes.

1–3 Years

Motor skills develop during this stage. Communication and language improve. Temper tantrums begin at this age. Children are less afraid of strangers and it is thus the right time to introduce the child to dentistry. At this age they are less afraid of the new people and the surrounding. This is also the appropriate time to begin any preventive procedures.

3–6 Years

Fear of separation and abandonment prevails in this age group. They think and feel that dentistry is a mode of punishment. Children of this age group benefit by the presence of parents in the operatory during dental treatment, particularly those less than 4 years. Children over 4 years of age begin to adapt and show no difference in behavior whether the mother was present or absent from the operatory.

The decrease in the fear may be due to:
* Realization that there is nothing to fear
* Social pressure to conceal fear
* Social limitation
* Adult guidance

During this period fantasy plays a role, and gains comfort and the courage to meet the real situation.

Intelligent children display more fear because of their greater awareness of danger and reluctance to accept verbal assurance.

6–12 Years

Children of this age group are very social. They are peer oriented and have their own groups in school. Achievement in school influences his self-esteem. Children with low self-esteem show behavior problems in dental clinic. Children learn faster during this age. They can reason and convey to the dentist when pain is being inflicted by gesture. They try to resolve real fears. Family support is important in understanding and overcoming his fears.

>12 Years

Adolescent period is characterized by uneven biologic, psycholoic and social development. They learn to tolerate unpleasant situation and have marked desire to be obedient. They develope considerable emotional control. They become concerned about their appearance. The dentist as motivation for seeking dental attention, can use this interest in cosmetic effect.

Methods to Deal with an Emotionally Upset Child

1. Understand the reason why the child is emotionally upset
2. Ignore inappropriate behavior that can be tolerated
3. Comment on the child's behavior when it is good.
4. Provide physical outlets and exercise, both at home and at school.
5. Take an interest in the child's activities. A child can be given activities that he/she enjoys. They should be appreciated for their effort.
6. Use humor. Jokes can often defuse most of the angry child.
7. Instill discipline. It includes setting limits, but being flexible when needed.
8. Choose the appropriate behavior guidance method

FACTORS INFLUENCING CHILD'S BEHAVIOR[6-9] (FIG. 5.1)

1. Factors involving the child
   A. Growth and development
   B. IQ of the child
   C. Past dental experience
   D. Social and adaptive skill
   E. Position of the child in the family
2. Factors involving the parents
   A. Family influence
   B. Parent-child relationship
   C. Maternal anxiety
   D. Attitude of parents to dentistry
3. Factors involving the dentist
   A. Appearance of the dental office
   B. Personality of the dentist
   C. Time and length of appointment
   D. Dentist's skill and speed
   E. Use of fear promoting words
   F. Use of subtle, flattery, praise and reward.

Factors Involving the Child

Growth and Development

Growth is defined as an increase in size, whereas the development is progression towards maturity. Both proceed in a relatively predictable logical step like sequential order. These processes are influenced by genetic, familial, cultural, interpersonal and psychic factors.

Most children demonstrate emotional maturation along with physical growth. During maturation the

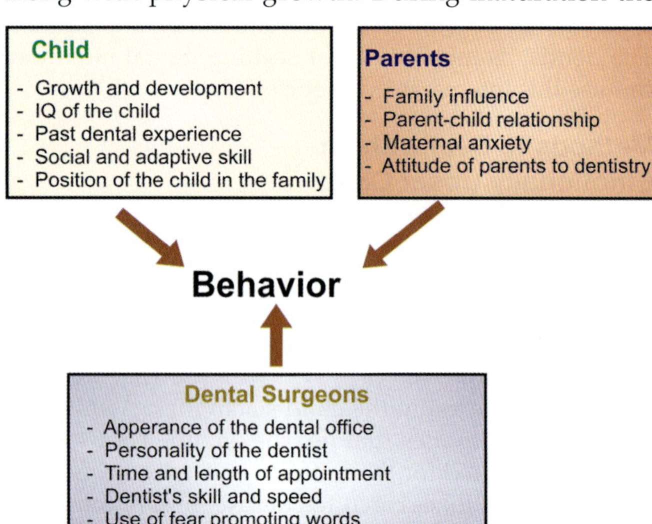

Fig. 5.1: Factors influencing child behavior

child's behavior is systematically affected by the inherent genetic makeup. With each new experience, a new behavior develops as directed by the child's internal system from his motivation and from the consequences of his behavior. Therefore parameters that influence behavior depends upon the biologic, cognitive, emotional, perceptual, personality, social and language development.

IQ of the Child

Intelligent quotient (IQ) is the method of quantifying the mental ability in relation to chronological age formulated by Alfred Binet in the early 1900's.

$$\text{Formula: IQ} = \frac{\text{Mental age}}{\text{Chronological age}} \times 100$$

It is measured by tasks, examining memory, spatial relationship, reasoning, etc. There are several other tests—For example, Wechsier preschool and primary scale of intelligence (WPPSI), Wechsier intelligence scale for children revised (WISC-R), etc.

Positive relationship exists between IQ and acceptance of dental treatment.

Past Dental Experience

A child entering the clinics may be either totally new to the dental experience or may have had an unhappy previous dental experience. Care has to be taken to make the first impression the best and acceptable experience for the child who is experiencing dental treatment for the first time. At the same time the child who already has previous painful experience needs to be reassured that things will be different now and thus retraining is required before one can accept a tolerable behavior.

Social and Adaptive Skill

An important aspect of the overall functioning is the level of the child's social and adaptive skills. It is important to consider how effective the child is in meeting the standards for personal independence and social responsibility in everyday situations.

It is very easy to communicate and manage a child who adapts and is friendly with the clinic staff. A child who is very introvert and socially not adjustable requires more than the routine behavior management techniques.

Postion of the Child in the Family and Child's Behavior (Ordinal—Position Syndrome)

1. First child: Uncertainty, mistrustfulness, insecurity, shrewdness, stinginess, dependence, responsibility, authoritarianism, jealousy, sensitive.

2. Second child: Independence, aggressive, extrovert, funloving, adventuresome
3. Middle child: Aggressiveness, easily distracted, inferiority and prone for behavior disorders.
4. Last child: Secure, confident, immature, envy, irresponsible, spontaneous good and bad behavior.

Factors Involving the Parents

Family Influence

The environment at home is an important factor in the development of a child's personality and his behavior patterns. Socioeconomic status of parents influences the behavior of the child and the way parents deal with the behavior. It is found that parents belonging to low socioeconomic status show authorization in controlling the child than middle and high-income group.

Mother's nutritional status and state of physical health can affect the neurologic as well as somatic development of the fetus which directly influences the children's mental, physical and emotional development.

Bell has termed the parent-child relationship as "one tailed", since parental characteristics are viewed as having a unilateral influences on those developing in the child. According to this theory, the child's characteristics including the personality, behavior and reaction to stressful situation are the direct product of various maternal characteristics. It was found that loving mothers tend to have calm, happy children, while hostile mothers tend to have children who are excitable and unhappy.

Parent-Child Relationship

Most of the relevant mother-child relationship falls into two broad categories:
1. Autonomy vs control
2. Hostility vs love

Maternal attitudes and behavior have been described and rated in relation to these two categories.

Mothers who allowed autonomy and who expressed affection had children who were friendly and cooperative. Conversely, punitive or depressed mothers and those who ignored their children did not exhibit these positive behavioral characteristics. Friendly, cooperative child will probably also exhibit these traits in the dental office.

Characteristics of parent child relationship that may influence child's behavior in dental clinic are:
1. Over-protective/over-anxious parents
2. Over indulgence
3. Under affection and rejection
4. Domination
5. Identification
6. Authoritarian

Over-protective/Over-anxious Parents

Factors responsible for maternal over protection may be:
- History of previous miscarriage
- Long delay in conception
- Family's financial condition
- Death of a sibling
- If mother is aware that she cannot have another child
- Serious illness or handicapped condition
- Parental absence by divorce or death.

Characteristics of the over-protective child
- Parents show undue concern for the child
- Child is always made to feel babyish
- The child is not permitted to play alone
- They are usually shy, timid and fearful
- Lack ability to make decisions
- Cooperative dental patients.

Over indulgence: The parents give the child whatever the child asks like toys, candies, etc. and they usually place very little restraint upon their child's behavior.

Characteristics of the over indulged child
- Spoiled child who is accustomed to getting his own way.
- His emotional development is impeded and he is aggressive, demanding and displays temper tantrums.
- In the dental office, when they cannot control the situation they may show bursts of temper.

Under affection and rejection: The extent of neglect may vary from mild detachment to total neglect.

Characteristics the child suffering from under affection and rejection
- The children appear well behaved.
- They usually develop resentment and become completely withdrawn to a shell.
- There is lack of love and affection and the child usually lacks a feeling of belonging or worthiness.
- Some children may show anxiety, cry easily and will resort to any behavior to attract attention. Such children are usually demanding.

Domination: Parents with this attitude demand from their children excessive responsibility, which is incompatible with their chronological age. They cannot accept the child as he is, but compare him with others.

Characteristics of the child having dominating parents
- Associated with resentment, evasion, submission and restlessness.
- They are fearful of resisting openly and will obey commands slowly. With kindness and consideration they generally develop into good dental patients.

Identification: Some parents try to relive their own lives in those of their children. They attempt to give the child every advantage denied to them. If the child does not respond favorably, the parent shows disappointment and the child has a feeling of guilt.

Characteristics of the child:
- The child cries easily and lacks confidence.
- These children should be handled kindly and with consideration.

Authoritarian: Such parents choose non-love-oriented techniques for controlling child behavior. Discipline takes the form of physical punishment or verbal ridicule. The mother feels that the child should follow her set of ideas.

Characteristics of the child with authoritative parents
- The response of the child will be submission, coupled with resentment and evasion.

Maternal Anxiety

Highly anxious parents tend to affect their child's behavior negatively. Children under the age of 4 years are affected greatly by mothers anxiety.

Attitude of Parents to Dentistry

Parents with positive dental attitude will develop the same in the child. Whereas a fearful parent may develop fear unknowingly in a child.

Factors Involving the Dentist

Appearance of the Dental Office

Since the child may enter the dental office with some fear, the first objective of the dentist is to put the child at ease. To achieve this, the reception room should be made as comfortable and warm as possible (Fig. 5.2A).

Children's chairs and tables with a small lamp and shade should be made available where they can sit and read. Small toys can be kept in the room to amuse very young child. A music player with chosen music helps to comfort the frightened child. An aquarium with colored fishes can be placed in one corner of the room. Cartoon characters can be hung on the wall. The assistant can make animals out of cotton wool, which can prove very amusing to children. Puzzles and story books suitable for different age group should be placed on a neat and attractive rack.

Try to avoid children seeing adults in pain. They can be made to leave the clinic through another door. It is important that the office assistant, receptionist and the dental hygienist also show enthusiasm, as the children are extremely sensitive to hidden emotions.

Personality of the Dentist

The approach of the dentist should be casual, confident and friendly towards the child (Fig. 5.2B). The dentist must be in command of the situation and modify any behavior that interferes with the dental treatment. The dental surgeon should never loose his temper as this will create a feeling of success in the mind of the child and will ruin the child for all future dental visits.

When approaching a new child patient, always call him by his or her nick name or at least the first name. All conversation should be directed towards him. Do not talk in a loud voice or shake hands vigorously. Approach the child with confidence in your voice.

The dentist's conversation must be directed to the subject of interest to the child and never underestimate the intelligence of the child.

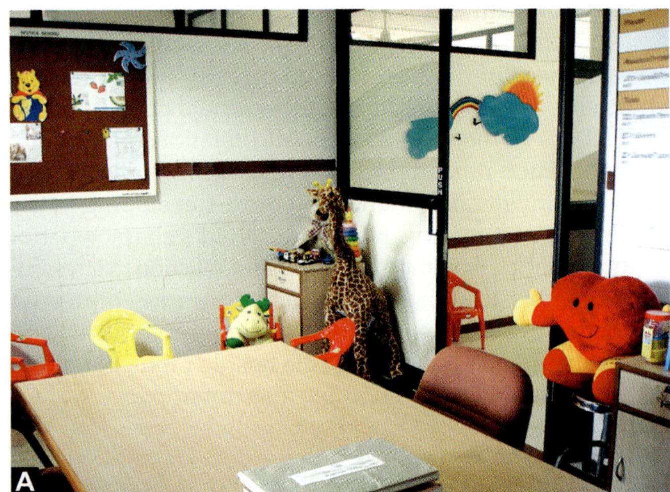

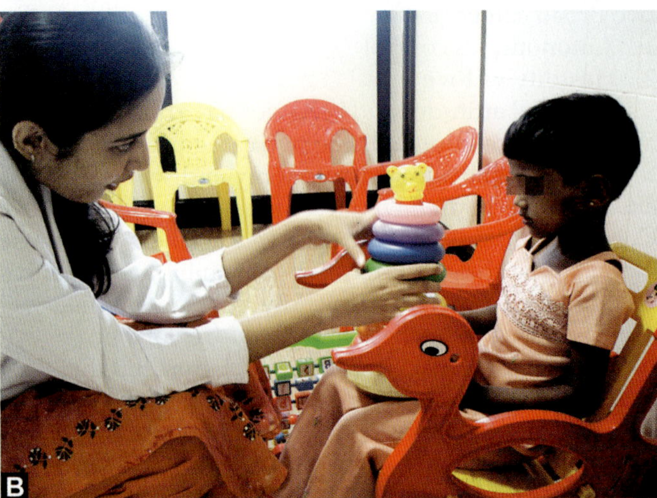

Figs 5.2A and B: (A) Colorful atmosphere of the reception eases the child's fear; (B) Doctors should be friendly and playful to make the child at ease

The dentist can help the child to display good behavior by:

- Gaining the confidence of the child that we are there to help.
- Permitting children to express their feeling and being a good listener onself.
- Making children feel that their reactions are understood.
- Comforting children when it is appropriate.
- Encouraging children when they show acceptable behavior.

Time and Length of Appointment

When dealing with children both the time and the length of appointment are important. Children cannot sit in one position for longer time and their threshold of tolerance is very low. Therefore they should not be kept in the chair for periods longer than half an hour. With longer appointment they tend to become less cooperative. Once a child looses his self-composure his cooperation is very difficult to regain.

Children should not be given appointment during their naptime or soon after some emotional experience such as birth of a sibling or death of some one close. At these times, cooperation may be difficult to secure and emotional difficulties are likely to be encountered.

Dentist's Skill and Speed

The dentist should perform his duties with dexterity, in a preplanned manner to avoid any loss of time. A child can endure discomfort if he knows it is soon going to end.

Avoiding the use of Fear Promoting Words[10]

The use of fear promoting words such as needle, injections, etc should be avoided. The words that can be used alternatively are called as euphemisms.

For example:	Euphemisms	Actual word
	Mosquito bite	needle prick
	Rain coat	rubber dam
	Tooth button	rubber dam clamp
	Coat rack	rubber dam frame
	Tooth paint	sealant
	Cavity fighter	fluoride
	Wind gun	air syringe
	Vacuum cleaner	suction
	Pudding	alginate
	Motor cycle	hand piece/bur

Use of Subtle, Flattery, Praise and Reward

One of the most important rewards sought by the child is the approval of the dentist. In praising a child, it is better to praise the behavior than the individual. Tiny gifts such as alphabet erasers, tiny gold stars, toys or stickers make good gifts. It is the recognition more than the material that makes the child happy. Flattery can also be used as a reward after the treatment. It can be a pat on the back, praise or a gift (Fig. 5.3).

PARENT COUNSELING

Parent education is very important to get a satisfactory rapport between the entire family and the dentist. Some points to be discussed are as follows:

- Parents should not voice their own personal fears in front of the child.
- Parents should never use dentistry as a threat or punishment.
- The parents should familiarize their child with dentistry by taking the child to the dentist along with sibling or themselves
- Parents should themselves be bold and display courage in dental clinic
- Importance of parental attitude and home environment in building confidence in a child.
- Regular dental care helps in preventing dental disease and also helps in the development of positive attitude towards dentistry.
- Discourage parents from bribing their children.
- The parent should be instructed never to scold, shame or ridicule to overcome the fear of dental treatment.
- Outsiders like friends or relatives should be discouraged from exhibiting their fear in front of the child.
- The parent should not promise the child what the dentist is not going to do. Lying only leads to disappointment and mistrust.
- Several days before the appointment, the parent should be instructed to convey to the child in a

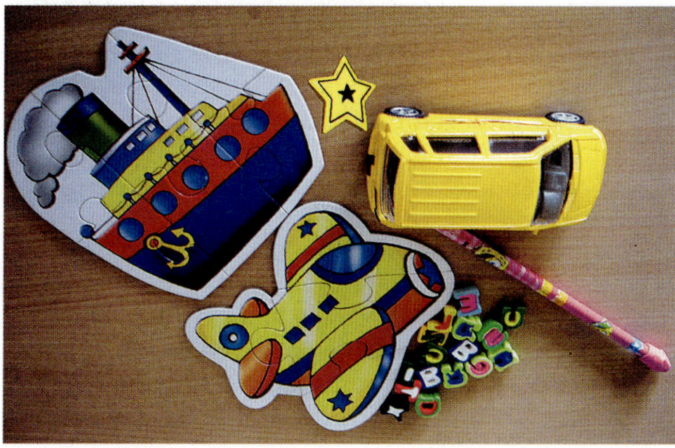

Fig. 5.3: Type of gifts that can be given to children

casual manner that they have been invited to visit the dentist.

CHILD-PARENT SEPARATION

The presence or absence of the parent sometimes can be used to gain cooperation for treatment. There are different opinions for the parental presence/absence during a treatment procedure. Some prefer their presence as the parent may assist in behavior management. On the contrary, parental presence may hinder communication between the dental surgeon and the patient if the parent is interfering. Some children behave well in the absence of their parents but it may be untrue if the child is very young as the child may prefer parental presence. For the clinician it may work both the ways and help to gain the patient's attention and improve compliance, avert negative or avoidance behaviors, establish appropriate dentist-child roles, enhance effective communication among the dentist, child, and parent and minimize anxiety and achieve a positive dental experience.[11]

The advantage of not allowing the parents in the operatory are:

1. Parents often repeat order, creating an annoyance for both dentist and child patient.
2. The parents inject orders which become a barrier to development of rapport between the dentist and child.
3. The dentist is unable to use voice control in the presence of the parent because the parent may be offended.
4. The child's attention is divided between parent and the dentist.
5. The dentist's attention is divided between parent and the child.

The advantage of allowing the parents in the operatory are:

1. A parent can be a major asset in supporting and communicating with the child, such as a handicapped child.
2. Another important exception is related to the age factor. Children below 2-3 years find it difficult to express and reach proper communication with the dentist and vice-versa.
3. Young children are prone to a number of fears, including fear of the unknown and of abandonment. They also lack the ability to adjust to a new situation or environment. The mother's presence can serve to reduce the fears of the young child and can offer emotional support during this experience.

CLASSIFICATION OF CHILDREN'S BEHAVIOR[12]

Wright's Classification of Behavior (1975)[12]

Cooperative Behavior

- Reasonably relaxed, have minimal apprehension and can be treated by a straight forward behavior shaping approach.
- Have or develop good rapport with the dentist and are interested in the dental procedure.
- Laugh and enjoy the situation.
- Allow the dentist to function effectively and efficiently.

Lacking Cooperative Behavior

- This behavior is contrast to cooperative child
- Includes very young child (<2½) or with specific debilitating or handicapping conditions
- They can pose major behavioral problems.

Potentially Cooperative Behavior

- Differs from a child lacking cooperative ability in that this child is able to cooperate and is physically and medically fit.
- When classified as potentially cooperative, the judgement is that the child's behavior can be modified. This group of children are the one who require behavioral modification procedures.
- Potentially cooperative group are further cate-gorized as follows:

Uncontrolled behavior

- Seen in 3-6 years.
- Tantrum may begin in the reception area or even before.
- This behavior is also called as 'incorrigible'.
- Tears, loud crying, physical lashing out and flailing of the hands and legs—all suggestive of a state of acute anxiety or fear.
- School aged children tend to model their behavior after that of adults.
- If it occurs in older children, there may probably be deep rooted reasons for it.

Defiant behavior

- Can be found in all ages, more typical in the elementary school group.
- Distinguished by "I don't want to" or "I don't have to" or "I wont".
- They protest when they are brought to the dental clinic against their will, as they do at home.

- Also referred to as "stubborn" or "spoilt."
- Once won over, these children frequently become highly cooperative.

Timid behavior

- Milder but highly anxious.
- If they are managed incorrectly, their behavior can deteriorate to uncontrolled.
- May shield behind the parent.
- Fail to offer great physical resistance to the separation.
- May wimper, but do not cry hysterically.
- May be from an overprotective home environment or may live in an isolated area having little contact with strangers.
- Needs to gain self-confidence of the child.

Tense cooperative behavior

- Border line behavior
- Accept treatment, but are extremely tense
- Tremor may be heard, when they speak
- Perspire noticeably

Whining behavior

- They do not prevent treatment, but whine through-out the procedure
- Cry is controlled, constant and not loud
- Seldom are there tears
- These reactions are at times frustrating and irritating to the dental team
- Great patience is required while treating such children.

Frankl's Behavior Rating Scale (1962)[11]

A. Rating No. 1
  - Definitely negative
    - Refuses treatment
    - Immature, uncontrollable
    - Defiant behavior
    - Crying forcefully
B. Rating No. 2
  - Negative
    - Reluctance to accept treatment
    - Immature, timid and whining
C. Rating No. 3
  - Positive
  - Accepts treatment
    - Tense cooperative
    - Whining and timid
D. Rating No. 4
  - Definitely positive
    - Good rapport,
    - Understanding and interested

Wright (1975)[12] Added Symbolic Modifications

Wright (1975)[12] added symbolic modifications to the Frankl's rating scale and made it more applicable and easier to understand child behavior

Rating no. 1 – definitely negative   (- -)
Rating no. 2 – negative   (-)
Rating no. 3 – positive   (+)
Rating no. 4 – definitely positive   (++)

Lampshire's Classification[6]

A. *Cooperative:* The child is physically and emotionally relaxed and is cooperative throughout the entire procedure.
B. *Tense cooperative:* The child is tensed, and cooperative at the same time.
C. *Outwardly apprehensive:* Avoids treatment initially, usually hides behind the mother, avoids looking or talking to the dentist. Eventually accepts dental treatment.
D. *Fearful:* Requires considerable support so as to overcome the fears of dental treatment.
E. *Stubborn/Defiant:* Passively resists treatment by using techniques that have been successful in other situations.
F. *Hypermotive:* The child is acutely agitated and resorts to screaming kicking, etc.
G. *Handicapped:* Physical or mental.
H. *Emotionally immature:* Emotionally handicapped.

Kopel's Classification (1959)[6]

- Very young patient
- Emotionally disturbed patient, such as:
  - Child from a broken or poor family
  - Pampered or spoiled child
  - Neurotic child
  - Excessively fearful child
  - Hyperactive child
- Physically handicapped child
- Mentally handicapped child
- Child with previous untoward medical or dental experience.

BEHAVIOR GUIDANCE

According to American Academy of Pediatric Dentistry (AAPD)[1] behavior guidance is based on scientific principles requiring skills in communication, empathy, coaching, and listening.

The goals of behavior guidance are to establish communication, alleviate fear and anxiety, deliver quality dental care, build a trusting relationship between dentist and child, and promote the child's positive attitude toward oral/dental health and oral healthcare.

Principles of behavior management technique is as following:

1. **Anticipation:** Explaining the child regarding the procedure and answering the question regarding dentistry and procedures. This can be done through tell show do approach, good communication, etc.
2. **Diversion:** Diverting the child's attention away from fear producing situation may calm the child and allow the dentist to perform the treatment without disturbance. Audioanalgesia, Hypnodontics, etc.
3. **Substitution:** It involves substituting unwanted behavior by an accepted behavior. This can be done by contingency management, modeling, etc.
4. **Restriction:** Restricting a child from exhibiting unwanted behavior. This can be achieved through physical restrains or pharmacological behavior management technique.

Objectives of Behavior Guidance

1. To establish effective communication with the child and the parent
2. To gain the confidence of both the child and the parent and the acceptance of dental treatment
3. To teach the child and the parent, the positive aspects of preventive dental care
4. To provide a relaxing and comfortable environment for the dental team to work in, while treating the child.

Techniques use to manage child behavior in the dental clinic:

Behavior Guidance Techniques

   a. Preappointment behavior modification
   b. Communication
   c. Behavioral shaping
      – Tell-show-do technique
      – Desensitization
      – Modeling
      – Contingency
   d. Other methods
      – Distraction/audioanalgesia
      – Voice control
      – Hypnodontics
      – Coping
      – Relaxation
      – Aversive conditioning techniques—HOME, implosion therapy.

Advanced Behavior Guidance Techniques

   a. Protective stabilization
   b. Sedation
   c. General anesthesia

Preappointment Behavior Modification

Behavior modification is the technique for modifying child's behavior using Learning Theory principles. It is aimed at preparing the child for a dental visit. Various methods used for pre appointment behavior modification includes audiovisual aids, letters, films and vidotapes. Children are explained the importance of maintaining the teeth in health. Video clipping may include other children undergoing dental treatment so that the child will feel the similarity and reproduce the behavior exhibited by the model. Preappointment behavior modification can also be performed with live patient as models such as siblings, other children or parents.

Mails can be sent addressed to the child that provides brief information regarding the procedure. It is called as preappointment mailing. Parents can also be given advice for preparing the child for their first dental visit.

Child's First Dental Visit

It is generally recommended that a child's first visit be made at about 3-4 years of age. The degree of co-operation exhibited by preschool children at their first appointment is high.

The first visit usually involves only examination, radiographic evaluation and if possible a prophylaxis and topical fluoride treatment unless the child presents with an acute dental problem.

It should be remembered that fear of abandonment is high in younger children and may lead to anxiety during taking of the radiograph leading to uncooperative behavior. It is advised that parent be present in the operatory during treatment in an very young child. Parents can also hold the radiograph in the child's mouth while taking the radiograph so that the child feels secure. Very young children should not be left alone on the dental chair.

Communication[12,13]

The hallmark of a successful dentist in managing child dental patient is his ability to communicate with them and win their confidence. The fears and the natural innate curiosity present in a child makes it important that explanation of a child predict that explanations must be given for new or different techniques and procedures. Communication forms one of the essential features of the tell-show-do technique.

Communication may be accomplished by a number of means but, in the dental setting, it is affected primarily through dialogue, tone of voice, facial expression, and body language.

The 4 "essential ingredients" of communication are: sender, the message, the context or setting in which the message is sent and the receiver.

The age of the child also dictates the level and amount of information that can be included in the communication. The dentist, therefore, must have a basic understanding of the cognitive development of children. Communication may also be impaired when the dentist's expression and body language are not consistent with the intended message. It is therefore important that the dentist shows no signs of uncertainty, anxiety, or urgency while communicating with a child.

Nonverbal communication/Multisensory communication: Nonverbal communication is the reinforcement and guidance of behavior through appropriate contact, posture, facial expression, and body language. It helps to enhance the effectiveness of other communicative management techniques and gain or maintain the patient's attention and compliance. The act of placing a hand on the child's shoulder conveys a feeling of warmth and friendship. Eye contact, alert listening is equally important.

Objectives of Communication

a. *Establishment of communication:* Communication helps the dentist to learn about the child and makes the child at ease and relaxed. But this should not be overdone. Some children realize that by controlling conversation, they can exert considerable influence over their environment.

b. *Establishment of the communicator:* Communicator may be any person in the clinic who can provide information. Initial communication is provided by the receptionist who welcomes the child and the parent with the smile. This initial communication is very important in building confidence and projecting the attitude of the clinic staff to the patient. The dental assistant should talk to the child during the transfer from reception room to operatory and during the preparation of the child in the dental chair. When the dentist arrives, the assistant usually takes a more passive role, as the child can listen to one person at a time.

c. *Message clarity:* Message content varies from a hearty good morning to relevant information and thank you. Message should be simple and easy to understand by a young child. Euphemisms can be used. While talking to a child it is important to remember certain points. They are:
   - The child may not respond to a question immediately. It takes more time for the question to 'sink in' than for adults
   - The command that are given should be simple and within the ability of the patient to obey

   - All command's should be given in a positive language since the negative approach may tend to stimulate fear. Example – "Do not move" is avoided and replaced by "I can't fix your teeth until you sit still."

Behavioral Shaping[14]

It is based on the stimulus-response theory and principles of social learning. The child is guided step by step until a desirable behavior is achieved. The child is explained about the procedure using euphemisms and age appropriate language. Tell-Show-Do Technique has been the main key to success and should be used for all the procedures and all age groups. Care should be taken that the child learns new desirable behavior and does not revert back.

Retraining may be required before initiating any other techniques in children who are preconditioned and are wrongly oriented towards dental treatment through previous dental visits or parents. Such children will be fearful or apprehensive and thus retraining helps the child perceive new concepts and understands that he/she is not going to be hurt. Nitrous oxide-oxygen sedation has also been found to be effective in abolishing the stimulus generalization and aid in retraining.

Different techniques used for behavior shaping are follows:
1. Tell-show-do technique
2. Desensitization
3. Modeling
4. Contingency management

> **The outline for a behavior management includes:**
> - State the general task to the child at the outset
> - Explain the necessity for the procedure
> - Divide the explanation for the entire procedure
> - Make all explanations at a childs level of understanding
> - Reinforce appropriate behavior.

Tell-show-do technique

This technique was introduced by Addleston in 1959.[15] The technique involves verbal explanations of procedures in phrases appropriate to the developmental level of the patient (tell); demonstrations for the patient of the visual, auditory, olfactory, and tactile aspects of the procedure in a carefully defined, nonthreatening setting (show); and then, without deviating from the explanation and demonstration, completion of the procedure (do) (Figs 5.4A to C).

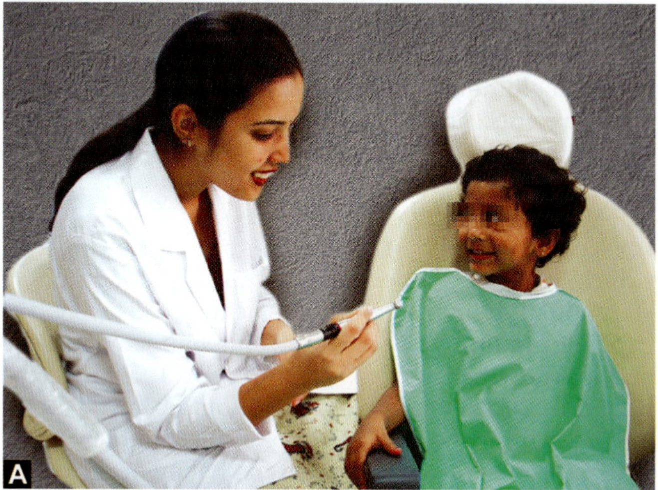

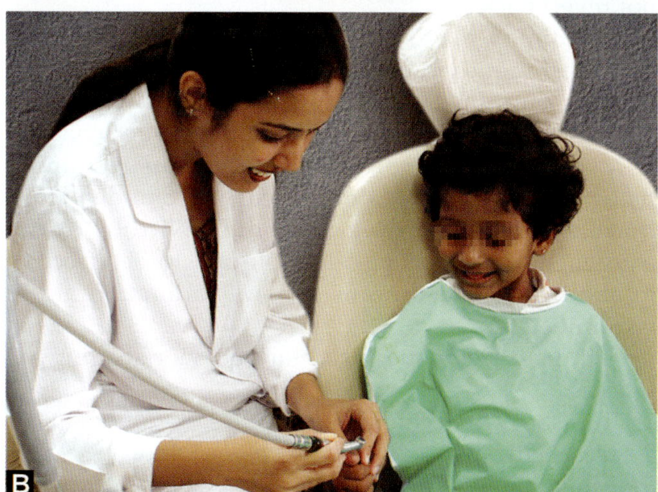

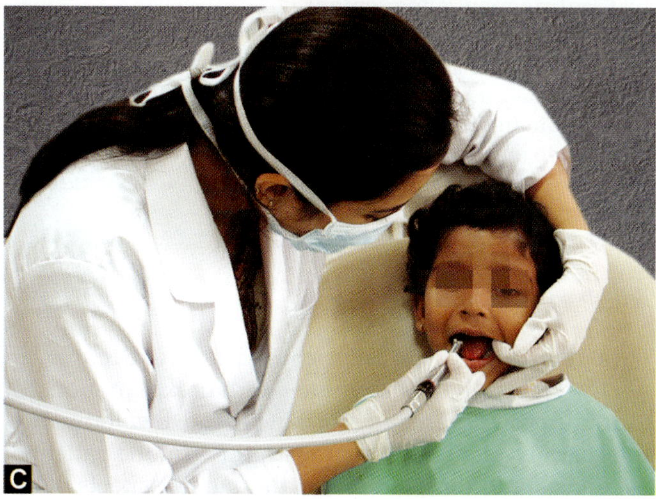

Figs 5.4A to C: Tell-show-do technique: (A) The handpiece is explained to the child; (B) The child is shown how it works and that water can be used to clean; (C) Then the handpiece is taken intraorally to do the restoration

The tell-show-do technique is used with communication skills (verbal and nonverbal) and positive reinforcement.

While taking radiographs the X-ray machine is introduced as a camera that takes the photo of the teeth. The child should be assured that it won't hurt him but only goes near the cheek.

This technique should be practiced every time a new instrument or a new procedure object is introduced to the child.

Demonstrations using tactile or olfactory stimulation (Tell-touch-Do or Tell-Smell-Do) will benefit a child who is visually impaired.

Desensitization

Desensitization propagated by Wolpe (1952) is a process for modifying the effects of phobias or fear. It is also called as reciprocal inhibition. It is a training procedure or steps taken to reduce the sensitivity of the patient to a particular anxiety producing situation or object. An hierarchy of fear promoting situation is first listed. Each situation or object is then introduced progressively starting from the least fear producing to more threatening stimuli.[6]

Technique involves three stages

1. Training the patient to relax
2. Constructing a hierarchy of fear producing stimuli related to the patient's principal fear.
3. Introducing each stimulus in the hierarchy in turn to the relaxed patient, starting with the stimulus that causes least fear and progressing to the next only when the patient no longer fear that stimulus.

Example

If the child is frightened of the restoration, desensitization might include successive introduction of the child to the:

- Reception
- Dentist
- Dental chair
- Oral examination
- Oral prophylaxis
- Restoration

This technique requires many appointments and visits.

Modeling

This was developed by Bandura[16] and follows the principle of social learning. This procedure involves, allowing a patient to observe one or more individuals (model) who demonstrate appropriate behavior in a particular situation. The patient will frequently imitate the model's behavior when placed in a similar situation. This technique is considered by some as one of the pre appointment behavior modification techniques.

Models can be live (other children present in the operatory) (Fig. 5.5).

• Filmed (symbolic or vicarious). A model can be used which is not present physically. For example, Mickey mouse undergoing dental treatment in picture or video format.

Steps in modeling as follows:

1. Obtaining the patients attention
2. The desired behavior is modeled
3. Physical guidance of the desired behavior may be necessary when the patient is initially expected to mimic the modeled behavior
4. Reinforcement of the required behavior

Modeling is a technique which yields significant benefit with minimum effort. Rather than waiting in the reception room, where they may be adversely influenced by maternal anxiety associated with the dental situation, children may be brought into an operatory immediately upon arrival to the office if a suitable model is being treated. When siblings act as model, less anxious sibling should be selected, making other one realize that there is nothing to fear and 'I too can'

To summarize, modeling aids in[17]

1. Stimulation of new behavior
2. Facilitation of behavior in an appropriate manner
3. Disinhibition of inappropriate behavior due to fear
4. Extinction of fear.

Contingency management

The presentation or withdrawal of reinforcers to modify a child's behavior is termed contingency management.

Reinforcers by definition always increases the frequency of a behavior. They can be of two types:

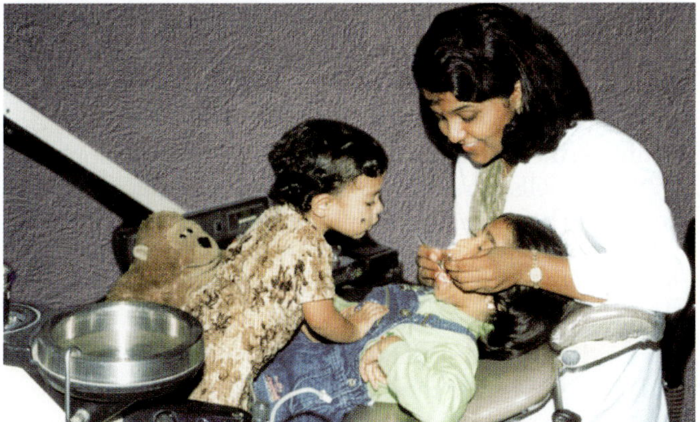

Fig. 5.5: Elder sibling can play the role of a model

1. *Positive reinforcers*—whose contingent presentation increases the frequency of a behavior. Positive reinforcement is an effective technique to establish desirable patient behavior by rewarding the desired behaviors thus, strengthening the recurrence of those behaviors.
2. *Negative reinforcers*—is one whose contingent withdrawal increases the frequency of a behavior.

Reinforcers can be material, social or activity.

Material: Most effective in children are small gifts.

Social: Represents the majority of all reinforcing events affecting human behavior. Praise, positive facial expression, nearness and physical contact are effective social reinforcers.

Activity: Involves the opportunity or privilege of participating in a preferred activity after performance of a preferred behavior. This is especially used at home. For example "first you work, then you play".

The anxious patient can be reassured with these reinforcers. Social reinforcers should be dispensed throughout each dental visit in a sincere manner, in response to appropriate patient behavior.

Distraction

Distraction is the technique of diverting the patient's attention from what may be perceived as an unpleasant procedure. Thus it helps to decrease the perception of unpleasantness and avert negative or avoidance behavior. Music in the back ground, television in front of the child may act as affective distractors. Sometimes giving the child a short break during a stressful procedure can be an effective use of distraction prior to considering more advanced behavior guidance techniques.

Audioanalgesia: It is also called as 'white noise'. This consists of providing a sound stimulus of such intensity that the patient finds it difficult to attend to anything else. The effect is due to distraction, displacement of attention and a positive feeling on the part of the dentist that it can help.

Voice control[18,19]

Voice control is a controlled alteration of volume, tone, or pace of the voice to influence and direct the patient's behavior. When normal communication tones and expression fails, voice control can be fundamental element in obtaining child's compliance and is prove to be an effective method for managing negatively behaving children. The dentist must exhibit an attitude of confidence for voice control to be successful.

Voice control in the form of sudden command to "stop crying and pay attention" is most effective when used in conjunction with other communication methods. Although voice control may appear as one of the means of communicative guidance, it may be considered aversive in nature by some parents. Parents unfamiliar with this technique may benefit from an explanation prior to its use to prevent misunderstanding.

Thus the purpose of voice control are to gain the patient's attention and compliance, avert negative or avoidance behavior and to establish appropriate adult-child roles. Voice control is contraindicated for children who are hearing impaired.

Hypnodontics

Use of hypnosis in dentistry is known as hypnodontics. Hypnosis is defined as a particular state of mind which is usually induced in one person by another—a state of mind in which suggestions are not only more readily accepted than in the waking state, but are also acted upon more powerfully than would be possible under normal conditions.

James Braid of England, first coined the term hypnosis and described the phenomenon as 'neurohypnosis'. Four main features of hypnosis are:
1. Discontinuity from normal waking experience but different from sleep.
2. A compulsion to follow the cues given by the hypnotist both during and after the hypnotic experience.
3. A potential for experiencing as real any distortions of perception, memory or feeling based on suggestions given by the hypnotist rather than on objective reality.
4. Ability to tolerate logical inconsistency that would normally be disturbing.

Coping

Patients differ not only in their perception and response to pain but also in their ways of dealing or coping with the stress associated with painful experiences. Same can be used to modify child's behavior in the dental clinic. Different coping mechanisms are:
1. Distraction or displacement of attention away from the threat is an ideal method of coping. This can be achieved by constantly talking and asking interesting questions to the child.
2. Allowing the child to verbalize fears to the dentist makes the child feel secure.
3. Allowing parents to be in the operatory. The child feels secure with the parent.

Relaxation

Relaxation usually involves a series of basic exercise that may take several months to learn and which require the patients to practice at home for at least fifteen minutes each day. This technique apparently works by reducing tension, well-known potentiator of pain.

HOME: Hand Over Mouth Exercise also Called as Hand Over Mouth Technique

It was first described in the 1920's by Dr Evangeline Jordan who wrote " if a normal child will not listen but continues to cry and struggle ... hold a folded napkin over the child's mouth ... and gently but firmly hold his mouth shut. His screams increase his condition of hysteria, but if the mouth is held closed, there is little sound, and he soon begins to reason".

Levitas[20] referred this procedure as hand-over-mouth exercise and Kramer[21] termed is as 'aversive conditioning'.

This method has been the most controversial one, with critics suggesting that it may be psychologically disturbing to the child.[22]

Indication of HOME technique

- For normal children who are momentarily hysterical, belligerent or defiant.
- Used for children with sufficient maturity to understand simple verbal commands.

Contraindication of HOME technique:

- Immature, frightened or the child with a serious physical, mental or emotional handicap.

Purpose

- Gain the child's attention and to stop his verbal outburst so that communication can be established.

Technique of HOME

The dentist gently but firmly places his hand over the child's mouth. With the verbal outburst completely stopped, the child is told that when he cooperates the hand will be removed (Fig. 5.6). When the patient indicates his willingness to cooperate, usually by a nod of the head and cessation of attempts to scream, the hand is removed and the patient is reevaluated. If the disruptive behavior continues, the dentist again places his hand over the child's mouth and tells him that he must cooperate. Once the child cooperates he must be complimented.

Other variants of hand over mouth technique

- Hand-over-mouth—airway unrestricted
- Hand-over-mouth and nose—airway restricted
- Towel held over mouth:
  - Dry towel held over the mouth and the nose
  - Wet towel held over the mouth and the nose

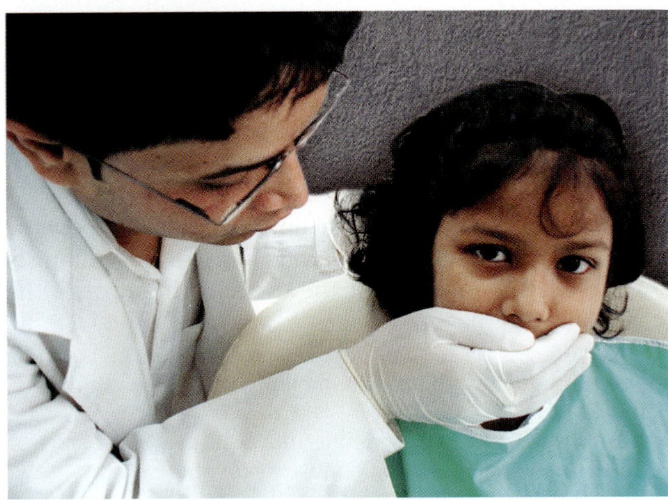

Fig. 5.6: HOME technique

But ideally airway should never be restricted and care should be taken that the child is not a mouth breather.

Implosion therapy

In this technique the patient is flooded with many stimuli. The child has no other choice but to face it until the negative behavior disappears. It comprises of HOME technique, voice control and physical restraints together.

Advanced Behavior Guidance

This technique is used in children who cannot cooperate due to lack of psychological or emotional maturity and/or mental, physical, or medical disability. The advanced behavior guidance techniques include protective stabilization, sedation, and general anesthesia. They are extensions of the overall behavior guidance continuum with the intent to facilitate the goals of communication, cooperation, and delivery of quality oral healthcare in the difficult patient.

Protective Stabilization

Protective stabilization is another term used for restraints. The restriction may involve an assistant, stabilization device, or a combination of both.

The objectives of patient stabilization are to reduce or eliminate untoward movement, protect patient, staff, dentist, or parent from injury and to facilitate delivery of quality dental treatment.

Indications

1. Patients who cannot cooperate due to lack of maturity or mental or physical disability
2. Sedated patients may require limited stabilization to reduce untoward movement.

Contraindications

1. Cooperative nonsedated patients
2. Patients who cannot be immobilized safely due to associated medical or physical conditions
3. Patients who have experienced previous physical or psychological trauma from protective stabilization.
4. Nonsedated patients requiring lengthy appointments.

Disadvantages

1. Physical or psychological harm, violation of a patient's rights.
2. Stabilization devices placed around the chest may restrict respirations and cause harm especially for patients with respiratory compromise.

Before deciding of protective stabilization, alternative behavior guidance modalities, dental needs of the patient, patient's emotional development and the patient's medical and physical status must be considered. The least restrictive, but safe and effective, protective stabilization must be preferred.

Due to the possible aversive nature of the technique, informed consent must be obtained and documented in the patient's record prior to the use of protective stabilization.

Some of the commonly used protective stabilization devices are:

For the body

- *Papoose board (Fig. 5.7):* It is simple to use and store and is available in different sizes to hold both large and small children. It has attached head stabilizers and is reusable. Its disadvantage is that it does not fit the contour of the dental chair and sometimes a supporting pillow is needed. An extremely resistant patient may develop hyperthermia if restrained for too long.
- *Triangular sheet:* Also called bed sheet technique described by Mink. It allows the patient to sit upright during radiographic examinations. Its disadvantages include the frequent need for strapping, to maintain the patient's position in the chair, the difficulty of its use on small patients and the possibility of airway impingement should the patient slip downward unnoticed.
- *Pedi wrap:* Does not have supports or a backboard and has mesh net fabric, and permits better ventilation, lessening the chances of the patient developing hyperthermia. It is strapped to the body and maintained in the dental chair.
- *Beanbag dental chair insert:* Helps accommodate the hypotonic and severely spastic persons who need more support and less restraining in the dental chair.

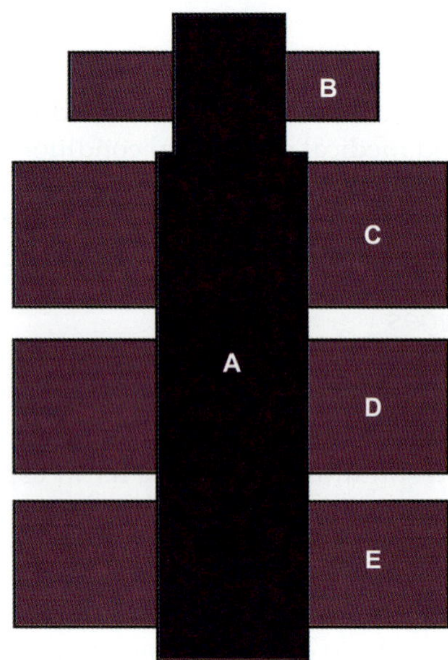

Fig. 5.7: Diagrammatic representation of a papoose board: The child is made to lie on the center board and straps that are present on either side of the board are wrapped over the child. (A) Center board; (B) Straps for the head; (C) Straps for the upper body; (D) Straps for the lower body; (E) Straps for the legs

- *Safety belt:* Velcro straps can be used to restrain the child to the dental chair.
- *Use of bed sheet:* Long sheets such as bed sheets can be used to wrap the child. This restricts the movement of the hands and the legs (Fig. 5.8).
- *Extra assistant:* Parents can help hold the child on the dental chair (Fig. 5.9). This also gives additional security to the child.

For the extremities

- Posey straps   Can be used if the movement of the
- Velcro straps   extremities are the only problem. They are fastened to the arms of the dental chair and allow limited movement of the patient's forearm and hand
- Towel and tape
- Forearm body support
- Extra assistance

For the head

- Head positioner
- Plastic bowl
- Extra assistant

For the teeth

- Padded and wrapped tongue blades (Fig. 5.10)—Can be used by the parents to aid with home care. Simple icecream sticks that are piled and wrapped in a gauze can be used as restrains for the teeth.

- Mouth prop or bite block (Figs 5.11A and B)—Used at times during injection to prevent children from closing their mouths or children who are fatigued from a long appointment, are stubborn or defiant or who constantly closed his mouth in order to interrupt treatment.
- Finger guard or interocclusal thimble—It is inexpensive and fits the dentist's finger. Its main disadvantage is the limited mobility of the dentist's hand once the splint is in place.

Two types of mouth prop are molt mouth prop and rubber block

Molt mouth prop—Available in adult and child sizes, allows accessibility to the opposite side of the mouth and operates on a reverse scissor action. Its disadvantages include the possibility of lip and palatal lacerations and luxation of teeth if it is not used correctly. The patient's mouth should not be forced opened beyond its natural limits.

Rubber bite blocks—They are available in different sizes and should have floss attached for easy retrieval if they become dislodged in the mouth.

Premedication

Premedication refer to a drug given to a patient before any procedure. Here in this chapter we are discussing the drugs that are given to reduce the anxiety before any dental procedure or induction of general anesthesia.

Guidelines for the use

1. Detailed medical history should be taken to prevent undesired drug interaction
2. Decision to use premedication—should be done before one resorts to sedatives, conscious sedation or general anesthesia.

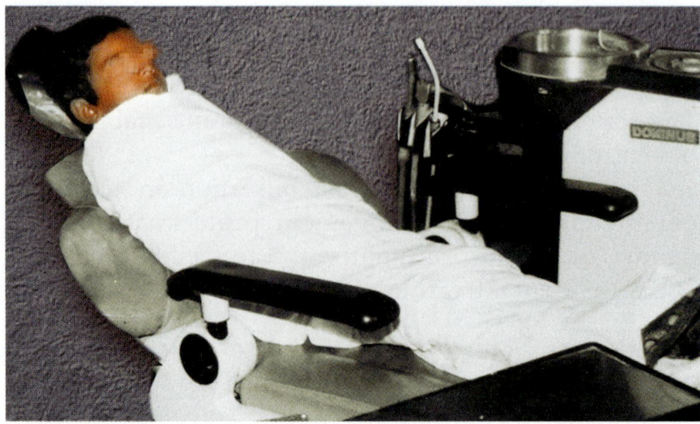

Fig. 5.8: A long sheet wrapped around the child restrains the body and the extremities

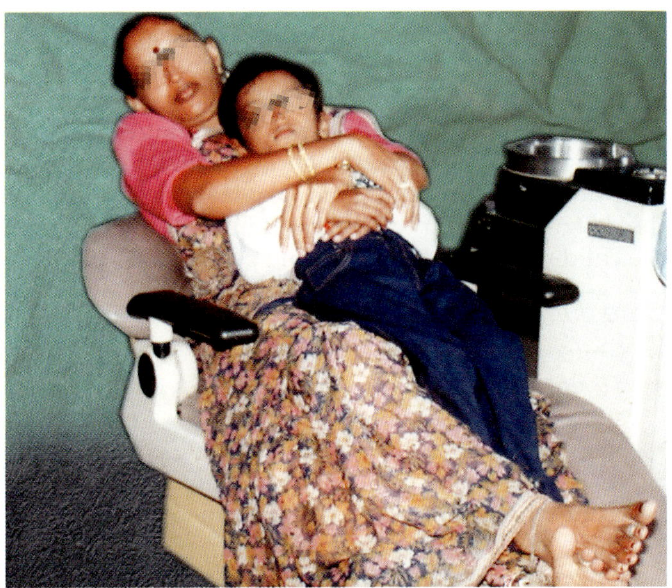

Fig. 5.9: Mother sits on the chair and the child lies over the mother. Mother holds the child's hands and her legs are crossed over the child's legs. If the child is small, one hand can be used to restrain both the child's hands and the other preferably the left can be placed on the forehead to restrain the head

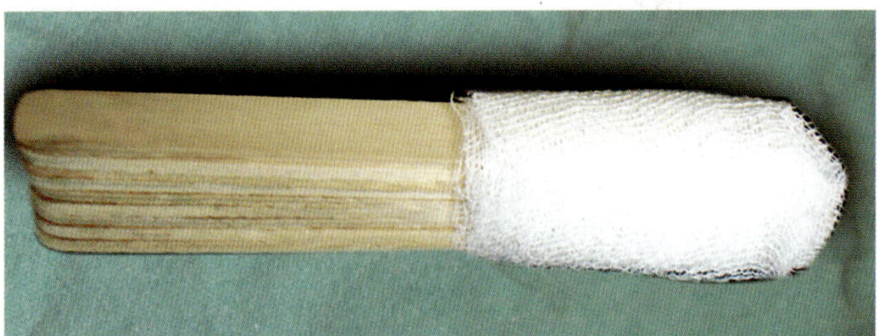

Fig. 5.10: Ice cream sticks wrapped with gauze can be used as restraint for the mouth

3. Selecting a premedication agent—depends upon the properties, effects, dosage, duration of action, hypersensitivity, etc. The type and dosage used should never impair the vital reflexes of the child.
4. Consent and preoperative instructions should be given before any procedure. This reduces parent anxiety. Instructions includes the method of administration of the drug, its safety precautions, side effects of the drugs, dietary precautions, etc. Parents should accompany the child.
5. High levels of personnel training is a must
6. Call for documentation of events during the treatment (vital signs, etc.)
7. Assistant other than the operatory must participate in the procedure to constantly monitor physiological parameters.
8. Postoperative care includes—discharge only when vital signs are stable, patient is alert, can walk with minimal assistance.

Agents used for Premedication for General Anesthesia

1. Anticholinergics:
   - Infants under 1 year: Atropine 0.02 mg/kg- IV during anesthesia or IM 30 min before
   - Healthy children 1-3 years of age: Atropine 0.02 mg/kg- IV during anesthesia or IM 30 min before
   - Healthy children over 3 years of age: Optimal psychological management
   - If indicated diazepam 4 mg/kg suspension.
2. Sedatives
3. Anti emetic: Hydroxyzine, metoclopramide.

Agents used for Premedication Sedation

They can be sedative hypnotics, antianxiety drugs or analgesics.
a. Sedatives—hypnotics
   • Primary action is sedation or sleepiness

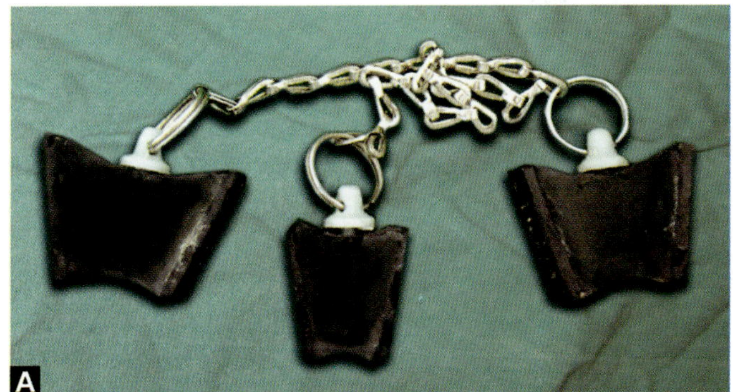

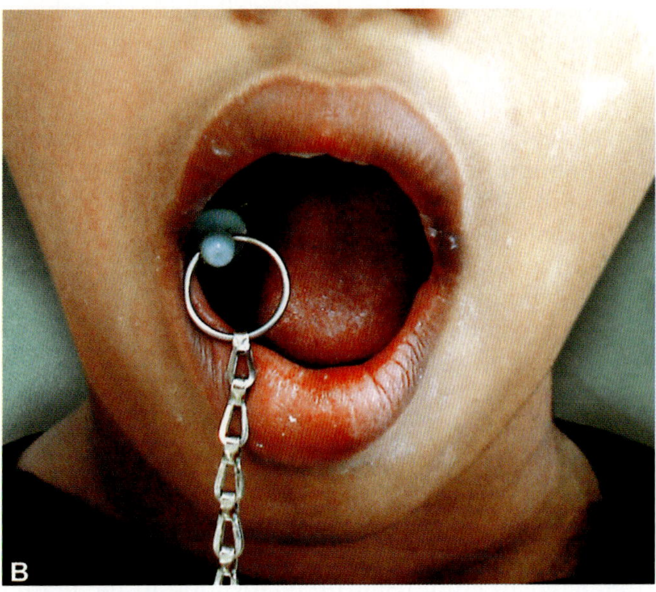

Figs 5.11A and B: Rubber bite blocks: (A) They are available in different sizes; (B) Bite block placed in between the teeth

- On increasing the dose it can lead to general anesthesia, coma and death.
- Site of action: Reticular activating system (normal dose), cortex (increased dose)
- Drugs: They are of two categories—barbiturates (Pentobarbital, secobarbital, etc) and nonbarbiturates (chloral hydrate and paraldehyde).

b. Anti-anxiety drugs
- Also called as mild tranqulizers
- Primary action is to decrease or remove anxiety
- Primary site of action: Limbic system (seat of emotions)
- Higher doses can cause sedation (recticular activating system) or sleep (Cortex)
- Drugs: Benzodiazepines (Diazepam, midazolam, etc.), hydroxyzine, diphenhydramine.

c. Analgesics
- Ideally analgesics relieve pain without altering consciousness.
- Analgesics can be of two types, non-narcotic and narcotic.

Non-narcotic Analgesic

- Act at the peripheral nerve endings
- Useful in case of mild to moderate pain
- Less toxic
- Less side effects
- Absence of drug dependence.

Narcotic Analgesics/Opoids

- Act in the central nervous system
- More efficient against severe acute pain
- Drugs used are: Natural opium alkaloids (Morphine, codeine), semisynthetic opiates (Heroine, pholcodiene), synthetic opioids (Pethidine, fentanyl, methadone, tramadol)
- Actions: Analgesia, Sedation, Cough suppression
- Contraindications
  - Bronchial asthma
  - Head injury
  - Hypotensive states
  - Hypothyroidism
  - Liver and kidney disease
- Adverse drug effects
  - Sedation
  - Respiratory depression
  - Dependence
  - Abuse.

Administration of Premedication

It is better to administer premedication in the dental office as the dentist can use routes other than oral and also accurate timing of the administration can be done. Frequently parents fail to observe the time of administration, or may fail to report vomiting or incomplete ingestion. Another advantage of office administration is that treatment can be begun at the time of optimum effect on the child who responds quickly to the drug, whereas if the drug is administered at home, the child may be in transit during peak drug activity.

Care during Premedication

- Child should never be left unattended
- To enhance drug efficacy the child's environment should be kept as quiet as possible.
- The child who is aroused before the medication has reached peak activity may remain excited and the child who receives additional premedication before peak activity is reached may be overmedicated. Once the desired level of sedation is obtained it is still essential to administer local anesthesia. A sedated child aroused by painful stimuli may display considerable agitation and confusion.

Postoperative Instruction

- After the completion of the treatment the child whether is asleep or awake, will be in a sedated condition.
- The child may sleep for many hours, depending on the drug and the dosage used.
- Upon awakening, the child may complain of hunger or thirst if the sleep has been prolonged. The mouth and pharynx may be dry, so it is better to start with little water and then to proceed with other food.
- Recovery period may be extended for several hours and should be under supervision.

Factors Influencing Dosage

A. **Age and weight:** Young's rule or Clarke's rule can be used to calculate the dosage.

B. **Emotional state and activity:** Extremely anxious or defiant child will required more premedication than will the mildly apprehensive child. The child who displays greater physical activity will usually require higher dosage than will a child who is more passive.

C. **Route of administration:** Drugs given intravenously will act more rapidly and are given in lower dose, whereas a drug given orally act more slowly and dosage requirement are higher. Intramuscular administration of drugs results in intermediate onset of action and dosage requirements.

D. **Environment:** Dosages required are generally lower when a drug is taken in a nonstress full (lying in a bed) environment and when the patient is expected to remain quite. Conversely the amount of drug required is usually higher when an anxious patient requires premedication in the dental office, where auditory, tactile and visual stimulation can be intense.

E. **Time of the day:** Dosage may sometimes be reduced if given during the time when the child usually takes a nap. Conversely dosages may have to be elevated if the drug is administered during the time when the child is usually engaged in active play.

General causes of premedication failure
- Prescription of an insufficient dose of drug
- Accidental or intentional reduction of dosage by the parents
- Failure of the child to co-operate in swallowing premedication
- Expectoration or vomiting of a portion of the medication
- Children with medical condition such as brain damage and other problems are often inadequately premedicated and may require increased doses or different drugs.

Sedation

Sedation can be used safely and effectively in patients who are unable to cooperate during dental treatment for reasons of age or mental, physical, or medical condition. Moderate sedation is usually preferred while performing treatment in dental clinic setup.

Moderate Sedation/Conscious Sedation

The term conscious sedation has been replaced by Moderate sedation[23] (AAPD). It helps achieve co-operation in a child by reducing their anxiety but maintaining the conscious state of the child. The child's response to verbal stimuli may be sluggish but responds and is cooperative.

Aides in:
- Erasing fear, anxiety and apprehension
- Helps to reduce patient motion
- Creates a semihypnotic state
- Increases tolerance for longer appointments
- Slightly raises the pain threshold
- Maintaining the conscious of the child.

Indications

1. Fearful, anxious patients for whom basic behavior guidance techniques have not been successful
2. Patients who cannot cooperate due to a lack of psychological or emotional maturity and/or mental, physical, or medical disability

3. Patients for whom the use of sedation may protect the developing psyche and/or reduce medical risk.

Contraindications
1. The cooperative patient with minimal dental needs
2. Predisposing medical conditions which would make sedation inadvisable, as follows:
   - Hypersensitivity to the agent
   - Chronic obstructive pulmonary disorder
   - Psychiatric patients
   - Cardiac patients
   - Epilepsy, bleeding disorder.

Advantages
- Patient is conscious
- Relative safety
- Least disturbs the metabolic process and general functions
- Has all vital reflex intact
- Can communicate and cooperate
- Quickly returns to normal state after few minutes
- Rapid onset and recovery time, because of very low plasma solubility
- Ease of dose control
- Lack of serious adverse effects
- Produces euphoric effect.

Disadvantages
- Weak agent— not so affective in moderate or severely anxious patients, as dose cannot be increased
- Lack of patient acceptance—some may not like it
- Inconvenience—when inhalation is used the mask may hinder exposure of the oral cavity especially in children
- Potential chronic toxicity—retrospective survey studies of dental office personnel who were exposed to trace levels of N_2O suggests a possible association with and increased incidence of spontaneous abortions, congenital malformations, certain cancer, liver disease, kidney disease and neurologic disease.

Objectives for Sedation in Pedodontic Practice[24]

Sedation facilitates provision of good quality care by minimizing extreme disruptive behavior.
- The needs of the child
  - Reduce fear and perception of pain during the treatment
  - Facilitate coping with the treatment
  - Prevent development of dental fear and anxiety
- The needs of the dentist
  - Facilitate accomplishment of dental procedures
  - Reduce stress and unpleasant emotions
  - Prevent "burn-out" syndrome.

Terms and definition

Sedative: A drug that subdues excitement and calms the subject without inducing sleep, though drowsiness may be produced. In a minimal or moderate sedation, patients retain the ability to maintain a patent airway independently and continuously and also respond to physical or verbal stimulus.

Deep sedation: Controlled state of depressed consciousness or unconsciousness from which the patient is not aroused easily. It may be accompanied by partial or complete loss of protective reflexes including the ability to maintain a patent airway independently and respond purposefully to physical stimulation or verbal command.

Moderate sedation/Conscious sedation: It is a minimally depressed level of consciousness in which the patient's ability to maintain a patent airway independently and continuously and to respond appropriately to physical stimulation or verbal command is retained. For definition purpose it is given separately, but American Academy of Pediatric Dentistry (AAPD) recognizes it as Moderate sedation.

Hypnotic: A drug that induces and/or maintains sleep, similar to normal arousal sleep.

Tranquilizer: It can be major tranquilizer (antipsychotics) or minor tranquilizer (anti-anxiety). Antipsychotics produce calmness, control symptoms of psychosis, cause reversible extrapyramidal symptoms and do not tend to cause habituation. Used for treatment of delusion, excited or psychotic states. Anti-anxiety agents produce calmness but to lesser degree, do not possesses antipsychotic properties or cause extrapyramidal symptoms. Used in the treatment of common psychoneurotic states such as nervous tension and mild depression.

General anesthesia: Controlled state of unconsciousness accompanied by loss of protective reflexes, including the ability to maintain airway independently and respond purposefully to physical stimulation or verbal command.

Requisites for Performing Treatement Under Sedation

1. The clinician should be formally trained and possess a thorough knowledge of the agent which is to be administered.
2. The decision should be made based on a careful analysis of the:
   - Actual need of the patient. Pharmacological management should be the choice when only other nonpharmacological techniques have failed.
   - The nature and extent of the treatment required
   - The risk-to-benefit ratio
   - Physical status of the patient
   - The economic feasibility of alternative choices.

3. There should be a well-documented informed consent. No sedation technique should be attempted unless the parent or guardian has been educated and informed consent obtained.
4. Dentist utilizing pharmacological management approaches should be trained in basic cardiac life support.
5. Strict information to parents regarding diet restriction.
6. Discharge: Before discharging, the child should be alert and oriented (or have returned to an age-appropriate base line). A responsible adult must be present to observe the child for complications after discharge. The adult must be given written and oral instructions on.
   - Appropriate diet
   - Medications
   - Management of possible postoperative bleeding
   - Level of activity.

Patient Monitoring[25-29]

Sedation of pediatric patients has serious associated risks, such as hypoventilation, apnea, airway obstruction, laryngospasm, and cardiopulmonary impairment making monitoring very important.

The reasons why children are at high-risk during sedation:
1. Smaller size—drug dosage should be exactly calculated
2. Immature system—drug reaction may vary than in adult
3. Higher basal metabolic rate
4. Increased oxygen demand and immature alveolar system associated with narrow nasal passage, increased secretions, enlarged tonsils and adenoids – so risk of poor ventilation leading to oxygen desaturation
5. More prone for bradycardia, decreased cardiac output and hypotension.
6. Retention of lipophilic drugs may be prolonged in obese children- increasing its duration of action.

The American Academy of Pediatrics (AAP) and American Academy of Pediatric Dentistry (AAPD)[30,31] have published a series of guidelines for the monitoring and management of pediatric patients during and after sedation for any procedure.

General Precautions

1. Patient Selection: Patients who are in ASA Classes I and II are selected for procedure under sedation
2. Dietary precautions
3. Adequate facilities to manage emergency must be readily available

4. Adequate documentation, including informed consent, instructions, observations, etc.

Specific Precautions

a. Continuous clinical observation
Children under sedation must be monitored continuously. It includes:
   - Observing breathing: movements of the thorax, passage of the air stream and respiratory frequency. The vast majority of sedation complications can be managed with simple maneuvers, such as supplemental oxygen, opening the airway, suctioning, and bag-mask-valve ventilation.
   - Observing skin color
   - Response by the patient to Physical stimulation and Verbal command (For Conscious Sedation).
b. Pulsoximetry
The use of pulseoximetry is required to monitor oxygen saturation of blood. Pulsoximetry is not deemed required for conscious sedation with nitrous oxide/oxygen sedation, but is preferred in benzodiazepin sedation.
c. Capnography
It measures the expired carbon dioxide, which is valuable to diagnose the simple presence or absence of respirations, airway obstruction, or respiratory depression.

Routes of Administration of the Drug

- Inhalation
- Oral
- Rectal
- Parental
  - Intramuscular
  - Submucosal
  - Intravenous

Inhalation sedation: Nitrous oxide is the gas that is used for moderation through nasal route.

Oral sedation: It is the most accepted route for administration of any drug. Absorption through this route is not consistent and depends upon the conditions of the stomach. Reversal is also not possible and recovery time is prolonged as the drug is slowly metabolized. Advantages of this route is the convenience cheaper and reduced toxicity.

Intramucular sedation: This route can be used in children who refuse taking drugs through oral route. Even in this route it is not possible to reverse the actions once the drug is injected. The site of injection in children is the upper outer quadrant of the gluteal region into the gluteus maximus muscle. Pheripheral vasoconstriction that occurs in children when they are anxious may delay the absorption of the drug from the site of injection.

Submucosal sedation: It involves deposition of the drug beneath the mucosa. Onset of action is fast compared to the intramuscular route. Caution should be exercised in selecting a drug as it should not irritate the delicate mucosa.

Intravenous sedation: This route is not used regularly and should be practiced only by persons qualified to provide intravenous sedation. Onset of action is about 20-25 seconds. The patient has to be closely monitored.

> **American society of anesthesiologists—risk assessment[32-33]**
>
> Cl I: No organic, physiological, biochemical or psychiatric disturbance
> Cl II: Mild to moderate systemic disturbance without significant physical limitation
> Cl III: Severe systemic disturbances with physical limitation (steroid depended asthama or severe mental retardation)
> Cl IV: Life-threatening disorder (renal disorder)
> Cl V: Moribund patient – Who has little chance of survival
> Cl I and Cl II are patients considered fit for receiving sedation in dental office.

Patient Consent

The parents or legal guardians must be agreeable to the use of conscious sedation for the child. They should be well informed regarding the risk, benefits and associated particulars. Written consent must be obtained prior to the procedure.

Instruction to the Parents

It includes information regarding the restriction of food and liquids intake prior to sedation administration. The main reason for this avoidance is to prevent aspiration of stomach contents if, at all, there is vomiting during the sedation procedure. Empty stomach also improves drug uptake when administered orally. According to American Academy of Pediatric Dentistry dietary instructions to be given are as follows:

1. Clear liquids: For example, water, fruit juice without pulp—up to 2 hours before the procedure.
2. Breast milk: up to 4 hours before the procedure.
3. Infant formula and nonhuman milk: upto 6 hour before the procedure.
4. Light meal: Up to 6 hours before the procedure.
   After the treatment, solid food should be given only after the clear fluid is tolerated.

Inhalation Sedation

The American Academy of Pediatric Dentistry (AAPD)[34] recognizes nitrous oxide/oxygen inhalation as a safe and effective technique to reduce anxiety, produce analgesia, and enhance effective communication between a patient and healthcare provider.

The patient responds normally to verbal commands. All vital signs are stable, there is no significant risk of losing protective reflexes, and the patient is able to return to preprocedure mobility.

The clinical effect of nitrous oxide/oxygen inhalation is said to be more predictable among the majority of the population.

Nitrous Oxide (N$_2$O)

It is the common inhalation agent used. It is a colorless, odorless, heavier than air (specific gravity 1.53), non-inflammable gas. It is absorbed quickly from the alveoli of the lungs and is physically dissolved in the blood with no chemical combination anywhere in the body. It is carried in the serum portion of the blood and excreted through lungs without any biotransformation. Small amount may be found in the body fluids and intestinal gas.

Nitrous oxide has multiple mechanisms of action. The analgesic effect of nitrous oxide appears to be initiated by neuronal release of endogeneous opioid peptides with subsequent activation of opioid receptors and descending Gamma-aminobutyric acid type A (GABAA) receptors and noradrenergic pathways that modulate nociceptive processing at the spinal level. The anxiolytic effect involves activation of the GABAA receptor either directly or indirectly through the benzodiazepine binding site.[35]

Actions (Pharmacodynamics) of Nitrous Oxide

- Creates an altered state of awareness without impaired motor function and is a central nervous system depressant
- Increases the respiratory rate and decreases the tidal volume
- Cardiac output is decreased and pheripheral vascular resistance is increased (important in cardiac patients)
- Rapid induction and reversal may induce vomiting.

Objectives of nitrous oxide/oxygen inhalation include:

1. Reduce or eliminate anxiety
2. Reduce untoward movement and reaction to dental treatment
3. Enhance communication and patient cooperation
4. Raise the pain reaction threshold
5. Increase tolerance for longer appointments

6. Aid in treatment of the mentally/physically disabled or medically compromised patient
7. Reduce gagging
8. Potentiate the effect of sedatives.

Indications for use of nitrous oxide/oxygen analgesia/anxiolysis include:

1. A fearful, anxious, or obstreperous patient
2. Certain patients with special healthcare needs
3. A patient whose gag reflex interferes with dental care
4. A patient for whom profound local anesthesia cannot be obtained
5. A cooperative child undergoing a lengthy dental procedure.

Absorption, metabolism and excretion

- Enters blood by crossing pulmonary epithelium and depends upon the concentration gradient
- During early phases of administration – brain, heart, liver and kidney absorbs the major portion of nitrous oxide from blood
- Expired through lungs.

Requirements of the equipment used for the induction of nitrous oxide[36]

1. Should have a continuous flow design with flow meters capable of accurate regulation
2. Automatic shutdown if oxygen level falls < 20%
3. Flush level for easy and immediate flushing of the system with 100% oxygen
4. Can be either mobile units or operating from a central supply
5. Good and efficient scavenger system
6. Nasal hood should be of adequate size—for the adults and children.

Techniques

Nitrous oxide/oxygen must be administered only by appropriately trained individuals, or under their direct supervision. Very important in the procedure for affective conscious sedation is the acceptance of the nosepiece by the patient. If the patient exhibits resistance, then this method is not advised for such children. This requires explanation at the youngster's level of comprehension, a slow approach and behavior shaping with positive reinforcement throughout. The sensation which the child is going to experience should be explained to the child before and during the procedure.

Selection of an appropriately sized nasal hood should be made. A flow rate of 5 to 6 L/min generally is acceptable to most patients. The flow rate can be adjusted after observation of the reservoir bag. The bag should pulsate gently with each breath and should not be either over- or underinflated. Introduction of 100% oxygen for 1 to 2 minutes followed by titration of nitrous oxide in 10% intervals is recommended. At concentration between 30–50%, the patient is relaxed and listens to instructions. During nitrous oxide/oxygen analgesia, the concentration of nitrous oxide should not exceed 50%. Nitrous oxide concentration may be decreased during easier procedures (e.g. restorations) and increased during more stimulating ones (e.g. extraction, injection of local anesthetic). During treatment, it is important to continue the visual monitoring of the patient's respiratory rate and level of consciousness. The effects of nitrous oxide largely are dependent on psychological reassurance. Therefore, it is important to continue traditional behavior guidance techniques during treatment. Once the nitrous oxide flow is terminated, 100% oxygen should be delivered for 3 to 5 minutes.[3] The patient must return to pretreatment responsiveness before discharge. Continuous clinical observation of the patient must be done during any dental procedure.

Informed consent must be obtained from the parent and documented in the patient's record prior to administration of nitrous oxide/oxygen. The practitioner should provide instructions to the parent regarding pretreatment dietary precautions, if indicated. In addition, the patient's record should include indication for use of nitrous oxide/oxygen inhalation, nitrous oxide dosage (i.e. percent nitrous oxide/oxygen and/or flow rate), duration of the procedure, and post-treatment oxygenation procedure.

Difference between Conscious Sedation and General Anesthesia

Conscious sedation	General anesthesia
Treatment done in several appointments	All procedures done in one appointment
Used in cooperative but anxious and fearful patient	Used in very uncooperative patient
Need for basic preoperative investigation	Requires thorough investigation and anesthetist's approval for fitness
Patient is conscious during the procedure	Patient is unconscious
Reflexes and airway maintained	Reflexes are lost and ventilation required
Patient need not be starving before procedure, but lighter stomach is preferred	Requires to be in empty stomach at least 6 hours before the procedure

Patient Symptoms Obtained at Various Nitrous Oxide Levels

Nitrous oxide	Symptoms
10-20%	Tingling feeling (paresthesia), sensation of warmth
20-40%	Numbness of the extremities, floating sensation, auditory changes (distant humming noise), analgesia and euphoria
40-60%	Dreaming, laughing or giddiness, sweating nausea and vomiting, uncoordinated movement, loss of eyelid reflex

Common Problems Associated with Nitrous Oxide[37-40]

Nitrous oxide/oxygen analgesia/anxiolysis has an excellent safety record. Nausea and vomiting are the most common adverse effects, occurring in 0.5% of patients. Fasting is not required for patients undergoing nitrous oxide analgesia/anxiolysis. The practitioner, however, may recommend that only a light meal be consumed in the 2 hours prior to the administration of nitrous oxide. Children desaturate more rapidly than adolescents, and administering 100% oxygen to the patient for 3 to 5 minutes once the nitrous oxide has been terminated is important.

1. Sleep: Patient may go into sleep during the procedure and frequent arousal or communication is required
2. Airway obstruction: Frequent repositioning of the head is needed to hyper extend the mandible so that the tongue is brought forward
3. Vomiting, this can be prevented by:
   - Using minimum effective concentration
   - Avoiding prolonged procedure
   - Empty stomach inhalation
   - Slow return to upright position
   - Aspiration is unlikely—so just ask the patient to vomit in a chairside emesis basin if there is vomiting.
4. Nitrous oxide may fill up middle ear space and in patients with otitis media can cause acute pain.
5. Diffusion hypoxia: As nitrous oxide is 34 times more soluble than nitrogen in blood, diffusion hypoxia may occur. It rapidly diffuses into alveoli and dilutes the alveoli air causing a fall in the partial pressure of oxygen in alveoli leading to headache and disorientation. 100% oxygen given for about 10 minutes will prevent this problem from occurring. It is also seen that this rarely occurs in an healthy individual.
6. Chronic exposure to nitrous oxide by clinic personnel, may lead to importence, neurotoxicity, renal and liver toxicity. Constant check on leakage, good

cross-ventilation and scavenging system will reduce the concentration of nitrous oxide in the ambient air. Devices such as infrared spectrophotometry or dorsimetry badges can be used to measure the exposures.

Other Drugs used for Sedation

1. Hydroxyzine
   - Rapidly absorbed from the gastrointestinal tract.
   - Clinical effect seen in 15 to 30 minutes, with peak levels at 2 hours.
   - Excreted by the liver with a mean half-life of 3 hours.
   - Administration is preferably by the oral route.
   - Intramuscular injections must be deep in a large muscle mass. Care must be exercised in the small child. It should not be injected subcutaneously or intravenously because of potential tissue necrosis and hemolysis.
   - Adverse reactions: Extreme drowsiness, dry mouth, and hypersensitivity
   - Dosage: Oral—0.6 mg/kg
     IM—1. 1 mg/kg

2. Promethazine (Phenergan)
   - Well-absorbed after oral ingestion.
   - Onset is within 15 to 60 minutes, with a peak at 1 to 2 hours and a duration of 4 to 6 hours.
   - Metabolized by the liver.
   - Any phenothiazine should be used with caution in children with a history of asthma, sleep apnea, or a family history of sudden infant death syndrome (SIDS). Phenothiazines lower the seizure threshold and should be avoided in seizure-prone patients.
   - Interactions: Potentiates other CNS depressants.
   - Adverse reactions: Dry mouth, blurred vision, thickening of bronchial secretions, mild hypotension, extrapyramidal effects.
   - Dosage: Oral/IM—0.5 to 1. 1 mg/kg.
     SC—not recommended
     Maximum recommended single dose is 25 mg.

3. Diphenhydramine (Benadryl)
   - Rapidly absorbed through the gastrointestinal tract,
   - Maximum effect in 1st hour and a duration of 4 to 6 hours.
   - Metabolized by the liver and completely excreted in 24 hours.
   - Produces a mild sedative effect but has additive effects with other CNS depressants.
   - Adverse reactions: Disturbed coordination, epigastric distress, and thickening of bronchial secretions

   - Dosage: Oral, IM, or IV—1.0 to 1.5 mg/kg. Maximum single dose is 50 mg

4. Diazepam (Valium)
   - It is lipid soluble and water insoluble.
   - It is rapidly absorbed from the gastrointestinal tract
   - Peak levels reaches at 2 hours.
   - Biotransformation of the drug occurs quite slowly, with a half-life of 20 to 50 hours. The drug has three active metabolites, and these are more anxiolytic than sedative.
   - Diazepam can be administered orally, rectally or parenterally. If the intravenous route is to be utilized, a large vein and slow administration is recommended because of the drug's propensity to cause irritation of the vein, with resultant thrombophlebitis. Additionally, rapid administration may result in apnea.
   - Ataxia and prolonged CNS effects are the only common adverse reactions that can be anticipated when diazepam is used for conscious sedation.

Doses

Children 4-8 years of age: 0.5-0.8 mg diazepam per kilogram. Maximum dose 15 mg.
Children over 8 years of age: 0.2-0.5 mg diazepam per kilogram. Maximum dose 15 mg.

> **Rebound effect of diazepam**
>
> After intravenous administration of diazepam, it is redistributed within 30 to 45 minutes, and the patient seems to be not sedated though free from anxiety. The patient should not be considered recovered from the drug. It has simply been redistributed. Later the stored drug can be redistributed to the CNS by a fatty meal some time later and the patient will suddenly be resedated. This is referred to as the 'Rebound effect.'

5. Midazolam
   - Midazolam is the preferred benzodiazepine and is similar to diazepam but with twice the potency.
   - Significant advantage of midazolam over diazepam is its high water solubility. Consequently, the possibility of thrombophlebitis is reduced to a minimum.
   - After intravenous administration, sedation occurs in 3 to 5 minutes. There is no rebound phenomenon from metabolites.
   - After oral administration the peak plasma concentration is reached within 20 minutes, faster via the rectal route in about 10 min. The sedative effect lasts for only 45 minutes and the elimination half time is 2 hours, thus the recovery is fast.

- Midazolam can also be effectively given intramuscularly.
- Recently the oral form and nasal spray has become available and holds great promise for pediatric conscious sedation. The drug is highly lipophilic, providing for rapid absorption from the gastrointestinal tract as well as rapid entry into brain tissue.
- Midazolam may produce respiratory depression with higher doses.
- Contraindications: It should not be given to children
  - Under the age of one year
  - With any form of acute disease
  - With neuromuscular diseases as myasthenia gravis
  - With allergy to BZD
  - With sleep apnea
  - With liver dysfunction
  - With hepatic dysfunction
- Side effects: Includes Paradoxical reaction, over sedation, hallucinations
- Dosage: Oral—0.25 to 1 mg/kg to a maximum single dose of 20 mg
  IM—0.1 to 0.15 mg/kg to a maximum dose of 10 mg

Oral: Children under 25 kilogram of weight shall have 0.3-0.5 mg midazolam per kilogram. Maximum dose 12 mg.

Children over 25 kilogram of weight shall have 12 mg midazolam.

Tablets are given 60 min before dental treatment, and oral mixtures given approximately 20-30 minutes before.

Rectal: Children under 25 kilogram of weight shall have 0.3-0.4 mg midazolam per kilogram bodyweight. Maximum dose 10 mg midazolam.

Children over 25 kilogram of weight shall have 10 mg midazolam.

Rectal solution is administered approximately 10 minutes before treatment starts.

Interactions: Contemporaneous intake of erythromycin, hypnotics, anxiolytics, antidepressants, antipsychotics, antiepileptics, antihistamines, opioids, grapefruit juice, clonidine and alcohol can enhance the effect. Drug interactions shall be followed in national databases.

6. Barbiturates
   Barbiturates can produce all levels of CNS depression, ranging from mild sedation to general anesthesia and deep coma.

The short-acting barbiturates, seconal and pento-barbital were previously recommended for pediatric oral conscious sedation, but it is not being used now due to the availability of sedative/hypnotics with fewer adverse effects.

7. Chloral hydrate
   Chloral hydrate is an extremely well-known and widely used drug for pediatric sedation.
   - It has an onset of action of 15 to 30 minutes when given orally.
   - The peak effect may not occur, however, for an hour or more.
   - It has a duration of action between 4 and 8 hours and a half-life of 8 to 11 hours as a result of active metabolites.
   - The primary metabolite of choral hydrate is trichloroethanol (TCE), which is responsible for most of the CNS effects that occur.
   - Chloral hydrate is irritating to gastric mucosa and unless diluted in a flavored vehicle will frequently cause nausea and vomiting.
   - Children will often enter a period of excitement and irritability before becoming sedated.
   - The drug causes prolonged drowsiness or sleep and respiratory depression. In large doses it will produce general anesthesia.
   - Large doses additionally depress the myocardium and can produce arrhythmias and thus should be avoided in patients with cardiac disease.
   - The lethal dose of chloral hydrate is stated to be 10 gm in adults, yet ingestion of 4 gm has caused death. Because the drug dose does not reliably produce sedation of a degree to permit operative procedures at lower doses, the tendency is to push the dosage higher to achieve the necessary sedation. With such a wide range of reported toxicity this choice may be unwise for many pediatric patients. It is recommended that young children receive not more than 1 gm. As a total dose. Risks are increased when chloral hydrate is combined with nitrous oxide, narcotics, or local anesthetic agents. At higher doses and in combinations, loss of a patent airway is a common problem
   - Dosage: Must be individualized for each patient and is about 25 to 50 mg/kg to maximum of 1 gm.

8. Meperidine
   It is a synthetic opiate agonist. It is very water soluble but is incompatible with many other drugs in solution.

- Meperidine may be administered orally or by subcutaneous, intramuscular, or intravenous injection.
- It is least effective by mouth. It is very bitter and requires masking by a flavoring agent.
- Peak effect will occur in 1 hour and last about 4 hours. Parenteral routes shorten the time of onset and duration.
- High doses lead to an accumulation of normeperidine, a primary metabolite of meperidine, resulting in seizures. Meperidine should be used with extreme caution in patients with hepatic or renal disease and history of seizures.
- Dosage: Oral, subcutaneous, or IM—1 to 2.2 mg/kg, not to exceed 100 mg.

9. Fentanyl
   - It is a very potent narcotic analgesic.
   - A dose of 0. 1 mg is approximately equivalent to 10 mg of morphine or 75 mg of meperidine.
   - Fentanyl has a rapid onset, and after a submucosal or intramuscular injection the onset will occur in 7 to 15 minutes, with duration of action upto 1 to 2 hours.
   - The drug is metabolized by the liver and excreted in the urine.
   - Respiratory depression is the same as with other narcotics.
   - In higher doses administered rapidly by vein, rigidity of skeletal muscle has been reported. This effect can be reversed by naloxone along with a skeletal muscle relaxant. Bradycardia also has been reported and atropine can be used to normalize heart rate.
   - Fentanyl can be administered by the intramuscular, intravenous, or submucosal route.
   - It is not recommended for use in children under 2 years of age.
   - Dosage: 0.002 to 0.004 mg/kg

> **Chloral hydrate:** It is the commonly used premedication
> - It is an hypnotic that stimulates sleep at the cortical level, with no loss of reflexes.
> - It is contraindicated in patients with marked hepatic or renal impairment, children receiving anticoagulant therapy.
> - Dosage: 500–750 mg for children aged 2–4 years.
> - Ill effects: Nausea and vomiting.

General Anesthesia

General anesthesia is preferred in children where behavior modification and conscious sedation have failed to improve the behavior.

General anesthesia is a controlled state of unconsciousness accompanied by a loss of protective reflexes, including the ability to maintain an airway independently and respond purposefully to physical stimulation or verbal command. The use of general anesthesia sometimes is necessary to provide quality dental care for the child.[41]

Some of the points that should be considered before deciding on general anesthesia are:
1. Alternative behavioral guidance modalities
2. Dental needs of the patient
3. The effect on the quality of dental care
4. The patient's emotional development
5. The patient's medical status

Prior to general anesthesia, appropriate documentation regarding informed consent, instructions provided to the parent, dietary precautions, and preoperative health evaluation should be completed.

Indications

1. Patients who cannot cooperate due to a lack of psychological or emotional maturity and/or mental, physical, or medical disability
2. The extremely uncooperative, fearful, anxious, or uncommunicative child or adolescent
3. Patients requiring significant surgical procedures
4. Patients requiring immediate, comprehensive oral/dental care.

Contraindications

1. A healthy, cooperative patient with minimal dental needs
2. Redisposing medical conditions which would make general anesthesia inadvisable.

Patient Indicated for Treatment under General Anesthesia

1. Patients with serious medical problems who may be compromised and pose a serious medical or anesthesia risk in an nonhospitalized environment
2. Patients requiring complex or extensive dental care that can be accomplished more safely and conveniently with a multidisciplinary team of health care professionals
3. Patients who are not able to cooperate in dental clinic due to their handicapping conditions or disorders
4. Very young children who do not understand or rationalize and hence unable to cooperate in normal outpatient setting.
5. Children who has to undergo hospitalization and treatment under general anesthesia for reasons other than dental problems. Dental treatment can be simultaneously done in the operation theater under general anesthesia.

Requirements of hospital set up for dental treatment:

1. An well equipped dental unit.
2. Experience, understanding and cooperative hospital staff.
3. Availability of adequate operating room time and patient beds.
4. Readily available pediatrician.
5. Close proximity to the dentist's private office.

Steps in Hospital Procedures

Step 1: Initial examination and parent discussion

At the time of the initial dental appointment, a complete examination is performed and a detailed treatment plan is made. The treatment plan is discussed with the parents. Parents are informed about the need to perform the treatment under general anesthesia, associated risks and expenses.

Steps 2: Consultations

Medical clearance for performing dental treatment under general anesthesia should be obtained after discussion with the child's physician.

Step 3: Patient admittance

Routinely treatment is performed in the morning and the patient can be admitted to the hospital the previous day evening. A consent form for anesthesia and dental procedure should be signed by the parents or guardian.

Step 4: Preoperative procedures

Personal and medical record entry in the case sheet should be verified. Review nursing notes in the chart. Check to ensure that the patient's medical history and physical examination has been performed by the child's physician and recorded in the case sheet.

Step 5: Preoperative preparation

All the equipment available in the hospital should be checked (Fig. 5.12). Any instruments or materials not provided or available for performing dental procedure must be brought by the dental team. All the instruments must be sterilized. Experienced dental surgery assistant should be present for assistance.

On the day of the dental operation the dentist and his team should arrive at the hospital at least 1hour before the scheduled dental operation. All the personnel should change their clothing and wear operator's gown, gloves, shoe covers or special shoes provided inside the premises, head cover and surgical mask (Fig. 5.13).

The instruments and materials should be pre-arranged (Figs 5.14A and B) on a trolley.

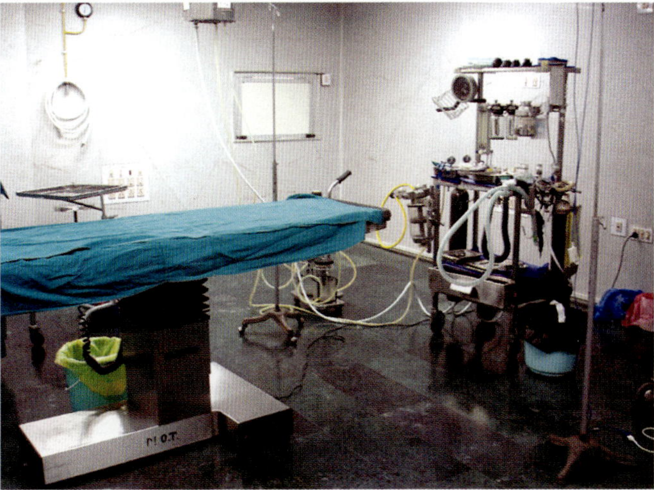

Fig. 5.12: Operation table, Boyle's apparatus and other necessary equipments in the operation theater

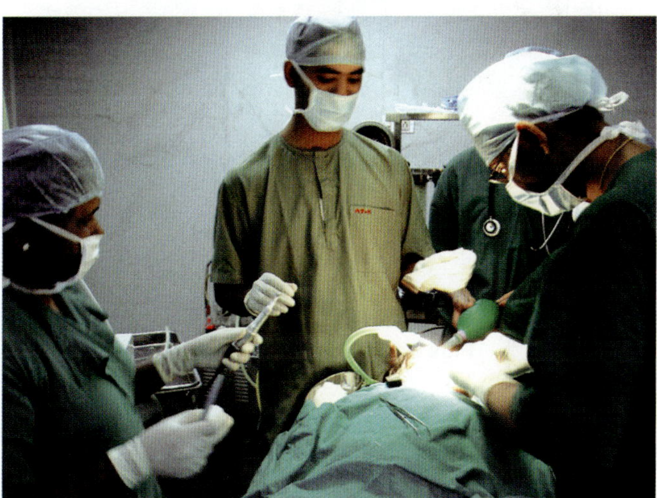

Fig. 5.13: Attire of the operating persons in the operation theater

Step 6: Anesthesia induction

The patient will be premedicated and may or may not be able to converse.

After the anesthesiologist are ready with the monitoring devices (Figs 5.15A to C) and intravenous route, induction begins. In younger children, induction may begin with a low percentage of anesthetic gases. In older children, a barbiturate may be used. Intravenous succinylcholine or a similar drug is administered to assist in the induction of the patient.

The dentist should request nasal intubation (Fig. 5.16) instead of oral intubation (Fig. 5.17) for maintenance of the anesthetic state. When the anesthesiologist has completed the placement of the nasal tube, the

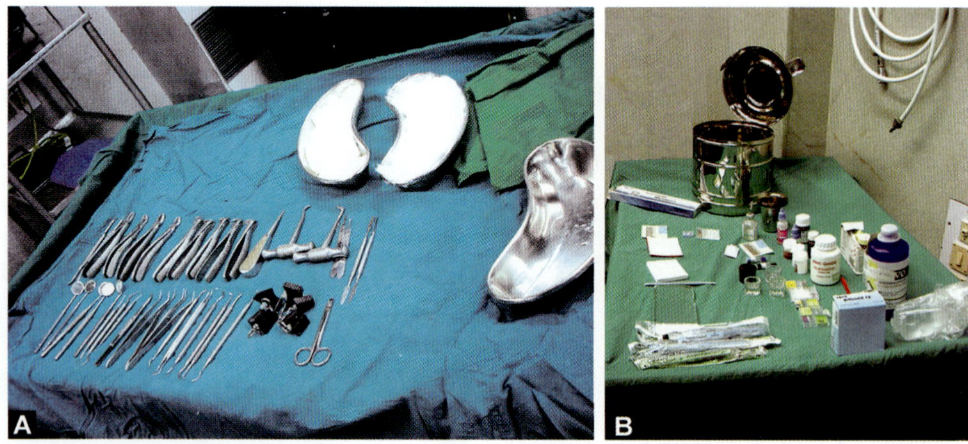

Figs 5.14A and B: Instruments and material should be arranged neatly on a trolley to be readily available

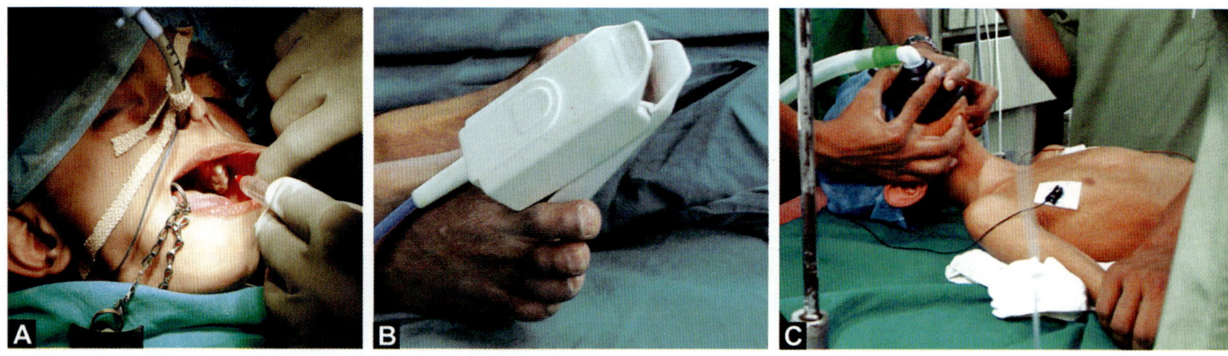

Figs 5.15A to C: Monitoring devices: (A) Intubation (Nasal); (B) Pulse oximeter; (C) Cardiac leads

tube should be taped in place on the child's face and nose. Some anesthesiologists will place an ophthalmic ointment in the eyes and then tape them shut to prevent conjunctivitis and entry of foreign bodies in the eyes.

Step 7: Dental treatment procedure

The dental surgery equipment is brought into place. A throat pack is a must and is carefully placed. The patient's lips are lubricated by petroleum jelly to avoid drying. Bite blocks (Fig. 5.18) should be used for mouth opening.

While selecting the type of treatment to be rendered to the patient following points should be remembered:
- Any two or more surfaces of caries should be restored with a stainless steel crown.
- Any incipient interproximal or developmental precarious lesions should be restored.
- There should be no heroic pulp therapy done where prognosis is a doubt.
- Indirect pulp capping and direct pulp capping procedures should be avoided

- When there is doubt as to pulpal status and the treatment choice perform the more radical one. For example when there is a doubt regarding the health of the radicular pulp perform pulpectomy instead of pulpotomy.

The anesthesiologist must be informed as to the anticipated finishing time because the amount of gaseous anesthesia can be reduced, and the patient will receive a high percentage of oxygen.

Rinse and thoroughly aspirate the mouth. Gently remove the throat pack and inspect the area for any debris. The anesthesiologist will use an aspirating tube to clear the nasal area, pharynx, and throat of debris and accumulated fluids.

Step 8: Postoperative procedures

Do not leave the operating room until the patient has recovered and reacting. Reassurance to the patient during this period is often very helpful for recovery.

The operative summary and postoperative instructions are entered in the patient's case chart.

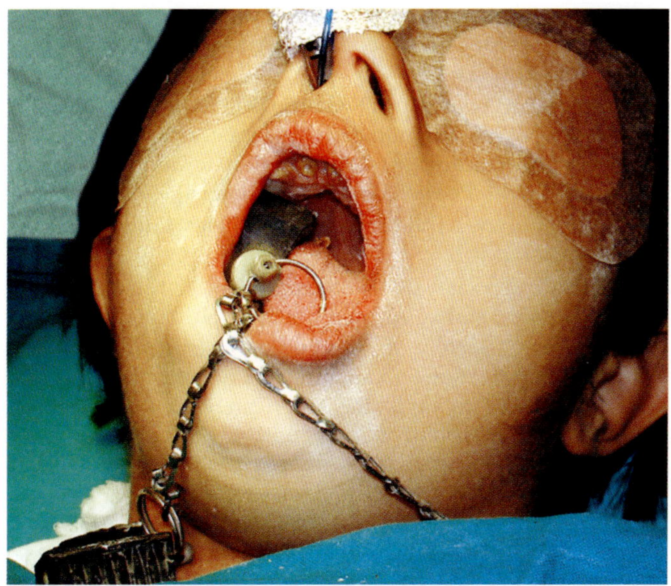

Fig. 5.16: Nasal intubation

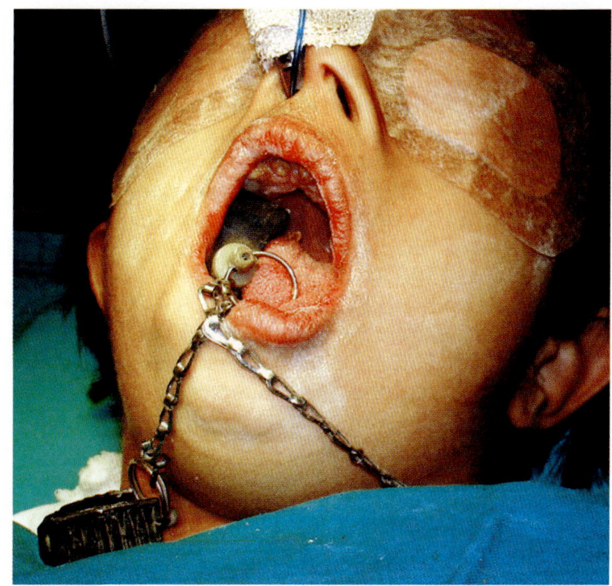

Fig. 5.18: Rubber bite blocks used to restrain the mouth

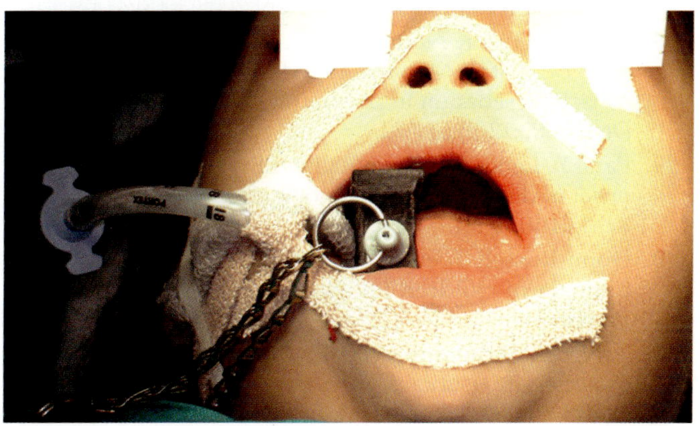

Fig. 5.17: Oral intubation. It may not be possible for nasal intubation in children less than 5 years

Step 9: Discharge and follow-up care

The patient's progress is reviewed and the patient is discharged. Discharge orders should be written after checking the nurse's notes and the patient has been evaluated by the attending anesthesiologist and physician. The discharge summary should include:

1. Patient's name, hospital number, age, sex, address
2. Date of admission and discharge
3. Diagnosis
4. Preoperative and postoperative comments
5. Procedure performed
6. Complications if any
7. Discharge status
8. Name of the anesthetist and operating person (Pedodontist)
9. Follow-up
10. Name of the person preparing the discharge summary with signature
11. Signature of the chief operating person.

Agent used for general anesthesia

1. Halothane
2. Enflurane
3. Isoflurane
4. Sevoflurane
5. Desflurane

REFERENCES

1. http://www.aapd.org/media/Policies_Guidelines/G_BehavGuide.pdf
2. Wright GZ, Stigers JI. Nonpharmacologic Management of Children's Behaviors. Dentistry for the child and adolescent, 9th Ed, Elsevier Mosby 2011;27-40.
3. Finn SB. Parent counseling and child behavior. In Clinical Pedodontics. 4th Ed. WB. Saunders Company, Philadelphia 1987.
4. Elsbach HG. Crying as a diagnostic tool. ASDC J Dent Child 1963;30:13-6.
5. Susan Mc Millan. Behavior of children and adolescents. Pediatric Dentistry, Scientific foundation and clinical practice, Stewart RE, Barber TK, Troutman KC, Wei SHY, 1982;150-64.
6. Wolpe J. Experimental neuroses as a learned behavior. Br. J Psychol 1952;43:243.
7. Braham RL, Morris ME. Text book of Pediatric Dentistry. 2nd Edition CBS Publishers, Delhi 1990;368-92

8. Binet A. New methods for the diagnosis of the intellectual level for subnormals, L'Annee Psycholgique 1905;12:191-244.

9. Forehand RS, Mc Mahon RJ. Helping the Non-Compliant Child: A Clinician's guide to parent training. New York, The Guilford Press, 166-71.

10. Lenchner V, Wright GZ. Nonpharmaco-therapeutic approaches to behavior management. In Wright, GZ Behavior management in Dentistry for children. Philadelphia. WB Saunders Co. 1975.

11. Frankl SN, Shiere FR, Fogels HR. Should the parent remain in the operatory? J Dent Child 1962;29:150-63.

12. Wright GZ. Behavior management in dentistry for children, Philadelphia, WB Saunders, 1975.

13. Chambers DW. Communicating with the young dental patient. J Am Dent Assoc 1976;93(4):793-9.

14. Peterson, GB. A day of great illumination: BF Skinner's discovery of shaping. Journal of the Experimental Analysis of Behavior, 2004;82:317-28.

15. Addleston H. Child patient training. CDS Rev 1959;38:7.

16. Bandura A. Principles of behavioral modification. New York: Holt, Rinehart and Winston, 1969.

17. Rimm DC, Masters JC. Behavior therapy: techniques and empirical findings, New York, Academic Press, 1974.

18. Pinkham JR. Voice control: an old technique reexamined. J Dent Child 1985;52:199-202.

19. Abushal MS, Adenubi JO. Attitudes of Saudi parents toward behavior management techniques in pediatric dentistry. J Dent Child 2003;70(2):104-10.

20. Levitas TC. HOME:hand over mouth exercise. J Dent Child 1974;41(3):23-25.

21. Kramer WS. Aversion-A method for modifying child behavior. J Nebr. Dent Assoc 1974;51:7.

22. Pinkhan JR. Patient management, Pediatric Dentistry, Infancy through Adolescence, 4th Edition, Elsevier Publications 2005;394-413.

23. http://www.aapd.org/media/Policies_Guidelines/G_Sedation.pdf

24. http://www.eapd.gr/dat/EE8559BA/file.pdf

25. Pediatric Dentistry. Guideline for monitoring and management of pediatric patients during and after sedation for diagnostic and therapeutic procedures: An update. Pediatr Dent 2006;28(suppl):115-32.

26. Pena BM, Krauss B. Adverse events of procedural sedation and analgesia in a pediatric emergency department. Ann Emerg Med 1999;34:483-91.

27. Coté CJ, Karl HW, Notterman DA, Weinberg JA, McCloskey C. Adverse sedation events in pediatrics: Analysis of medications used for sedation. Pediatrics 2000;106:633-44.

28. Benusis KP, Kapaun D, Furnam LJ. Respiratory depression in a child following meperidine, promethazine, and chlorpromazine premedication: Report of case. J Dent Child 1979;46:50-53.

29. Wilson S. Pharmacological management of the pediatric dental patient. Pediatr Dent 2004;26:131-6.

30. American Academy of Pediatrics, Committee on Drugs. Guidelines for monitoring and management of pediatric patients during and after sedation for diagnostic and therapeutic procedures: Addendum. Pediatrics, 2002;110:836-8.

31. American Academy of Pediatric Dentistry. Guidelines on the elective use of minimal, moderate, and deepsedation and general anesthesia for pediatric dental patients. Chicago, Ill. Pediatr Dent 2004;26(suppl):95-105.

32. http://www.aapd.org/media/Policies_Guidelines/G_Sedation.pdf

33. American Society of Anesthesiologists. New classification of physical status. Anesthesiol 1963;24:111.

34. American Society of Anesthesiologists. Practice guidelines for sedation and analgesia by nonanesthesiologists: An updated report by the American Society of Anesthesiologists task force on sedation and analgesia by nonanesthe-siologists. Anesthesiology 2002;96:1004-17.

35. Emmanouil DE, Quock RM. Advances in understanding the actions of nitrous oxide. Anesth Prog 2007;54(1):9-18.

36. Bennett RC. Sedation in dental practice. 2nd ed. St. Louis, CV Mosby Co. 1978.

37. Kupietzky A, Tal E, Shapira J, Ram D. Fasting state and episodes of vomiting in children receiving nitrous oxide for dental treatment. Pediatr Dent 2008;30(5):414-9.

38. Hosey MT. UK National Clinical Guidelines in Paediatric Dentistry. Managing anxious children: The use of conscious sedation in paediatric dentistry. Int J Paediatr Dent 2002;12(5):359-72.

39. Patel R, Lenczyk M, Hannallah RS, McGill WA. Age and onset of desaturation in apnoeic children. Can J Anaesth 1994;41(9):771-4.

40. Dunn-Russell T, et al. Oxygen saturation and diffusion hypoxia in children following nitrous oxide sedation, Pediatr Dent 1993;15(2):88-92.

41. American Academy of Pediatric Dentistry. Guideline on use of anesthesia care providers in the administration of in-office deep sedation/general anesthesia to the pediatric dental patient. Pediatr Dent 2006;28(suppl):133-5.

FURTHER READING

1. Alwin N, Murray JJ, Niven N. The effect of children's dental anxiety on the behaviour of a dentist. Int J Paediatr Dent 1994;4(1):19-24.

2. American Academy of Pediatric Dentistry Clinical Affairs Committee—Behavior Management Subcomittee; American Academy of Pediatric Dentistry Council on Clinical Affairs—Committee on Behavior Guidance.: Guideline on behavior guidance for the pediatric dental patient. Pediatr Dent 2005-2006;27 (7 Reference Manual):92-100.

3. Blankstein KC. Low-dose intravenous ketamine: an effective adjunct to conventional deep conscious sedation. J Oral Maxillofac Surg 2006;64(4):691-2.

4. Brill WA. Child behavior in a private pediatric dental practice associated with types of visits, age and socioeconomic factors J Clin Pediatr Dent 2000 Fall;25(1):1-7.

5. Cathers JW, Wilson CF, Webb MD, Alvarez ME, Schiffman T, Taylor S. A comparison of two meperidine/hydroxyzine sedation regimens for the uncooperative pediatric dental patient. Pediatr Dent 2005;27(5):395-400.

6. Chowdhury J, Vargas KG. Comparison of chloral hydrate, meperidine, and hydroxyzine to midazolam regimens for oral sedation of pediatric dental patients. Pediatr Dent 2005;27(3):191-7.

7. Collado V, Hennequin M, Faulks D, Mazille MN, Nicolas E, Koscielny S, Onody P. Modification of behavior with 50% nitrous oxide/oxygen conscious sedation over repeated visits for dental treatment a 3-year prospective study. J Clin Psychopharmacol 2006;26(5):474-81.

8. Efron LA, Sherman JA. Five tips for managing pediatric dental anxiety. Dent Today 2005;24(6):104-5.

9. Efron LA, Sherman JA. Tips for managing children with attention deficit hyperactivity disorder in the dental setting. NY State Dent J 2005;71(3):18-20.

10. Foster T, Perinpanayagam H, Pfaffenbach A, Certo M. Recurrence of early childhood caries after comprehensive treatment with general anesthesia and follow-up. J Dent Child (Chic) 2006;73(1):25-30.

11. Fox C, Newton JT. A controlled trial of the impact of exposure to positive images of dentistry on anticipatory dental fear in children. Community Dent Oral Epidemiol 2006;34(6):455-9.

12. Greenbaum PE, Turner C, Cook EW 3rd, Melamed BG. Dentists' voice control: effects on children's disruptive and affective behavior. Health Psychol 1990;9(5):546-58.

13. Guidelines for behavior management of The American Academy of Pediatric Dentistry. Va Dent J 1994; 71(1):20-5.

14. Hijazi OM, Haidar NA, Al-Eissa YA. Chloral hydrate. An effective agent for sedation in children with age and weight dependent response. Saudi Med J 2005; 26(5):746-9.

15. Hosey MT, Makin A, Jones RM, Gilchrist F, Carruthers M. Propofol intravenous conscious sedation for anxious children in a specialist paediatric dentistry unit. Int J Paediatr Dent 2004;14(1):2-8.

16. Hosey MT. Anxious children: coping in dental practice. Dent Update 1995;22(5):210-5.

17. Kotsanos N, Arhakis A, Coolidge T. Parental presence versus absence in the dental operatory: a technique to manage the uncooperative child dental patient. Eur J Paediatr Dent 2005;6(3):144-8.

18. Lal S. Consent in dentistry. Pac Health Dialog 2003; 10(1):102-5. Review.

19. Leitch J, Lennox C, Robb N. Recent advances in conscious sedation. Dent Update 2005;32(4):199-200, 202-3.

20. Loyola-Rodriguez JP, Aguilera-Morelos AA, Santos-Diaz MA, Zavala-Alonso V, Davila-Perez C, Olvera-Delgado H, Patino-Marin N, De Leon-Cobian I. Oral rehabilitation under dental general anesthesia, conscious sedation, and conventional techniques in patients affected by cerebral palsy. J Clin Pediatr Dent 2004; 28(4):279-84.

21. Malviya S, Milgrom P, Moore PA, Shampaine G, Silverman M, Williams RL, Wilson S. Balancing efficacy and safety in the use of oral sedation in dental outpatients. J Am Dent Assoc 2006;137(4):502-13.

22. Meyer S, Grundmann U, Gottschling S, Kleinschmidt S, Gortner L. Sedation and analgesia for brief diagnostic and therapeutic procedures in children. Eur J Pediatr. 2007;166(4):291-302. Epub 2007 Jan 5.

23. Murray JJ, Niven N. The child as a dental patient. Curr Opin Dent 1992;2:59-65. Review

24. Nash DA. Engaging children's co-operation in the dental environment through effective communication. Pediatr Dent 2006;28(5):455-9.

25. Newton JT, Shah S, Patel H, Sturmey P. Non-pharmacological approaches to behaviour management in children. Dent Update 2003;30(4):194-9.

26. Palmer NO, Fleming P, Randall C. Pharmaceutical prescribing for children. Part 6. The management of medical emergencies in children in dental practice. Prim Dent Care 2007;14(1):29-33.

27. Peretz B, Gluck G. Magic trick: a behavioural strategy for the management of strong-willed children. Int J Paediatr Dent 2005;15(6):429-36.

28. Piedalue RJ, Milnes A. An overview of non-pharmacological pedodontic behaviour management techniques for the general practitioner. J Can Dent Assoc 1990; 56(2):137-44.

29. Pike AR. Prevention of anxiety during the first dental visit of a three-year-old child. Gen Dent 1995;43(5):448-51.

30. Primosch RE, Guelmann M. Comparison of drops versus spray administration of intranasal midazolam in two- and three-year-old children for dental sedation. Pediatr Dent 2005;27(5):401-8.

31. Rakaf HA, Bello LL, Turkustani A, Adenubi JO. Intra-nasal Midazolam in conscious sedation of young Pediatric dental patients. Int J Pediatr Dentist 2001;11:33-40.

32. Riley JL 3rd, Gilbert GH. Childhood dental history and adult dental attitudes and beliefs. Int Dent J 2005; 55(3):142-50.

33. Roberts JF. How important are techniques? The empathic approach to working with children. ASDC J Dent Child 1995;62(1):38-43. Review.

34. Samra-Quintero PA, Bernardoni-Socorro C, Borjas AM, Fuenmayor NR, Estevez J, Arteaga-Vizcaino M. Changes in blood pressure in children undergoing psychological treatment before dental procedures. Acta Odontol Latinoam 2006;19(1):9-12.

35. Shashikiran ND, Reddy SV, Yavagal CM. Conscious sedation—an artist's science! An Indian experience with midazolam. J Indian Soc Pedod Prev Dent. 2006;24(1):7-14.

36. Soares F, Britto LR, Vertucci FJ, Guelmann M. Interdisciplinary approach to endodontic therapy for uncooperative children in a dental school environment. J Dent Educ 2006;70(12):1362-5.

37. Ten Berge M, Veerkamp J, Hoogstraten J. Dentists' behavior in response to child dental fear. ASDC J Dent Child 1999;66(1):36-40, 12.

38. Ten Berge M, Veerkamp JS, Hoogstraten J, Prins PJ. On the structure of childhood dental fear, using the Dental Subscale of the Children's Fear Survey Schedule. Eur J Paediatr Dent 2002;3(2):73-8.

39. Tsai CL, Tsai YL, Lin YT, Lin YT. A retrospective study of dental treatment under general anesthesia of children

with or without a chronic illness and/or a disability. Chang Gung Med J 2006;29(4):412-8.

40. Wilson KE, Girdler NM, Welbury RR. A comparison of oral midazolam and nitrous oxide sedation for dental extractions in children. Anaesthesia 2006;61(12):1138-44.
41. Wilson S. Pharmacological management of the pediatric dental patient. Pediatr Dent 2004;26(2):131-6.
42. Yamada CJ. New challenges in management of the anxious pediatric dental patient. Hawaii Dent J. 2006;37(5):14-6.

QUESTIONS

1. Define fear and what are the different types of fear?
2. Describe the factors influencing child's behavior.
3. Explain the parent-child relationship in terms of child behavior.
4. Child parent separation.
5. Enumerate different classification of children's behavior and discuss any two of them in detail.
6. What is behavior guidance? Explain the principles of behavior guidance technique.
7. What are the different techniques of behavior guidance?
8. Child's first dental visit.
9. Role of communication in behavior guidance.
10. What is behavioral shaping?
11. Explain tell-show-do and contingency management technique.
12. Discuss in detail the hand over mouth exercise (HOME).
13. What are the different protective stabilization methods?
14. What are the guidelines for the use of premedication in dental practice?
15. Define conscious sedation. Describe in detail inhalation conscious sedation.
16. Enumerate the differences between conscious sedation and general anesthesia.
17. Define general anesthesia. Explain the indications, contraindications and requirements of hospital set-up for dental treatment under general anesthesia?

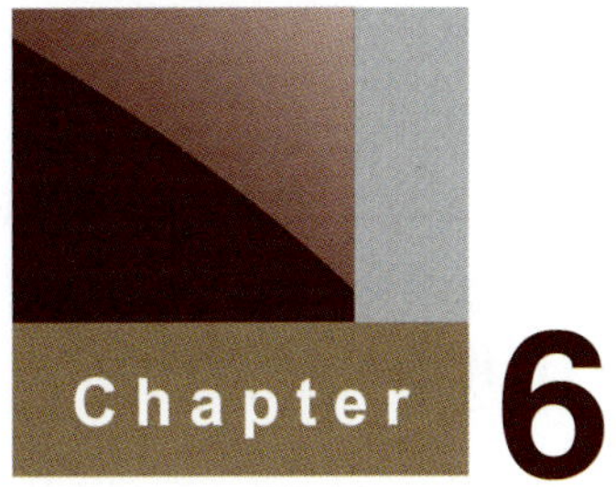

Preventive and Interceptive Orthodontics

INTRODUCTION

Monitoring the developing dentition and guiding the eruption during the primary, mixed, and permanent phase is an integral component of comprehensive oral healthcare. The purpose of this is to achieve a stable, functional, and esthetically acceptable occlusion. Early diagnosis and successful treatment of developing malocclusions can have both short-term and long-term benefits while achieving the goals of occlusal harmony and function and dentofacial esthetics. Pedodontists are in an advantageous position in identifying a developing malocclusion, thus reducing or eliminating the need for corrective therapy in later adult life. Management of orthodontic problems includes the recognition and diagnosis of possible risk factors and appropriate treatment of dentofacial abnormalities.[1-4]

According to revised American Association of Pediatric Dentistry (AAPD)[5] guidelines, a thorough clinical examination, appropriate records, differential diagnosis, sequential treatment plan are necessary to manage any condition affecting the developing dentition.

Clinical examination should include:
1. Facial analysis to:
    a. Identify adverse transverse growth patterns including asymmetries
    b. Identify adverse vertical growth patterns
    c. Identify adverse sagittal (anteroposterior) growth patterns and dental anteroposterior occlusal disharmonies
    d. Assess esthetics and identify orthopedic and orthodontic interventions that may improve

esthetics and resultant self-image and emotional development.

2. Intraoral examination to:
   a. Assess overall oral health status
   b. Determine the functional status of the patient's occlusion.
3. Functional analysis to:
   a. Determine functional factors associated with the malocclusion
   b. Detect deleterious habits
   c. Detect temporomandibular joint dysfunction, which may require additional diagnostic procedures.

Diagnostic records include:

1. Extraoral and intraoral photographs to:
   a. Supplement clinical findings with oriented facial and intraoral photographs
   b. Establish a database for documenting facial changes during treatment
2. Diagnostic dental casts to:
   a. Assess the occlusal relationship
   b. Determine arch length requirements for intra-arch tooth size relationships
   c. Determine arch length requirements for inter-arch tooth size relationships
   d. Determine location and extent of arch asymmetry
3. Intraoral and panoramic radiographs to:
   a. Establish dental age
   b. Assess eruption problems
   c. Estimate the size and presence of unerupted teeth
   d. Identify dental anomalies/pathology
4. Lateral and anteroposterior cephalograms to:
   a. Produce a comprehensive cephalometric analysis of the relative dental and skeletal components in the anteroposterior, vertical, and transverse dimensions
   b. Establish a baseline growth record for longitudinal assessment of growth and displacement of the jaws
5. Other diagnostic views (e.g. magnetic resonance imaging, computed tomographic scans) for hard and soft tissue imaging as indicated by history and clinical examination.

A child should be seen by his dentist as early as 2½ years and should include thorough clinical examination with diagnostic records like the X-rays, study models and photographs.

By the time the child is 5 years. The child should be placed on a definite schedule for obtaining longitudinal records.

GUIDELINES FOR MONITORING DURING EACH PHASE OF DENTITION

1. *Primary dentition stage:* Evaluation of primary teeth includes identification of:
   a. All anomalies of tooth number and size
   b. Anterior and posterior crossbites
   c. Presence of habits along with their dental and skeletal sequelae.

   Radiographs are taken based upon risk assessment/history. Habits and posterior crossbites should be diagnosed and addressed as early as feasible. Parents should be informed about findings of adverse growth and developing malocclusions. Interventions/treatment can be recommended if diagnosis can be made, treatment is appropriate and possible, and parents are supportive and desire to have treatment done.

2. *Early mixed dentition stage:* Palpation for unerupted teeth should be part of every examination. Panoramic, occlusal, and periapical radiographs, as indicated at the time of eruption of the lower incisors and first permanent molars, provide diagnostic information concerning:
   a. Anomalies of tooth numbers (e.g. missing, supernumerary, fused, gemination).
   b. Tooth size and shape (e.g. peg or small lateral incisors).
   c. Positions (e.g. ectopic first permanent molars).

   Space analysis can be done to evaluate arch length/crowding at the time of incisor eruption. Treatment should address: (1) habits; (2) arch length shortage; (3) intervention for crowded incisors; (4) intervention for ectopic molars and incisors; (5) holding of leeway space; (6) crossbites; and (7) adverse skeletal growth. Treatment should take advantage of high rates of growth and prevent worsened adverse dental and skeletal growth.

3. *Mid-to-late mixed dentition stage:* Ectopic tooth positions should be diagnosed, especially canines, bicuspids, and second permanent molars. Intervention for ectopic teeth may include extractions and space maintenance to aid eruption and reduce the risk of need for surgical bracket placement and orthodontic traction. Intervention for treatment of skeletal disharmonies and crowding may be instituted at this stage.

4. *Adolescent dentition stage:* If not instituted earlier, orthodontic diagnosis and treatment should be planned for Class I crowded, Class II, and Class III malocclusions as well as posterior and anterior crossbites. Third molars should be monitored as to

position and space, and parents should be informed. In full permanent dentition, final orthodontic diagnosis and treatment can provide the most functional occlusion.

Preventive and interceptive orthodontics are the two phases of orthodontics that is best practiced in a developing stage.[6]

Preventive orthodontics: According to Graber "is the action taken to preserve the integrity of what appears to be a normal occlusion at a specific time". The procedures that are done are aimed to prevent the development of any risk factors that would probably cause malocclusion. Hence preventive orthodontics are undertaken before the actual malocclusion develops, thus preventing the development of future malocclusion.

Interceptive orthodontics "is employed to recognize and eliminate potential irregularities and malpositions in the developing dentofacial complex".

Difference between preventing and intercepting depends on the timing of the service that is rendered.

PREVENTIVE ORTHODONTICS

It involves taking radiographs and use of study models to identify any risk factors that may lead to malocclusion in the later life. It also involves counseling parents regarding these risk factors and other needs of the child so as to achieve good oral health.

Indication of future malocclusion

- Deviation from the normal growth and development.
- Disharmony between the skeletal, muscle and dental structures, as in oral habits.
- Premature loss of deciduous teeth.
- Extensive carious lesions, especially involving the proximal sides.

Role of Radiographs in Preventive Orthodontics

To identify:
- Congenital missing teeth
- Supernumerary tooth
- Deviation in eruptive and resorptive patterns
- Caries and other pathology.

Role of Study Models in Preventive Orthodontics

- As permanent records
- For measurement of arch length and arch width
- To estimate space adequacy
- To study growth changes through serial study casts.

Prenatal Advice to Mother as a Part of Preventive Orthodontics

- Regarding healthy diet and nutrition that will aid in normal growth and development of the fetus.
- Proper nursing technique which will influence the functional and psychological development of the child
- Relation of mother's health and the tooth development of the child.

Postnatal Care as a Part of Preventive Orthodontics

- Care of the deciduous teeth, such as early detection of caries, oral hygiene instructions, fluoride therapy and space maintenance
- Removal of supernumerary tooth, as it can cause impaction or midline diastema
- Removal of retained deciduous tooth, as it may deviate the path of eruption of the successor
- Removal of ankylosed tooth, if the successor is present
- Correction of premature contact
- Oral habit correction
- Use of mouth protector
- Correction of abnormal frenal attachment.

INTERCEPTIVE ORTHODONTICS

It includes all procedures undertaken to reduce the severity of malocclusion, so that normal occlusion can progress in future. It includes:
- Serial extraction
- Occlusal equilibration—like removal of premature contact and correction of minor malocclusion
- Control of abnormal habits
- Muscle exercise
- Frenum correction
- Removal of supernumerary teeth, ankylosed teeth or any soft or hard tissue that form barriers for eruption of permanent teeth.
- Space regaining following premature loss of deciduous tooth/teeth leading to space closure.

Aims of Preventive and Interceptive Orthodontics

The aim is to achieve:
1. Permanent dentition with all teeth in good alignment and contacts anatomically compatible with a healthy periodontium.
2. Dental arches well related in all three planes of space with an optimal intercuspation that is substantially identical in both centric occlusion and centric relation.
3. Dentition in harmony with esthetics in frontal and profile appearance.

4. Stability between skeletal, dental and muscular components.

SERIAL EXTRACTION

Gross tooth size arch length discrepancy problems are those in which there is a significant difference between the size of all the permanent teeth and the space available for them within the alveolar housing. As no clinically useful correlation has been established till date regarding the size of primary teeth and that of the permanent teeth, cases of tooth material excess cannot be diagnosed until early mixed dentition. Depending on the age at which the problem is first observed, the protocol and rationale for the treatment of a case of gross discrepancy varies. It may be treated early with sequential removal of certain deciduous teeth followed by permanent teeth in the mixed dentition or with premolar extractions and subsequent fixed appliance therapy in the permanent dentition. The goal of early treatment is to create space in the mixed dentition for the eruption of permanent teeth into more favorable positions over basal bone to prevent or reduce the complexity of future orthodontic treatment in the permanent dentition.

The early treatment of space deficiency in mixed dentition by way of sequential removal of certain teeth is commonly known as serial extraction therapy. It is an interceptive orthodontic procedure done to guide the eruption of permanent teeth into a favorable occlusion in order to intercept/reduce the severity of a developing malocclusion.

Historical Perspective

It was always recognized that the removal of one or more irregular teeth would improve the appearance of the remaining teeth. Bunon in his ' Essay on Diseases of the Teeth', published in 1743, made the first reference to the removal of deciduous teeth to achieve a better alignment of the permanent teeth. Though the procedure was introduced to the profession 250 years ago, it has been grossly misunderstood.

The term serial extraction was introduced by Kjellgren of Sweden in 1929. The term serial extraction embraced all planned extraction of any teeth in order to take advantage of eruption and natural drifting. Unfortunately, Kjellgrens's phrase resulted in indiscriminate removal of teeth by individuals who understood the procedure simply as the removal of teeth serially.

Hotz of Switzerland, however, referred to the procedure as guidance of eruption. This term was more suited to the procedure as it involved an understanding of the growth and development of the erupting dentition.

Dale and Dale suggested the use of term guidance of occlusion as it is the final occlusion and not mere the presence of well aligned dentition which is of concern to the clinician.

In addition to Kjellgren and Hotz, Heath of Australia and Nance, Loyd, Dewel and Mayne of the United States also contributed immensely to the development of the serial extraction therapy. Nance, who presented clinics on his method of "progressive extraction" in the 1940's has been called the "father" of serial extraction philosophy in the United States.

Indications

Serial extraction therapy is indicated in cases presenting with deficient space in the transitional dentition as shown by the mixed dentition analysis; provided there is a harmonious facial skeleton anteroposteriorly, transversely and vertically.

The space deficiency might manifest as any one or a combination of the following:

1. Premature unilateral loss of a deciduous canine with resultant midline shift to the same side.
   This may be due to the pressure of the erupting crown of a permanent lateral incisor against the root of deciduous canine. As soon as it is lost, the incisors will shift into the space created, relieving the pressure on the remaining canine.
2. Premature bilateral loss of deciduous canines in the lower arch resulting in lingual collapse of incisors
3. Lingual eruption of lateral incisors/canines erupting mesially over the lateral incisors.
   Either of the situation is suggestive of arch length deficiency.
4. Mesial drift of buccal segments. Rotation and tipping of permanent molars in either arch are usually a sign of mesial drift of buccal teeth. If the molars are rotated/tipped excessively, case should be considered for comprehensive orthodontic therapy.
5. Abnormal eruption direction and eruption sequence.
6. Flaring of incisors especially in the lower arch.
7. Ectopic eruption/abnormal resorption.
8. Labial stripping or gingival recession, usually of a lower incisor. The gingival recession and alveolar destruction on labial surface of one or several of mandibular incisors is indicative of an arch length deficiency.

General Rules

The extraction of permanent teeth should be never taken casually; it should never be done by clinicians unless they have the technical skills to correct all the sequelae of those extractions. Though some of the extraction space will be utilized for the spontaneous alignment of the crowded teeth, comprehensive precision appliance therapy is needed to close the remaining space, parallel the roots, establish the occlusal plane and to get a good intercuspation.

Eisner has suggested the following rules as an insurance against unwanted complications.

Rule 1: There must be a Class I molar relationship bilaterally.

Rule 2: The facial skeleton must be balanced anteroposteriorly, vertically and mediolaterally.

Rule 3: The discrepancy must be atleast 5 mm in all four quadrants.

Rule 4: The dental midlines must coincide.

Rule 5: There must be neither an open bite nor a deep bite.

The more the case satisfies the above requirements, easier it is to treat the case and better will be the results.

Diagnostic Records

Along with the routine diagnostic records like case history and clinical examination, one needs to obtain a set of study models and a complete series of long cone technique periapical radiographs or a panoramic radiograph.

The study models are necessary to do the mixed dentition analysis and to calculate the amount of crowding existing in the arches.

The radiographs help in evaluating the following:

1. Evaluation of dental age of the patient including status of eruption of the permanent teeth and resorption of roots of deciduous teeth.
2. Congenital absence of teeth.
3. Presence of supernumerary teeth.
4. Detection of any abnormal position or eruptive pathway of the permanent teeth in the alveolar bone.
5. Detection of any pathologic condition in the early stages.

Cephalometric radiographs help one to assess the relationship between the various craniofacial structures and the dentoalveolar structures. It is useful for the following:

1. Evaluation of sagittal and vertical jaw positions including the vertical facial proportions.
2. Incisor inclinations there by helping in total space analysis.
3. Classification of facial patterns.

Technique of Serial Extraction

There is no single technique for serial extraction which can guarantee success in all patients. The treatment is initiated based on a tentative diagnosis and it may be necessary to re-evaluate these tentative decisions and change them several times during the tenure of the treatment.

The serial extraction therapy is usually done in three stages with each of the stages accomplishing a specific purpose.

1. *Removal of deciduous canines between 8-9 years of age*: The immediate purpose of extraction of deciduous canines is to permit the optimal alignment of the erupting lateral incisors. It prevents the palatal eruption of the maxillary incisors in crossbite and lingual eruption of the mandibular incisors. The correct position of the lateral incisors prevents the mesial migration of the canines into unfavorable positions which might warrant complicated fixed mechanotherapy at a later date. One should also understand that the space for the erupting canine is compromised by allowing the optimal alignment of lateral incisors. This step is well suited for the maxillary arch as the first premolars erupt ahead of the canines.

   In the mandibular arch where the canines erupt ahead of the premolars, this step needs to be modified. In such cases, the deciduous canines are maintained in their position and the first deciduous molars are extracted to hasten the eruption of the first premolar.

2. *Removal of the first deciduous molars about 12 months after the extraction of deciduous canines:* The purpose of the extraction of the first deciduous molars is to accelerate the eruption of the first premolars ahead of the canines. It is dicey in the mandibular arch where the normal sequence is for the canine to erupt ahead of first premolar. Hence, this maneuver is seldom successful in the lower arch.

   In cases with Class I malocclusions where first premolar is locked below the permanent canine and the second deciduous molar, it is preferred to extract the first deciduous molars ahead of the deciduous canines so as to accelerate the eruption of first premolar. Sometimes the enucleation of unerupted premolar is done, so as to obtain the optimal benefits of the procedure. Second deciduous molars which interfere with the eruption of the first premolars (owing to a convex mesial bulge) may have to be removed to facilitate the eruption of premolars. But this might necessitate the placement of a space maintainer to prevent the mesial drift of the first permanent molar.

3. *Removal of the erupting first premolars:* The purpose of extraction of the first premolars is to allow the canine to drift distally into the space created by the extraction. Bulging canine eminences have been

observed to move distally on their own into the extraction sites. It is seen more often in the maxillary arch as the maxillary premolar erupts ahead of the lower first premolar.

Alternative Methods

There are no hard and fast rules or cook book approaches which can be applied to all the cases indicated for serial extraction therapy. Though the procedure is initiated when the patient is about 8 years of age with an interval of 6-12 months between each step, there are a number variables which can affect the choice of teeth and timing of extraction. These variables include dental age of the patient, sequence of eruption and the response to the already initiated treatment procedure.

Since the teeth tend to tip into the extraction site of the 1st premolars there is a tendency for the bite to deepen which can be prevented by placement of an acrylic bite plane. Cases showing excessive mesial drifting of the posterior teeth can be managed by use of a removable appliance which could be used in retraction of canines. A lingual holding arch in the mandible might be needed in cases with severe space deficiency to prevent the uprighting of the incisors (especially in cases showing deep bite tendency). Maxillary molars showing a mesio-lingual rotation requires a maxillary holding arch.

PROBLEMS ENCOUNTERED IN PRIMARY AND MIXED DENTITION PERIODS AND ITS MANAGEMENT

The most common problems encountered in primary and mixed dentition periods are:
1. Crossbite, diastema and deep bite
2. Developing malocclusions
3. Space management
4. Oral habits

CROSSBITE MANAGEMENT[7-12]

Anterior and posterior crossbites are malocclusions which involve one or more teeth in which the maxillary teeth occlude lingually with the antagonistic mandibular teeth. If the midlines undergo a compensatory or habitual shift when the teeth occlude in crossbite is termed as functional shift. A crossbite can be of dental or skeletal origin or a combination of both.

Anterior Crossbite

A simple anterior crossbite is of dental origin if the molar occlusion is Class I and the malocclusion is the result of an abnormal axial inclination of maxillary anterior teeth.

This condition should be differentiated from a Class III skeletal malocclusion where the crossbite is the result of the basal bone position.

Dental crossbites result from the tipping or rotation of a tooth or teeth. The condition is localized and does not involve the basal bone. Skeletal crossbites involve disharmony of the craniofacial skeleton.

Treatment Considerations

Crossbites should be considered in the context of the patient's total treatment needs.
Anterior crossbite can lead to:
1. Attrition of tooth/teeth
2. Altered skeletal growth
3. Decreased arch perimeter
4. Thinning of the labial plate of the alveolar bone and gingival recession in relation to the lower teeth
5. Poor esthetics

A simple anterior crossbite can be aligned as soon as the condition is noted, if there is sufficient space; otherwise, space needs to be created first.

Appliances Used for Correction of Anterior Crossbite

A. Tongue blade
B. Inclined plane
C. Composite plane
D. Reverse stainless steel crown
E. Hawley's appliance with Z spring
F. Use of screws embedded in acrylic

Tongue Blade Therapy (Fig. 6.1)

It is used while the incisors are still erupting and when single tooth is in crossbite. The tongue blade is inserted at an angle between the teeth and the patient is asked to bite firmly for 5 seconds followed by rest. This is repeated 25 times for 3 times a day. It is discontinued if unsuccessful even after 2 weeks. The main disadvantage with this is that the patient cooperation is required.

Inclined Plane (Figs 6.2 and 6.3)

It is used when more than one teeth are in crossbite. The appliance is made of acrylic and produces a forward sliding motion of the maxillary incisors on closure. This appliance should not be worn for more than 4 weeks as it may cause supraeruption of the posterior teeth, leading to anterior open bite.

The child may experience temporary discomfort in speech and food intake.

Composite Plane

An inclined plane is fabricated on the lower incisors with composite instead of acrylic.

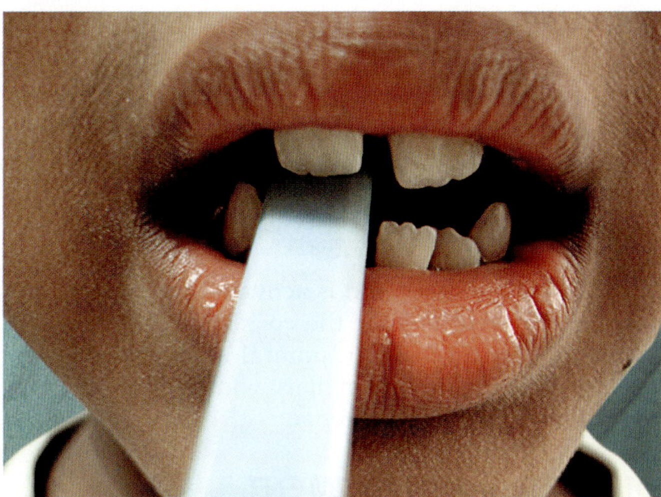

Fig. 6.1: Tongue blade in position

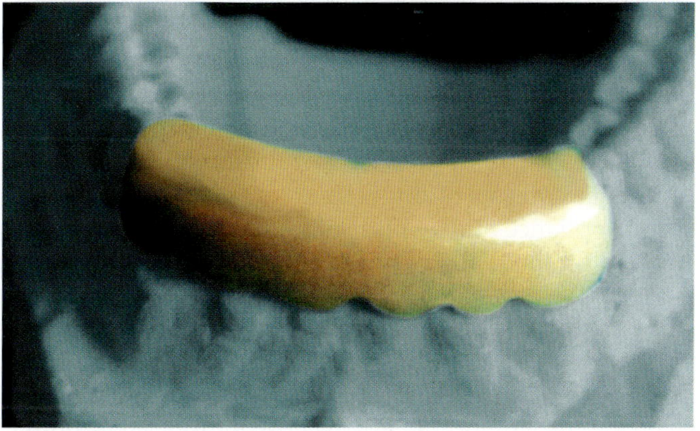

Fig. 6.2: Inclined plane for the correction of anterior crossbite

Reverse Stainless Steel Crown (Fig. 6.4)

It is used when there is a single tooth crossbite. The crown is cemented backward on the maxillary incisor. This forces the upper tooth to move out towards the lip as the child bites down on the lower teeth. The crossbite can be corrected in 2-4 weeks.

Maxillary Appliances with Z' Springs and Posterior Bite Plane (Figs 6.5A and B).

It is used when many teeth are in crossbite along with posterior bite plane. The posterior bite plane is used to keep the anterior teeth out of occlusion, so that the incisors can jump the bite.

Screws Embedded in Acrylic (Fig. 6.6)

The appliance consists of jackscrew inserted in a palatal acrylic appliance. It is a removable, slow expansion device. Every turn (1/4) opens the midline by 0.25 mm and is activated every week. A total of 4.5 mm expansion can be achieved. It is activated by a small pin. The same appliance can be used as retainer for 3-6 months. Since it is a removal appliance oral hygiene maintenance is easier.

Posterior Crossbite

Early correction of unilateral posterior crossbites has been shown to improve functional conditions significantly and largely eliminate morphological and positional asymmetries of the mandible.

Functional shifts should be eliminated as soon as possible with early correction to avoid asymmetric growth.

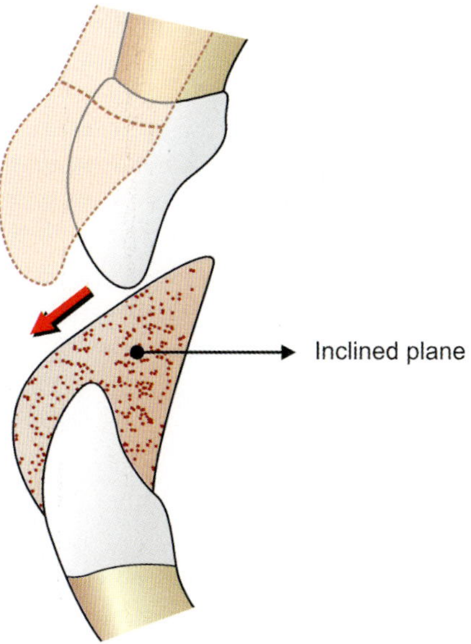

Fig. 6.3: Diagram of the slope of inclined plane showing 45° slope, over which the upper incisors slide in a downward and forward direction

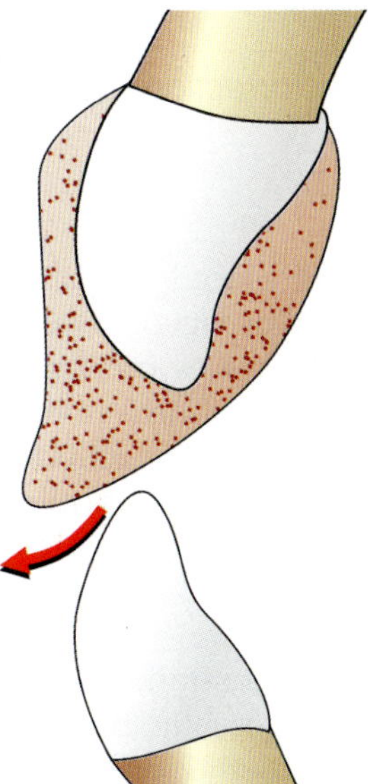

Fig. 6.4: Reverse stainless steel crown cemented on the upper incisor for the correction of anterior crossbite

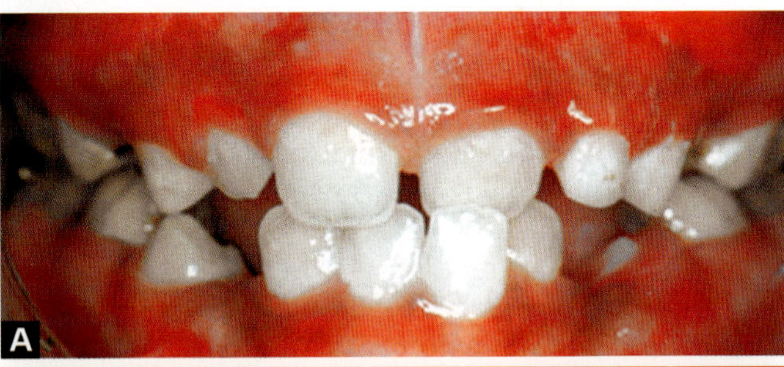

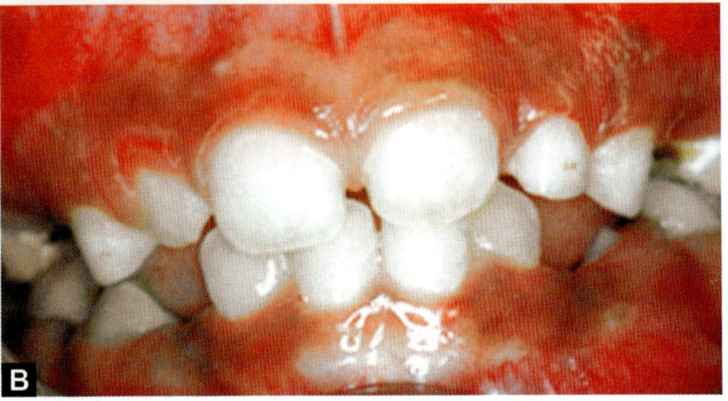

Figs 6.5A and B: Crossbite correction with Z' springs:
(A) Pretreatment; (B) Post-treatment

Treatment decisions depend on the:
1. Amount and type of movement (tipping vs bodily movement, rotation, or dental vs orthopedic movement)
2. Space available
3. Anteroposterior, transverse, and vertical skeletal relationships
4. Growth status
5. Patient cooperation.

Appliance Used for Correction of Posterior Crossbite

Cross Elastics

Bands with hooks are placed on the palatal aspect of upper tooth and buccal aspect of lower tooth that are in crossbite. Orthodontic elastics are engaged in the hooks and worn for 24 hours/day. Correction may take 3 weeks to 3 months. More change will be reflected in the position of the maxillary molars due to cancellous nature of the maxillary alveolar bone.

Jack Screw

The appliance design is similar to the one used for correction of anterior crossbite, but the position of the screw is more posterior in the midline. There are chances of dentoalveolar tipping of posterior teeth and requires patient cooperation and constant evaluation.

Fixed Porter Arch or Quad Helix Appliance

It is a fixed device with molar bands cemented of the first permanent molar. The disadvantage is that it is difficult to fabricate and adjusting is done without removal from the mouth. It is adjusted once a month and requires 3 to 4 months for correction.

Rapid Palatal Expansion Appliance

It is a fixed appliance and is activated twice daily. It is worn for 2 months after the correction for retention. There is splitting of midpalatal suture producing orthopedic increase in maxillary width reflected by the formation of midline diastema.

DIASTEMA MANAGEMENT

Etiology of diastema can be due to ugly duckling stage, large frenum, mesiodens, habits, peg shaped lateral incisors, loss of tooth resulting in drift, discrepancies between tooth size and jaw size. Management is aimed at removal of the etiological factor. Removal or fixed appliance can be used to correct the diastema. Removal appliance consists of finger springs or a split labial bow. Fixed appliance utilizes elastics engaged on to the brackets bonded on the labial surface of the central incisors.

DEEP BITE MANAGEMENT

Usually seen due to infraeruption of posterior teeth and overclosure of mandible. Also seen in temporomandibular joint (TMJ) dysplasias due to imbalance caused by temporalis and lateral pterygoid. Anterior bite plane can be given that allows eruption of premolars and relieves the muscle spasm.

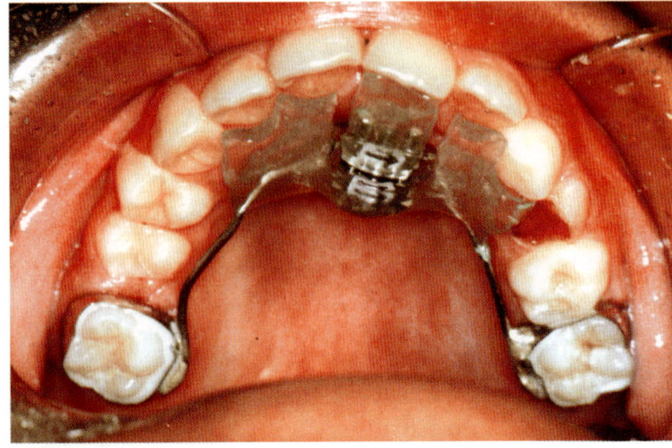

Fig. 6.6: Appliance with screw for the correction of crossbite

DEVELOPING MALOCCLUSIONS IN CHILDREN

Class II Malocclusion (AAPD)[5]

Class II malocclusion (distocclusion) may be unilateral or bilateral and involves a distal relationship of the mandible to the maxilla or the mandibular teeth to maxillary teeth. It may be due to dental, skeletal or combination factors.

Factors to consider when planning orthodontic intervention for Class II malocclusion are:
a. Facial growth pattern
b. Amount of anterior posterior discrepancy
c. Patient age
d. Projected patient compliance
e. Space analysis
f. Anchorage requirements
g. Patient and parent acceptance.

Treatment modalities include:
a. Extraoral appliances (headgear)
b. Functional appliances
c. Fixed appliances
d. Tooth extraction and interarch elastics
e. Orthodontics with orthognathic surgery.

Class III Malocclusion

Class III malocclusion (meso-occlusion) may be unilateral or bilateral and involves a mesial relationship of the mandible to the maxilla or mandibular teeth to maxillary teeth. It may be due to dental, skeletal or combination factors.

The etiology of Class III malocclusions can be hereditary, environmental, or both.

Factors to consider when planning orthodontic intervention for Class III malocclusion are:
1. Facial growth pattern
2. Amount of anteroposterior discrepancy
3. Patient age
4. Projected patient compliance
5. Space analysis
6. Anchorage (headgear)
7. Functional appliances
8. Fixed appliances
9. Tooth extraction
10. Interarch elastics
11. Orthodontics with orthognathic surgery

Tooth Size/Arch Length Discrepancy and Crowding[13-17]

Arch length discrepancies include inadequate arch length and crowding of the dental arches, excess arch length and spacing, and tooth size discrepancy, often referred to as a Bolton discrepancy.

These arch length discrepancies may be found in conjunction with complicating and other etiological factors including missing teeth, supernumerary teeth, and fused or geminated teeth. Inadequate arch length with resulting incisor crowding is a common occurrence with various negative sequelae and is particularly common in the early mixed dentition.

Initial assessment may be done in early mixed dentition, when mandibular incisors begin to erupt utilizing appropriate radiographs. Comprehensive diagnostic analysis and evaluation of maxillary and mandibular skeletal relationships, direction and pattern of growth, facial profile, facial width, muscle balance, and dental and occlusal findings including tooth positions, arch length analysis, and leeway space is required.

Treatment considerations include:
1. Making space for permanent incisors to erupt and become straight naturally through primary canine extraction and space/arch length maintenance.
2. Orthodontic alignment of permanent teeth as soon as it erupts, expansion and correction of arch length as early as feasible.
3. Utilizing holding arches in the mixed dentition until all permanent premolars and canines have erupted.
4. Extractions of permanent teeth.
5. Maintaining patient's original arch form.

Well-timed early intervention can:
1. Prevent crowded incisors.
2. Increase long-term stability of incisor positions.
3. Decrease ectopic eruption and impaction of permanent canines.
4. Reduce orthodontic treatment time and sequelae.
5. Improve gingival health and overall dental health.

APPLIANCE USED TO INTERCEPT DEVELOPING SKELETAL MALOCCLUSION

Preorthodontic Jaw Trainer[18]

The flexibility as well as inherent memory effects of silicone which is a nonthermoplastic polyurethane material is used to fabricate preorthodontic jaw trainer. This appliance brings about tooth guidance and as well as functional effects.

Design of Preorthodontic Jaw Trainer (Figs 6.7A and B)

• The appliance is soft and shaped in the form of the normal parabolic shape of the dental arches.
• It has channels for the maxillary and mandibular teeth.

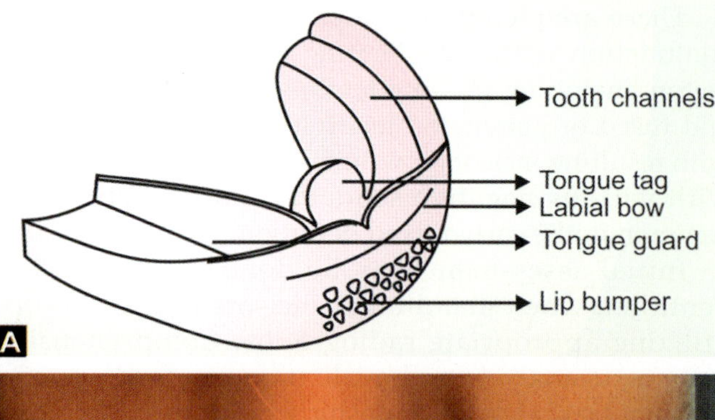

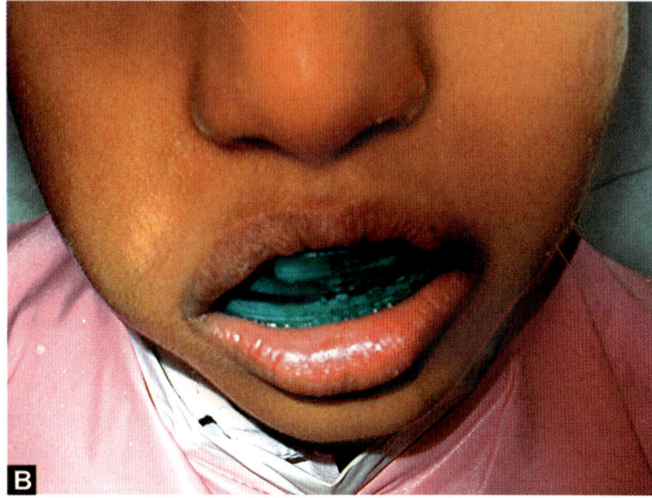

Figs 6.7A and B: (A) Parts of a preorthodontic trainer;
(B) Preorthodontic trainer in patients mouth

- The labial/buccal screen has premolded condensations of the material, which act as labial bow. This allows the irregular teeth to get aligned and the tooth channels further guide the teeth into the normal arch form.
- The oral screen like structure enveloping the teeth buccally/labially help in treating the mouth breathing or thumb sucking habits. This allows for the child to shift from oral to nasal breathing, which in turn allows the nasal passages to develop and the palate to descend.
- The maxillary arch, therefore, tends to develop into a shallow and a U' shaped arch due to the parabolic shape of the appliance.
- Promotion of development of a U' shaped arch allows an increase in the inter-canine dimensions of the maxilla, which in turn allows an increase in the inter-canine dimensions of the mandible, thereby allowing resolution of mandibular anterior crowding.
- Small projections on the labial aspect of the oral screen like structure in the region relating to the mandibular anteriors, behaves as a lip bumper,

thereby allowing a mandibular anterior arch to develop into a rounded one and thereby increasing arch perimeter.
- It also allows the perioral group of muscles to become normotonic thereby ensuring a lip seal.
- A tongue tag has also been incorporated in the maxillary palatal aspect, which is used to train aberrant tongue habits such as retained infantile or tongue thrust cases.

Method of Use

These are used in two phases:
1. The softer blue preorthodontic trainer is use first and allows for correction of aberrant muscle movements and mild tooth movements. This is generally worn for about 6 months.
2. It is followed by the firmer pink preorthodontic trainer, which exerts slightly greater forces for the alignment of teeth and has to be worn for about 12 months.

The Cad/Cam process has allowed the appliance to be developed in such a way that a single size is applicable to all the patients. The only adjustments required are in case of the distal aspects, which can be easily trimmed.

The appliance should be inserted for a minimum of one hour daily during the day and also be worn while sleeping. Initially, the appliance may fall out while sleeping at night, this would decrease over a couple of weeks and finally the appliance would not fall out in sleep, as the aberrant muscular forces become normal.

Initially it may be worn for at least one hour, so as to unlearn the old habits and learn the correct habits at the conscious levels. A clinical review once every month is important to review as well as motivate the child to wear the appliance. The appliance is kept clean by brushing the same with lukewarm soft soapy water everyday.

Indications of Preorthodontic Jaw Trainer

1. Mandibular anterior crowding
2. Class II division 1 and 2
3. Anterior open bite
4. Deep bite
5. Mild class III/pseudo class III
6. Tongue thrusting, thumb sucking and mouth breathing habits.

Contraindications of Preorthodontic Jaw Trainer

1. Posterior crossbite
2. Severe class III
3. Complete nasal obstruction
4. Noncooperative child/parent.

SPACE MANAGEMENT

Space management or maintenance is aimed at preserving the space required for the eruption and alignment of permanent dentition.

Premature loss of tooth is one of the most frequent etiological cause for space loss in children, other causes being interproximal caries, ectopic eruption of first permanent molars, delayed eruption, ankylosis of primary molars, disproportionate tooth size, etc.

Regardless of the cause, loss of space results in arch length reduction and loss of structural balance and functional efficiency.

Definitions

Space Maintenance

"Defined as the measures or procedures that are brought into use following premature loss of deciduous tooth/teeth, to prevent loss of space and improve arch development."

Space Management

"It includes the measures that diagnose and prevent or intercept situations, so as to guide the development of dentition and occlusion."

CHANGES FOLLOWING PREMATURE[19-20] TOOTH LOSS (FIGS 6.8 AND 6.9)

A tooth is maintained in its correct relationship in the dental arch as a result of the action of a series of forces, e.g. second deciduous molar is held in correct relationship by:
1. Mesial force exerted by the first permanent molar
2. Distal force exerted by the first deciduous molar
3. Tongue on lingual side
4. Cheek on buccal side
5. Alveolar process and periodontal tissue producing an upward force
6. Teeth in the opposing arch extending a downward force.

If one of the forces are removed or altered, changes in the relationship of adjacent teeth will occur and will result in drifting of teeth and development of space problems.

ETIOLOGY OF SPACE CLOSURE/ CONTRIBUTING FACTORS

1. *Inclination of the long axis of permanent molars:* If two teeth contact each other in occlusion and each tooth is

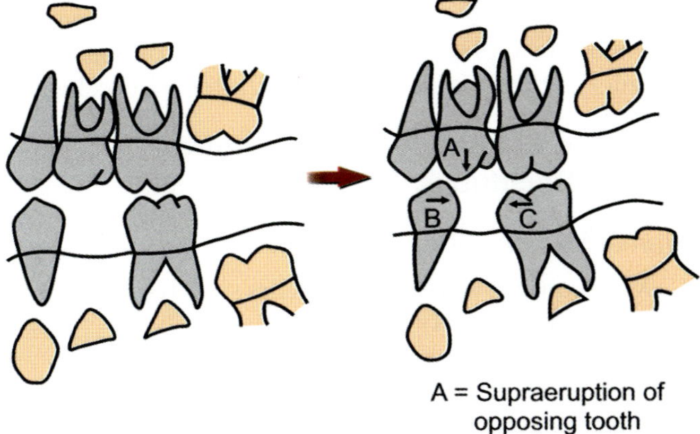

Fig. 6.8: Change occurring due to premature loss of lower first deciduous molar

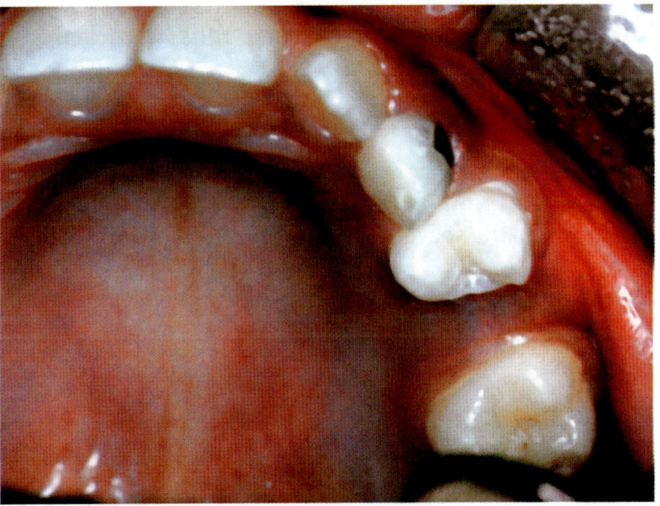

Fig. 6.9: Closure of space following premature loss of second deciduous molar

inclined in a mesial direction, there will be created a mesial component of force which will tend to tip these teeth further and will transmit a mesial force to the contacting adjacent tooth. This factor is more significant in permanent dentition than primary dentition because the later are more vertically positioned.
2. *Path of least resistance:* Teeth tend to move in the direction of the path of least resistance as created by loss of support following extraction of an adjacent tooth.
3. *Influence of buccal musculature:* The buccinator that wraps the posterior teeth may exert mesial force on posterior teeth.
4. *Effect of the position of the center of rotation of the mandible:* Smyd[21] (1955) pointed out that more the

axis of mandibular rotation is lowered in respect to the occlusal plane, the less the amount of horizontal anterior thrust is transmitted to the teeth in occlusion.

Resulting Effects due to Premature Loss of Deciduous Teeth

Premature Loss of Anterior Teeth

- Main concern is based on esthetics speech and function
- Space loss is rarely observed.

Premature Loss of First Deciduous Molar

- Effect depends on the stage of occlusal development
- If it is lost before the eruption of first permanent molar, strong eruptive forces of the erupting tooth will tip the second deciduous molar into the space required for the first premolar.
- Distal drifting of deciduous canine especially during active eruption of later incisor.

Premature Loss of Second Deciduous Molar

- Before eruption of the first permanent molar there is complete chance of permanent molar erupting into the space due to loss of contact guidance causing impaction of second premolar
- After the eruption of the first permanent molar, it may drift into the space resulting in reduced arch perimeter.

PLANNING FOR SPACE MAINTENANCE,[20,22] FACTORS INVOLVED

Time Lapse Since Loss

Maximum closure occurs within the first 6 months after extraction. Therefore, it is best to insert an appliance as soon as possible after extraction.

Dental Age of the Patient

It is a general rule that the teeth erupt when 3/4th of the root is developed, regardless of the child's chronological age. Thus the length of the developing root of the succedaneous tooth gives an indication the time required for the tooth to erupt into the oral cavity. But experience tells us that the tooth can erupt even before less than half of the root has developed (Fig. 6.10).

Amount of Bone Covering the Unerupted Tooth

Space maintainer is required when there is sufficient thickness of bone over the erupting succedaneous tooth. An erupting premolar usually requires 4-5 months to erupt or move through 1 mm of bone as measured on a bite wing radiograph. When the bone covering is

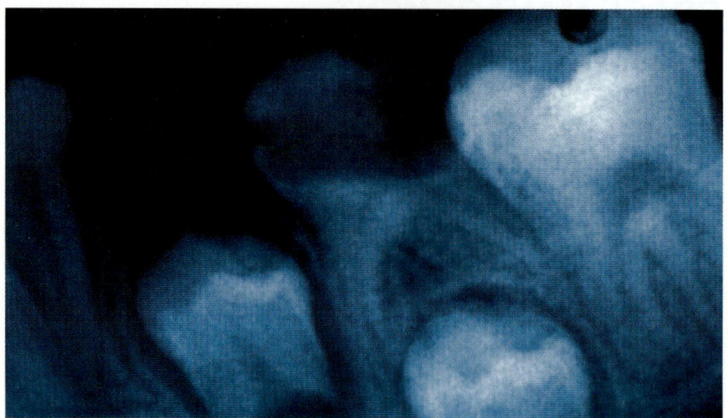

Fig. 6.10: Premolar seen erupting with less than half root formation

destroyed by infection (Figs 6.11A and B), eruption is accelerated and the teeth may even sometimes erupt with minimum of root formation.

Sequence of Eruption of Teeth

The relationship of developing and erupting teeth adjacent to the space created has to be considered. For example, if the second deciduous molar is lost prematurely and second permanent molar is ahead of eruption of the second premolar, then there is possibility that second permanent molar will exert a strong force on the first permanent molar causing it to drift mesially and to occupy some of the space required by the second premolar.

Type of Tooth Lost

Loss of maxillary second deciduous molar results in the maximum amount of space loss (up to 8 mm). This is followed by mandibular second deciduous molar (up to 4 mm). Loss of first deciduous molar with retention of second deciduous molar shows less space loss.

Delayed Eruption of Permanent Tooth

Delay in eruption of permanent teeth may be due to impaction or deviation in the eruptive path. In such cases it is necessary to extract the primary teeth and construct a space maintainer and allow the permanent tooth to erupt and assure its normal position.

Congenital Absence of Permanent Tooth

It has to be decided whether to hold the space and provide fixed prosthesis later or allow space closure where consultation with orthodontist is necessary for the tilted tooth may require orthodontic tooth repositioning.

Presence of Oral Habits

Abnormal forces are exerted on the dental arches. So in such condition space maintainers has to be given immediately.

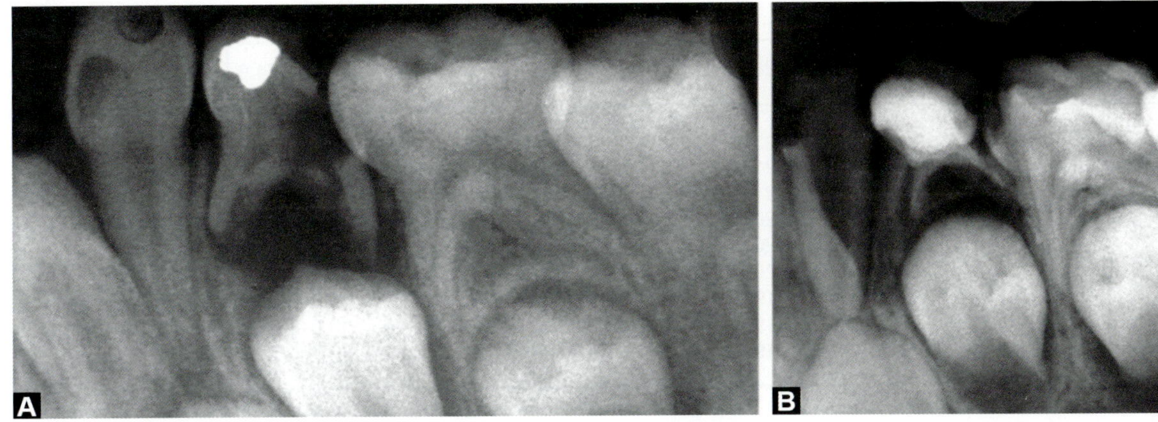

Figs 6.11A and B: Since there is no bone over the erupting premolar in both the cases removal of the grossly decayed first deciduous molar will result in early eruption of the premolar

Existing Malocclusion

Arch length inadequacy and other forms of malocclusion particularly the Class II div 1 progressively become severe after the untimely loss of mandibular primary teeth.

SPACE ANALYSIS

It is done to estimate the space adequacy for the succedaneous tooth and to fairly predict how much space will be required for eruption and proper alignment in the dental arch.

Various analysis used for estimating space adequacy are:

Moyer's Mixed Dentition Analysis[23]

The greatest mesiodistal width of the lower incisors are measured with Boley's gauge.

The amount of space needed for the alignment of the incisors is determined as follows—Boley's gauge is set to a value obtained by measuring the greatest mesiodistal width of the lower incisors. One point is placed at the midline and the other point lies along the dental arch on the right side. This point is marked on the cast and represents the point where the distal surface of the lateral incisor will be when aligned properly. The same thing is repeated on the left side of the arch. The space that is available for permanent canine and premolar is determined. The distance from the point marked on the cast, to the mesial surface of the permanent first molar is measured. This distance is the space available for eruption and alignment of the permanent canine, and two premolars. The combined width of mandibular canine and premolar is predicted with the aid of the probability chart (Fig. 6.12). The estimated canine and premolar size value is substracted from the measured space, to obtain the extra space available.

Johnson and Tanaka's Analysis[24]

This analysis includes two steps:

First step: Determine the available arch length from the mesial of the permanent first molar on one side to the same of the contralateral side.

Second step: Measure the widths of the mandibular permanent four incisors and add them together. This is the space required in the arch for ideal alignment.

The estimated width of the maxillary and mandibular canine and premolar is calculated by adding 10.5 mm and 11.0 mm, respectively to the half of the sum of the width of the mandibular permanent incisors.

Third step: Substract the width of the lower incisors and the two times the calculated premolar and canine width (both sides) from the total arch length approximation. If the result is positive, there is more space available in the arch than needed. Conversely if the result is negative, the unerupted teeth require more space than that available to erupt.

This method does not require additional radiographs. But it tends to over predict slightly the widths of the unerupted premolar.

Radiographic Method

IOPA of the unerupted teeth and of the overlying primary teeth are taken. The enlargement ratio for each unerupted permanent tooth is computed by measuring the nearest erupted tooth first in the mouth and then in the radiograph.

The equation used is:

$$\frac{\text{Erupted tooth size in the mouth}}{\text{Erupted tooth size in X-ray}} \times \text{Unerupted tooth}$$

$$\text{size in X-ray} = \text{Correct tooth size}$$

Maxilla:

Width of mandibular incisors	19.5	20.0	20.5	21.0	21.5	22.0	22.5	23.0	23.5	24.0	24.5	25.0
95%	21.6	21.8	22.1	22.4	22.7	22.9	23.2	23.5	23.8	24.0	24.3	24.6
85%	21.0	21.3	21.5	21.8	22.1	22.4	22.6	22.9	22.2	23.5	23.7	24.0
75%	20.6	20.9	21.2	21.5	21.8	21.0	22.3	22.6	22.9	23.1	23.4	23.7
65%	20.4	20.6	20.9	21.2	21.5	21.8	22.0	22.3	22.6	22.8	22.1	23.4
50%	20.0	20.3	20.6	20.8	21.1	21.4	21.7	21.9	21.2	22.5	22.8	23.0
35%	19.6	19.9	20.2	20.5	20.8	20.0	21.3	21.6	21.9	22.1	22.4	22.7
25%	19.4	19.7	19.9	20.2	20.5	20.8	21.0	21.3	21.6	21.9	22.1	22.4
15%	19.0	19.3	19.6	19.9	20.2	20.4	20.7	20.0	20.3	21.5	21.8	22.1
5%	18.5	18.8	19.0	19.3	19.6	19.9	20.1	20.4	20.7	21.0	21.2	21.5

Mandible:

Width of mandibular incisors	19.5	20.0	20.5	21.0	21.5	22.0	22.5	23.0	23.5	24.0	24.5	25.0
95%	21.1	21.4	21.7	22.0	22.3	22.6	22.9	23.2	23.5	23.8	24.1	24.4
85%	20.5	20.8	21.1	21.4	21.7	22.0	22.3	22.6	22.9	23.2	23.5	23.8
75%	20.1	20.4	20.7	21.0	21.3	21.6	21.9	22.2	22.5	22.8	23.1	23.4
65%	19.8	20.1	20.4	20.7	21.0	21.3	21.6	21.9	22.2	22.5	22.8	23.1
50%	19.4	19.7	20.0	20.3	20.6	20.9	21.2	21.5	21.8	22.1	22.4	22.7
35%	19.0	19.3	19.6	19.9	20.2	20.5	20.8	21.1	21.4	21.7	22.0	22.3
25%	18.7	19.0	19.3	19.6	19.9	20.2	20.5	20.8	21.1	21.4	21.7	22.0
15%	18.4	18.7	19.0	19.3	19.6	19.8	20.1	20.4	20.7	21.0	21.3	21.6
5%	17.7	18.0	18.3	18.6	18.9	19.2	19.5	19.8	20.1	20.4	20.7	21.0

Fig. 6.12: Probability chart used for Moyers mixed dentition analysis

Hixon and Oldfather[25]

It involves summing of the maximum mesiodistal diameter of one permanent central incisor and one lateral incisor, with the diameter of the unerupted first and second bicuspids measured on the radiograph taken by the paralleling technique. The following prediction chart can be used:

Modification of Hixon and Oldfather method measures lower incisor widths and the widths of the unerupted premolars measured from radiographs to predict permanent tooth size.

Measured Value	Estimated Tooth Size
23 mm	18.4 mm
24 mm	19.0 mm
25 mm	19.7 mm
26 mm	20.3 mm
27 mm	21.0 mm
28 mm	21.6 mm
29 mm	22.3 mm
30 mm	22.9 mm

SPACE MAINTAINERS

Definition of Space Maintainers

Space maintainers are devices used to maintain or regain the space following the loss of deciduous tooth/teeth. The goal of space maintenance is to prevent loss of arch length, width, and perimeter by maintaining the relative position of the existing dentition.[26]

Requirements of a Space Maintainer[27]

1. Should maintain the desired proximal dimensions of the space created by the loss of tooth.
2. Should be functional.
3. Should not interfere with eruption of occluding teeth.
4. Should not interfere with the eruption of the replacing permanent teeth.
5. Should not interfere with speech, mastication or functional movement of mandible.
6. Should be simple and strong.
7. Should not impose excessive stress on adjacent tooth.
8. Easily cleansable.
9. Should not restrict the normal growth and function.

Indications of a Space Maintainer

1. Generally indicated when the forces acting upon the teeth are unbalanced and the space analysis indicates a possible space inadequacy for the succedaneous teeth, as when there is malocclusion or abnormal oral habits.
2. When a malocclusion exists that would be further compounded with loss of space.
3. Maximum closure occurs within the first 6 months after extraction. Therefore, it is best to insert an appliance as soon as possible after extraction.
4. The teeth erupt when 3/4th of the root is developed, regardless of the child's chronological age, it is advisable to place a space maintainer if the tooth is not ready for eruption.
5. An erupting premolar usually requires 4-5 months to erupt or move through 1 mm of bone as measured on a bite wing radiograph. This should be kept in mind while advising a space maintainer.
6. Disorder in the sequence of eruption of teeth.
7. Delayed or altered eruption of permanent tooth.
8. Congenital absence of permanent tooth.

Containdications of a Space Maintainer

1. When there is no alveolar bone overlying the crown of erupting tooth and there is sufficient space for its eruption.
2. When space left is excess of the mesiodistal dimensions required for the eruption and space loss is not expected.
3. When there is gross space discrepancy requiring future extractions and orthodontic treatment.
4. When permanent succeeding tooth is congenitally absent and space closure is desired.

Adverse Effects Associated with Space Maintainers[28-30]

1. Dislodged, broken, and lost appliances
2. Plaque accumulation
3. Caries
4. Interference with successor eruption
5. Undesirable tooth movement
6. Inhibition of alveolar growth
7. Soft tissue impingement
8. Pain

Classification of Space Maintainers

1. According to Hitchcock[31]
   a. Removable, fixed or semifixed
   b. With bands or without bands
   c. Functional or nonfunctional
   d. Active or passive
   e. Certain combinations of the above
2. According to Raymond C Throw
   a. Removable
   b. Complete arch
      – Lingual arch
      – Extraoral anchorage
   c. Individual tooth space maintainer
3. According to Heinrichsen
   a. Fixed space maintainer
      – Class I —— Nonfunctional
         1. Bar type
         2. Loop type
         ——Functional
         1. Pontic type
         2. Lingual arch type
      – Class II ——Cantilever type
         (distal shoe, band and loop)
   b. Removable space maintainer

Removable Space Maintainers (Figs 6.13 to 6.15)

They are space maintainers that can be removed and reinserted into the oral cavity by the patient. It can be functional or nonfunctional, and are bilateral most of the time.

Indications of Removable Space Maintainer

- Bilateral loss of posterior teeth in the mandibular arch before the eruption of the permanent incisors
- Missing anterior teeth where it is made functional
- Cases where patient cooperation is not a major criteria
- When space maintenance is required for a short period of time.

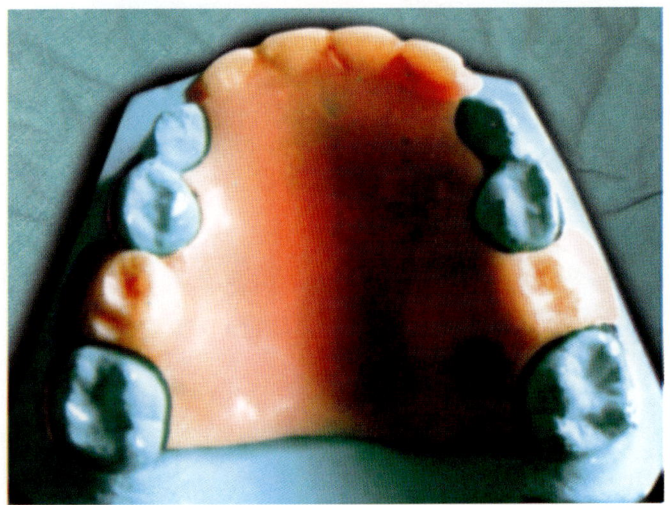

Fig. 6.13: Bilateral removable functional passive space maintainer

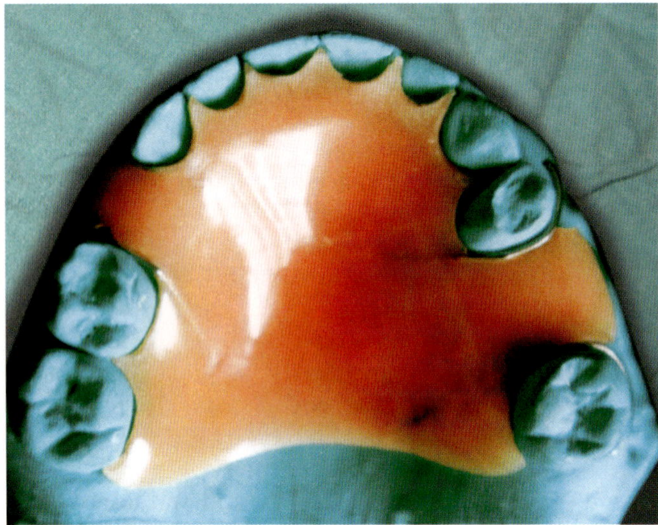

Fig. 6.14: Bilateral removable nonfunctional passive space maintainer

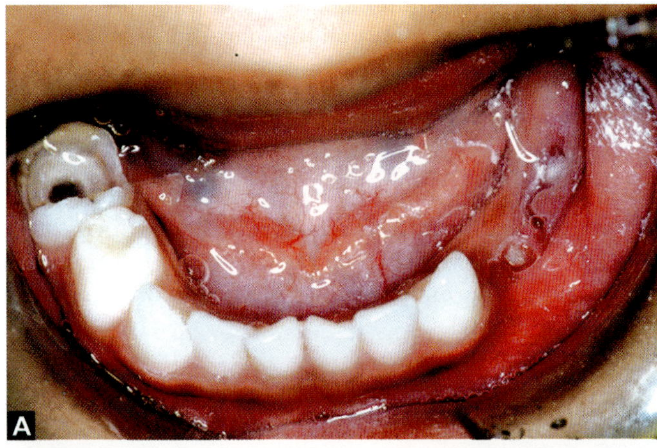

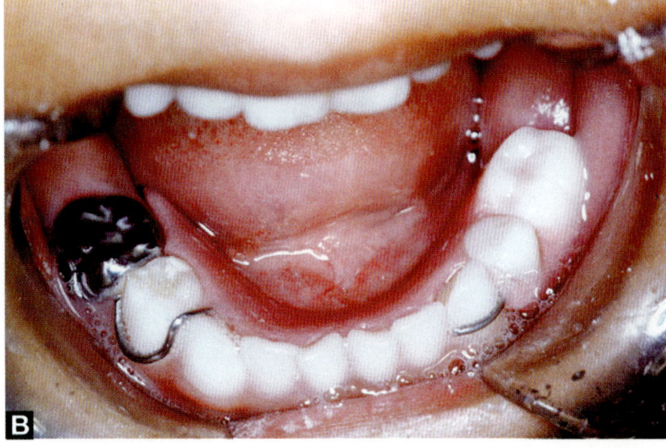

Figs 6.15A and B: Removable function space maintainer: (A) Pretreatment; (B) Post-treatment

Contraindications of Removable Space Maintainer

- Uncooperative patient
- Patients allergic to acrylic
- Epileptic patient

Advantages of Removable Space Maintainer

1. Easily cleansable—both the teeth and appliance.
2. Maintains vertical dimensions when made functional.
3. Can be used in combinations with other preventive or interceptive procedures, such as habit reminders.
4. Can be worn partime—allowing free blood circulation.
5. Can be made esthetically desirable.
6. Facilitates chewing and speaking when it is made functional.
7. Stimulates eruption of permanent teeth.
8. Keep the tongue in bounds.
9. Band contruction is not necessary, thus reducing the chair side time.
10. Room may be made for erupting teeth without making a new appliance.

Disadvantages of Removable Space Maintainer

1. May be lost or broken.
2. Patient cooperation is important.
3. Restrict lateral growth of jaw if clasps are made incorrectly.
4. May irritate the soft tissues.

Types of Removable Space Maintainers

1. Acrylic partial denture.
2. Complete denture—given when there is loss of all the teeth as in rampant caries or ectodermal dysplasias.
3. Removable distal shoe space maintainer—acts as acrylic immediate partial denture with distal shoe extension into the alveolus. It is used when fixed distal shoe cannot be placed due to many missing teeth.

Ideal Requirements of Removable Space Maintainer

1. It should restore or improve masticatory function.
2. It should restore and improve aesthetics and facial contours.
3. It should not interfere with normal growth of the dental arches.
4. Its bulk should not be an impediment to good speech.
5. Its design should allow the patient to insert and remove it easily.
6. The design should permit easy adjustment and alterations if required.
7. It should be cleaned easily.

8. Its design should require minimal or no preparation of the abutment teeth.
9. It should prevent over eruption of opposing teeth or drift of the adjacent teeth.
10. Be noncariogenic and nonirritating to the supporting tissues.

Fixed Space Maintainer

They can be unilateral or bilateral, functional or nonfunctional, active or passive space maintainers that are designed to be cemented on to the tooth and thus cannot be removed by the patient.

Advantages of Fixed Space Maintainer

1. Patient cooperation is not required.
2. Jaw growth is not hampered.
3. Succedaneous teeth are free to erupt, depending on the design.
4. Masticatory function is restored if pontics are placed.

Disadvantages of Fixed Space Maintainer

1. Elaborate instrumentation is required.
2. Increased risk of caries.
3. Some designs interfere with eruption of successor, as with band and bar spacemaintainer.

Types of Fixed Space Maintainer

1. Band and loop/crown and loop/band and bar space maintainer.
2. Lingual arch space maintainer.
3. Transpalatal bar space maintainer.
4. Nance palatal arch space maintainer.
5. Fiber reinforced composite.
6. Distal shoe space maintainers.

Band and Loop Space Maintainers (Figs 6.16 and 6.17)

- They are unilateral, fixed, nonfunctional and passive space maintainer.

Indications of band and loop space maintainer

- Used when single tooth is missing in the posterior segment.
- It can also be given in bilateral posterior tooth loss, before the eruption of permanent anteriors in the mandible, where two band and loop space maintainer can be given instead of removable space maintainer.

Contraindications of band and loop space maintainer

- High caries activity
- Marked space loss
- More than one adjoining teeth missing.

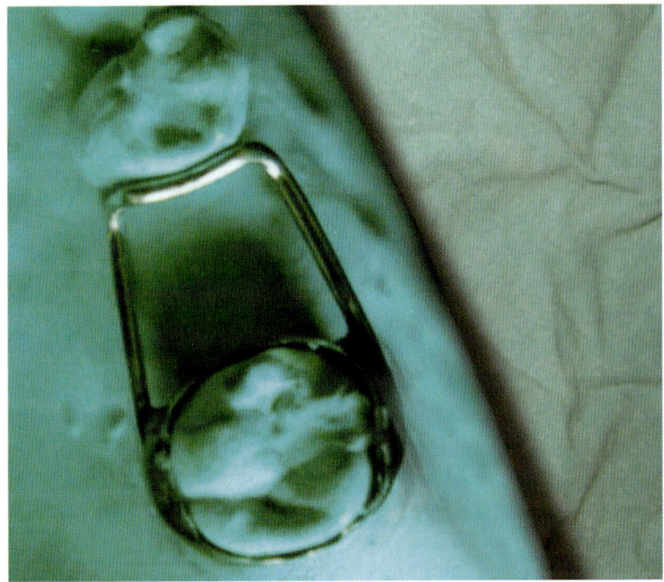

Fig. 6.16: Band and loop space maintainer

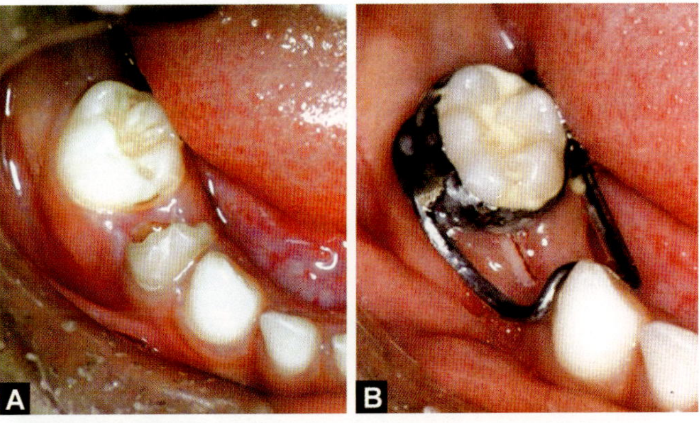

Figs 6.17A and B: Band and loop space maintainer: (A) Pretreatment; (B) Post-treatment

Disadvantages of band and loop space maintainer

- Nonfunctional
- Does not prevent continued supraeruption of opposing tooth
- Caries check is difficult
- Oral hygiene maintenance is difficult
- The loop may slip from the position and impinge on the gingiva. Occlusal rests given to the loop that rests on the occlusal surface of the mesial abutment tooth prevents this disadvantage.

Design of band and loop space maintainer

- It consists of a band fabricated from 0.005″ steel band and a loop that extends from the band to the distal surface of the anterior abutment tooth. The loop is placed 1 mm from the gingival surface. It should not be very wide that it may interfere with the cheek and tongue movements.

- Occlusal rest may be given on the loop that rests on the occlusal surface of the tooth, to prevent gingival tipping of the loop.

Construction of band and loop space maintainer

- Stainless steel band can be of two types, the preformed and custom made (Figs 6.18A and B). Preformed steel bands are available in different sizes and correct size has to be selected according to the size of the patients tooth. Custom made band are made by taking the required amount of band material from the spool and pinching them to form the band. Custom made bands are fabricated using various pliers (Figs 6.19A to C). They are adapted such that cervically it extends 1 mm subgingivally, occlusally it should not extend up to the occlusal surface as it may interfere with the occlusion (Fig. 6.20).
- *Preformed bands:* They are readily available in different sizes. Correctly fitting band is selected and is pushed into place with finger pressure. Upper band is rocked from buccal over to the lingual surface and an lower band from lingual to buccal surface. A band pusher

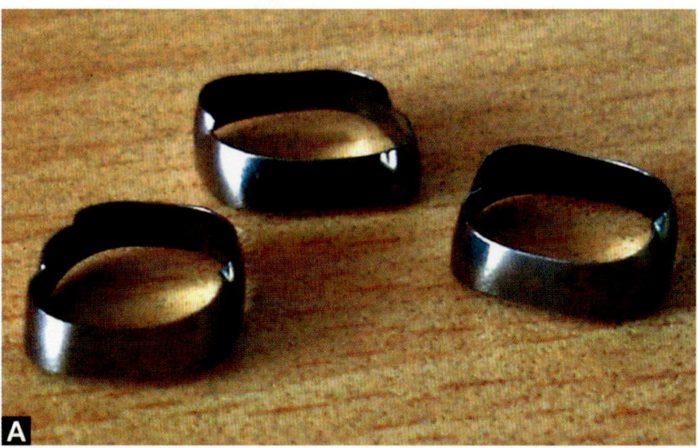

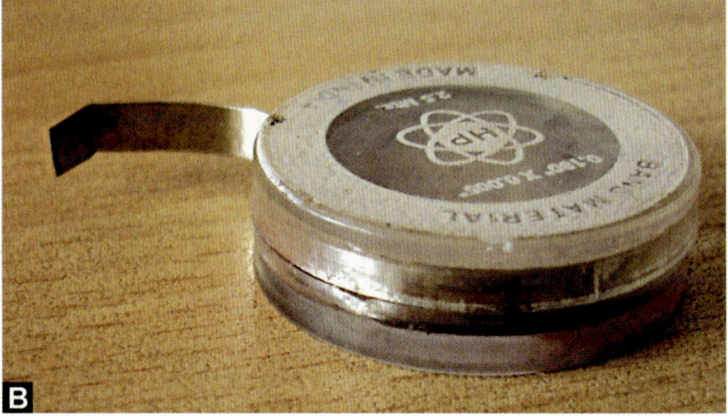

Figs 6.18A and B: Band used for space maintainer: (A) Preformed bands; (B) Band material available in spool

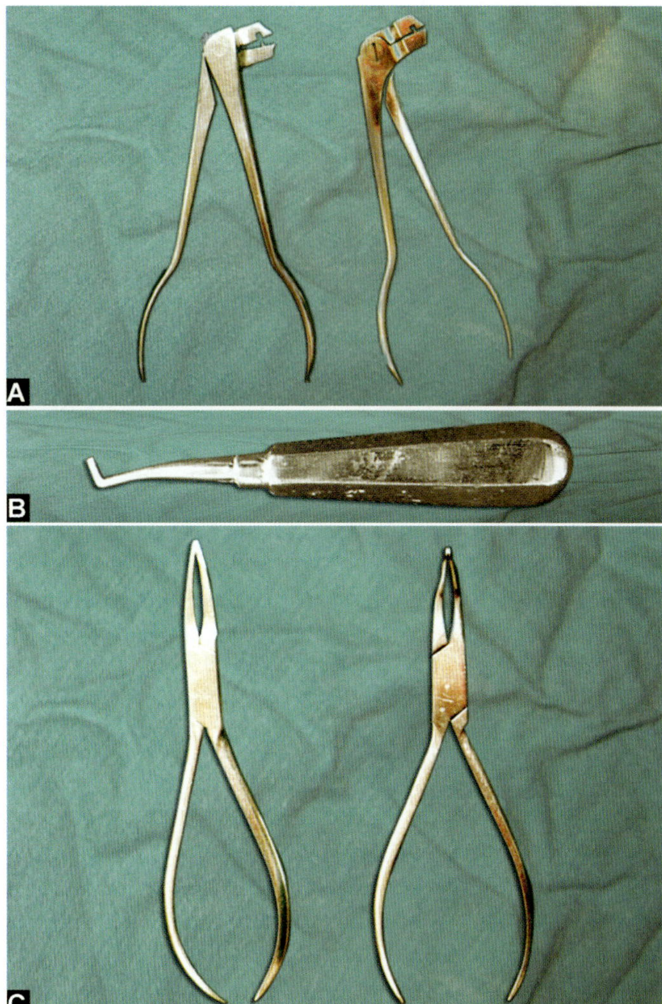

Figs 6.19A to C: Pliers used for construction of band and loop space maintainer: (A) Beak pliers; (B) Band adaptor; (C) Howe's plier (Straight and curved)

or amalgam condenser should be used to burnish the band into buccal and lingual grooves. The gingival portion of the band can be contoured for good retention using a contouring plier.[32]

- Impression of the arch is made with alginate and the band is removed from the tooth and placed in the impression (Fig. 6.21) with occlusal portion of the band facing towards the alginate and secured with wax or pins (Fig. 6.22). Cast is prepared with dental stone.
- Cast is obtained with the band secure on the tooth.
- Loop is prepared with 0.9 mm hard round stainless steel wire (Fig. 6.23). The loop extends from the middle of the band from its either side to reach the distal surface of the anterior abutment tooth just below the contact point and above the gingival margin.
- The loop is then soldered to the band.

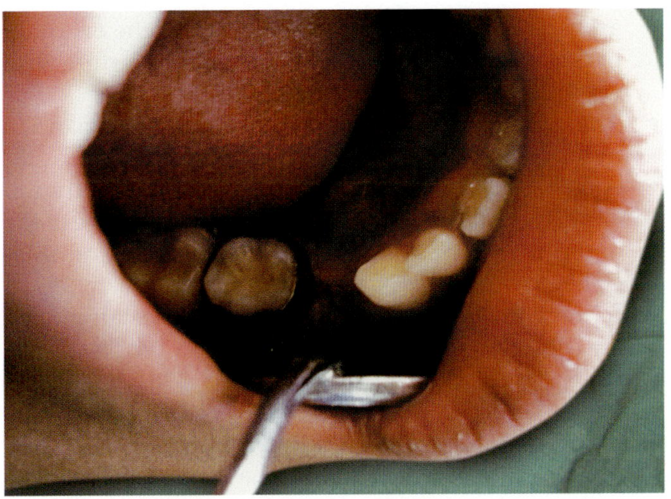

Fig. 6.20: Band adapted on the tooth

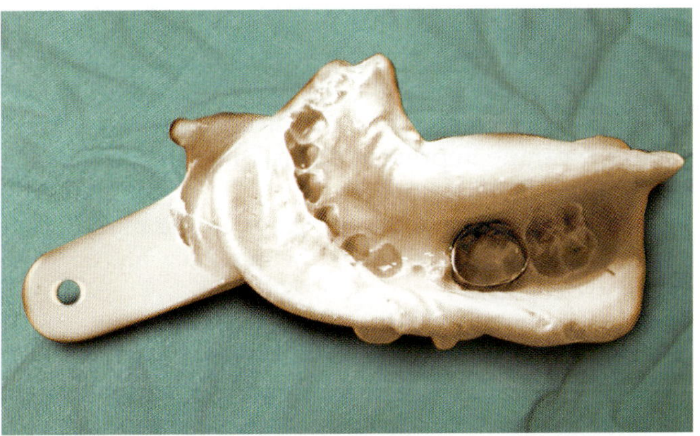

Fig. 6.21: Band place in the impression, occlusal margin facing towards the impression

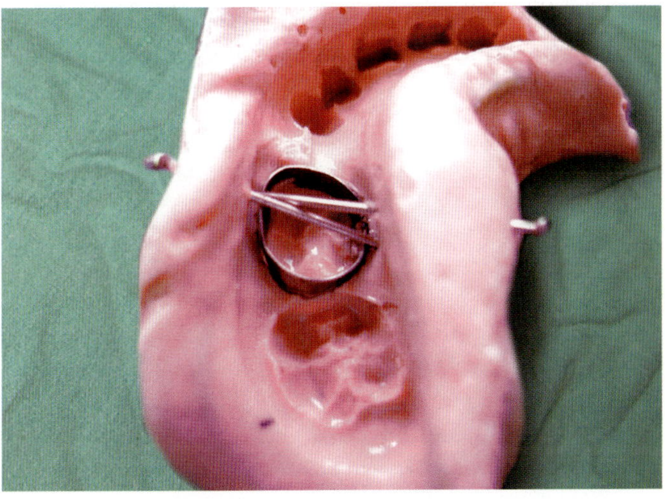

Fig. 6.22: Band secured in the impression with pins

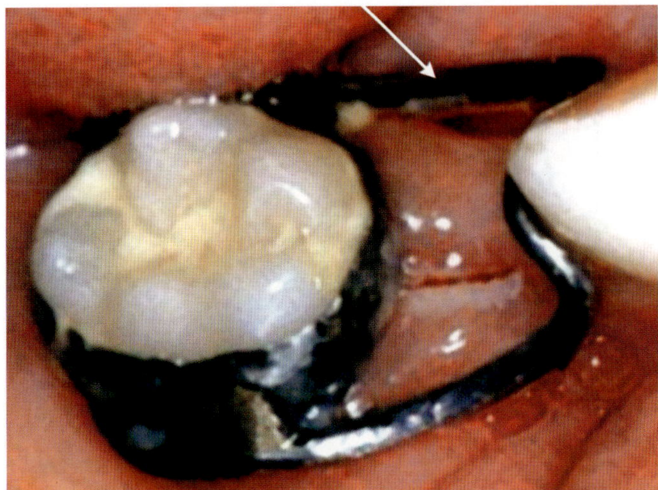

Fig. 6.23: Loop that is soldered to the band

- The joint is finished and polished using white stone and rubber wheel.
- The band is cemented with glass ionomer cement, polycarboxylate or zinc phosphate cement. Glass ionomer cement is the material of choice.

Modifications of Band and Loop Space Maintainers

1. *Crown and loop space maintainer (Figs 6.24 and 6.25):* Crown is replaced instead of a band. It is done when the abutment tooth requires the placement of crown for reasons such as gross caries, hypoplastic tooth or on a RCT treated tooth.
2. *Reverse crown/band and loop (Fig. 6.26):* If the distal abutment tooth cannot be banded or crowned then the mesial abutment tooth is banded or crowned and loop is extended distally. This situation usually arises when the distal abutment tooth is not fully erupted.
3. *Band and bar space maintainer (Fig. 6.27):* Instead of a cantilever design both the abutment teeth are banded and a bar placed in between them instead of a loop. It is sturdier but may interfere with the eruption of the permanent tooth as the bar is positioned on the center of the ridge.
4. *Bonded space maintainer:* In this design no band is placed. The loop that is similar to band and loop design is bonded with resin on the buccal and lingual surface of both the abutment teeth. The wire passes from one abutment to the other crossing the alveolar ridge.

Lingual Arch Space Maintainer (Fig. 6.28)

- It is a bilateral, fixed or semifixed, nonfunctional, passive space maintainer.
- Indicated when there is bilateral loss of molars after the eruption of the permanent incisors in the lower

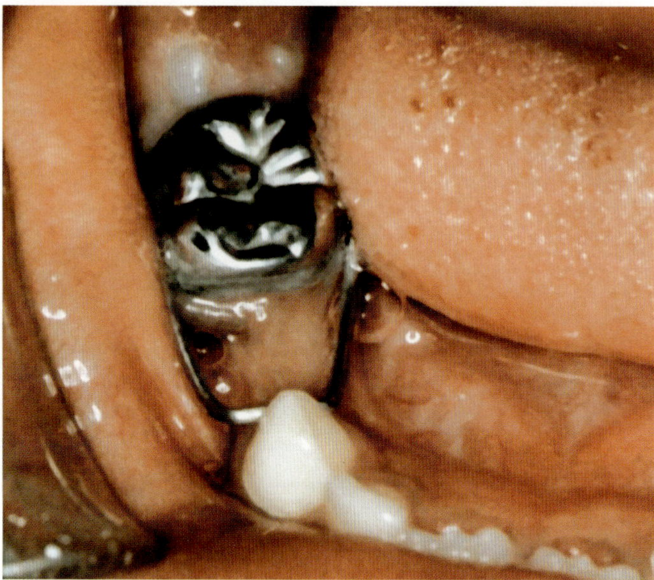

Fig. 6.24: Crown and loop space maintainer

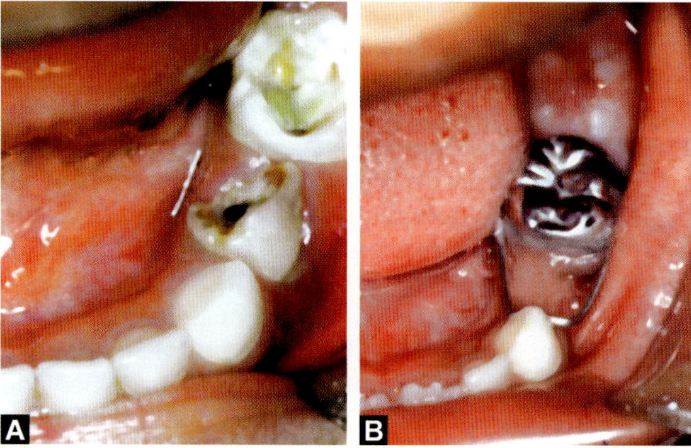

Figs 6.25A and B: Crown and loop space maintainer:
(A) Pretreatment; (B) Post-treatment

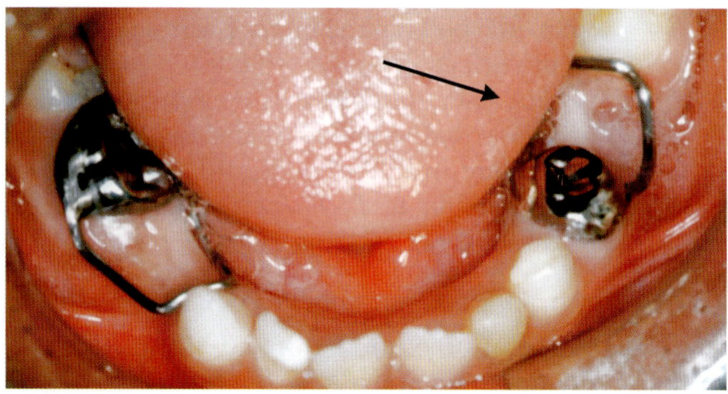

Fig. 6.26: Reverse crown and loop space maintainer
on the right lower quadrant

arch. If the lingual arch is given before the eruption of the permanent lower incisors it may interfere with the eruption of the permanent incisors.

- The right and left first permanent molars are banded in the lower segment.
- A 'U' shaped arch wire extends from the lingual surface of the molar bands to the lingual surface of the anterior teeth. They are placed above the cingulum of the lower incisors.
- It prevents the mesial movement of the posterior teeth and collapse of the anterior segment.

Modifications of lingual arch

- It can be made semifixed by welding a molar tube one on each of the bands on the lingual aspect. The arch wire is passed into the tube instead of soldering to the band. Part of the design (band) is fixed and the other part (arch wire) is removable.
- A 'U' loop can be incorporated in the arch wire to make it active, which aids in distalizing the molar and proclination of the collapsed incisors (Fig. 6.29A).
- Spurs can be added to the arch wire at the distal end of the canine to prevent distal collapse of the canine (Fig. 6.29B).
- Lingual arch is commonly given in the mandibular arch, but it can be given in the maxillary arch if there is no deep bite.

Transpalatal Bar Space Maintainer (Fig. 6.30)

- It is a bilateral, fixed, passive and nonfunctional space maintainer
- The first permanent molars are banded
- The arch wire extends from the palatal aspect of the band to cross the midline transversly at right angles to the midpalatine raphe
- It prevents the mesiolingual rotation of the permanent molar around the palatal root and prevents mesial movement of molars

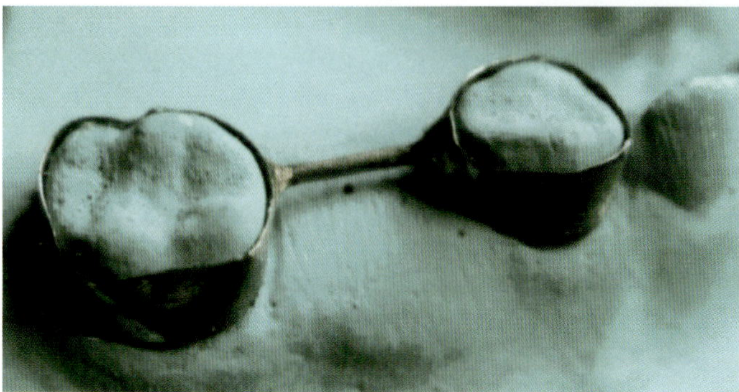

Fig. 6.27: Band and bar space maintainer

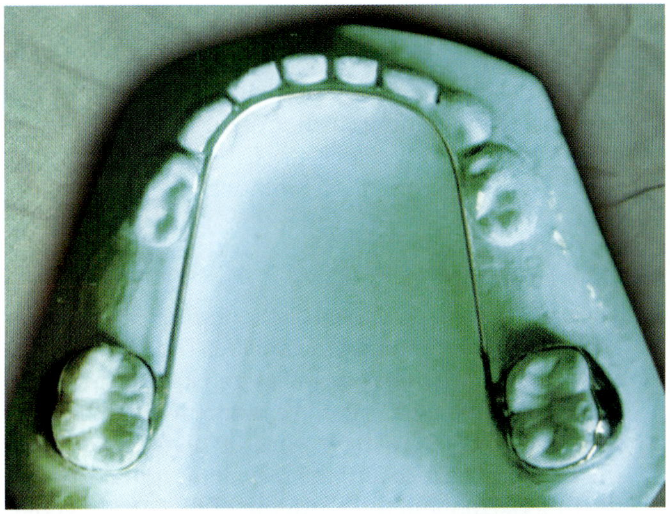

Fig. 6.28: Lingual arch space maintainer

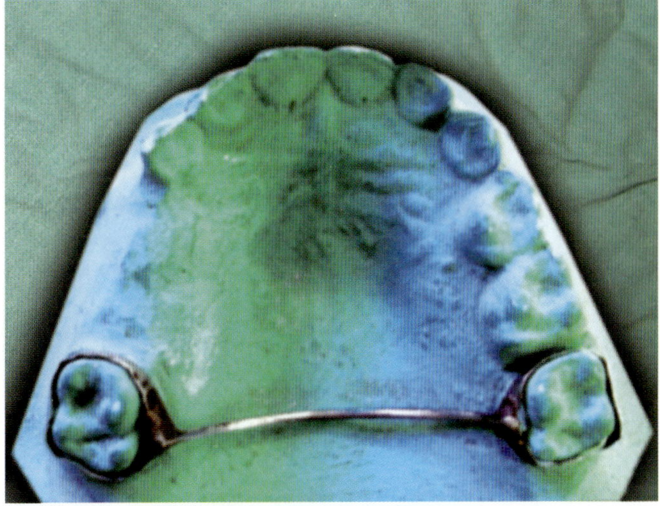

Fig. 6.30: Transpalatal bar

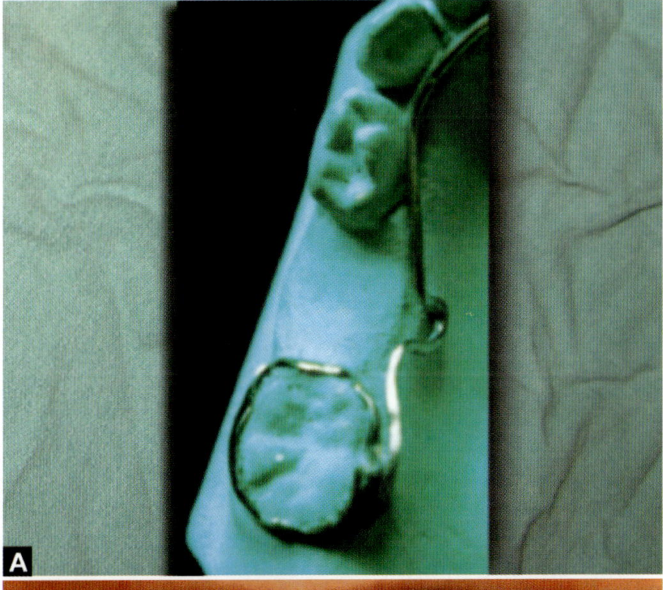

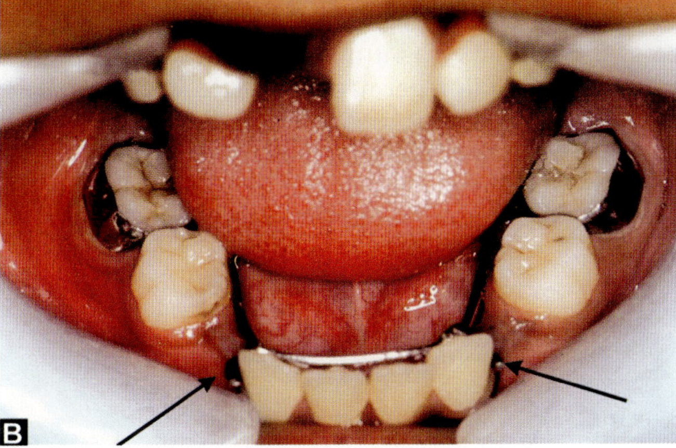

Figs 6.29A and B: Modification of lingual arch space maintainer: (A) Lingual arch space maintainer with 'U' loop; (B) Lingual arch space maintainer with canine spurs

- It is used when there is unilateral loss of deciduous molars. If given in a bilateral missing case, then both the permanent molars can move mesially simultaneously.

Nance Palatal Arch[33] (Figs 6.31 and 6.32)

- It is a bilateral, fixed, passive and nonfunctional space maintainer
- The first permanent molars are banded
- The arched wire extends from the palatal surface of one molar band to the other. Anteriorly it extends up to the rugae area and is embedded in an acrylic button. The acrylic button that is firmly placed on the rugae provides good anchorage
- Indicated when there is bilateral missing deciduous molars in the upper arch
- It can be made active by incorporating 'U' loop to the wire. Opening the loop causes distalization of the first permanent molar
- The acrylic button may irritate the soft tissues and this appliance may not be suitable for patients allergic to acrylic.

Distal Shoe Space Maintainers[34-37] (Fig. 6.33)

Early version of distal shoe space maintainer was called as Willet's distal shoe and was made of cast gold. It was very expensive and difficult to fabricate, so it was modified to the present design. It is called as Roche's modified distal shoe appliance.

It is a unilateral, fixed, nonfunctional and passive space maintainer. It is an intra-alveolar appliance, in which a portion of the appliance is extending into the alveolus.

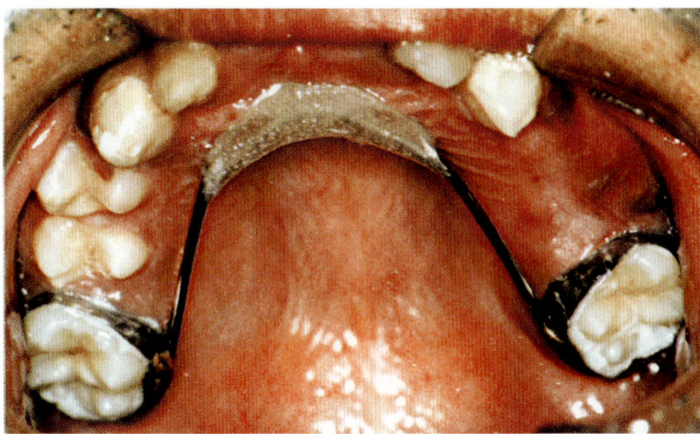

Fig. 6.31: Nance palatal arch space maintainer

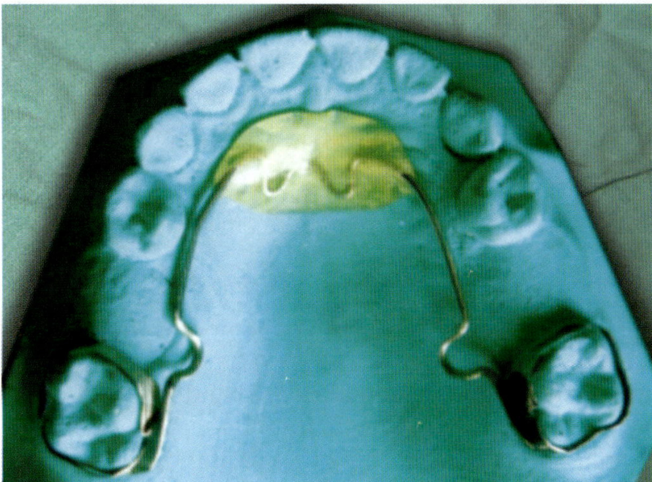

Fig. 6.32: Nance palatal arch space maintainer with 'U' loop

Distal shoe space maintainer is normally not indicated in a maxillary arch. This is because the maxillary permanent molars have a distally inclined path of eruption initially. As they erupt they become more horizontally positioned. In such a situation the mesial migration of the erupting tooth is very rare.

Indications of distal shoe space maintainer

- It is indicated when there is premature loss of second deciduous molar before the eruption of the first permanent molar.
- Used only when one tooth is lost on one quadrant as the strength of the appliance is limited. So when both the first and second deciduous molars are missing in the same quadrant, removable distal shoe is preferred.

Contraindication of distal shoe space maintainer

- Inadequate abutments due to multiple loss of teeth
- Poor oral hygiene

- Missing permanent first molar
- Lack of patient and parent cooperation
- Presence of medical conditions such as blood dyscrasias, congenital cardiac defect predisposing to subacute bacterial endocarditis, history of rheumatic fever, diabetes, general debilitation.

Construction of distal shoe space maintainer (Figs 6.34A to F)

- The band/crown is adapted on the first deciduous molar and an alginate impression is made. The band/crown is removed from the tooth and placed in the impression and cast is prepared with the band/crown on the cast.
- An IOPA is taken to determine the distance between the alveolar surface and the mesial marginal ridge of the first permanent molar (depth of the intra-alveolar extension) and also to measure the distance between the distal surface of the first deciduous molar and the mesial surface of the first permanent molar (space required for the eruption of the second premolar).
- On the cast the position of the mesial surface of the first permanent molar is marked with the help of a divider, from the distal surface of the first deciduous molar.
- A 'V' shaped notch is made at the marked point. The depth of the notch is such that it extends to about 1 mm below the mesial marginal ridge of the first permanent molar, as per the measurements made on the radiograph.
- A loop is fabricated that extends from the band/crown on the first deciduous molar up to the slot and then bends at right angles into the slot prepared. The space in between the two portions of the loop can be filled with solder.
- The loop is then soldered to the band, finished and polished. The appliance is sterilized before trying in the patient's mouth.
- It is advised to extract the tooth just before cementation of the appliance as it minimizes the risk of mesial migration of first permanent molar.
- The band/crown is tried in the patient's mouth after the extraction of the mandibular second molar. The intra-alveolar portion of the loop extends into the extraction socket. An IOPA is taken to confirm the

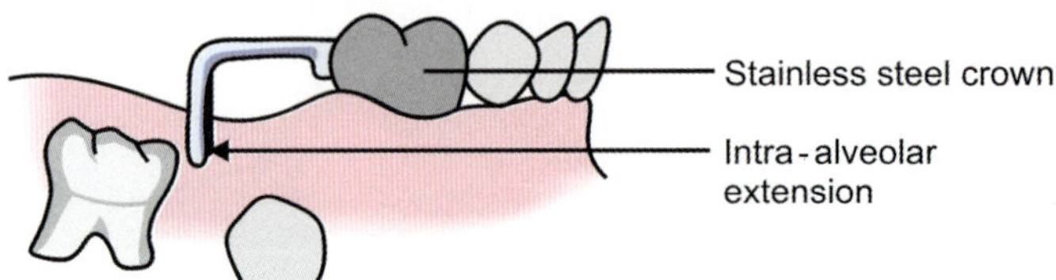

Fig. 6.33: Intra-alveolar extension of distal shoe space maintainer

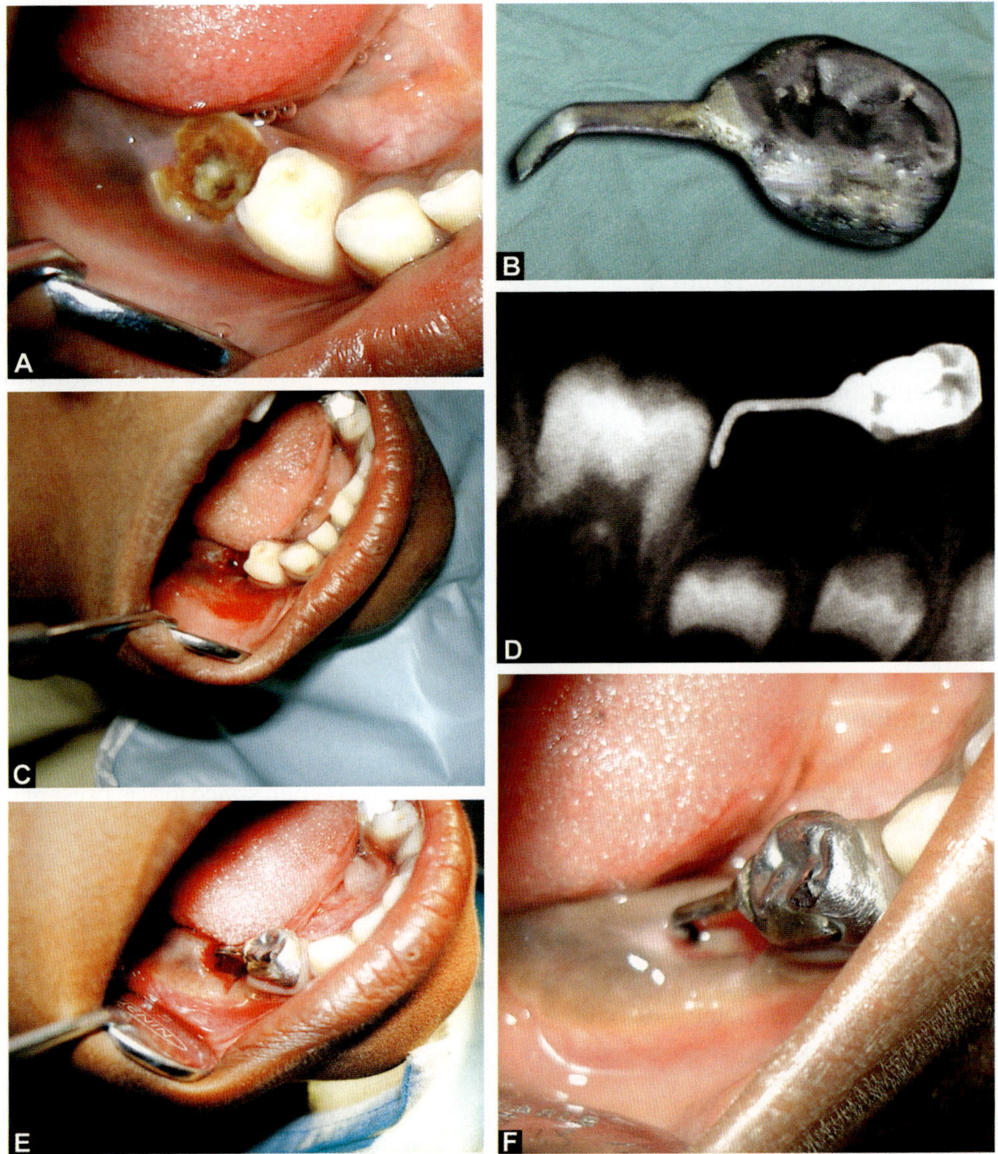

Figs 6.34A to F: Placement of distal shoe space maintainer: (A) Second deciduous molar is advised for extraction; (B) Distal shoe is prepared. The intra-alveolar extension is soldered to the crown; (C) Second deciduous molar is extracted; (D) The distal shoe is placed on the tooth and radiograph is taken to confirm the position of the intra-alveolar extension with respect to the erupting first permanent molar; (E) The appliance is cemented in place; (F) Postoperative healing seen at the extraction site

position of the intra-alveolar extension. It should lie 1 mm below the mesial marginal ridge of the first permanent molar.

- The band/crown is then cemented and patient kept on recall until the permanent molar erupts. Then the intra-alveolar extension is cut and the appliance acts as a band and bar space maintainer till the second premolar erupts. The intra-alveolar portion is never totally lined by epithelial tissues and is associated with a chronic inflammatory response.

- *Modification:* A crown can be cemented on the abutment tooth and band for the distal shoe adapted on the crown. This provides stability to the design.

Situations where distal shoe is contraindicated, 2 options of management are:
1. Allow drifting of the first permanent molar followed by regaining the space with the active space maintainer.
2. Use of removable appliance that do not penetrate the tissue, but applies pressure on the ridge mesial to the unerupted first permanent molar.

Fiber Reinforced Composite as Space Maintainers (Fig. 6.35)

Classification of fibers

Based on the material used[38,39]

1. Ultrahigh molecular weight polyethylene fibers—ribbond and connect.
2. Glass fibers—GlasSpan and fiber Splint ML
3. Fibers preimpregnated with resin—Vectris, StickNet, and FiberKor.

Based on the fiber orientation[40]

1. Unidirectional
2. Braided
3. Woven

Besides being used for space maintenance, fiber reinforced composites are used for splinting of traumatized tooth/teeth (Please refer the chapter 'Trauma and its Management'), as endodontic posts and also in fabrication of prosthesis.

Active Space Maintainers/Space Regainers

This type of space maintainer as the name suggests is active and brings about the movement of the tooth/teeth. It can be a removable or fixed, unilateral or bilateral appliance.

The goal of space regaining intervention is the recovery of lost arch width and perimeter and/or improved eruptive position of succedaneous teeth. Space regained should be maintained until adjacent permanent teeth have erupted completely and/or until

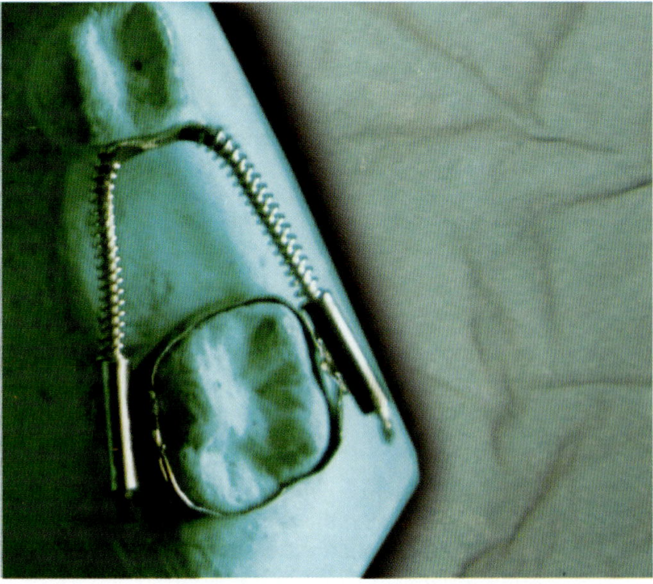

Fig. 6.35: Gerber space regainer

a subsequent comprehensive orthodontic treatment plan is initiated.

Indication of Active Space Maintainers

- When there is a need to re-establish about 3 mm or less of space.

Factors to be Considered before Planning for Active Space Maintainer

- It is easy to regain space in maxilla than in mandible, due to increased anchorage provided by the palatal vault and possibility of extraoral anchorage. Also the bone in maxilla is cancellous compared to the compact bone of mandible.
- Space loss by tipping can be regained when the crown of the tooth is tipped back
- Space loss by bodily movement of the adjacent tooth should be regained by moving the tooth back bodily.

Removable Space Regainer

- It consists of retentive components like the Adams clasp, an active component such as springs or screws and a acrylic base plate.
- It is used when space loss is present on one quadrant only.
- It takes about 3-4 months to regain 3 mm of space
- Screw design has the advantage that the tooth to be moved can also be clasped to help retain the appliance.
- Single or double cantilever spring can be used with adequate anchorage.
- Extraoral force can be applied by the use of headgear. It consists of a face bow, extraoral bow and intraoral arch wire, neck pad and elastic band. 14-16 hours of wearing is required per day and generates 100-200 gm of force.

Free end loop space regainer

It utilizes a labial arch wire for stability and retention, with a back-action loop spring constructed with 0.025 wire. The base of the appliance is made of acrylic resin. Movement of the permanent molar is achieved by activating the free end of the wire loop at specific intervals.[41]

Split saddle/split block space regainer

It differs from the free end spring type in that the functional part of the appliance consists of an acrylic block that is split buccolingually and joined by a wire in the form of a bucal and lingual loop. The appliance is activated by periodic spreading of the loops. The activator block is split with a disk after the appliance has been processed.

Sling shot space regainer

It consists of a wire elastic holder with hooks instead of a wire spring that transmits a force against the molar to be distalized. This is called sling shot appliance, since the distalizing force is produced by the elastic stretched on the middle of the lingual surface of the molar to be moved. The other is arranged in the same position on the buccal surface of the molar. The elastic are changed once each day.

Jack screw

It is another type of removable appliance used for space regaining which will incorporate an expansion screw in the edentulous space. Space is opened by expanding the plates anteroposteriorly.

Fixed Space Regainer

It is a fixed, unilateral, nonfunctional and active space maintainer.

Indicated when there is space closure following the premature loss of deciduous molar by mesial drifting of the first permanent molar.

Types of fixed space maintainer

1. Gerber space regainer
2. Jackscrew space regainer

Gerber Space Regainer
(Open Coiled Space Regainer) (Fig. 6.35)

It consists of band adapted on to the tooth and an open coil inserted into a U' shaped wire. The wire is inserted into the molar tube on the band and whole assembly is cemented on the tooth.

Fabrication of Gerber space regainer

- The band is adapted on the tooth, generally the permanent first molar that is to be distalized to regain space.
- The buccal and lingual tubes are soldered to the adapted band with the help of a spot welder. These tubes are about 0.25 inches long and have flanges for spot welding.
- The tubes should be parallel to one another in all planes and their lumen should be aimed in between the contact point of crown and the gingiva of the mesial abutment tooth.
- An impression of the band and tubes is taken with the band seated on the tooth and the band is then removed.
- The holes in the tube are plugged with carding wax to prevent them from getting blocked by stone plaster.
- The band is then seated in the impression and stone plaster is poured after stabilizing the same.

- A 0.7 mm stainless steel wire is then bent to a U' shape, which will fit passively in both the buccal and lingual tubes.
- The anterior part of the U' shaped wire should have a reverse bend where it contacts the distal outline of the first premolar. The wire will contact the distal surface of the first premolar below its greatest convexity.
- At the junction of the straight part and the curved part of the wire, both buccal and lingually, solder is flowed to make a stop.
- Then open coil spring is cut enough, so as to extend from the stop to a point about 2 mm distal to the anterior limit of the tube on the molar band.
- The coil spring is slipped on the wire. The wire is then put in the tubes. The band with the wire and compressed springs is cemented on the molar.
- The compressed spring will try to recoil and exert reciprocal pressure mesially to the premolar and distally to the permanent molar.

Jackscrew Space Regainer

The jackscrew space regainer is used to recover the loss of space caused by drifting of tooth into an edentulous area.

It consists of 2 banded adjacent teeth and a threaded shaft with a screw and a locknut. This is activated regularly to exert a consistent force against the banded teeth. This appliance produces rapid results.

Fabrication of jackscrew space regainer

- Band is fabricated and impression made
- The cast is poured after transferring the bands on the impressions.
- A 0.036" buccal tube is welded to the molar band.
- The tube should be centered in the middle one-third of the band and aligned with the other banded abutment tooth.
- A jackscrew unit as received from the manufacturer consists of one adjustment nut and one lock nut on a threaded shaft. Slide the threaded end of the shaft into the molar tube.
- The mesial end of the shaft is trimmed and contoured to the premolar band surface and soldered onto the premolar band.
- End of the shaft should be trimmed, so that it extends 2 mm from the distal end of the tube.
- It is then cemented into the patient's mouth.

Space Maintainers that can be Used for Premature Loss of Deciduous Molars

1. Maxillary anterior teeth
   - Removable functional space maintainer
   - Fixed cantilever prosthesis

2. Mandibular anterior teeth
   – Removable functional space maintainer
   – Fixed cantilever prosthesis
3. Maxillary first deciduous molar
   Unilateral loss
   a. Band and loop space maintainer
   b. Transpalatal arch space maintainer
   c. Removable functional space maintainer
   Bilateral loss
   a. Nance palatal arch
   b. Two band and loop space maintainer
   c. Removable functional space maintainer
4. Maxillary second deciduous molar
   Unilateral loss
   a. Band and loop space maintainer
   b. Transpalatal arch space maintainer
   c. Removable functional space maintainer
   Bilateral loss
   a. Nance palatal arch
   b. Two band and loop space maintainer
   c. Removable functional space maintainer
5. Mandibular first deciduous molar
   Unilateral loss
   a. Band and loop space maintainer
   b. Removable functional space maintainer
   Bilateral loss
   a. Lingual arch space maintainer—after the eruption
      of the permanent incisors
   b. Two band and loop space maintainer
   c. Removable functional space maintainer
6. Mandibular second deciduous molar
   Unilateral loss, before the eruption of first permanent
   molar:
   a. Distal shoe space maintainer
   Unilateral loss, after the eruption of first permanent
   molar:
   a. Band and loop space maintainer
   b. Removable functional space maintainer
   Bilateral loss, before the eruption of first permanent
   molar:
   a. Two distal shoe space maintainer, one on each side
   Bilateral loss, after the eruption of first permanent molar:
   a. Lingual arch space maintainer—after the eruption
      of the permanent incisors
   b. Two band and loop space maintainer
   c. Removable functional space maintainer
7. Maxillary first and second deciduous molars
   Unilateral loss
   a. Transpalatal arch space maintainer
   b. Removable functional space maintainer
   Bilateral loss
   a. Nance palatal arch
   b. Removable functional space maintainer

8. Mandibular first and second deciduous molars
   Unilateral loss
   a. Removable functional space maintainer
   Bilateral loss
   a. Lingual arch space maintainer
   b. Removable functional space maintainer
   Before the eruption of permanent first molars
   a. Removable functional space maintainer.

Soldering Procedure

Soldering is a process of joining two or more metal components by heating them to a temperature below their solidus temperature and filling the gap between them using a molten metal with a liquidus temperature below 450°C.

The soldering process involves:
1. Substrate metals to be joined
2. *A filler metal (usually called solder):* The filler metal must be compatible with the oxide-free substrate metal, but it does not necessarily have a similar composition.

Primary properties of filler metal required are:

- Sufficiently low flow temperature
- Ability to wet the substrate metal
- Sufficient fluidity at the flow temperature
- Adequate hardness, strength, tarnish and corrosion resistance
- An acceptable color

3. *A flux:* Flux is a compound applied to metal surfaces that dissolves or prevents the formation of oxides and other undesirable substances that may reduce the quality or strength of a soldered area.
4. *Heat source:* The portion of the flame used to heat the soldering assembly is at the tip of the reducing zone, because this produces the most efficient burning process and the most heat. An improperly adjusted torch or improperly positioned flame can lead to oxidation of the substrate or filler metal and may result in a poor solder joint.

All are equally important, and the role of each must be taken into consideration.

Fluxes may be divided into the following three types, according to their primary purpose:
Type I: Surface protection—Covers the metal surface and prevents access to oxygen so that no oxides can form.
Type II: Reducing agent—Reduces any oxides present and exposes clean metal.
Type III: Solvent—Dissolves any oxides present and carries them away.

Technical Procedures

The soldering technique involves several critical steps:
1. Cleaning and preparing the surfaces to be joined.
2. Assembling the parts to be joined.
3. Preparing and fluxing the gap surfaces between the parts.
4. Maintaining the proper position of the parts during the procedure.
5. Controlling the proper temperature.
6. Controlling the time to ensure adequate flow of solder and complete filling of the solder joint.

> Flow temperature is that temperature at which the filler metal wets and flows on the substrate metal and produces a bond. The flow temperature of the filler metal should be lower than the solidus temperature of the metals being joined. A general rule is that the flow temperature of the filler metal should be at least 55.6°C (100°F) lower than the solidus temperature of the substrate metal.

REFERENCES

1. Kanellis MJ. Orthodontic treatment in the primary dentition. In: Bishara SE (Ed) Textbook of Orthodontics. Philadelphia, Pa: WB Saunders Co; 2001; pp. 248-56.
2. Woodside DG. The significance of late developmental crowding to early treatment planning for incisor crowding. Am J Orthod Dentofacial Orthop. 2000;117(5):559-61.
3. Kurol J. Early treatment of tooth-eruption disturbances. Am J Orthod Dentofacial Orthop. 2002;121(6):588-91.
4. Sankey WL, Buschang PH, English J, et al. Early treatment of vertical skeletal dysplasia: The hyperdivergent phenotype. Am J Orthod Dentofacial Orthop. 2000; 118(3):317-27.
5. http://www.aapd.org/media/Policies_Guidelines/G_DevelopDentition.pdf
6. Premkumar S. Graber's Textbook of Orthodontics: Basic Principles and Practice. Elsevier India Pvt. Ltd; 2009.
7. Nanda RS. Basics of undergraduate orthodontics. Oklahoma City: Oklahoma University Health and Science Center Press; 1993.
8. Mathewson RJ, Primosch RE. Fundamentals of Pediatric Dentistry, 3rd edition. USA: Quintessence Publishing Co. Inc; 1995.
9. Graber TM, Swain BF. Orthodontics: Current Principles and techniques. St. Louis: The CV Mosby Company; 1985.
10. Currier GF, Austerman JB. Fabrication of appliances for preventive, interceptive and adjunctive orthodontics. Oklahoma City: Oklahoma University Health Science Center Press; 1992.
11. Sonnesen L, Bakke M, Solow B. Bite force in preorthodontic children with unilateral crossbite. Eur J Ortho. 2001; 23(6): 741-9.
12. Pinto AS, Bushang PH, Throckmorton GS, et al. Morphological and positional asymmetries of young children with functional unilateral posterior crossbites. Am J Orthod Dentofacial Orthop. 2001;120(5):513-20.
13. Bolton WA. The clinical application of a tooth-size analysis. Am J Orthod. 1962;48:504-29.
14. Dugoni SA, Lee JS, Varela J, et al. Early mixed dentition treatment: Postretention evaluation of stability and relapse. Angle Orthod. 1995;65(5):311-20.
15. Foster H, Wiley W. Arch length deficiency in the mixed dentition. Am J Orthod. 1958;68:61-8.
16. Little RM, Riedel RA, Stein A. Mandibular arch length increase during the mixed dentition: Postretention evaluation of stability and relapse. Am J Orthod Dentofacial Orthop. 1990;97(5):393-404.
17. Little RM. Stability and relapse of mandibular anterior alignment: University of Washington studies. Semin Orthod. 1999;5(3):191-204.
18. Singh G. Textbook of orthodontics. New Delhi: Jaypee Brothers Medical Publishers; 2004.
19. Lundström A. The significance of early loss of deciduous teeth in the etiology of malocclusion. Am J Orthod 1955; 41:819.
20. Owen DG. The incidence and nature of space closure following the premature extraction of deciduous teeth, a literature review, Am J Orthod. 1971;59:37.
21. Smyd ES. Dentistry in Biophysics. D Digest. 1955;61:482-90.
22. Brothwell DJ. Guidelines on the use of space maintainers following premature loss of primary teeth. J Can Dent Assoc. 1997;63(10):753-66.
23. Moyers RE. Handbook of Orthodontics. Chicago: Year Book Medical Publishers Inc; 1973.
24. Tanaka MM, Johnston LE. The prediction of the size of unerupted canines and premolars in a contemporary orthodontic population. JADA. 1974;88(4):798-801.
25. Staley RN, Kerber PE. A revision of the Hixon and Oldfather mixed dentition prediction method. Am J Orthod. 1980;78:296.
26. Ngan P, Alkire RG, Fields HW Jr. Management of space problems in the primary and mixed dentitions. J Am Dent Assoc. 1999;130(9):1330-9.
27. Anderson AW, Bonus HW. A Handbook of Clinical and Laboratory Pedodontics. College of Dentistry. University of Illinois: Chicago; 1972. pp. 1-2.
28. Dincer M, Haydar S, Unsal B, et al. Space maintainer effects on intercanine arch width and length. J Clin Pediatr Dent. 1996;21(1):47-50.
29. Qudeimat MA, Fayle SA. The longevity of space maintainers: A retrospective study. Pediatr Dent. 1998;20(4):267-72.
30. Cuoghi OA, Bertoz FA, de Mendonca MR, et al. Loss of space and dental arch length after the loss of the lower first primary molar: A longitudinal study. J Clin Pediatr Dent. 1998;22(2):117-20.
31. Hitchcock PH. Preliminary steps in preventive orthodontics. In: Finn SB (Ed). Clinical Pedodontics, 4th edition: WB Saunders Company; 1987.
32. Nance HN. The limitations of orthodontic treatment. Am J Orthod. 1947;33:253.
33. Willet RC. Premature loss of deciduous teeth. Angle Orthod. 1929;16:389.

34. Hicks EP. Treatment planning for the distal shoe space maintainer. Dent Clin North Am. 1973;17:135-50.
35. Brill WA. The distal shoe space maintainer: chairside fabrication and clinical performance. Pediatr Dent. 2002;24:561-5.
36. Mayhew MJ, Dilley GJ, Dilley DC, et al: Tissue response to appliances in monkeys. Pediatr Dent. 1984;6:148-52.
37. Braham RL, Morris ME. Textbook of Pediatric Dentistry. 2nd edition. Delhi: CBS Publishers; 1990.
38. Ganesh M, Tandon S. Versatility of Ribbond in Contemporary Dental Practice. Trends Biomater. Artif. Organ. 2001;20:53-8.
39. Kargul B, Çaglar E, Kabalay U. Glass Fiber-reinforced Composite Resin as Fixed Space Maintainers in Children: 12-month Clinical Follow-up. J Dent Child. 2005;72:109-12.
40. Premnath K, Sharmila MR, Kalavathy N. Bonding with ribbond—single visit fixed partial denture. SRM University Journal of Dental Sciences. 2010;1:134-6.
41. Barbería E, Lucavechi T, Cárdenas D, et al. Free-end space maintainers: design, utilization and advantages. J Clin Pediatr Dent. 2006;31:5-8.

FURTHER READING

1. Ak G, Sepet E, Pinar A, et al. Reasons for early loss of primary molars. Oral Health Prev Dent. 2005;3(2):113-7.
2. Al-Dashti AA, Cook PA, Curzon ME. A comparative study on methods of measuring mesiodistal tooth diameters for interceptive orthodontic space analysis. Eur J Paediatr Dent. 2005;6(2):97-104.
3. American Academy of Pediatric Dentistry. Clinical guideline on management of the developing dentition in pediatric dentistry. Pediatr Dent. 2004;26(7):128-31.
4. Barberia E, Lucavechi T, Cardenas D, et al. Free-end space maintainers: design, utilization and advantages. J Clin Pediatr Dent. 2006 Fall;31(1):5-8.
5. Battagel JM. The aetiological factors in Class III malocclusion. Eur J Orthod. 1993;15(5):347-70.
6. Bayardo RE. Anterior space maintainer and regainer. ASDC J Dent Child. 1986;53(6):452-5.
7. Bijoor RR, Kohli K. Contemporary space maintenance for the pediatric patient. N Y State Dent J. 2005;71(2):32-5.
8. Brill WA. The distal shoe space maintainer chairside fabrication and clinical performance. Pediatr Dent. 2002; 24(6):561-5.
9. Brothwell DJ. Guidelines on the use of space maintainers following premature loss of primary teeth. J Can Dent Assoc. 1997;63(10):753, 757-60, 764-6.
10. Butani Y, Levy SM, Nowak AJ, et al. Overview of the evidence for clinical interventions in pediatric dentistry. Pediatr Dent. 2005;27(1):6-11.
11. Choonara SA. Orthodontic space maintenance—a review of current concepts and methods. SADJ. 2005;60(3):113, 115-7.
12. Cozza P, Marino A, Lagana G. Interceptive management of eruption disturbances: case report. J Clin Pediatr Dent. 2004;29(1):1-4.
13. Dincer M, Haydar S, Unsal B, et al. Space maintainer effects on intercanine arch width and length. J Clin Pediatr Dent. 1996;21(1):47-50.
14. Durward CS. Space maintenance in the primary and mixed dentition. Ann R Australas Coll Dent Surg. 2000;15:203-5.
15. Kokich VG, Kokich VO. Congenitally missing mandibular second premolars: clinical options. Am J Orthod Dentofacial Orthop. 2006;130(4):437-44.
16. Kupietzky A. Clinical technique: removable appliance therapy for space maintenance following early loss of primary molars. Eur Arch Paediatr Dent. 2007;8 (Suppl) 1:30-4.
17. Lin YT, Lin WH, Lin YT. Immediate and six-month space changes after premature loss of a primary maxillary first molar. J Am Dent Assoc. 2007;138(3):362-8.
18. Magalhaes M, Araujo L, Chiaradia C, et al. Early dental management of patients with Mobius syndrome. Oral Dis. 2006;12(6):533-6.
19. Melo L, Ono Y, Takagi Y. Indicators of mandibular dental crowding in the mixed dentition. Pediatr Dent. 2001;23(2):118-22.
20. Qudeimat MA, Fayle SA. The longevity of space maintainers: a retrospective study. Pediatr Dent. 1998; 20(4):267-72.
21. Rajab LD. Clinical performance and survival of space maintainers: evaluation over a period of 5 years. ASDC J Dent Child. 2002;69(2):156-60,124.
22. Simsek S, Yilmaz Y, Gurbuz T. Clinical evaluation of simple fixed space maintainers bonded with flow composite resin. J Dent Child (Chic). 2004;71(2):163-8.
23. Stahl F, Grabowski R. Orthodontic findings in the deciduous and early mixed dentition--inferences for a preventive strategy. J Orofac Orthop. 2003;64(6):401-16.
24. Tulunoglu O, Ulusu T, Genc Y. An evaluation of survival of space maintainers: a six-year follow-up study. J Contemp Dent Pract. 2005;6(1):74-84.
25. Wong ML, Che Fatimah Awang, Ng LK, et al. Role of interceptive orthodontics in early mixed dentition. Singapore Dent J. 2004;26(1):10-4.
26. Yilmaz Y, Kocogullari ME, Belduz N. Fixed space maintainers combined with open-face stainless steel crowns. J Contemp Dent Pract. 2006;7(2):95-103.

QUESTIONS

1. Define space maintenance and space management.
2. What are the factors responsible for closure of space following premature loss of tooth/teeth?
3. Explain the factors to be considered while planning for space maintenance.
4. What is space analysis? Explain in detail Moyer's mixed dentition analysis.
5. What are the requirements of space maintainer?
6. Classify space maintainers and describe removable space maintainers.
7. Band and loop space maintainers.
8. Discuss the space maintainers that can be indicated for a premature loss of tooth/ teeth in maxilla.
9. What are space regainers and explain any one in detail.

PERNICIOUS ORAL HABITS

Pernicious oral habits are habits which are abnormal and results due to lack of harmony between the child and his environment.

Most of the oral habits produce harmful effects on the development of the maxillofacial complex, leading to unbalanced pressure exerted on the immature and highly malleable alveolar ridges and potential changes in the position of the teeth and occlusion.

The habit can be acquired by imitation from others or may infuse a certain sense of security and comfort, as the child seems to retire to his world of fantasy, thus becoming cut out to any situation which otherwise promotes a feeling of fear and distress.

DEFINITION

Pernicious means tending to a fatal issue.

"Habit is defined as an automatic response to a specific situation acquired normally as the result of repetition and learning. At each repetition the act becomes less conscious and if repeated often enough, may enter the realm of unconscious habit."

When the habit involving the oral cavity becomes fatal, that is when the habit causes defects in orofacial structures it is termed as pernicious oral habit.

FACTORS THAT MAKE A HABIT—PERNICIOUS

A habit is considered to be pernicious when they interfere with the child's physical, emotional or social functioning. The severity of the ill-effects of a habit depends upon the frequency, intensity and duration for which the habit is practiced.

Frequency—How often the habit is performed (number of times per day).

Intensity—How vigorously is it practiced?

Duration—Total number of years/months/weeks/days since the habit is being performed.

CLASSIFICATION OF PERNICIOUS ORAL HABITS[1,2]

Pernicious oral habits can be classified as follows:

By Earnest Klein
a. Intentional habits (meaningful)
b. Unintentional habits (empty)

A habit can be either meaningful or empty, e.g. let us assume that a 5 years old child is left in the care of a baby sitter for a period of 3 months, while the parents are away for a vacation. The child is horrified by the belief that his parents have deserted him. He is lonesome and develops feeling of insecurity and resorts to thumb sucking. Under these circumstances sucking the thumb becomes an 'meaningful habit', where there is direct cause and effect relationship. This habit becomes an 'empty habit', if the child continues to suck his thumb after his parents return home, because now the cause is removed but the effect remains.

By Brash
a. Purely muscular, e.g. tongue thrusting, lip sucking.
b. Combined activity of the muscles of jaw, mouth and thumb, e.g. thumb sucking.
c. Muscular action combined with introduction of passive object into the mouth, e.g. pencil chewing.
d. Habits in which muscles of the mouth and jaw take no active part, the effect on the position of the teeth are produced by extraneous pressure, e.g. abnormal pillowing.
e. Functional disturbance, e.g. mouth breathing.

By Morris and Bohana
a. Pressure habits—thumb sucking, tongue thrusting, etc.
b. Nonpressure habits—mouth breathing, etc.
c. Biting habits—pencil biting, etc.

By Sydney Finn
a. *Noncompulsive:* Habits which are easily added or dropped from the child's behavior pattern as he/she matures.
b. *Compulsive:* It is acquired and express a deep seated emotional need.

By William James
a. Useful habits, e.g. nasal breathing
b. Nonuseful habits/harmful habits, e.g. mouth breathing.

> Points to be considered before treatment of oral habits:
> 1. Is the habit normal for that age? For example, tongue thrusting or thumb sucking in an infant is normal.

Contd...

Contd...

2. Why has the child acquired the habit? Can it be a meaningful or empty habit?
3. Is the habit self-correcting, damaging or persisting? For example, thumb sucking is normal in infants and self-correcting with the advancing age.
4. What is the correct time of interception for correction?
5. Is the habit potentially harmful to the mouth or the paraoral structures? Intensity, duration, and frequency are the index of severity of the habit should also be considered.
6. Psychological implication for allowing or not allowing the child to continue the habit, especially in an meaningful habit.
7. First the psychological problem should be treated then the habit as such.
8. What is the appropriate means of correction of the habit?

THUMB SUCKING HABIT

It is observed that most of the children below 3 years suck their thumb or finger. Thumb sucking in infants is common and is meant to meet both psychological and nutritional needs. It is a spontaneous activity that develops soon after birth. Between birth and 3 months of age, its intensity increases until the age of 7 months and then gradually declines. Most of the children discontinue the habit by 3-4 years of age. If the habit continues beyond this period there are definite chances that it may lead to dentofacial changes, and the severity depending on the frequency, duration and intensity of the habit.[3,4]

Definition of Thumb Sucking

According to Gellin[5] "it is the placement of thumb or one or more fingers in varying depths into the mouth".

Classification of Thumb Sucking[6,7]

According to Cook (Figs 6.36A and B)

1. *α group:* The thumb pushes the palate in a vertical direction and displays only little buccal wall contractions. Here the thumb applies pressure on the palate but sucking action is minimum or nil. Characteristic features, therefore, seen will be a deep palate with no posterior crossbite.
2. *β group:* Strong buccal wall contractions are seen and a negative pressure is created resulting in posterior crossbite.
3. *γ group:* Alternate positive and negative pressure is created. Posterior crossbite may be a feature in some cases depending on the frequency and duration of habit.

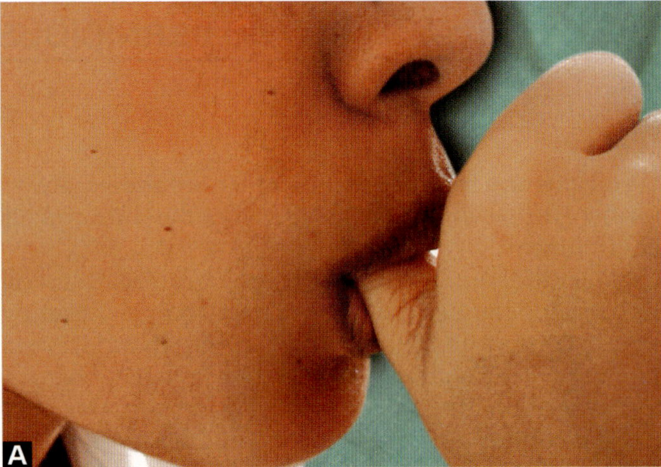

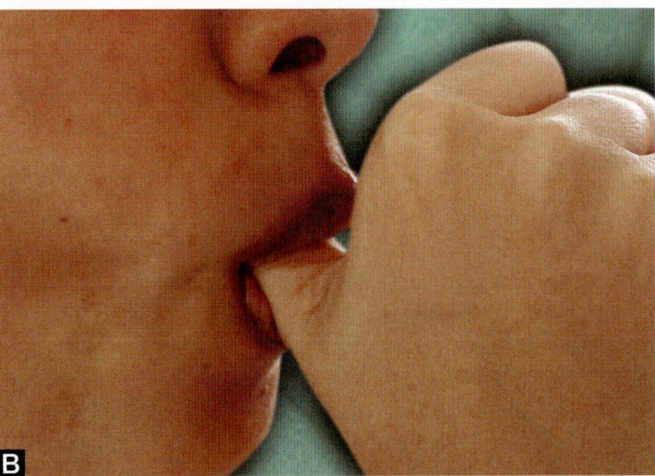

Figs 6.36A and B: Position of the thumb as per Cook's classification: (A) Little or no buccal wall contraction; (B) Buccal wall contraction seen during thumb sucking habit

According to Subtleny (Figs 6.37A to D)

1. *Group I:* Thumb is inserted beyond the first joint, pressing against the palatal mucosa and alveolar tissue. Lower incisors press against the thumb.
2. *Group II:* The thumb extends up to the first joint or just anterior to it. No palatal contact. Contact is present with only the anterior teeth.
3. *Group III:* Thumb is placed fully into the mouth in contact with the palate as in group I but the lower incisors do not contact the thumb.
4. *Group IV:* The thumb does not progress appreciably into the mouth. The lower incisors contact the thumb at the nails.

Theories Explaining Thumb Sucking Habit[8-10]

Various theories have been discussed to explain the development of thumb sucking habit. They are:

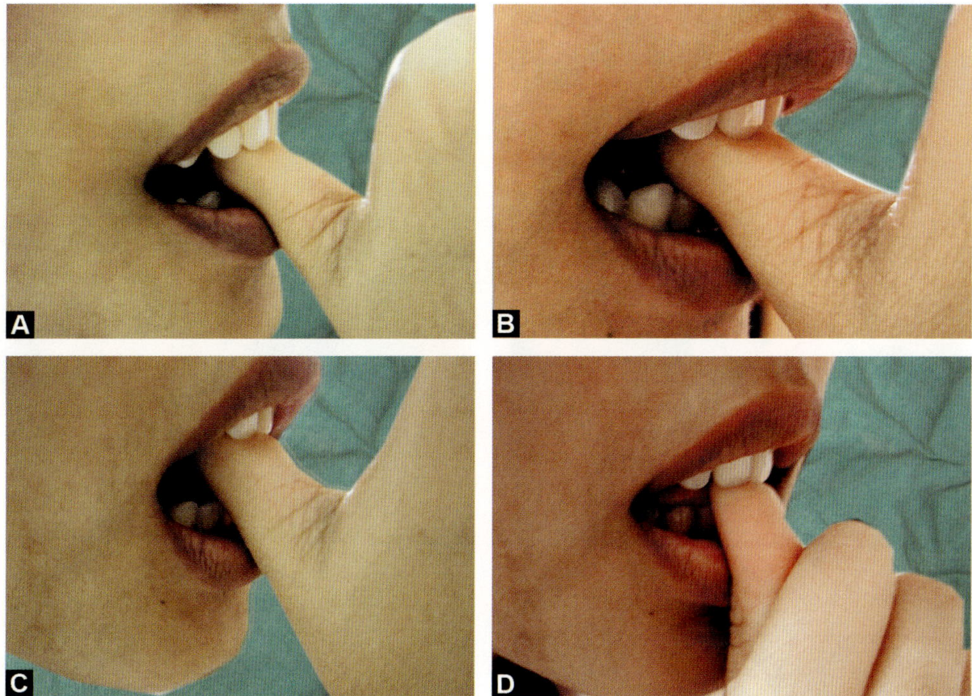

Figs 6.37A to D: Position of the thumb as per Subtleny's classification: (A) Thumb is inserted beyond first joint and lower incisors presses over the thumb; (B) Thumb is inserted slightly anterior to the first joint but contact is made only with incisors; (C) Thumb is inserted beyond first joint but lower incisors do not contact the thumb; (D) The lower incisors contact the thumb at the nails

Psychosexual/Psychoanalytical Theory

Formulated by S Freud, according to which thumb sucking habit evolves from an inherent psychosexual drive where the child derives pleasure during sucking the thumb. It views continuation of the habit as the manifestation of an underlying psychological disturbance and therefore as a mechanism for stress management. Elimination of the habit may cause it to be substituted by other antisocial activities.

Oral Drive Theory

It is formulated by Sears and Wise. According to this theory prolongation of nursing strengthens the oral drive and child begins thumb sucking.

Benjamin's Theory

According to this theory thumb sucking arises from the rooting reflex common to all mammalian infants. This primitive reflex is maximal during the first 3 months of life. If it persists into later life it can lead to an abnormal habit.

Rooting reflex—is the movement of an infant's head and tongue towards a stimulus touching an infant's cheek.

Learning Theory

According to this theory habit stems from an adaptive response and assumes no underlying psychological cause and aquired as a result of learning.

Clinical Features of a Child Practicing Thumb Sucking

When a thumb is sucked, it can be positioned in varying positions inside the mouth as explained in the classification and the other fingers are most of the time rolled into a fist or curled over the bridge of the nose or (Figs 6.38A and B). The type of malocclusion seen is dependent on the position of the digit, the associated contraction of the musculature, mandibular position, facial skeletal pattern along with the duration, intensity and frequency of the habit.[3]

Changes Seen in Orofacial Structures (Figs 6.39A and B)

1. Labial flaring of maxillary anterior teeth
2. Lingual collapse of mandibular anterior teeth
3. Increased overjet
4. Hypotonic upper lip and hyperactive lower lip
5. Tongue placed inferiorly leading to posterior crossbite due to maxillary arch contraction

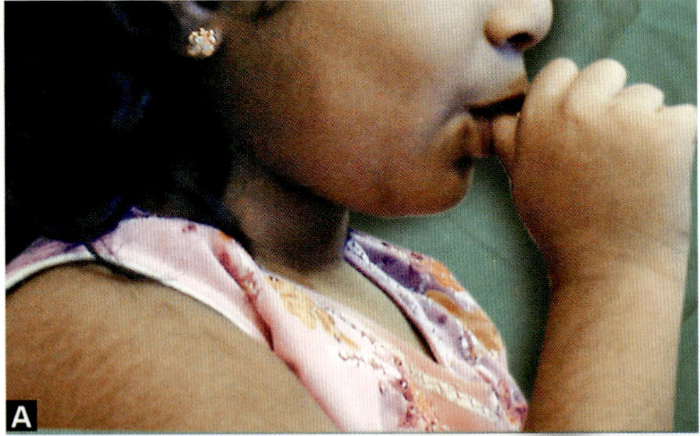

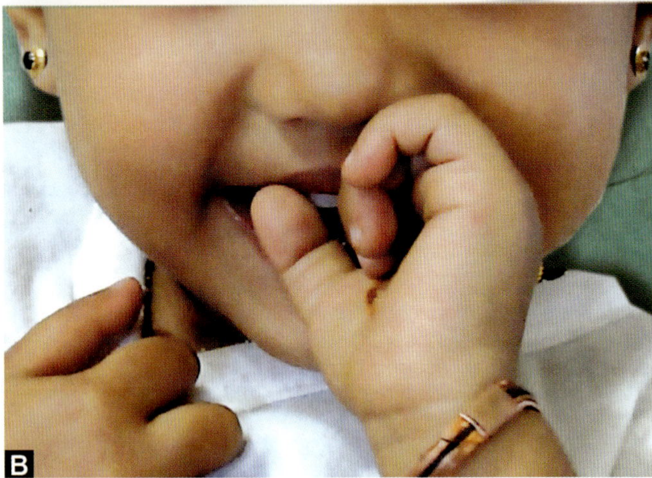

Figs 6.38A and B: Thumb or any finger (Digit sucking) can be used for sucking: (A) Fingers are rolled into a fist while thumb sucking; (B) Index finger is used for sucking

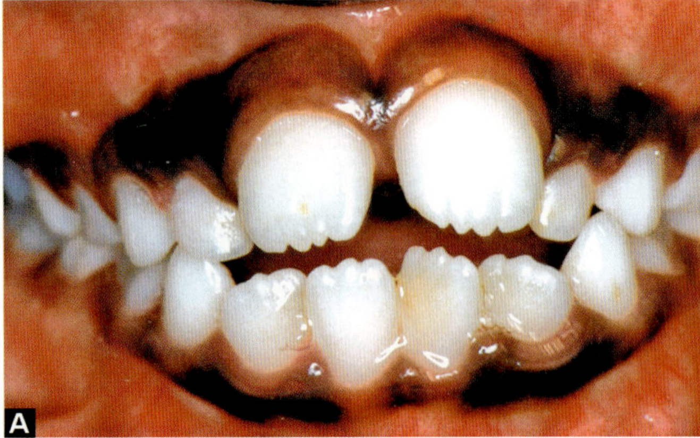

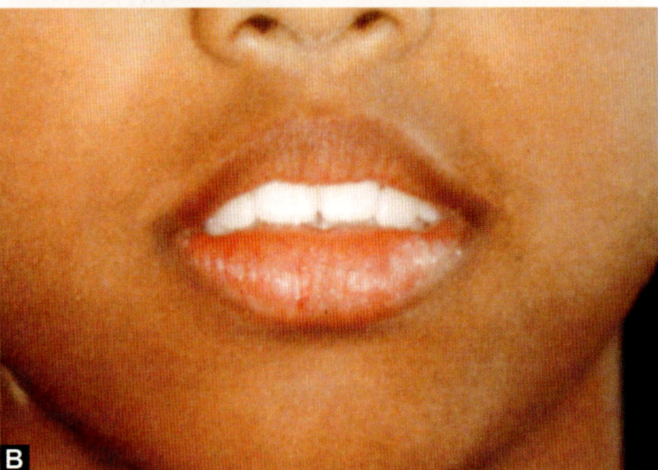

Figs 6.39A and B: Clinical features of thumb sucking: (A) Labial flaring of maxillary anterior teeth; (B) Hypotonic upper lip

6. Associated with simple tongue thrust, which is an adaptive response to open bite
7. Narrow nasal floor and high palatal vault
8. Some craniofacial skeletal changes may also be seen
9. Fungal infection, keratotic lesions—on the thumb
10. Thumb nail exhibits dish pan (concave) appearance.

Factors Influencing the Severity of Dental Defects due to Thumb Sucking[4]

The type of malocclusion depends upon:
1. *Position of the digit:* The effect of thumb sucking depends whether the thumb is placed just at the entrance of the oral cavity or is it placed very inside touching the palate. If the thumb is placed just at the entrance there may not be any palatal changes observed.
2. *Associated orofacial muscle contraction:* Whether the child is actively involving orofacial muscles. When there is associated muscle contraction the intensity of the defects greatly increases.

3. *Position of mandible during sucking:* When the mouth is kept open the tongue is carried down along with the lower jaw. Thus during swallowing there is only buccal muscle contraction (As the thumb is inside the mouth most of the time) and thus the force applied on the molars is one sided. The tongue being in a lowered position fails to exert reciprocal force from the lingual side. This may cause posterior crossbite.
4. *Facial skeletal morphology:* Straight profile withstands the effects of thumb sucking better than typical Class II facial skeleton. Therefore, a mild habit may be more detrimental in some faces than a severe one in others.
5. *Duration, intensity and frequency of the habit:* Increase in all the three factors results in severe changes in orofacial structures.

Three Distinct Phases of Development of Thumb Sucking Habit

The development of thumb sucking can be divided into three distinct phases:

Phase 1: Extends from birth to 3 years normal and subclinically significant sucking. This period is considered normal and does not require any intervention. It should be kept in mind at the end of this stage that any vigorous thumb sucking may be carried into the next phase which then becomes abnormal. So preventive measures can be instituted and thumb substituted by physiological pacifiers.

Phase 2: Extends from 3 to 6-7 years. It is associated with clinically significant sucking. The habit may be meaningful or empty. It is necessary to manage or correct the habit at this stage.

Phase 3: Intractable sucking. When the habit proceeds into phase 3, problem becomes more serious and may require psychotherapy.

Management of Thumb Sucking Habit[11]

Steps in the management of thumb sucking habit:

Discussion with the Child

- The first step in the treatment of the habit is to make the child understand that the habit is going to cause problem to him/her and needs to be stopped. Any measure to stop the habit is possible only when the child fully cooperates.
- Second important step is to differentiate whether the habit is a meaningful or an empty habit. Meaningful habit is managed by treating the etiology first and then the practice or ill effects of habit.
- No threats or shamming should be done. Friendly attempts made to learn about child's attitude towards the habit
- Photographs, video or casts of other child before and after treatment is shown.
- *Dunlop β hypothesis:* The patient is made to sit in front of the mirror and asked to suck his thumb. This will make him realize, how awkward he looks and wants to stop sucking his thumb.
- Child is given a card to score the number of times he has sucked his thumb. After 2 weeks it is assessed to study the severity of the habit. The process of keeping the record will tend to reduce the number of times the child sucks the thumb.
- Be supportive and let the child know that you want to help him.

Discussion with the Parents

- The habit should not be made the topic of discussion at home and the child should not be ridiculed.
- Most of the children will loose the habit by the end of this phase.

Use of Rewards

When the child agrees to stop the habit, he/she is asked to maintain a calendar. The child marks the dates when he/she refrains from the habit. The child is then rewarded based on the number of marks.

Use of Habit Reminders

- This method is used when the reward system fails and the child is finding it difficult to stop the habit by himself.
- Bitter substance/nail polish applied on the thumb can also be used as reminders to withdraw or prevent the thumb from entering into the mouth.
- Habit reminders: It is also advocated in children who are aware of the ill effects and want to discard the habit. Patient cooperation is very important. Habit reminders reminds the child of the habit whenever he puts his thumb into the mouth. Thumb guard made of acrylic or gauze (Figs 6.40A and B) will remind the child as the thumb is taken to the mouth and also the child does not derive any pleasure sucking the thumb guard. Other appliance that can be used as reminders which are inserted onto the tooth are palatal bar, hay rake, etc. (Figs 6.41A and B). These appliances can be removable or fixed.
- Bluegrass appliance: It incorporates a six sided roller instead of a rake and spins around a 0.045″ stainless steel wire.[12]
- If there is nocturnal component, an elastic bandage may be wrapped loosely from the middle of the forearm to

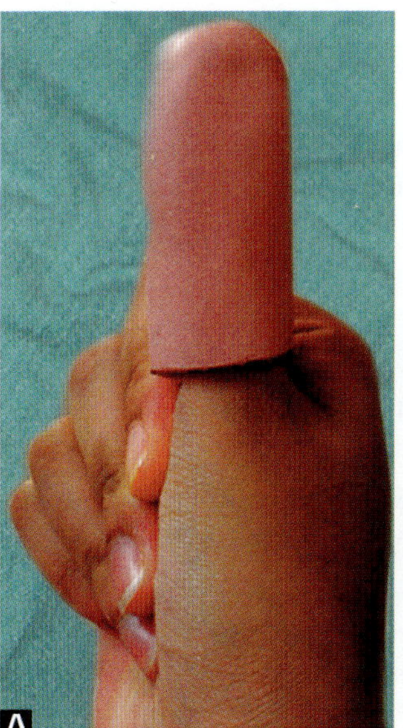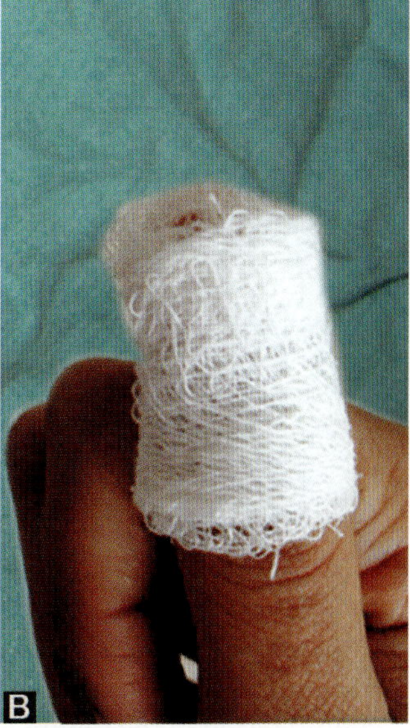

Figs 6.40A and B: (A) Acrylic guard; (B) Gauze wrapped around the thumb acts as a guard

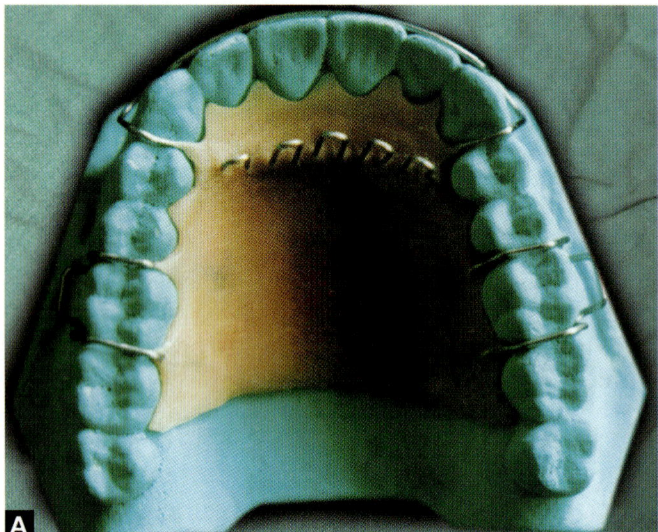

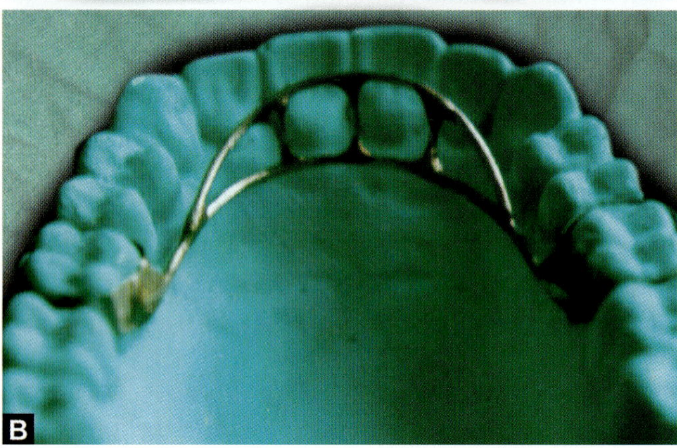

Figs 6.41A and B: Habit reminder with palatal rake: (A) Removable; (B) Fixed

the biceps area to prevent the thumb reaching the mouth (Fig. 6.42). The child (and not the parent) can also place thumb bandage at night as reminder.

> **Ideal appliance for correction of thumb sucking should:**
>
> - Offer no restraint to normal muscular activity
> - Have no shame attached to its use
> - Not or minimally involve parents for placement and removal
> - Well adapted, out of the way of normal oral functioning

> The habit will usually be broken by the end of 3 weeks and the child must be rewarded at the end. Habit reminders should be left in the mouth for 6 months as retainer. Next 3 months are needed to correct posterior crossbite with quad helix and 3 months are required for stabilization.

TONGUE THRUSTING HABIT

Definition

Norton and Gellin defined tongue thrust "as a condition in which the tongue protrudes between the anterior or posterior teeth during swallowing with or without affecting tooth position".

Tongue thrusting can be either anterior or posterior. Anterior tongue thrust is associated with forceful anterior thrust of the tongue and posterior tongue thrust is associated with lateral thrust of the tongue usually seen when there is any missing tooth/teeth.

Different Types of Tongue Thrusting Habits[10,13-15]

According to Moyer

A. Normal swallow: (a) Infantile swallow, (b) Adult swallow
B. Simple tongue thrust
C. Complex tongue thrust
D. Retained infantile swallow.

Features of Infantile Swallowing Pattern

- Almost all infants thrust their tongue while swallowing and the tongue lies between the gum bads.
- Mandible is stabilized by obvious contraction of facial muscles especially the buccinator.
- Seen in neonate and gradually disappears with eruption of teeth and growth of mandible.
- It is due to the differential growth of tongue and jaws. The growth of the tongue is nearing completion at birth

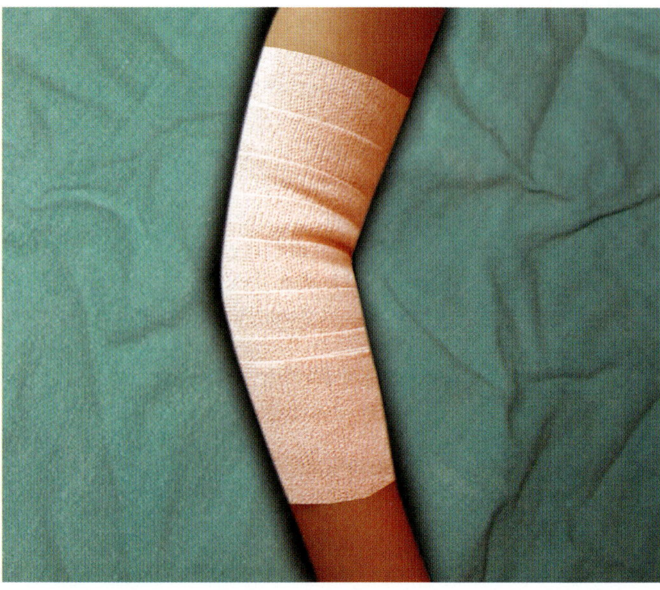

Fig. 6.42: Elastic bandage wrapped around the arm and forearm

compared to the jaws thus the tongue is relatively bigger to be accommodated in a smaller jaw. Later as the jaw grows it can accommodate the tongue explaining the lower incidence of tongue thrusting with age.

Features of Adult Swallowing Pattern

- As a person swallows the tip of the tongue contacts the palatal rugae posterior to the maxillary anterior teeth, midportion contacts the hard palate and the posterior aspect assumes a 45° angulation against the posterior pharyngeal wall to permit the bolus of food to move into the digestive tract.
- Facial expression muscles are passive but mandibular elevators are contracted. Thus during a normal adult swallow there is no contraction of muscles of facial expression including the lips and cheek.

Features of Swallow Associated with Simple Tongue Thrusting (Fig. 6.43A)

- Simple tongue thrusting is associated with teeth together swallow
- There is associated contraction of lip, mentalis and mandibular elevators. So when the child swallows tight pursing of the lips with pluckering of the chin due to mentalis contraction is seen
- Well-circumscribed anterior open bite is the characteristic malocclusion observed
- It may also be due to some adaptive mechanism as observed in thumb sucking habit, which is associated with anterior open bite. When the child want to swallow the anterior open bite is sealed by the tongue to create a vaccum so as to complete the act of swallowing resulting in anterior tongue thrusting
- Posterior teeth are in stable interdigitation.

Features of Swallow Associated with Complex Tongue Thrusting (Fig. 6.43B)

- The teeth do not occlude when the child swallow and is termed as teeth apart swallow.
- Poor occlusal interdigitation with generalized anterior open bite is characteristic.
- Combined lip, facial and mentalis contraction is observed.
- Lack of contraction of mandibular elevators
- Tongue thrusts in between the teeth
- Likely to be mouth breathers.

Features of Retained Infantile Swallow (Fig. 6.43C)

- Seen due to undue persistence of the infantile swallow.
- Usually occlude on one molar in each quadrant.
- Strong contraction of facial muscles during swallowing.

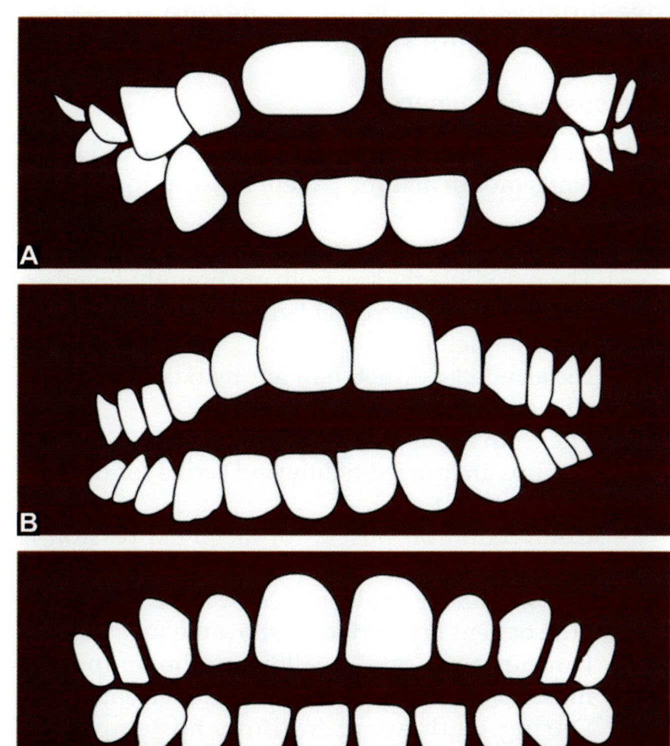

Figs 6.43A to C: Dental defect seen in different types of tongue thrusting habit: (A) Swallow associated with simple tongue thrusting; (B) Swallow associated with complex tongue thrusting; (C) Retained infantile swallow

- Tongue protrudes markedly and is held between all the teeth during the initial stages of the swallow.
- Expressionless face.
- Children restrict themselves to soft diet.

Reasons for the Prevalence of Tongue Thrusting Habit in Children

It may be due to:

1. The comparative largeness of the tongue within a retrognathic not fully developed mandible causing the tongue to protrude out.
2. Enlarged adenoid and palatine tonsils: It is very common in children and results in blockage of nasopharynx leading to mouth breathing. This inturn may lead to tongue thrust during swallowing
3. As associated with thumb sucking habit: Thumb sucking may result in anterior open bite leading to tongue thrust associated swallowing pattern.
4. Malocclusion: The incidence of tongue thrusting during swallowing has been reported to be higher in children with malocclusion than in children with good occlusion.

Investigative Methods for Identifying Tongue Thrusting Habit[10]

Methods of Examination

A. Patient is seated upright: A little water is placed in the patient's mouth and the patient is asked to swallow it.

   During normal swallowing pattern:
   – The mandible rises as teeth are brought together
   – The lips touch each other lightly showings scarcely any contraction
   – Facial muscles do not show any marked contraction

   During abnormal swallowing:
   – The teeth are apart
   – The lips are pursed tightly and active contraction is seen
   – Contraction of muscles of facial expression is clearly seen

B. Examiners hand is lightly placed over the temporalis and the patient is asked to swallow the water
   – During the normal swallowing the temporalis muscle contracts as the mandible is elevated
   – During teeth apart swallow, no temporalis contraction can be felt.

C. The lower lip is lightly held with thumb and finger and the patient is asked to swallow the water
   – During the normal swallowing process, the patient is able to swallow normally
   – In the abnormal swallowing pattern, the swallow will be inhibited, as strong mentalis and lip contractions are needed for mandibular stabilization and the water will spill out of the mouth.

General Clinical Features of Tongue Thrusting Habit (Figs 6.44A to C)

1. Proclination and flaring of incisors resulting in midline diastema.
2. Anterior open bite
3. Short and flaccid upper lip
4. Posterior crossbite.

Prognosis		
Simple tongue thrust	—	Excellent
Complex tongue thrust	—	Good
Retained infantile swallow	—	Very poor

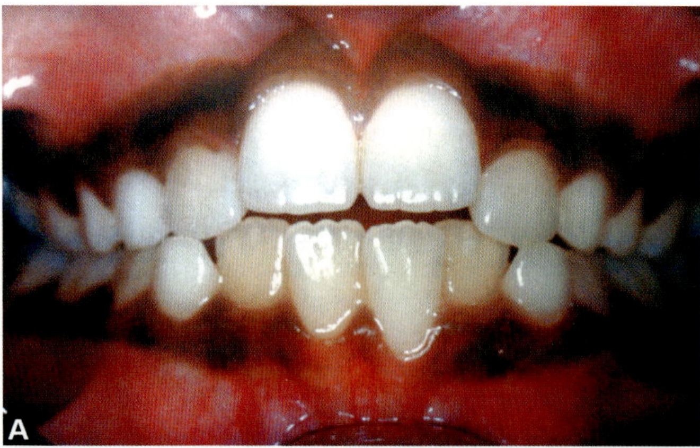
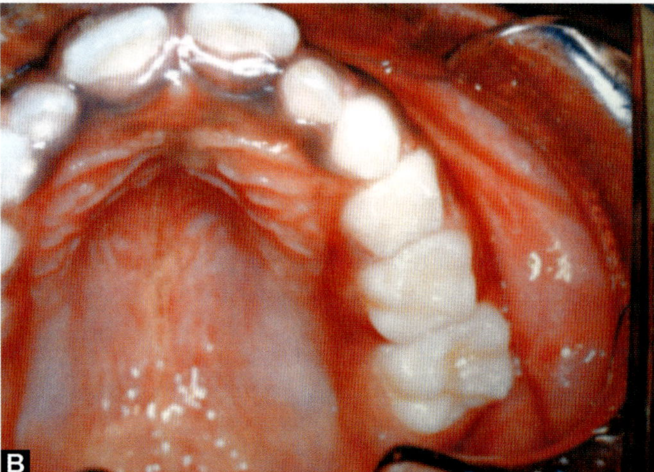
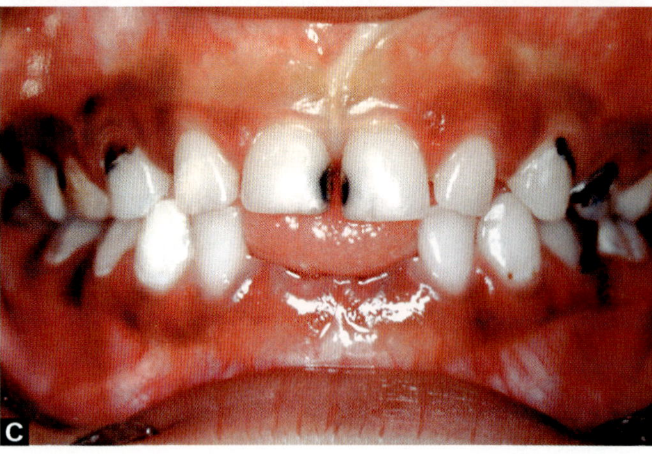

Figs 6.44A to C: Features of tongue thrusting habit: (A) Anterior proclination; (B) Narrow palate; (C) Tongue is seen thrusting into the edentulous space cause due to exfoliation of the incisors

Management of Tongue Thrusting Habit

The management of tongue thrusting habit is aimed at teaching the child the correct positioning of the tongue. This can be done by:

1. The patient is instructed to put the tip of the tongue at the correct position and swallow with lips pursed and teeth in occlusion. This helps the patient to learn a new reflex on the conscious level (40 times/day in 2-3 sessions).

2. A flat sugarless fruit drop can be placed on the back of the tongue and it is held against the palate in the correct position until it completely dissolves. This is practiced once or twice a day.
3. When the patient learns normal tongue position this has to be reinforced and made into an unconscious act.

The appliance therapy is initiated for children above 9 years.

Appliances used can be either fixed with bands and palatal rake or removable with Adam's clasp and Jackson's crib.

MOUTH BREATHING HABIT

Mouth breathing can be defined as habitual breathing through mouth instead of the nose. Breathing can be achieved through nose or mouth. A nasal breather can quickly change the mouth breathing during the strenuous exercises. Thus a mouth breather is one who breathes orally even in relaxed and stressful situation.

Etiology of Mouth Breathing Habit

It is estimated that 85% of the mouth breathers suffer from some degree of nasal obstruction while 20% are habitual mouth breathers.

Etiology can be due to:
- Anatomic (e.g. short upper lip, DNS),
- Pathological (enlarged adenoid, nasal polyps, etc.)
- Habitual.

Clinical Features Seen in Mouth Breathing Habit[16]

Facial appearance of a child with mouth breathing habit is termed as 'Adenoid Facies' and is characterized by:
- Long narrow face, narrow nose and nasal passage
- Flaccid and short upper lip
- Dolichofacial skeletal pattern
- Nose tipped superiorly
- Expressionless face
- Narrowed maxillary arch
- Labial flaring of the maxillary incisors
- Mouth breathing gingivitis
- Anterior open bite
- Increased caries incidence in maxillary anterior teeth.

Examination of a Child for Mouth Breathing Habit[17]

Examination is done as follows:
1. Observe the patient unknowingly while at rest,
   In a nasal breather: The lips touch lightly
   But in a mouth breather: The lips are kept apart
2. Patient is asked to take deep breath
   Nasal breather keeps the lips tightly closed
   Mouth breather takes a deep breath, keeping the mouth open.
3. Ask the patient to close the lips and take a deep breath through the nose.
   Nasal breather: It demonstrates good control of alar muscles which control the size and shape of external nares. So dilatation and contraction of nares is present
   Mouth breather: It may be capable of breathing through nose, but do not change the size or shape of the external nares.
4. *Butterfly test:* Take a piece of cotton and shape it into a butterfly. Place it on the philtrum and check for the movement of the cotton fibers. If they are moving in a direction towards the nose then the patient is a mouth breather.
5. *Two surface mirror test:* A double sided mouth mirror is taken. It is kept on the philtrum. If the fog if formed on the mirror facing the mouth, then the patient is a mouth breather.
6. *Water test:* The patient is asked to hold a mouthful of water for few minutes without swallowing. If the patient is a mouth breather he/she will not be able to hold the water in the mouth for long period.

Management of a Child with Mouth Breathing Habit

Management includes:
1. Identification and correction of nasal obstruction.
2. Physical exercise
   - Respiratory exercise
   - Lip exercise—horn and flute
   - Stretching and twisting of upper lip
3. Mechanical—oral screen.

Oral Screen/Vestibular Screen (Fig. 6.45)

- It is a myofunctional appliance that is easy to fabricate and easy to wear.
- It is curved corresponding to the curvature of the arch and is made of acrylic.
- It works on the principle of both force application and force elimination.
- Posterior crossbite can be corrected utilizing the principle of force elimination by providing a spacer between the teeth and the screen.
- Anterior teeth proclination can be corrected utilizing the principle of force application. This is possible by making the screen come in contact with the proclined teeth, so that the forces from the lips are transmitted directly to the proclined teeth through the screen.

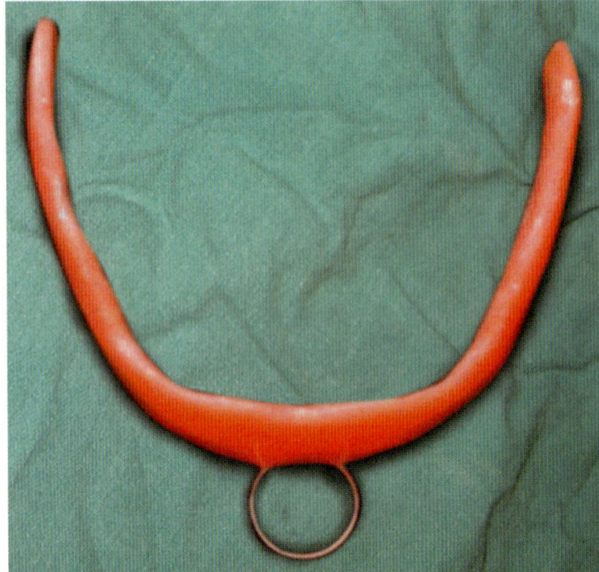

Fig. 6.45: Oral screen

- Oral screen can be used for the correction of mouth breathing, thumb sucking, lip biting or cheek biting habits.
- Lip exercises are possible with oral screen, which improves the tonicity of the lips.
- *Construction:* Upper and lower impressions are made and cast prepared. The casts are occluded in centric occlusion and sealed. Posteriorly the appliance will extend up to the distal margin of the last erupted teeth. The upper and lower borders will extend to the full depth of the sulcus. The modeling wax of about 2-3 mm is adapted over the labial, buccal and alveolar surface. Window in the wax is made over the incisal one third of the proclined anterior teeth, so that the acrylic will touch the teeth directly. The appliance is then fabricated with self-cure or heat cure acrylic. The wax spacer is removed. The appliance is finished and polished.
- The appliance has to be worn for 2-3 hours during the day and during the sleep at night.
- When the appliance is worn there is a space between the buccal surface of the posterior teeth and the oral screen. In the anterior region the oral screen touches the proclined incisors.
- Patient is taught few lip exercises to improve the tonicity of the lip. The child holds the ring and tries to pull the oral screen out of the mouth. Simultaneously the lips are tightly pursed, so that the appliance does not come out of the mouth. This improves their tonicity and increases their length. During these lip exercises the forces exerted by the lip is transmitted to the proclined teeth through the oral screen. Posteriorly the buccal musculatures are kept away from the teeth and

are prevented from exerting force on the teeth. This helps in arch expansion by the constant force applied by the tongue from the palatal aspect.
- *Modifications:*
  - If the patient feels difficult to breathe, then multiple holes can be made that are closed one by one over a period of time.
  - A metallic ring is made and placed in the midline of the appliance which will help to hold the oral screen (Hotz modification).
  - Double oral screen can be given with a similar additional lingual screen in tongue thrusting habit.

BRUXISM[17-19]

Definition

It can be defined as 'habitual grinding of teeth when the individual is not chewing or swallowing'.[17]

The habit may occur only during sleep, during the wakening hours or both. About 15% of children and young adults practice bruxism.

Etiology

Causes are:
1. Psychic tension associated with any kind of stress.
2. Occlusal interference due to faulty restoration, malocclusion, etc.
3. Intestinal parasites, subclinical nutritional deficiency, allergy and endocrine disturbance.

Features

They are as follows:
1. Occlusal surfaces are worn considerably with exposing dentin or even the redness of dental pulp may show through dentin. Rarely is there any pulp exposures as there is formation of secondary dentin.
2. Masticatory muscle soreness
3. TMJ pain
4. Trauma to the periodontium.

Management

Management of bruxism can be categorized as:

1. *Adjunctive Therapy*
   a. *Psychotherapy:* Aimed at lowering emotional or psychic tension
   b. *Autosuggestion and hypnosis:* Where the patient becomes conscious of his nervous habit and understands the possible consequence
   c. *Relaxing exercise and physiotherapy:* Serve to decrease muscle tension and bruxism. Exercise and massage may relieve pain

d. *Elimination of oral pain and discomfort:* Pain associated with periodontal disease, lip and cheek should be eliminated.

2. *Occlusal Therapy*
   a. *Occlusal adjustments:* Bite raising crowns, splints and elimination of occlusal interference
   b. *Bite plates and splints:* The purpose is to stop bruxism by elimination of occlusal interference, to avoid occlusal wear, to restrict the jaw movements and break the habit
   c. Occlusal reconstruction and prosthesis
   d. *Bite guard:* Prevents continual abrasion of teeth.
   Tranquilizers have been helpful in overcoming bruxism.

LIP BITING AND MENTALIS HABIT

Normal lip anatomy and function are important for speaking, eating and maintaining a balanced occlusion. Lip biting may or may not be associated with mentalis habit.

Features of Lip Biting and Mentalis Habit

Lip biting habit may take on many forms. Two extreme types extends from mild wetting the lips with the tongue to pulling the lips into the mouth between the teeth (Figs 6.46A and B).

Mentalis Habit

The vermillion border of the lower lip is often everted with the lingual aspect elevated into the mouth along with the appearance of sublabial contracture line between the lip and chin.

Changes Seen due to the Lip Biting Habit

- Labial placement of maxillary incisors
- Collapsed lower incisors
- Increased overjet
- Reddened, irritated and chapped area below the vermillion border and is usually seen in the lower lip
- Can be associated with mentalis habit.

Management of Lip Biting Habit

Management includes:
1. Visual education
2. Lip bumper (Fig. 6.47) makes it difficult to draw the lower lip between the teeth
3. Correction of the overjet
4. Oral screen.

NAIL BITING HABIT

Features and Management

Nail biting habit is found among children, with marked increase from ages 3 to 6 years. From 7 to 10 years the

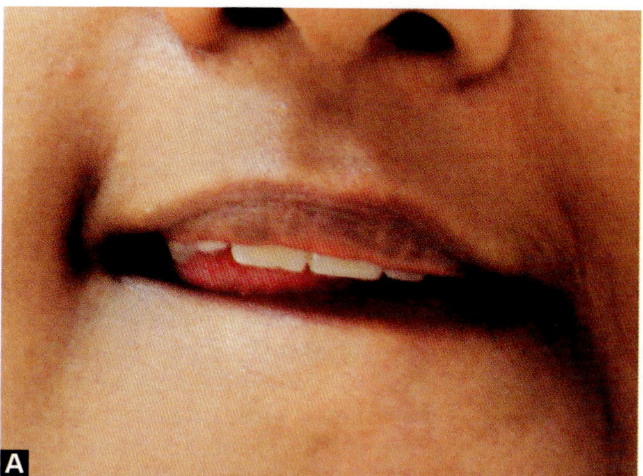
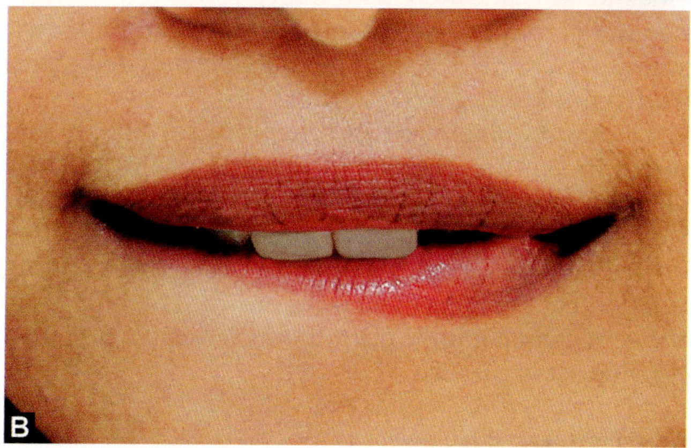

Figs 6.46A and B: Different types of lip biting: (A) Mild wetting of the lip by the tongue; (B) Biting of the lip

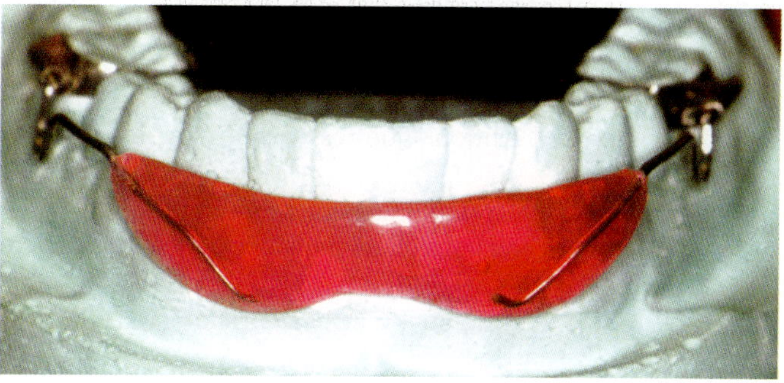

Fig. 6.47: Lip bumper

incidence remains relatively constant and again rises at 10 years. About 40% of the adolescents are nail biters. It may be a reflection of anxiety or personal adjustment.

Nail biting does not significantly harm the occlusion and the children are self-conscious and embarrassed about the habit themselves. The effective treatment consists of identifying the cause and its correction. In some instances, mesial rotation and notching of the central incisors may be observed.

Treatment

Management is similar to thumb sucking, that is:
1. Discussion with the child
2. Discussion with the parents
3. Habit reminders.

SELF-DESTRUCTIVE ORAL HABITS/MASOCHISTIC HABITS

Self-injurious habits are defined as deliberate harm done to one's own body without suicidal intent.[20] They include hitting the head with fist, banging the head against the wall, picking at the gingiva with fingers and finger nails, chewing the inside of the cheek, lip or tongue, etc. It has been associated with many conditions such as mental retardation, psychoses, sensory neuropathy and certain syndromes such as Lesch-Nyhan and de Lange's syndromes.[20-24]

Dental management includes in preventing from injury to the lip, cheek and other tissue of the oral cavity. Oral shields made of acrylic, lip bumpers have been suggested as a method to prevent such injuries. Other methods includes restraints, protective padding, sedation, etc.[25-27] If the habit is the outward manifestation of deeper psychological problems, consultation with psychiatrist is advised.

REFERENCES

1. Klein ET. The thumb-sucking habit: Meaningful or empty? Am J Orthod. 1971;59:283-9.
2. Brash JC. The Aetiology of Irregularity and Malocclusion of the Teeth. London: Dental Board of the United Kingdom; 1929. pp. 212.
3. Mathewson RJ, Primosch RE. Fundamentals of Pediatric Dentistry, 3rd edition. Quintessence Publishing Co. Inc; 1995.
4. Sorokolit CA, Nanda RS. The influence of function on the development and correction of malocclusion. J Okla Dent Assoc. 1989;80:22-31.
5. Gellin ME. Thumb sucking: Pediatricians' Guidelines. Clinical. Pediatrics. 1978;28:438-40.
6. Cook JE. Intraoral Pressures Involved in Thumb and Finger Sucking, MS thesis, University of Michigan, June, 1958.
7. Subtelny JD, Subtelny JD. "Oral Habits—Studies in Form, Function, and Therapy". Angle Orthod. 1973; 43(4):347-83.
8. Sears R, Wise G. Relation of cup feeding in infancy to thumb sucking and the oral drive. Am J Ortho psychiatry 1950;20:123.
9. Benjamin L. Non-nutritive sucking and dental malocclusion in the deciduous and permanent teeth of rhesus monkey. Child Dev. 1962;3:29.
10. Moyers RE. Etiology of molocclusion. In: Mayers RE (Ed). Handbook of Orthododontics, 4th edition. Chicago: Year Book Medical Publishers Inc; 1988.
11. Haskell BS, Mink JR. An aid to stop thumb sucking—the "Bluegrass" appliance. Pediatr Dent. 1991;13:83-5.
12. Melson B, Stensgaard K, Pedersen J. Sucking habits and their influence on swallowing pattern and prevalence of malocclusion. Eur J Orthod. 1979;1:271-80.
13. Moyers RE. The infantile swallow. Rep congr Eur orthod Soc. 1964;40:180-7.
14. Moyers RE. Postnatal development of the orofacial musculature in patterns of orofacial growth and development. Am Speech & Hearing Assoc Report 6, Washington DC; 1971.
15. Linder-Aronson S. Adenoids—their effect on mode of breathing and nasal air flow and their relationship to characteristics of the facial skeleton and the dentition. Acta Otolaryngol Suppl. 1970;265:3-132.
16. Moyers RE. Analysis of the orofacial and jaw musculature. In: Moyers RE. Handbook of Orthododontics, 4th edition. Chicago: Year Book Medical Publishers Inc; 1988.
17. Ramfjord SP. Bruxism, a clinical and electromyographic study. J Am Dent Assoc. 1961;2:62.
18. Attanasio R. An overview of bruxism and its management. Dent Clin North Am. 1997;41:229-41.
19. Lobbezoo F, Lavigne GJ. Do bruxism and temporomandibular disorders have a cause-and-effect relationship? Journal of Orofacial Pain. 1997;11:15-23.
20. Chen LR, Liu JF. Successful treatment of self-inflicted oral mutilation using an acrylic splint retained by a head gear. Pediatr Dent. 1996;18:408-10.
21. Hyman SL, Fisher W, Mercugliano M, et al. Children with self-injurious behavior. Pediatrics. 1990. 85(3 Pt 2):437-41.
22. Rasmussen P. The congenital insensitivity-to-pain syndrome (analgesia congenita): report of a case. Int J Paediatr Dent. 1996;6:117-22.
23. Saemundsson SR, Roberts MW. Oral self-injurious behavior in the developmentally disabled: Review and a case. ASDC J Dent Child. 1997;64:205-9.
24. Loschen EL, Osman OT. Self-injurious behavior in the developmentally disabled: pharmacologic treatment. Psychopharmacol Bull. 1992;28:439-49.
25. Wood AJ. A tongue shield appliance: design, fabrication, and case report. Spec Care Dentist. 1991;11:12-4.
26. Cehreli ZC, Olmez S. The use of a special mouthguard in the management of oral injury self-inflicted by a 4-year-old child. Int J Paediatr Dent. 1996;6:277-81.
27. Polyzois GL. Custom mouth protectors: an aid for autistic children. Quintessence Int. 1989;20:775-7.

FURTHER READING

1. Afzelius-Alm A, Larsson E, Löfgren CG, et al. Factors that influence the proclination or retroclination of the lower incisors in children with prolonged thumb-sucking habits. Swed Dent J. 2004;28(1):37-45.

2. Al-Emran S, Al-Jobair A. An assessment of a new reminder therapy technique for ceasing digit sucking habits in children. J Clin Pediatr Dent. 2005;30(1):35-8.

3. Aznar T, Galan AF, Marin I, et al. Dental arch diameters and relationships to oral habits. Angle Orthod. 2006;76(3):441-5.

4. Barberia E, Lucavechi T, Cardenas D, et al. An atypical lingual lesion resulting from the unhealthy habit of sucking the lower lip: clinical case study. J Clin Pediatr Dent. 2006 Summer;30(4):280-2.

5. Baydas B, Uslu H, Yavuz I, et al. Effect of a chronic nail-biting habit on the oral carriage of Enterobacteriaceae. Oral Microbiol Immunol. 2007;22(1):1-4.

6. Bishara SE, Warren JJ, Broffitt B, et al. Changes in the prevalence of nonnutritive sucking patterns in the first 8 years of life. Am J Orthod Dentofacial Orthop. 2006;130(1):31-6.

7. Bosnjak A, Vucicevic-Boras V, Miletic I, et al. Incidence of oral habits in children with mixed dentition. J Oral Rehabil. 2002;29(9):902-5.

8. Eslamian L, Leilazpour AP. Tongue to palate contact during speech in subjects with and without a tongue thrust. Eur J Orthod. 2006;28(5):475-9.

9. Flutter J. The negative effect of mouth breathing on the body and development of the child. Int J Orthod Milwaukee. 2006;17(2):31-7.

10. Fraser C. Tongue thrust and its influence in orthodontics. Int J Orthod Milwaukee. 2006;17(1):9-18.

11. Germec D, Taner TU. Lower lip sucking habit treated with a lip bumper appliance. Angle Orthod. 2005;75(6):1071-6.

12. Guaba K, Ashima G, Tewari A, et al. Prevalence of malocclusion and abnormal oral habits in North Indian rural children. J Indian Soc Pedod Prev Dent. 1998;16(1):26-30.

13. Herrera M, Valencia I, Grant M, et al. Bruxism in children: effect on sleep architecture and daytime cognitive performance and behavior. Sleep. 2006;29(9):1143-8. Erratum in: Sleep. 2006;29(11):1380.

14. Josell SD. Habits affecting dental and maxillofacial growth and development. Dent Clin North Am. 1995;39(4):851-60.

15. Kharbanda OP, Sidhu SS, Sundaram K, et al. Oral habits in school going children of Delhi: a prevalence study. J Indian Soc Pedod Prev Dent. 2003;21(3):120-4.

16. Molina OF, dos Santos J, Mazzetto M, et al. Oral jaw behaviors in TMD and bruxism: a comparison study by severity of bruxism. Cranio. 2001;19(2):114-22.

17. Monroy PG, da Fonseca MA. The use of botulinum toxin-a in the treatment of severe bruxism in a patient with autism: a case report. Spec Care Dentist. 2006;26(1):37-9.

18. Peng CL, Jost-Brinkmann PG, Yoshida N, et al. Comparison of tongue functions between mature and tongue-thrust swallowing—an ultrasound investigation. Am J Orthod Dentofacial Orthop. 2004;125(5):562-70.

19. Schneider PE, Peterson J. Oral habits: considerations in management. Pediatr Clin North Am. 1982;29(3):523-46.

20. Shetty SR, Munshi AK. Oral habits in children—a prevalence study. J Indian Soc Pedod Prev Dent. 1998;16(2):61-6.

21. Trawitzki LV, Anselmo-Lima WT, Melchior MO, et al. Breast-feeding and deleterious oral habits in mouth and nose breathers. Braz J Otorhinolaryngol. 2005;71(6):747-51

22. Vazquez-Nava F, Quezada-Castillo JA, Oviedo-Trevino S, et al. Association between allergic rhinitis, bottle feeding, non-nutritive sucking habits, and malocclusion in the primary dentition. Arch Dis Child. 2006;91(10):836-40.

23. Wu E, Viegas SF. Finger sucking and onycholysis in an infant. J Hand Surg Am. 2005;30(3):620-2.

QUESTIONS

1. Define pernicious oral habits.
2. Classify oral habits and explain each of them.
3. Explain the methods of diagnosis and management of thumb sucking habit.
4. Describe in detail the clinical features of mouth breathing habits.
5. What are the different types of tongue thrusting habits and how will you differentiate them from each other?
6. What are masochistic habits?

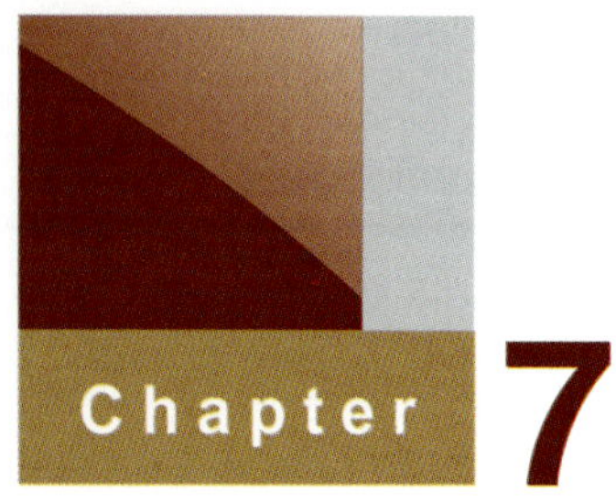

Dental Caries and its Management

DENTAL CARIES

DEFINITION

Dental caries can be defined as an infectious micro-biological disease of the teeth that results in localized dissolution and destruction of the calcified tisues. It is derived from Latin word meaning to 'Rot' or 'Decay.'[1]

Pits and fissures on the tooth surface are at the highest risk for the development of caries as they provide excellent areas of retention for microorganisms. The appearance of Streptococcus in the pits and fissures is usually followed by caries 6 to 24 months later.

Interproximal areas are also at risk as they are not exposed to tongue movements, salivary flow and the effects of mastication of food.

The facial and lingual surface, below the height of contour is not cleaned daily during the process of mastication. Therefore these surfaces are habitats for caries producing mature plaque.

ETIOLOGY OF CARIES

Caries is a multifactorial disease with interplay of many factors. Key's triad[2] (Fig. 7.1) explains the interplay of the host (the tooth and saliva) microflora and substrate (food). Many modifications of this interplay have evolved. One such modification considers saliva as a separate unit and involves an addition of time factor (Fig. 7.2).[3,4]

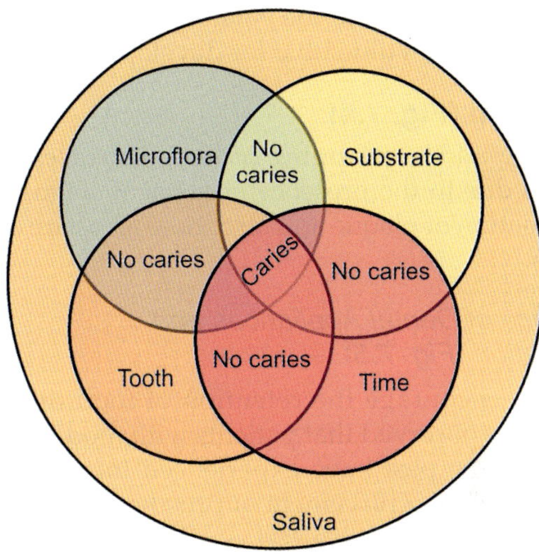

Fig. 7.2: Modification of Key's triad

Role of Tooth in the Etiology of Caries

It depends upon:
- Anatomic characteristics of the teeth
- Arch form
- Presence of dental appliances and restoration
- Composition.

Anatomic Characteristics of the Teeth (Fig. 7.3)

The teeth require additional 2-3 years for post-eruptive maturation through exposure to saliva. Permanent

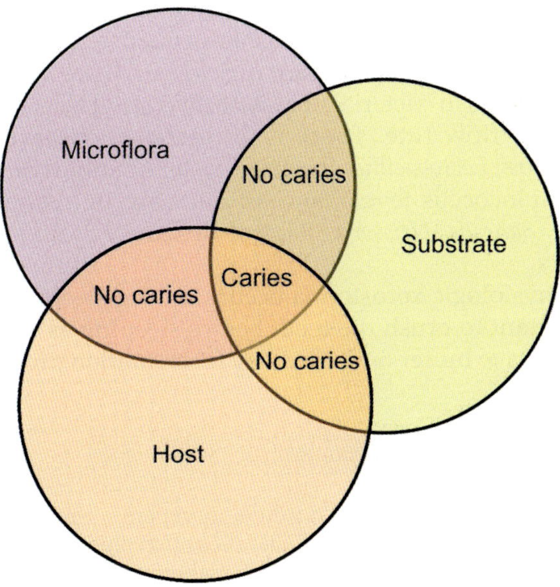

Fig. 7.1: Key's triad

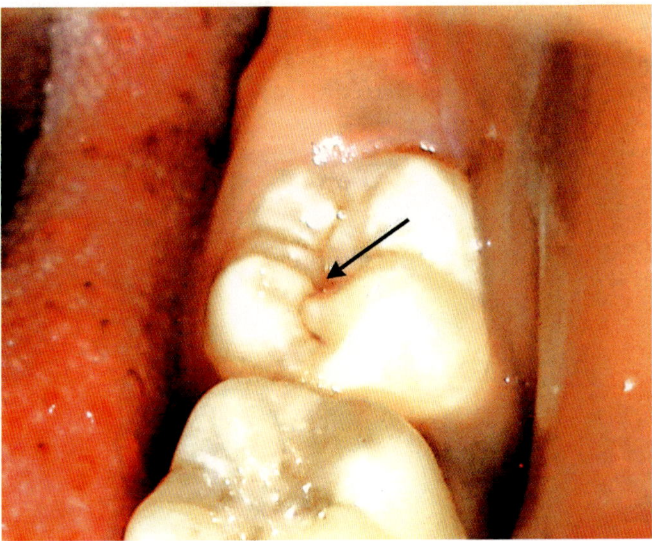

Fig. 7.3: Deep pits and fissures are at increased risk for caries

molars have incompletely coalesced pits and fissures that allow the dental plaque material to be retained at the base of the defect in contact with exposed dentin. The palatal pits of the maxillary molars, the buccal pit of the mandibular molars and the palatal pits on the maxillary incisors are very vulnerable for development of caries.

Arch Form (Fig. 7.4)

Crowding and overlapping of teeth increases the risk of caries due to the presence of areas of stagnation for accumulation of plaque and also these areas are difficult to clean.

Presence of Dental Appliances and Restoration (Fig. 7.5)

All these encourage the retention of food debris and plaque. It is observed that patients with moderate caries activity in the past have experienced increased caries activity following placement of prosthesis.

Composition of the Teeth

Surface zone of enamel is more resistant to caries compared to the inner layers due to the presence of:
- Dicalcium phosphate dihydrate (DCPD) and fluor-appatite
- Increased mineral and less organic matter
- Decreased water content
- Increased fluoride, chloride, zinc, lead and iron
- Decreased carbonate, and magnesium.

Role of Saliva in the Etiology of Caries

It depends upon the following properties of saliva:
- Composition
- Flow rate
- Salivary buffers
- Viscosity
- Antibacterial property

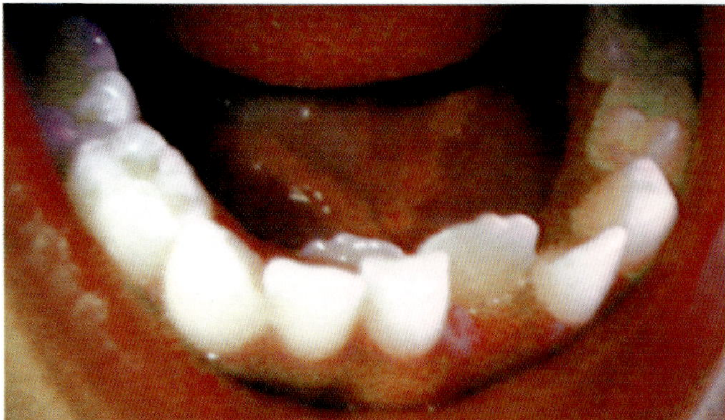

Fig. 7.4: Areas of overlap or crowding are at risk for developing caries

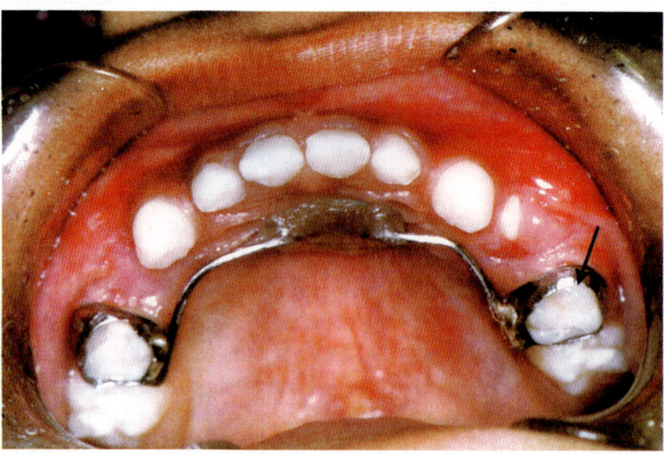

Fig. 7.5: Margins of the appliance help in retention of plaque

Composition of Saliva

There seems to be existing a direct relationship between caries prevalence and salivary amylase, urea, ammonia, calcium, phosphate, pH, etc.

Saliva of caries immune persons exhibit increased ammonia content which helps in neutralizing acids. Increased ptyalin in the parotid secretions is also associated with low caries due to its amylolytic activity.

> Submandibular secretion has 50% more calcium than parotid (6.8 mg/100 ml and 4.1 mg/100 ml respectively), so increased calculus is seen in mandibular anterior teeth.

Flow Rate of Saliva

Decreased salivary flow is associated with increased caries activity. Xerostomia is associated with cervical caries similar to the rampant caries.

Changes in bacterial flora is observed with decreased salivary flow rate. There is an increase observed in *S. mutans*, *Lactobacillus* species, yeasts, Actinomyces and Staphylococcus levels, and a decrease in *Veillonella*, *Strep. Sanguis*, *Neisseria*, Bacteroides and *Fusobacterium species*.

Physiologic xerostomia occurs during sleep, so it is important to brush the teeth before sleeping as there is no saliva to buffer or wash away fermentation products.

> **The etiology of xerostomia**
>
> Sarcoidosis, Sjögren's syndrome, therapeutic irradiation, surgical removal of salivary glands, anticholinergic drugs, antihistamins, antidepressants, diabetes mellitus, viral disease of the gland, etc.

Salivary Buffers

Chief buffer systems present in the saliva are mainly bicarbonates. Carbonic acid and phosphates to certain extent and ammonia to a lesser extent act as buffers.

> Critical pH[5] is that pH at which any particular saliva ceases to be saturated with calcium and phosphate. Below this value the inorganic material of the tooth may dissolve. The critical pH is 5.5.

> HCO_3 is more effective because
> - It can buffer rapidly by losing carbondioxide
> - Its pH is close to that encountered in plaque, so it is effective in that range
> - Increased flow results in increased bicarbonate release but less phosphate.

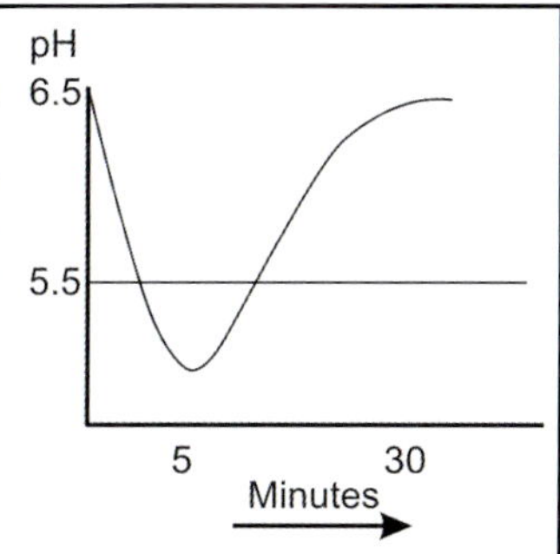

"Stephan's Curve."[6] There is a sudden fall in salivary pH from about 6.5 to 5.0 following intake of fermentable carbohydrates. The pH later returns to the normal resting value in about 15-40 minutes. This when plotted on a graph forms a curve and is termed as 'Stephan's Curve'.

Viscosity of Saliva

High caries incidence is associated with thick mucinous saliva as the saliva lacks its 'washing effect'.

Antibacterial Property

The antibacterial property of saliva is due to the presence of the following components.

Lysozyme—more in sublingual and submandibular saliva. Increased lysozyme activity is seen in caries free children.

Salivary lactoperoxidase system—peroxidase and thiocyanate act on hydrogen peroxide to produce hypothiocyanate. This in turn inactivates various bacterial enzymes and temporarily inhibit growth.

Immunoglobulin—secretory IgA is secreted in the saliva and has antibacterial property.

Microflora

Bacterial Colonization in the Oral Cavity

The type of bacteria seen in the oral cavity varies with age.

- Within hours of birth;
  S. salivarius, S. mitior form about 70%
- 1st year of life;
  a. *Dominant: Staphylococcus, Veilonella and Neisseria*
  b. *Less frequent: Actinomyces, Lactobacillus, Nocardia, Fusobacteria*
  c. *Sporadic: Bacteroids, Candida and Coliform*
  d. *Shortly after tooth eruption: S. sanguis followed by S. mutans.*

The notion that dental caries is an infectious, transmissible disease was first demonstrated by Keyes.[2] *Streptococcus mutans* and *Lactobacilli* produce greater amount of acid (aciduric) and can tolerate acidic environment (aciduric) and thus is more cariogenic than other bacteria in the oral cavity. Eight *Streptococcus mutans* serotypes have been identified and are collectively termed as *mutans streptococcus* (MS). *Mutans streptococcus* are most strongly associated with the onset of caries, whereas *Lactobacilli* are associated with active progression of cavitated lesions.[7,8]

Infants do not harbor this organism until sometime after teeth emerge. The initial acquisition of *S. mutans* in infants occurred during a well-delineated age range which is designated as the 'Window of infectivity'. This period ranges between 19 and 31 months with median age of 26 months.[9] Attempts to introduce these bacteria outside of this "window" result in markedly less colonization or caries activity. From the clinical point of view it must, therefore, be understood that this period is crucial and complete care must be taken to prevent or at least lessen the colonization of *S. mutans* during this period.[10] There has been observed a direct relationship between the numbers of bacteria in the mother's and child's mouth.[11,12] It is thus realized that reducing the bacterial count in mothers can postpone the colonization of bacteria in the child.

Bacteria Responsible for Smooth Surface, Fissure and Root Caries Varies

- Smooth surface caries—*S. mutans, S. salivarius*
- Fissure caries—*S. mutans, S. salivarius, S. sanguis, S. mitior, S. faecalis, A. viscosus, A. naeslundi, L. acidophilus, L. casei*
- Root caries—*S. mutans, S. salivarius, A. viscosus, A. naeslundi*

Streptococcus Mutans (S. mutans)[11,13-15]

S. mutans is the most common microorganism to cause caries. Clark in 1924 isolated a streptococcus strain that predominated in human carious lesions and he named them as *S. mutans*. For the next 40 years *S. mutans* was ignored and was rediscovered in 1960's.

Strepto: means arranged in chains

Coccus: means they are round in appearance

The cell wall is made of carbohydrate of either rhamose, glucose and galactose or galactose and rhamose or glucose and rhamose, which contribute for the antigenic properties.

Antigen responsible for group specificities are present on the cell wall.

S. mutans synthesize an extracellular polysaccharide (mutans) from sucrose using the enzyme glucosyl transferase. This material is composed of α (1-3)-linked glucose and aids in bacterial adhesion and provides energy source when extraneous carbohydrate is lacking. *S. mutans* also produces Lipo Teichoic Acid (LTA) which binds directly to enamel surface, facilitating colonization.

Characteristic features of streptococcus mutans

1. Spherical, 0.8-1.0 µ in diameter
2. Gram +ve cocci in short or medium chain
3. Nonmotile, encapsulated, nonsporing, facultative anaerobes and catalase –ve
4. On Mitis-Salivarius agar medium they grow as highly convex to pulvinate (cushion shaped) colonies, that are opaque with surface resembling frosted glass
5. Human salivary concentration of *S. Mutans* range from undetectable to 10^6-10^7 CFU/ml. Mothers with > 10^5 CFU/ml of salivary *S. Mutans* concentration are likely to infect their infants.
6. Produce α (green) hemolysis on blood agar
7. In solid media, colony morphology is rough, smooth or mucoid
8. Grow over a relative wide temperature range of 10-42°C, optimum being 37°C
9. Chief fermentation product is lactic acid. Small amount of formic acid, acetic acid and ethylalcohol are formed
10. When cultured with sucrose, they produce polysaccharide that are insoluble or can be precipitated with one part ethanol
11. Ferments mannitol and sorbitol
12. Uses NH_4 as the source of nitrogen, which gives them ecological advantage
13. Cultural characteristics:
    - Can be cultured in the presence of noninhibition concentration of sulfonamide, which helps in isolation of particular bacteria.
    - Grown on Mitis-Salivarius agar containing 20% sucrose and 0.2 units/ml bacitracin, which supresses other bacterial growth.

Properties of S. mutans

1. It can induce caries in experimental animals fed with high sugar diets

2. It is rarely found outside the mouth and appears to require a solid surface on which they colonize
3. They synthesize extracellular polysaccharide from sucrose using enzyme glucosyl transferase
4. Produce considerable amount of lipoteichoic acid
5. More aciduric than other streptococci
6. Produce acid in greater amount in solid media
7. Contain lysogenic bacteriophage
8. It is a homofermentative lactic acid former.

Plaque

Dental plaque may be readily visualized on teeth after 1-2 days with no oral hygiene measures. It is typically seen in areas where they are not debrided mechanically or by the movement of food over the teeth. Such areas include gingival one third of the tooth surface. Plaque is also deposited in cracks, pits and fissures and on the restorations, etc.

The location and rate of plaque formation vary among individuals and determining factors include oral hygiene, diet factors and salivary composition and flow rate.

It begins to form within 2 hours after teeth are brushed.[16] Within 5 hours microcolonies develop and by 24 hours 30% of coccus bacteria are present.

Plaque may be detected by running a periodontal probe or explorer along the gingival third of the tooth or by the use of disclosing solution.

It appears as white, grayish or yellow accumulation of variable thickness depending on its location and the extent and frequency of oral hygiene.

The time required for remineralization to replace the hydroxyapatite lost during demineralization is dependent on the age of the plaque. Younger the plaque, less time is required to neutralize the effects. Therefore, in the presence of recent plaque (about 12 hours or less) saliva will take about 10 minutes to remineralize following demineralization that occurs with single exposure of sucrose. But on the contrary it may take a period of 4 hours for the saliva to repair the same damage in the presence of plaque that is 48 hours or more old.[17]

Definitions of Plaque[1,18-20]

According to Wei—"Plaque is a complex mixture of dense microbial elements enmeshed within a gel like matrix of bacterial polysaccharide, salivary portiens and cellular components of the oral mucosa."

According to Sturdevant—"Plaque is a soft translucent and tenaciously adherent material accumulating on the surface of teeth."

According to Loe—"Plaque is a soft, non-mineralized, bacterial deposits which forms on teeth and dental prosthesis that are not adequately cleaned."

According to Glickman—"Plaque is a soft deposits that form the biofilm adhering to the tooth surface or other hard surfaces in the oral cavity, including removable and fixed restorations."

Facultative aerobes—pertaining to the ability to adjust to particular circumstances
Obligate aerobes—pertaining to or characterized by the ability to survive only in a particular environment.

Structure of plaque
Based on the location, plaque can be divided into supragingival and subgingival plaque.
Supragingival plaque
It is found at or above the gingival margin. When in direct contact with the gingival margin it is referred to a marginal plaque.
Supragingival plaque is made of 4 layers.
1. Plaque tooth interface
2. Condensed microbial layer
3. Body of the plaque
4. Plaque surface
Subgingival plaque
In children subgingival plaque may appear as either
1. Loose arrangement of mostly cocci
2. Condensed arrangement of cocci and rods or
3. Dense arrangement of cocci covered by a layer of filamentous organisms.

Composition of plaque
Plaque is composed primarily of microorganisms. One gram of plaque (wet weight) contains approximately 2×10^{11} bacteria. It has been estimated that > 325 different bacterial species may be found in plaque. Nonbacterial microorganisms found in plaque include mycoplasma species, yeasts, protozoa and viruses.
The intercellular matrix forms 20-30% of the plaque mass. It consists of organic and inorganic materials derived from saliva, gingival crevicular fluid and bacterial products.

Mean generation time, that is the time taken for the bacteria to double their number on an average is about 3 hours. So one microorganism during the first 24 hours multiply to a total of 256 microorganisms.

Hypothesis concerning etiology of caries:[21]
i. Nonspecific plaque hypothesis—says all plaque is cariogenic
ii. Specific plaque hypothesis—recognizes plaque as pathogenic only when signs of associated disease are present.

Pathogenic Constituents of Plaque

a. Substances producing/inducing direct tissue damage
For example, organic acids, ammonia, hydrogen sulfide, protease, collagenase, hyaluronidase, neuramindase, etc.
b. Inflammation inducing substance
For example, chemotactic substances like polypeptide, activators of complement cascade, histamine, etc.
c. Substances inducing indirect tissue damage by host immunological response.
For example, endotoxin, peptidoglycan, polysaccharide, bacterial antigen, etc.

Formation of Plaque[1]

The process of plaque formation can be divided into three phases.
1. Formation of the pellicle coating on the tooth surface
2. Initial colonization by bacteria
3. Secondary colonization and plaque maturation.

Acquired pellicle is an acellular, essentially bacteria free film that deposits on the teeth soon after eruption. It is derived from components of saliva and crevicular fluid. It can be of 3 types globular, fibrillar and granular.

Newly formed (2 hours) pellicle is fairly uniform in thickness (100-700 nm).

Diet and Dental Caries

Improper dieting has been related to various systemic disorders like atherosclerotic diseases, CVS disorders, certain cancer and last but not the least in relation to our profession is the dental caries.
Caries is a multifactorial disease and role of diet specifically carbohydrates is well established in the initiation of caries and is related to the type, frequency and mode of consumption.

Definition of Diet

"Diet refers to the customary allowance of food and drink taken by any person from day to day."

Cariogenicity of a Food

The absolute cariogenic potential of food is influenced by many factors:
A. Its fermentable carbohydrate content
B. Cariostatic factors in food—includes protein (protect against demineralization and reduce the rate of crystal dissolution), fat (shown to reduce caries in rats), calcium, phosphate and fluoride, phytates in cereals and cocoa.

C. Food retention—duration of presence of carbohydrate in oral cavity influence the period of time acid remains in contact with the tooth.
D. Eating pattern—sequence of food intake is very important. The acid produced by eating pears or sucrose was neutralized if they were eaten with cheese or peanuts.
E. Frequency—frequency of eating is also important and is found that in between meal snacking of carbohydrate containing food increases caries prevalence.
F. Cooking and processing also will affect the carbohydrate portion of the food. Starch that undergoes heating and cooling cycles develops some resistance and a small percentage (2-5%) becomes resistant to amylase of saliva. At temperatures used for cooking, carbohydrates interact with proteins. This reduces the bioavailability of the sugar and aminoacids. Sucrose which is a nonreducing sugar does not react in this way.
G. Other factors include detergent quality, texture, effect of mixing foods and pH of the food.

Eating Habits in Children

A direct relationship exists between caries prevalence and the frequency of in between meal snack consumption.

The basic initial diet of a child depends on the diet of the family, the positive reinforcement of healthy diet by parents, socioeconomic condition, etc.

Children prefer food that is sweet and attractive to look. Preschooler may be very fussy about choosing the type of food and also they may find it difficult to adjust in the new environment when they are sent to baby sitters, day care centers, etc. Their food habits may change from the routine home habits as they eat food from outside in the day time.

Television also plays an important role in affecting the likings of a child. Parents, teachers and caretakers must be educated about the kind of snack that is good for the child.

Family atmosphere especially at meal times also influences the dietary habit of a child. A friendly congenial atmosphere at meal times without threats will help the child attain a positive dietary practices.

An adolescent has adventurous lifestyles. They are more influenced by television, peers or idols and it is very difficult to convey messages and convince teenagers to accept them. One good thing about this age is that there is a strong desire to look attractive. Since mouth is the center of the face, having good set of teeth is also important.

Dietary modification are definitely indicated in patients who have active lesions in the developing permanent dentition or had caries in primary dentition.[22,23]

Role of Sugar in the Etiology of Caries[22-23]

Sucrose has been labeled the arch criminal of dental caries.[24] The extracellular polysaccharide produced by the bacteria utilizing sucrose, functions in a dual role as a structural matrix of the dental plaque and as a reservoir of substrate for the plaque organisms between meals. Some bacteria synthesize glucans, the polymers of glucose while others form levans from fructose. Patients on a soft protein- fat diet developed a thin structure less plaque after few days. When sucrose was included in the diet a striking difference in the appearance of the plaque became noticeable as it attained a considerable size and grew to form a voluminous and turgid mass.

EPIDEMIOLOGICAL STUDIES RELATING SUCROSE TO DENTAL CARIES

There are many important epidemiological studies done to correlate diet and caries.

Some of the important studies are:

Vipeholm Studies[25]

It was a study done in a mental institution in Sweden by Gustafsson et al from 1945-1953. The institution diet was nutritious which contained little sugar with no provision for between meal snacks. The dental caries rates in the inmates were relatively low.

The inmates were grouped into 7 groups as follows and caries incidence was compared:
1. Control group
2. Sucrose group—300 gm initially and later 75 gm
3. Bread group—345 gm, i.e. 50 gm of sugar
4. Chocolate group—65 gm
5. Caramel group—22 caramels, i.e. 70 gm of sugar
6. 8 toffee group—6 gm of sugar
7. 24 toffee group—120 gm of sugar.

Conclusion

- Increased carbohydrate mainly sugar increased caries
- Increased caries were seen when sugar is consumed in the form that will be retained on teeth surface
- In between meal snacks increased caries
- Caries activity varies widely
- Upon withdrawal of the sugar rich foods, the increased caries activity rapidly disappears
- Clearance time of the sugar correlated closely with caries activity.

Hope Wood House Study[26]

It is the home for orphans in Australia. The children were brought up from infancy. They were on vegetarian diet with occasional serving of egg yolk. Sugar and other refined carbohydrates were excluded from the children's diet. The dental caries prevalence in young children in the primary dentition was almost negligible and that of permanent teeth was 1/10th of the average Australian child. Oral hygiene was extremely poor and about 75% had gingivitis. When these children left the institution and exposed to routine diet, there was a sharp rise in caries rate.

Hereditary Fructose Intolerance

It is an autosomal recessive disorder of fructose metabolism associated with reduced activity of the enzyme fructose-1-phosphate aldolase by 2-5% in liver, renal cortex and small bowel. This enzyme is required for the metabolism of fructose. Following fructose intake, the patient experiences nausea, vomiting, excessive sweating, malaise, tremor, coma and convulsions. Such patients tend to avoid all sweats, cakes, candies and most fruits. They eat glucose, galactose, lactose and starch containing foods. It has been noted that their teeth are in extraordinary good condition. Caries when present is limited to pits and fissures and is usually not found in smooth surface. The low caries prevalence indicates that starchy foods do not produce decay whereas sugary foods do.[24]

Turku Sugar Studies[27]

This was done to test the effects of chronic consumption of sucrose, fructose and xlylitol on dental and general health. There was a dramatic reduction in caries incidence after 2 years of xylitol consumption. Fructose was found to be as cariogenic as sucrose for the first 12 months. Frequent inbetween meals chewing of xylitol gum produced anticariogenic effect.

PROTECTIVE FACTORS IN FOOD THAT HELP REDUCE CARIES[28]

1. Phosphates
2. Glycyrrhizinic acid
3. Fats and protein
4. Trace elements

Phosphates

Different Types of Phosphates that are Protective

- Inorganic phosphates—helps in remineralization or reduces dissolution and is a good buffer
- Trimetaphosphates is also protective
- Sodium metaphosphate appears to be the most effective.
- Calcium sucrose phosphate—by adsorbing on the tooth surface, it prevents enamel dissolution

- Organic phosphates (phytates, glycerophosphates) phytates—adsorb readily and firmly on enamel surface and prevent dissolution of enamel by acids.

Glycyrrhizinic Acid

It prevents caries by reducing enamel dissolution, inhibiting gycolysis and increasing plaque buffering power.

Fats and Protein

- Fats reduce the cariogenecity by providing a greasy layer. They also serve as anionic surfactant
- Proteins adsorb onto enamel surface and form a barrier
- Inclusion of milk solids reduced the cariogenecity of sugar containing foods.

Time

The time of contact between all the etiologic factors is the most crucial factor. If the food is washed off from the tooth surface through brushing, it is not available for the bacteria and thus reduces the risk of developing caries.

Trace Elements[29]

Trace element in diet can be cariostatic or caries promoting. They are thus grouped into:

Cariostatic—Fl, P
Mildly cariostatic—Mo, V, Cu, Sr, B, Li, Au, Fe
Doubtful cariostatic—Be, Co, Mn, Sn, Zn, Br, I, Y
Caries inert—Ba, Al, Ni, Pd, Ti
Caries promoting—Se, Mg, Cd, Pt, Pb, Si

Trace elements are variously defined depending upon the field of chemical, physical, or biologic sciences being discussed. In the field of biology, elements that are present in only minute quantities in animal tissues are called trace elements, regardless of their abundance in nature.

The trace elements can be divided into two categories:
1. Those that have well-defined human requirements, namely, iron, zinc, iodine, copper and fluorine.
2. Those that are integral constituents or activators of enzymes, namely, manganese, molybdenum, seleni-um, chromium and cobalt.

Trace elements in dental enamel of permanent teeth

Concentration range ppm	Elements
> 1000	Na, Cl, Mg
100–1000	K, S, Zn, Is, Sr, F
10–100	Fe, Al, Pb, B, Ba
1–10	Cu, Rb, Br, Mo, Cd, 1, Ti, Mn, Cr, Sn
0.1–0.9	Ni, Li, Ag, Ng, Sc, Be, Zr, Co, W, Sb, Hg
< 0.1	As, Cs, V, Au, La, Ce, Pr, Nd, Sm, Tb, Y
Not detected	Sc, Ga, Ge, Ru, Pb, In, Te, Eu, Gd, Dy Ho, Er, Tm, Lu, Hf, Ta, Re, Os, Ir, Pt, TI Bi, Rh

Possible Mechanism of Trace Element Action on Dental Caries

Effect of trace elements on dental caries is probably by altering the resistance of the tooth itself or by modifying the local environment at the plaque-tooth enamel interface. Like fluoride, other elements can modify the chemical and physical composition of the teeth thus affecting the solubility of the enamel to acid attacks.

The trace elements may also influence the microbial ecology of plaque to either inhibit or promote the growth of caries-producing bacteria.

MECHANISM OF DENTAL CARIES

Caries begins as a subsurface demineralization of the enamel which progresses along the enamel prisms to the DEJ, where the caries spreads laterally and centrally into the underlying dentin assuming a conical configuration with the apex towards the pulp.

Various Theories Put Forward to Explain the Mechanism of Caries[30-36]

1. *Worms:* According to ancient Sumerian text, tooth ache was caused by a worm that drank the blood of the teeth and fed on the roots of the jaws—5000 BC.
2. *Humors:* Persons physical and mental constitution was determined by 4 elemental fluids—blood, phlegm, black bile and yellow bile corresponding to 4 humors—sanguine, phlegmatic, melancholic and choleric. Diseases could be explained by an imbalance of these humors.
3. *Endogenous/vital theory:* Regards dental caries as originating within the tooth itself.
4. *Chemical theory:* Parmly said that a chemical agent was responsible. Foods putrified on tooth surface and dissolved the tooth material, 1819.
5. *Parasitic/septic theory:* According to Erdl (1843) there are filamental parasites on the surface membrane of the teeth. Ficinus called them denticolae.
6. *Sucrose chelation theory:* According to Eggers and Lura, sucrose itself causes enamel dissolution by forming unionized calcium saccharates, which requires inorganic phosphate.
7. *Glycogen theory:* According to Egyedi, susceptibilty to caries is related to a high carbohydrate intake during the period of tooth development, resulting in the deposition of excess glycogen and glycoprotein in tooth structure which are inturn degraded to acids by plaque bacteria.
8. *Autoimmune theory, (Burch and Jackson):* According to which the genes determine the caries susceptibility of tooth.
9. *Acidogenic/chemicoparasitic theory (Miller 1882):* Described dental decay as a chemicoparasitic disease consisting of two distinctly marked stages—the decalcification and dissolution. The acid formed is recognized as lactic acid.
10. *Proteolytic theory (Gottlieb, 1944):* Described enamel matrix as the key to caries formation, involving protein splitting microorganisms followed by physical and or acid dis-solution of the inorganic salts
11. *Proteolysis chelation theory (Schwartz and Martin 1955):* Involves 2 interrelated simultaneously occuring reactions
    - Microbial destruction of the largely proteinaceous organic matrix
    - Loss of apatite through dissolution by organic chelators

    Substances having chelating properties are peptides, aminoacids, citrate, lactate, hydroxyesters, ketoesters, polyphosphates, carbohydrates, etc.
12. *Theory of demineralization and remineralization:* Caries is actually the combined process of demineralization and remineralization. The ratio between demineralization and remineralization is very crucial that determines the hardness and strength of tooth structure. A fall in the pH of oral cavity results in demineralization and the oral environment becomes undersaturated with mineral ions, relative to a tooth's mineral content. Fall in the pH is due to the organic acids (lactic acid) that are produced by the action of plaque bacteria in the presence of dietary carbohydrates. This dissolution continues until the pH returns to normal level. If the demineralization phase continues for a longer period it results in excessive loss of minerals resulting in loss of enamel structure and cavitation, which is the typical feature of dental caries. Conversely, when the pH rises the reverse takes place resulting in deposition of mineral back to the tooth leading to remineralization. The process of remineralization is enhanced with agents such as fluoride, casein phosphopeptide (CPP), Novamin, Hydroxyapatite, etc. They are discussed in detail in 'Preventive Dentistry' section.

MICROSCOPIC STRUCTURE (FIGS 7.6A AND B)[1,37]

The microscopic structure of enamel caries are divided into four zones:

Zone 1: Translucent zone seen at the advancing front of the lesion

Zone 2: Dark zone (positive zone), lie deep to the area of visible radioluecency

Zone 3: Body of the lesion, area of greatest demineralization, and forms largest portion of carious enamel

Zone 4: Surface zone, that is relatively unaffected layer. It is radiopaque, due to partial demineralization may be present which can be explained by "Moreno Model."

Moreno model[38]—According to this model, bacterial acids dissolve the surface as well as the subsurface enamel. The calcium and phosphate ions produced from the subsurface dissolution diffuse outward toward the surface and reprecipitate on the surface, making the enamel surface appear unaltered. Thus, this surface zone is in an equilibrium with mineral being lost into the plaque due to low pH but being remineralized from the ions diffusing out from the subsurface lesion. If the cariogenic environment continues, eventually the rate of transfer from the surface enamel into plaque becomes greater than the rate of precipitation and the surface enamel collapses leading to cavity.

Microscopic Structure of Dentinal Caries (Fig. 7.7)

- On reaching the dentin, the carious lesion spreads laterally along the dentinoenamel junction often undermining the enamel, following the direction of dentinal tubules. The resulting lesion is cone shaped with base at DEJ and apex towards the pulp.
- Affected dentin displays different degrees of discoloration from brown to dark brown or almost black.

Zones from normal dentin to the lesion are as follows:

- *Normal zone:* Normal tubular structure with odontoblasts
- *Sub transparent zone:* Layer of demineralization of intertubular dentin and initial crystal formation in the tubule without bacterial invasion
- *Transparent zone:* Softer dentin, large crystals seen and no bacteria seen
- *Turboid zone:* Distortion and widening of dentinal tubules with bacterial invasion. Collagen is irreversibly denatured.
- *Infected zone:* Decomposed dentin filled with bacteria. There is no recognizable dentinal structure.

Destruction of dentin is usually more advanced along the incremental lines of growth producing transverse clefts. This is why carious dentin can be excavated by hand instruments in a plane parallel with the DEJ.

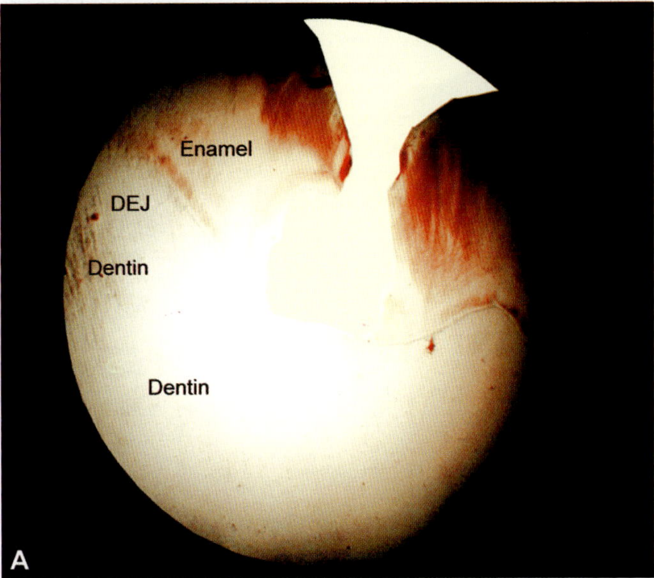

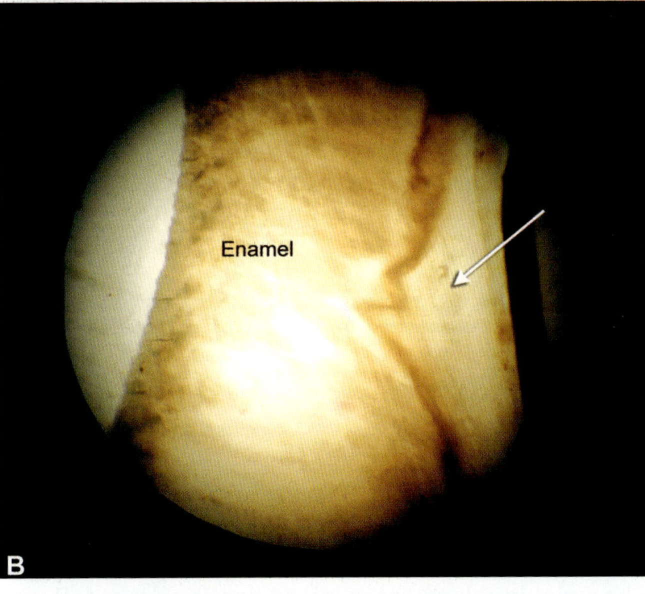

Figs 7.6A and B: Ground section of enamel caries: (A) Pit and fissure caries; (B) Smooth surface caries

AREA SUSCEPTIBILITY FOR CARIES[1,39-40]

The caries involvement in primary dentition is as follows:

- Mandibular molars, maxillary molars and maxillary anteriors are commonly involved. Mandibular incisors are affected only in rampant caries.
- Mandibular posterior teeth are more susceptible than their maxillary counterparts.
- First molar is less susceptible than second molar.

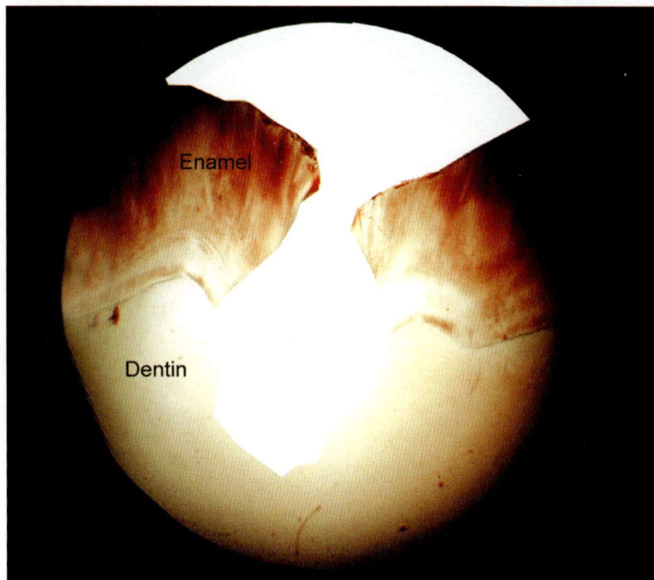

Fig. 7.7: Ground section of caries extending into dentin

- By 8 years—50% of second molar and 20% of first molar would have occlusal caries.
- Interproximal caries usually develops after the proximal contacts develop.
- Proximal caries progress more rapidly than occlusal caries and causes a higher percentage of pulp exposures.

Surface by surface comparison of the teeth		
Tooth	*Maxilla*	*Mandible*
Second molar	Occlusal+palatal	Occlusal+buccal
First molar	Occlusal	Occlusal+buccal
Canine	Buccal	Buccal
Incisors	Mesial	Not commonly involved

The caries involvement in mixed dentition is as follows:
- First permanent molars are at high-risk for development of caries as soon as they erupt.
- It is found that by 7 years, 25% of mandibular I molar had caries on the occlusal surface, 12% of maxillary I molar had occlusal caries. By 9 years 50% had caries in mandibular I molar and 35% in maxillary I molar. By 12 years, 70% had caries in mandibular I molar and 52% in maxillary I molar.
- The distal surface of deciduous second molar is a common site for caries, after the eruption of the first permanent molar.
- At 8 years, approximately 1% of the maxillary incisors will be carious and by 12 years, 15% of them will be carious.

The caries involvement in permanent dentition is as follows:
- Rise in caries attack rate continues with the eruption of the second permanent molars and premolars.
- Mandibular II molars are at high-risk for occlusal surface caries compared to the maxilla.
- The buccal groove in the mandibular molar and palatal groove in the maxillary molars are sites for morphologic defects and incomplete enamel formation.

CLASSIFICATION OF CARIES[41,42]

- **Based on the location**
  - Pit and fissure caries
  - Smooth surface caries
- **Based on the severity**
  - Acute caries
  - Chronic caries
  - Arrested caries
- **Based on the extension**
  - *Enamel caries:* Caries limited to enamel
  - *Dental caries:* Caries extending to dentin
  - *Root caries:* Usually not seen in children
- **Based on chronology**
  - Early childhood caries such as nursing bottle caries
  - Teenage caries such as rampant caries
  - Adult caries such as root caries which is common in adults
- **Based on the origin**
  - Primary (virgin) caries
  - Secondary (recurrent) caries

Enamel Caries—Early Features
- Small opaque white region, called as 'white spot' (Fig. 7.8) forms the initial feature.
- Enamel overlying this white spot is hard and shiny with no morphologic changes from the sound enamel.
- The outer enamel is more resistant to demineralization than the inner portion. Therefore, the greatest amount of mineral loss is seen 10-15 mm beneath the outer surface continuation of this process leads to the formation of white spot or subsurface enamel caries. This is the zone of demineralization that can be remineralized until the outer surface is intact.
- It may also appear brownish –'brown spot lesion' and the discoloration is due to exogeneous stain.

Pit or Fissure Caries (Fig. 7.9)
- Pit or fissure caries develops in the occlusal surface of molars and premolars, in the buccal and lingual

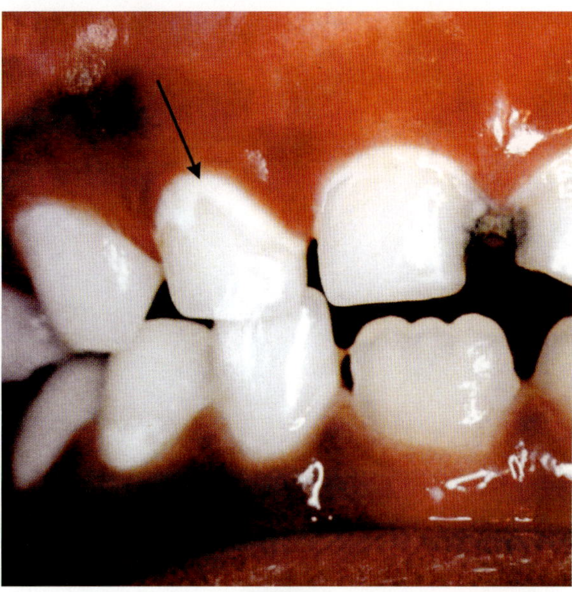

Fig. 7.8: Opaque white area seen on the cervical border of upper lateral incisor indicating early caries

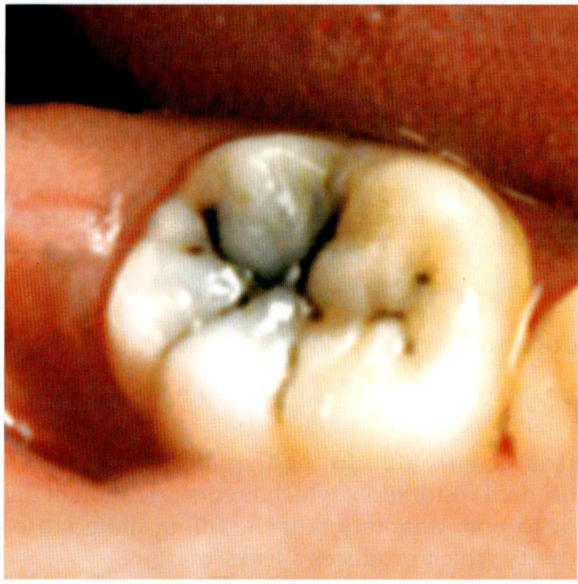

Fig. 7.9: Caries on the pits and fissures of posterior teeth

surface of the molars and in the lingual surfaces of the maxillary incisors.

- Carious lesion more often starts at both sides of the fissure wall, penetrating nearly perpendicular towards the DEJ. Enamel rods flare laterally in the bottom of the pit where caries follows the direction of enamel rods, characteristic triangular shaped base directed towards the dentin.
- Pits or fissures with high steep walls and narrow bases are those most prone to develop caries.

- They favor the retention of food debris and micro-organisms and caries may result from fermentation of this food and formation of acids.
- Pits and fissures affected by early caries may appear brown or black and will feel slightly soft and "catch" a fine explorer point.
- The enamel bordering the pit or fissure may appear opaque bluish white as it becomes undermined. This undermining occurs through lateral spread of the caries at the DEJ. Thus, there may be a large carious lesion with only a tiny point of opening.
- Pits and fissures can be of two types:[43]
  1. Shallow, wide V (34%) or U (14%)—shaped fissures that are self cleansing.
  2. Deep, narrow I shaped fissures (19%) that are constricted having a narrow slit like opening. They may also have lateral branches making it appear as K (26%), Y or Inverted Y shaped (7%) (Figs 7.10A and B).
- Since the pits and the fissures form a niche for plaque accumulation and also the bristles of the tooth brush cannot reach the area, these areas are highly susceptible for caries development.

Smooth Surface Caries (Figs 7.11A and B)

- Smooth surface caries develops on the proximal surfaces of the teeth or on the gingival third of the buccal and lingual surfaces.
- Smooth surface caries is generally preceded by the formation of a microbial or dental plaque.
- Proximal caries usually begins just below the contact point and appears in the early stage as a faint white opacity of the enamel without apparent loss of continuity of the enamel surface.
- The early white chalky spot becomes slightly rough-ened, owing to superficial decalcification of the enamel.
- As the caries penetrates the enamel, the enamel surrounding the lesion assumes a bluish white appearance. This is particularly apparent as lateral spread of caries at the DEJ occurs.
- Cervical caries usually extends from the area opposite the gingival crest occlusally to the convexity of the tooth surface. Thus the typical cervical carious lesion is a crescent shaped cavity beginning as a slightly rough-ened chalk area which gradually becomes excavated.

Acute Dental Caries (Fig. 7.12)

- It is that form of caries which runs a rapid clinical course and results in early pulp involvement by the carious process.
- The process is so rapid that there is little time for the deposition of secondary dentin.

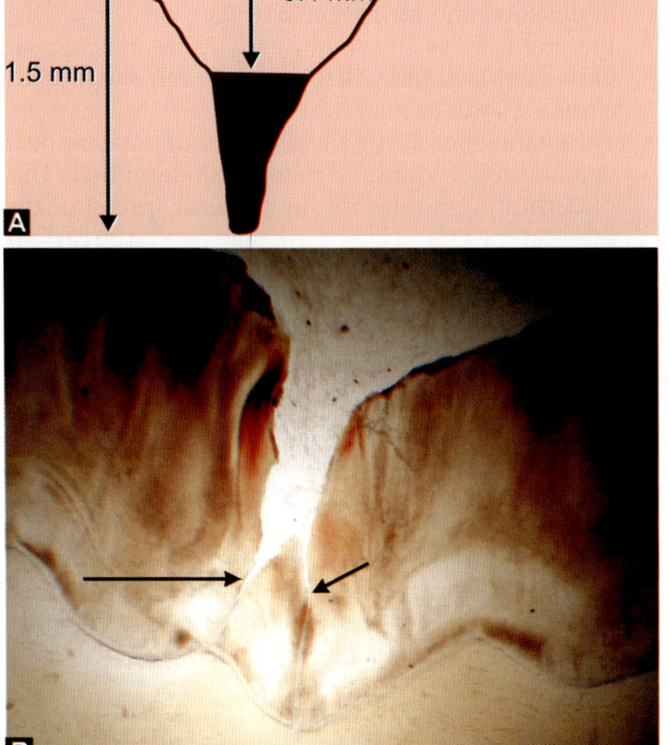

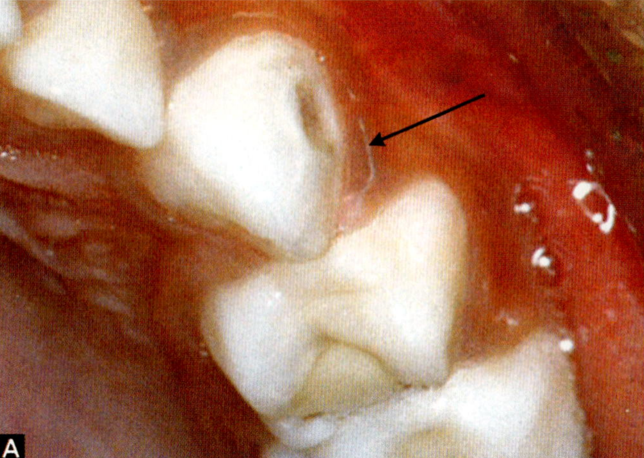

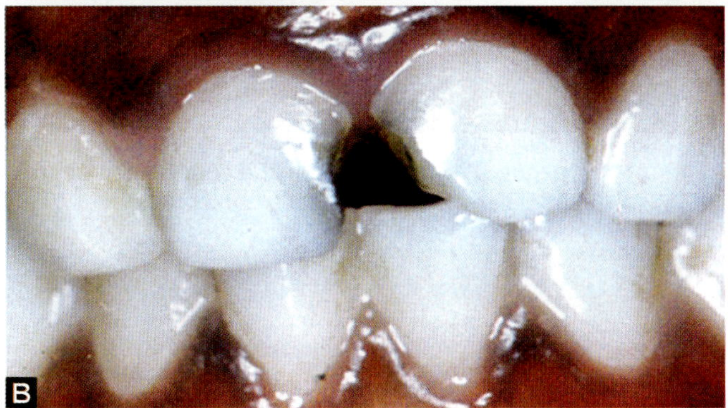

Figs 7.10A and B: Normal Fissure;
(A) Diagrammatic representation of a deep fissure
- Total depth of the fissure: 1.5 mm
- Depth to which a bristle can reach (Arrow): 0.4 mm
- Depth of the fissure that cannot be cleaned (Darkened area): 1.1 mm;

(B) Ground section of the normal fissure (Arrows) indicating the narrow fissures bifurcating into a inverted 'Y' shaped deep fissure

- The dentin is usually stained a light yellow.
- Nursing bottle and rampant caries are a type of acute caries that is fast spreading.

Chronic Dental Caries (Fig. 7.13)

- It is that form of caries which progresses slowly and tends to involve the pulp much later than acute caries.
- The slow progress of the lesion allows sufficient time for deposition of secondary dentin in response to the adverse irritation.
- The carious dentin often stains deep brown.
- The cavity is generally a shallow one with a minimum softening of dentin.
- There is little undermining of enamel and pain is not a common feature.

Figs 7.11A and B: Smooth surface caries: (A) Seen on the labial surface of lateral incisor; (B) Involving the proximal surface of central incisors

Recurrent Caries

- It is that type of caries that occurs in the immediate vicinity of a restoration.
- It is usually due to inadequate extension of the original restoration, which favors retention of debris or to poor adaptation of the filling material to the cavity which produces a leaky margin.
- The renewed caries follows the same general pattern as primary caries.

Arrested Caries (Fig. 7.14)

- It has been described as caries which becomes static or stationary and does not show any tendency for further progression.
- It occurs almost exclusively in caries of occlusal surfaces and is characterized by a large open cavity in which there is lack of food retention and in which, the superficially softened and decalcified dentin is

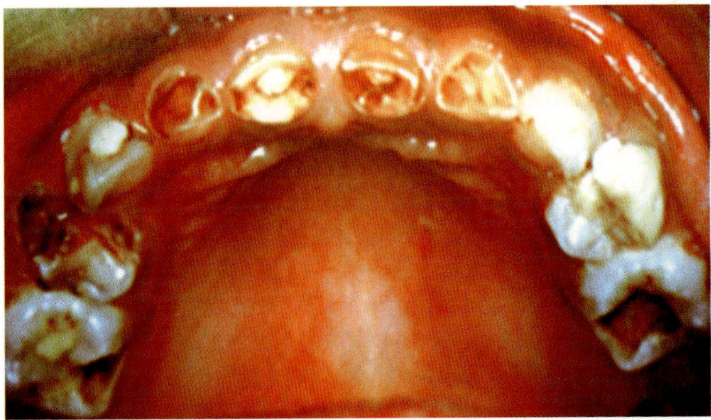

Fig. 7.12: Acute dental caries

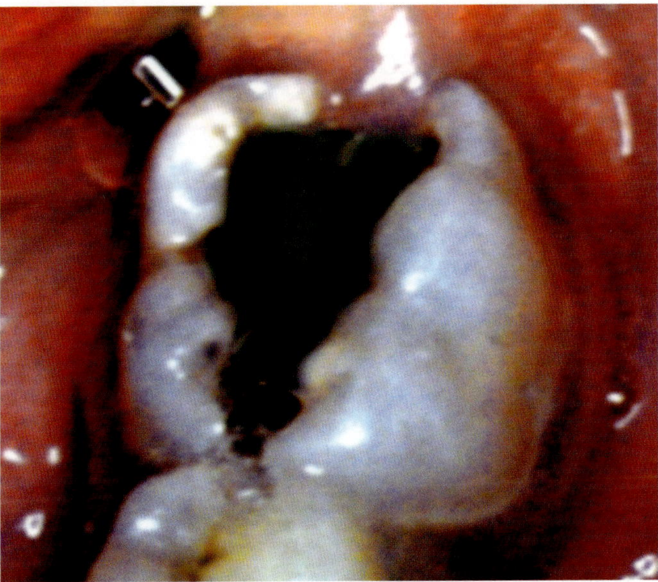

Fig. 7.13: Chronic dental caries

gradually burnished until it takes on a brown stained, polished appearance and is hard. This has been referred to as "Eburnation of dentin."

- Another form of arrested caries is that sometimes seen on the proximal surfaces of teeth in cases in which the adjacent approximating tooth has been extracted.

Rampant Caries

Rampant caries or fast spreading caries in children is very common but most difficult to treat. It can appear in teeth that were sound for many years suggesting a serious imbalance in oral environment as the reason. Young teenagers are particularly susceptible to rampant caries, due to their sudden change in eating and oral hygiene habits. Stress and emotional disturbance are related to rampant caries. Noticeable salivary deficiency that is seen in tense, nervous or disturbed persons and associated abnormal diet (excessive consumption of sweets) may be the reason for the development of rampant caries (Figs 7.15 and 7.16).

Definition

According to Massler (1945)[44]: "Rampant caries is defined as suddenly appearing, widespread, rapidly burrowing type of caries, resulting in early involvement of pulp and affecting those teeth usually regarded as immune to ordinary decay."

According to Winter (1966)[45]: "Rampant caries are caries of acute onset involving many or all of the teeth in areas that are usually not susceptible and are associated with rapid destruction of the crowns with frequent involvement of the dental pulp."

Management of rampant caries is the same as management of any caries but requires vigorous and persistent preventive and therapeutic effort. Management of the etiology (stress, etc.) needed to be done first. The next most important step is prevention of rapid destruction of remaining tooth structure. So all the carious teeth need to be excavated as early as possible to gain control over the rate of spread. This should be followed by rehabilitation in the subsequent appointments.

Early Childhood Caries

Early childhood caries was historically attributed to inappropriate and prolonged use of sweetened liquid in the bottle. Hence the older terms of "baby-bottle tooth decay" and "nursing caries."[41] Any practice that allows

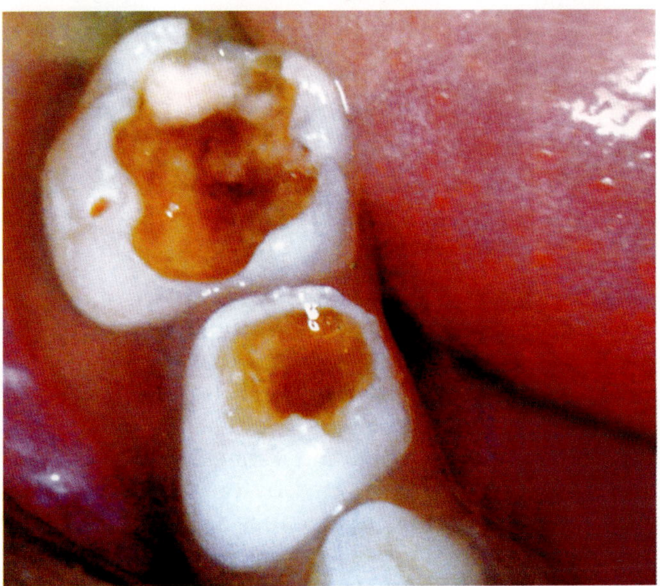

Fig. 7.14: Arrested caries

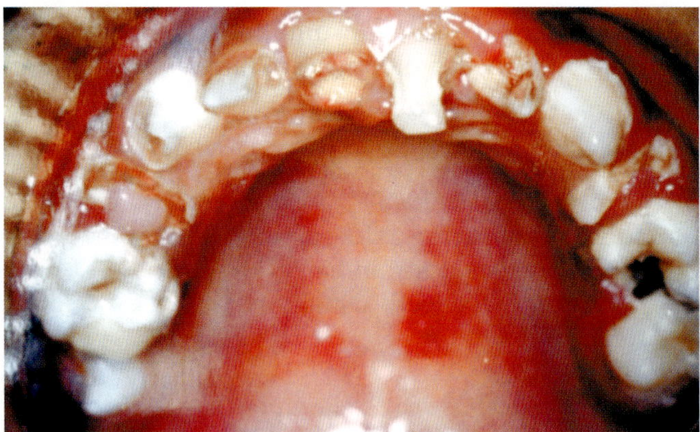

Fig. 7.15: Rampant caries

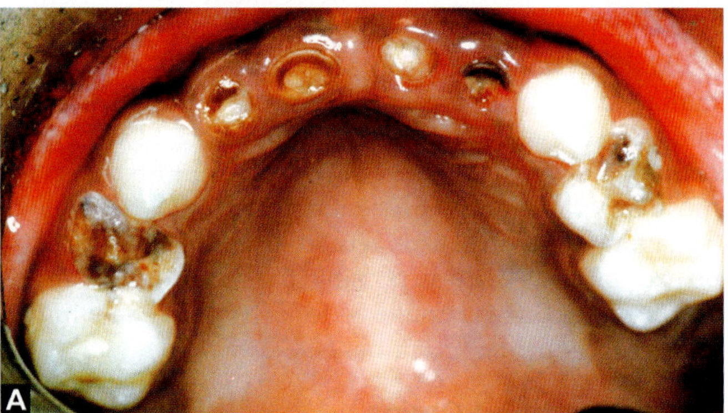

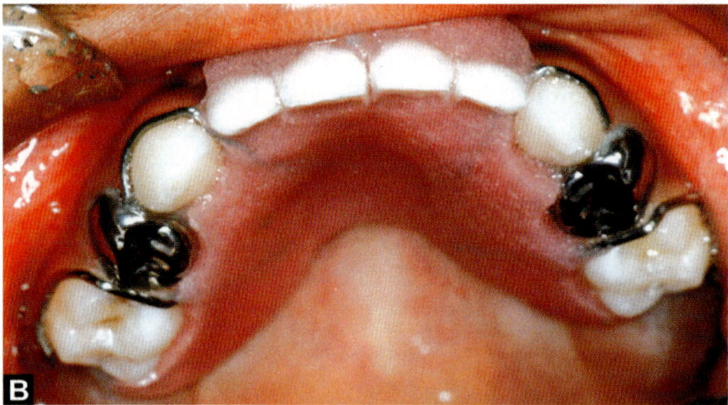

Figs 7.16A and B: Rampant caries and its management:
(A) Pretreatment; (B) Post-treatment

frequent sugar consumption in the presence of mutans streptococci may result in caries formation. Common contributing etiological practices in children include propped bottles containing sweetened liquids, frequent consumption of sweetened liquids from infant and toddler size "sippy" cups, and frequent snacking.

The caries risk generated by on-demand breast-feeding is unclear, but because lactose is poorly metabolized by mutans streptococci, other concomitant inappropriate dietary practices (e.g. frequent juice consumption or snacking) are more likely to be the culprits. Irregular oral hygiene habits also contribute for development of early childhood caries.[46-48]

Early childhood caries (AAPD 2008) is a specific type of caries that affects infants and young children. It is the presence of 1 or more decayed (noncavitated or cavitated lesions), missing (due to caries), or filled tooth surfaces in any primary tooth in a child 71 months of age or younger.

In children younger than 3 years of age, any sign of smooth-surface caries is indicative of severe early childhood caries (S-ECC). From ages 3 years through 5, 1 or more cavitated, missing (due to caries), or filled smooth surfaces in primary maxillary anterior teeth or a decayed, missing, or filled score of $\geq$ 4 (age 3), $\geq$ 5 (age 4), or $\geq$ 6 (age 5) surfaces constitute severe ECC.[49-51]

Classification of ECC[52]

Type I (Mild to Moderate ECC)

Isolated carious lesion (s) involving molars and/or incisors. They are found in 2-5 years old children. Cause of this caries is usually combination of cariogenic food and poor oral hygiene.

Type II (Moderate to Severe ECC)

Labiolingual caries lesion affecting maxillary incisors with or without involving the molars. The mandibular incisors are not affected. The cause is usually inappropriate bottle feeding habits and poor oral hygiene. It is found as soon as the teeth erupt into the oral cavity.

Type III (Severe ECC)

Caries involving almost all the teeth including the lower incisors. This is found in 3-5 years old children.

Features of ECC

* Early caries involvement of the maxillary anterior teeth, the maxillary and mandibular posterior teeth and mandibular canines is seen.
* Mandibular incisors are unaffected due to the protection by the tongue.
* Seen as white or dark brown collar of caries around the neck of the incisors, which develops into faciolingual caries and may also fracture the tooth.
* The main etiology is that the child is put to bed with a nursing bottle containing milk or sugar containing beverages. The child falls asleep and the milk or sweetened liquid becomes pooled around the maxillary anterior teeth. This provides an excellent culture medium for acidogenic microorganisms. Salivary flow is reduced during sleep and clearance of the liquid from the oral cavity is slowed.

Management thus includes advising that the infant be held while feeding. The child who falls asleep while nursing should be woken up, burped, mouth washed and then placed in bed. In addition the parents should start brushing the child's teeth as soon as they erupt and discontinue nursing bottles as soon as the child can drink from a cup, i.e at approximately 12-15 months of age.

Management includes parent counseling, provis-ional restorations, diet assessment, caries activity tests, and constant re-evaluations, fluoride therapy followed by restorations and recall once in 2-3 months.

Stages in the development of nursing bottle caries		
Stage	*Age (month)*	*Clinical appearance*
Initial	10-20	Maxillary anterior teeth—opaque white demineralization in the cervical or interproximal region
Damaged	16-24	Maxillary anterior teeth—yellow-brown discoloration. Cervical or interproximal superficial defects Maxillary first molars– will be in first stage
Deep lesions	20-36	Maxillary anterior teeth—marked enamel defect and pulpal irritation. Maxillary first molars are in second stage Mandibular first molars are in first stage.
Traumatic	30-48	Maxillary anterior teeth—loss of large enamel or dentin parts, crown fractures. Maxillary first molars are in third stage. Mandibular first molars are in second stage

Management of Dental Caries

Caries management is the combination of preventive and restorative dentistry. The concept is to restore all the existing carious lesions and prevent new caries from establishing. Preventive Dentistry thus aims at identifying the risk factors and providing customized preventive care to the child. Prevention of dental caries is explained in the "Prevention of Dental Caries" section and restoration of caries in the 'Pediatric Restorative Dentistry' section.

REFERENCES

1. Roberson TM. Cariology: the lesion, etiology, prevention and control, in Roberson TM, Heymann HO, Swift EJ. Sturdevant's Art and Sciences of Operative Dentistry, 5th Ed. Mosby 2006;65-134.
2. Keyes P, Fitzgerald RJ. Dental caries in the syrian hamster, Arch Oral Biol 1962;7:267-77.
3. Krasse B, Newbrun E. Objective methods of evaluating caries activity and their application, Pediatric Dentistry, Scientific foundation and clinical practice, Stewart RE, Barber TK, Troutman KC, Wei SHY. The CV Mosby Co. 1982;610-6.
4. Newbrun E. Cariology, Baltimore. The Williams and Wilkins Co. 1978.
5. Dawes C. What is the critical pH and why does a tooth dissolve in acid? J Can Dent Assoc 2003;69(11):722-4.
6. Stephan RM. Changes in the hydrogen ion concentration on tooth surfaces and in carious lesions. J Am Dent Assoc 1940;27:718.
7. Gibbons RJ, van Houte J. Dental caries. Ann RevMed 1975;26:121-35.
8. Loesche WJ, Rowan J, Straffon LH, Loos PJ. Association of Streptococcus mutans with human dental decay. Infect Immun 1975;11:1252-60.
9. Caufield PW, Cutter GR, Dasanayake AP. Initial acquisition of mutans streptococci by infants: Evidence for a discrete window of infectivity. J Dent Res 1993; 72(1):37-45.
10. Ooshima T, Sumi N, Izumitani A, Sobue S. Matemal transmission and dental caries induction in Sprague-Dawley rats infected with *Streptococcus mutans*. Microbiol Immunol 1998;32:785-94.
11. Loesche WJ. Role of *Streptococcus mutans* in human dental decay, Microbiol Rev 1986;50:353-80.
12. Brown JP, Junner C, Leiw V. A study of *Streptococcus mutans* level in both infants with bottle caries and their mothers. Aust Dent J 1985;30:96-8.
13. Clarke JK. On the bacterial factor in the etiology of dental caries. Brit J Exp Pathol 1924;5:141-7.
14. Loesche WJ. Microbiology of dental decay and periodontal disease. In: Baron's medical microbiology (Baron S et al., eds.) (4th ed.). Univ of Texas Medical Branch, 1996.
15. Kohler B, Andreen I, Jonsson B. The effect of caries-preventive measures in mothers on dental caries and the presence of the bacteria Streptococcus mutans and lactobacilli. Arch oral Biol 1984;29:879-83.
16. Eastcott AD, Stallard RE. Sequential changes in developing human dental plaque as visualized by scanning electron microscope. J Periodontol 1973;44:218-24.
17. Mc Donald RE, Avery DR, Stookey GK, Chin JR, Kowolik JE. Dental caries in the child and adolescent. Dentistry for the child and adolescent 9th Edition, Elsevier Mosby, 2011;177-204.
18. Wei SHY. Pediatric Dentistry. Total Patient care. Lea & Febriger, Philadelphia, 1988
19. Loe H. Human research model for the production and prevention of gingivitis. J. Dent Res 1971;50:256.
20. Newman MG, Takai HH, Carranza FA. Carranza's clinical periodontology. Saunders 9th Ed.
21. Loesche WJ. Clinical and microbiological aspects of chemotherapeutic agents used according to the specific plaque hypothesis. J. Dent Res 1979;58:2404.

22. Weiss RL, Trihart AH. Between meal eating habits and dental caries experience in preschool children. Am. J. Public Health 1960;50:1097.
23. Steinman RR, Woods RW. Hereditary, environment, diet and caries in children. J South Calif State Dent Assoc 1964;32:163.
24. Newbrun E. Sucrose, the arch criminal of dental caries. J Dent Child 36: 239, 1969. 2003, Philadelphia.
25. Gustafsson B, Quensel CE, Lanke L, et al. The Vipeholm dental caries study, the effect of different carbohydrate intake on caries activity in 436 individuals observed for five years. Acta Odontol Scand 1954;11:232.
26. Sullivan HR, Harris R. Hopewood House study, 2. Obeservations on oral conditions. Aust Dent J 1958;3:311.
27. Scheinin A, Makinen KK, and Ylitalo K. Turku sugar studies V. Final report on the effect of sucrose, fructose and xylitol diets on the caries incidence in man. Acta Odontol Scand 1975;33:(Suppl 70).
28. Wei SHY. Diet and Dental Caries. Pediatric dentistry, scientific foundation and clinical practice, Stewart RE, Barber TK, Troutman KC, Wei SHY, 1982;576-89.
29. Losee F I, Ludwig TG. Trace Elements and Caries. J Dent Res 1970;49:1229-35.
30. Newburn E. History and early theories of etiology of caries, Current concepts of caries etiology, Histopathology of dental caries, Cariology, 3rd edition, Quintessence Publication Co. 1989.
31. Eggers- Lura H. The nonacid complexing theory of dental caries. Holbaek, Denmark, 1967.
32. Egyedi H. Experimental Basis of the Glycogen theory of enamel caries. D. Items Interest 1953;75:971.
33. Burch PRJ, Jackson D. Periodontal disease and dental caries, some new etiological consideration. Br Dent J 1966;120:127-34.
34. Miller WD. The microorganisms of the human mouth. Philadelphia, SS White Dental Manufacturing Company, 1890.
35. Gottlieb B. Histopathology of enamel caries. J Dent Res 1944;23:379.
36. Schwartz A, Martin JJ. Speculation on lactobacilli and acid as possible anticaries factors. NY State Dent J 1955;21:367.
37. Silverstone LM. Dental caries pathogenesis, Pediatric Dentistry, Scientific foundation and clinical practice, Stewart RE, Barber TK, Troutman KC, Wei SHY, 1982; 535-47.
38. Moreno EC, Zahradnik RT. Chemistry of dental subsurface demineralization *in vitro*. J Dent Res 1974; 53:226.
39. Hennon DK, Stookey GK, Muhler JC. Prevalence and distribution of dental caries in preschool children J Am Dent Assoc 1969;79:1405.
40. National Center for Health Statistics: Plan and operation of the third National Health and Nutrition. Examination Survey 1988-94, Vital Health Stat 1994;1:32.
41. Gilmore HW, et al. Operative dentistry. 4th Ed. St. Louis, Mosby 1982.
42. Roberson TM. Fundamentals in tooth preperation, In, Roberson TM, Heymann HO, Swift EJ. Sturdevant's Art and Sciences of operative dentistry, 5th Ed. Mosby 2006; 281-321.
43. Hicks J, Flaitz CM. Pit and Fissure Sealants and Conservative Adhesive Restorations: Scientific and Clinical Rationale. Pediatric Dentistry, Infancy through Adolescence, 4th Edition, Elsevier Saunders 2005;520-76.
44. Massler JN. Teenage caries, J Dent Child 1945;12:57-64.
45. Winter GB, Hamilton MC, James PMC. Role of the comforter as an etiological Factor in rampant caries of the deciduous dentition arch. Dis. Child 1966;41:207.
46. Johnsen DC. Baby bottle tooth decay: A preventable health problem in infants. Update Pediatr Dent 1988;2:1.
47. Ripa L. Nursing caries: A comprehensive review. Pediatr Dent 1988;10:268.
48. Erickson PR, Mazhari E. Investigation of the role of human breast milk in caries development. Pediatr Dent 1999;21:86-90.
49. Drury TF, Horowitz AM, Ismail AI, et al. Diagnosing and reporting early childhood caries for research purposes. J Public Health Dent 1999;59:192.
50. Kaste LM, Drury TF, Horowitz AM, et al. An evaluation of NHANES III estimates of early childhood caries. J Public Health Dent 2000;59:198.
51. Ismail AI, Sohn W. A systematic review of clinical diagnostic criteria of early childhood caries. J Public Health Dent 1999;59:171.
52. Wyne AH. Early childhood caries nomenclature and case definition. Community Dent Oral Epidemiol 1999; 27:313-5.

QUESTIONS

1. Explain the etiology of caries in respect to Keye's triad.
2. What is Stephan's curve?
3. Role of *Streptococcus mutans* in caries formation.
4. Relation of diet and dental caries.
5. Theory of demineralization and remineralization in caries formation.
6. Classify caries.
7. Define rampant caries and what is the line of management of rampant caries?
8. What is ECC? Give its clinical features and management.

PREVENTIVE DENTISTRY

INTRODUCTION

Preventive dentistry has been defined as "The efforts which are made to maintain normal development, physiologic function and to prevent diseases of the mouth and adjacent parts."

According to WHO expert committee, prevention denotes a procedure or course of action that prevents the onset of disease.

PRINCIPLES AND OBJECTIVES OF PREVENTIVE DENTISTRY

1. To influence the lifestyle of individuals, families and communities, so that oral health is promoted or maintained.
2. To make provision of required treatment available to those individuals who have developed oral disease, so that the disease process is arrested at the earliest and loss of function is prevented.
3. To make children loose fear of dental procedures by education, experience and conscious efforts of care providers.

SCOPE

The main emphasis of modern oral health care practice is prevention of dental disease. This is because:
1. Dental diseases are common
2. Incidence of dental disease is on an increase
3. Primary prevention of dental diseases is possible due to sufficient knowledge of etiopathology and epidemiology
4. Most of the dental disease are initially symptom less
5. Secondary prevention of dental disease is also possible
6. Dental diseases are not self curing.

MINIMAL INTERVENTION DENTISTRY

The concept of minimal intervention dentistry (MID) has evolved as a consequence of our increased understanding of the caries process and the development of adhesive restorative materials.

Caries is now not treated just as a symptom but as a disease. Hence a medical approach is instituted which includes caries risk assessment besides restoration of the cavity.

Minimal invasive treatment or minimal invasive dentistry or microdentistry all form the minimal intervention dentistry. It is concerned with ultra conservation treatment of infected and affected oral tissues and aimed at preserving maximum amount of oral tissues by providing least invasive intervention often regarded by patient's as painless and atraumatic. It also aims at management of caries through risk assessment (CAMBRA, acronym used for "caries management by risk assessment).[1-4]

Aim's and Objectives of Minimal Intervention Dentistry[5]

1. The disease should be treated first
2. The surgical approach should be undertaken only as a last resort, with minimal removal of natural tooth material
3. Management begins with identification and elimination of the disease
4. Restoration per se will not prevent or eliminate disease
5. Caries is a bacterial infection and until the microflora is controlled the risk of further demineralization in the remaining tooth structure continues.

According to FDI World Federation, the Principles of Minimal Intervention Dentistry[6]

1. *Modification of the oral flora:* This can be achieved through adequate plaque control and reduced carbohydrate intake.
2. *Patient education:* It should include information regarding the etiology of dental caries and the methods of prevention. Dietary modification and oral hygiene maintenance should be stressed.
3. *Remineralization of noncavitated lesions of enamel and dentine:* Caries is a process of demineralization and remineralization. Early carious lesion can be revered through remineralization. Saliva plays a critical role in this process. Assessment of saliva for its quantity and quality forms an important aspect.
4. *Minimal operative intervention of cavitated lesions:* Restoration of cavitated lesions should be as conservative as possible with the aim of preserving the natural tooth followed by restoration with adhesive materials such as glass-ionomer cement and/or resin composite.
5. *Repair of defective restorations:* Since removal of old restorations results in removal of sound tooth

structure, repair should be considered as an alternative to replacement whenever possible.

Concepts of Minimal Intervention Dentistry

The three main concepts of MID are:
1. Identification of the risk factors
2. Prevention
3. Control

Concept of Identification

1. Caries risk assessment
   - Evaluation of saliva
   - Evaluation of caries activity (Caries activity tests)
   - Assessing the occlusion and tooth factor
   - Understanding the patients environment such as socioeconomic status, education status, etc.
   - Diet analysis
2. Anticipatory guidance and health education

Concept of Prevention

Prevention of caries forms the next phase by formulating plans to check the etiological factors. The three part strategy developed to prevent caries includes:

A. Combating caries inducing microorganisms[7-9]
   - The bisguanide antiseptics, chlorhexidine: At high concentration it acts as a detergent damaging the cell membrane and causing the loss of cytoplasmic constituents. At low concentrations it inhibits sugar transport and glycolytic rate and membrane bound ATPase activity.
   - Triclosan: It is a nonionic antibacterial agent against gram +ve bacteria. It is compatible with fluoride and hence can be used in dentrifices.
   - Delmopinol hydrochloride: It is a highly surface active substance which has shown to reduce the amount of plaque formation.
   - Caries vaccine: It can be active or passive immunization. But it is of less significance due to the involvement of many bacteria and factors in the etiology of caries.
   - Replacement therapy: In this method cariogenic bacteria are replaced by noncariogenic bacteria. But practically it is difficult to achieve.
B. Modifying caries promoting ingredients of diet and use of sugar substitutes—this is done through diet counseling.
C. Increasing the resistance of teeth to decay
   - Remineralizing agents such as fluorides, CPP, novamin, hydroxyapatite, etc.
   - Pit and fissure sealants.
   - Laser
   - Augmenting host resistance—protective system in saliva can be produced by recombinant DNA technology.

Concept of Control

It aims at treatment of caries and maintenance of restored tooth. Restoration or treatment of caries is aimed at removing only the active caries where remineralization is not possible. The tooth is then restored with an adhesive fluoride releasing material. Continued professional oral prophylaxis is important to maintain the restoration in good condition to reduce the risk of secondary caries. Special means of caries control includes:
1. Ozone application
2. Atraumatic restorative technique (ART)
3. Preventive resin restoration (PRR)
4. Chemomechanical caries removal concepts.

Components of Preventive Dentistry

- Caries risk assessment
- Dental home and anticipatory Guidance
- Professional Care: Includes special care given by the clinician such as pit and fissure sealant, PRR, fluoride therapy, etc.
- Home care: Includes tooth brushing, flossing, rinsing and other procedures done by patient and parents at home.

Caries-risk Assessment[10-17]

Caries risk assessment is used to determine the patient's relative risk for caries development. Assessment of risk forms the key element in preventing any diseases and it guides the practitioner to institute appropriate preventive strategies. There are various methods of caries risk assessment. American Academy of Pediatric Dentistry (AAPD) have developed CAT (Caries Risk Assessment Tool) which assesses the risk based on clinical condition, environmental factors and general health of the individual. Based on this, each child can be categorized as being at low, moderate or high risk for development of caries (Table 7.1) Risk assessment should be repeated at regular intervals as the child's risk for developing dental disease can change over time due to changes in habits (e.g. diet, home care), oral microflora, or physical condition.

Risk assessment of an individual child can be made by identifying the factors that cause the disease. It includes:
- Evaluation of saliva and other host factors (Caries susceptibility test)
- Evaluation of caries activity (Caries activity tests)

Table 7.1: Categorizing risk based on caries risk assessment tool (AAPD 2002)

Caries risk indicator	Low risk	Moderate risk	High risk
Clinical condition	No caries in past 24 months No enamel demineralization (white spot lesions) No visible plaque or gingivitis	Carious teeth in the past 24 months One area of white spot lesion Gingivitis	Carious teeth in the past 12 months More than one area of white spot lesions Visible plaque on anterior teeth Radiographic evidence of enamel caries High titer of mutans streptococci Wearing dental or orthodontic appliances Enamel hypoplasia
Environmental characteristics	Optimal systemic and topical fluoride exposure Consumption of simple sugars or foods strongly associated with caries initiation primarily at meal time High socioeconomic status Regular use of dental care in an established dental home	Suboptimal systemic fluoride and optimal topical fluoride exposure Occasional in between meal exposure of simple sugars or foods strongly associated with caries Midlevel socioeconomic status of caregiver Irregular use of dental services	Suboptimal topical fluoride exposure Frequent in between meal exposure of simple sugars or foods strongly associated with caries Low level socioeconomic status of caregiver No usual source of dental care Active caries present in the mother
General health conditions			Children with special health care needs Conditions impairing saliva secretion/composition

- Understanding the patient's environment such as socioeconomic status, education status, etc.
- Health and education
- Diet assessment, analysis and counseling.

Dental Home[18-29]

Definition (AAPD 2010)

The dental home is the ongoing relationship between the dentist and the patient, inclusive of all aspects of oral health care delivered in a comprehensive, continuously accessible, coordinated, and family-centered way. Establishment of a dental home begins at less than 12 months of age and includes referral to dental specialists when appropriate.

The dental home is inclusive of all aspects of oral health that result from the interaction of the patient, parents, nondental professionals, and dental professionals. This concept is derived from the American Academy of Pediatrics (AAP) definition of a medical home which states pediatric primary health care is best delivered where comprehensive, continuously-accessible, family-centered, coordinated, compassionate, and culturally effective care is available and delivered or supervised by qualified child health specialists.

Since physicians, nurses, and other healthcare professionals see new mothers and infants earlier than dentists, it is essential that they be aware of the infectious etiology and associated risk factors of early childhood caries, make appropriate decisions regarding timely and effective intervention, and facilitate the establishment of the dental home.

Children who have a dental home are more likely to receive appropriate preventive and routine oral health care. Referral by the primary care physician or health provider has been recommended, based on risk assessment, as early as 6 months of age, 6 months after the first tooth erupts, and no later than 12 months of age.

Furthermore, subsequent periodicity of reappointment is based upon risk assessment. This provides time-critical opportunities to implement preventive health practices and reduce the child's risk of preventable dental/oral disease.

Every infant should receive an oral health risk assessment from his/her primary health care provider or qualified health care professional by 6 months of age. This initial visit should consist of the following:
- Assessing the patient's risk of developing oral disease using a caries risk assessment
- Providing education on infant oral health
- Evaluating and optimizing fluoride exposure.

The following should be accomplished by 12 months of age:

- Recording thorough medical and dental histories
- Completing a thorough oral examination
- Assessing the infant's risk of developing caries and determining an appropriate prevention plan and interval for periodic re-evaluation based upon that assessment
- Providing anticipatory guidance regarding dental and oral development, fluoride status, non-nutritive sucking habits, teething, injury prevention, oral hygiene instruction, and the effects of diet on the dentition
- Planning for comprehensive care and periodicity schedules for oral health
- Referring patients to the appropriate health professional if intervention is necessary.

AAPD Recommendation for a Dental Home

1. The AAPD encourages parents and other care providers to help every child establish a dental home by 12 months of age.
2. A dental home should provide:
   a. Comprehensive oral health care including acute care and preventive services
   b. Comprehensive assessment for oral diseases and conditions
   c. Individualized preventive dental health program based upon a caries-risk assessment and a periodontal disease risk assessment
   d. Anticipatory guidance about growth and development issues (i.e. teething, digit or pacifier habits)
   e. Plan for acute dental trauma
   f. Information about proper care of the child's teeth and gingivae. This would include the prevention, diagnosis, and treatment of disease of the supporting and surrounding tissues and the maintenance of health, function, and esthetics of those structures and tissues.
   g. Dietary counseling
   h. Referrals to other specialists when care cannot directly be provided within the dental home
   i. Education regarding future referral to a dentist knowledgeable and comfortable with adult oral health issues for continuing oral health care; referral at an age determined by patient, parent, and pediatric dentist.
3. The AAPD advocates interaction with early intervention programs, schools, early childhood education and child care programs, members of the medical and dental communities, and other public and private community agencies to ensure awareness of age-specific oral health issues.

Preventive management of caries risk patients	
Risk category	**Preventive options**
Low	1. Dental health education 2. Reinforcement of good oral hygiene 3. Use of fluoride tooth paste 4. Maintained on recall visits
Moderate	1. Pit and fissure sealant 2. Dietary counseling 3. Fluoride mouth rinse 4. Professional topical fluoride 5. Use of dental floss especially when at risk for proximal caries 6. Maintained on recall visits
High	1. Preventive procedure are practiced more rigorously. 2. Recalled every 2-3 months 3. Continuous monitoring of *S. mutans* level 4. Chemical caries control

Anticipatory Guidance[30-34]

Anticipatory guidance is defined as proactive counseling of parents and patients about developmental changes that will occur in the interval between health supervision visits that includes information about daily caretaking specific to that upcoming interval.

Anticipatory guidance should follow risk assessment. In the simple words, anticipatory guidance is warning or guiding the parent and the child that the child is vulnerable for the development of disease due to the presence of risk factors and also informing and guiding them about the methods to prevent the future disease.

The scope for anticipatory guidance can be any diseases/disorder of the oral cavity such as caries, trauma, habits, etc.

Oral Health Instructions as a Part of Anticipatory Guidance

For the Mother/Caregiver)

- *Oral hygiene:* Toothbrushing and flossing by the mother on a daily basis
- *Diet:* Dietary education for the parents
- *Fluoride:* Using fluoridated toothpaste and rinsing every night with an alcohol-free, 0.05% sodium fluoride have been suggested to help reduce plaque levels and help enamel remineralization.
- *Caries removal:* Routine professional dental care for the mothers can help to keep their oral health in optimal

condition and minimize the potential of transfer of MS to the infant, thereby decreasing the infant's risk of developing ECC.

- *Delay of colonization:* Education of the parents, especially mothers, on avoiding saliva-sharing behaviors (e.g. sharing spoons and other utensils, sharing cups, cleaning a dropped pacifier or toy with their mouth) can help prevent early colonization of *Streptococcus mutans* in their infant's mouth. This can also be achieved by advising mothers to use xylitol chewing gum. Evidence demonstrates that this can reduce the *S. mutans* level and thus prohibit the transmission of these bacteria.

For the Child

- *Oral hygiene:* Oral hygiene measures should be implemented no later than the time of the eruption of the first primary tooth. Cleansing the infant's teeth as soon as they erupt with either a clean cloth or soft toothbrush will help reduce bacterial colonization. AAPD (2010) recommends that children's teeth should be brushed twice daily with fluoridated toothpaste and a soft, age-appropriate sized toothbrush. A "smear" of toothpaste is recommended for children less than 2 years of age, while a "pea-size" amount of paste is recommended for children 2-5 years of age.
- Flossing should be initiated when adjacent tooth surfaces cannot be cleansed with a toothbrush.
- *Diet counseling:* High-risk dietary practices appear to be established early, probably by 12 months of age, and are maintained throughout early childhood. Frequent night time bottle feeding, extended and re-peated use of a sippy or no-spill cup, frequent consumption of snacks or drinks containing fermentable carbohydrates increases the child's caries risk.
- *Fluoride:* Professionally-applied fluoride or other agents that aid in remineralization such as Casein Phosphopeptides (CPP) should be considered for children at high caries risk based upon caries risk assessment.
- *Injury prevention:* Age-appropriate injury prevent-ion counseling for orofacial trauma should be done.
- *Non-nutritive habits:* Non-nutritive oral habits (e.g. digit or pacifier sucking, bruxism, abnormal tongue thrust) may apply forces to teeth and dentoalveolar structures. It is important to discuss the need for early sucking and the need to wean infants from these habits before malocclusion or skeletal dysplasias occur.

Adolescent Oral Health Care

AAPD recognizes adolescent patient as having distinctive needs due to:

1. A potentially high caries rate
2. Increased risk for traumatic injury and periodontal disease
3. A tendency for poor nutritional habits
4. An increased esthetic desire and awareness
5. Complexity of combined orthodontic and restorative care
6. Dental phobia
7. Potential use of tobacco, alcohol, and other drugs
8. Pregnancy
9. Eating disorders
10. Unique social and psychological needs.

Thus a vigorous need based oral care instructions should be given to adolescents. Frequent evaluation and motivation is also important (Table 7.2).

> **Anticipatory guidance can include for all the dental diseases and related problems. Some of them are as follows:**
>
> 1. Growth and development: With regards to development of future malocclusion
> 2. Oral habits: Persistent habits that can lead to malocclusion
> 3. Trauma: Presence of risk factor is the indicator for serious injury during trauma
> 4. Medical illness: With regards to the relation and the problems associated with the existing illness and dental development and management.

Caries Activity Tests[35-37]

Caries activity is defined as the speed with which teeth are destroyed by caries, which includes new carious lesions and enlargement of the existing cavities during a certain period. Accurate analysis of the activity is important for treatment planning, selection of restorative material and recall appointments and for initiating preventive procedures.

Ideal Requisites of a Caries Activity Test

- Should have a sound theoretical basis
- Show maximal correlation with clinical status
- Be accurate with respect to duplication of results
- Be simple
- Be inexpensive
- Take less time to perform
- Should possess validity, reliability and feasibility.

> 1. Caries activity test means measuring the level of activity of bacteria for producing caries. e.g. lactobacillus colony count, Snyder test
> 2. Caries susceptibility test means measuring the level of vulnerability of host for caries activity. e.g. salivary reductase test, Buffer capacity test
> But both are routinely referred to as caries activity tests.

Table 7.2: AAPD Recommendations for periodic examination, preventive dental care and other treatments					
Procedure	Age				
	6-12 months	12-24 months	2-6 years	6-12 years	12+ years
Oral examination	✓	✓	✓	✓	✓
Assessment of growth and development	✓	✓	✓	✓	✓
Caries risk assessment	✓	✓	✓	✓	✓
Radiographic assessment	✓	✓	✓	✓	✓
Prophylaxis and topical fluoride	✓	✓	✓	✓	✓
Fluoride supplementation	✓	✓	✓	✓	✓
Anticipatory guidance counseling	✓	✓	✓	✓	✓
Oral hygiene counseling	Parent	Parent	Parent/Patient	Parent/ Patient	✓
Dietary counseling	✓	✓	✓	✓	✓
Injury prevention counseling	✓	✓	✓	✓	✓
Counseling for non-nutritive habits	✓	✓	✓	✓	✓
Counseling for speech and language development	✓	✓	✓	✓	✓
Substance abuse counseling				✓	✓
Counseling for intraoral/perioral piercing				✓	✓
Assessment and treatment developing malocclusion			✓	✓	✓
Assessment for pit and fissure sealants			✓	✓	✓
Assessment and /or removal of third molars					✓
Transition to adult dental care					✓

Some of the Caries Activity Tests

1. Lactobacillus colony count
2. Snyder test
3. Salivary reductase test
4. Saliva tongue blade method
5. Rapid caries activity test by resazurin disk.

Lactobacillus Colony Count[38,39]

- Introduced by Hadley in 1933
- It estimates the number of acidogenic and aciduric bacteria in patient's saliva, done by counting the number of colonies appearing on tomato peptone agar plates or Rogasa's medium.
- Saliva is collected after having the patient chew paraffin before breakfast.
- Saliva is diluted to 1:100 dilution
- 0.4 ml of this is spread on the surface of an agar plate and are incubated at 37°C for 3-4 days
- A count of the number of colonies is then made by using Quebec counter.

Disadvantages

- Results are available after few days
- Counting the colonies is a very tedious process

- Requires complex equipments and personnel with bacteriological training
- High cost
- Repeated sampling is required.

Results

Number of lactobacillus/ml	Caries activity of saliva
0-1000	Little or no activity
1000–5000	Slight activity
5000–10,000	Moderate activity
> 10,000	Marked activity

Snyder Test[40]

- It measures the rapidity of acid formation, when a sample of stimulated saliva is inoculated into glucose agar whose pH is adjusted to 4.7-5 and with bromocresol green as color indicator.
- Saliva is collected and shaken vigourously for 3 minutes.
- 0.2 ml is pipetted into the tube of agar and mixed.
- Agar is allowed to solidify and incubated at 37°C.
- Color change of the indicator is observed after 24, 48 and 72 hours.

Advantages

- Simple
- Requires simple equipments
- Moderate cost
- Found a high correlation between the snyder test and lactobacillus count test and clinical caries activity.

Results

Color change	Time	Caries activity
Yellow (pH $\leq$ 3.8)	24 hours	Marked activity
	48 hours	Definite activity
	72 hours	Limited activity
Green (pH 5.4)	24 hours	Continue test
	48 hours	Continue test
	72 hours	Inactive

Salivary Reductase Test[41]

- It measures the enzyme reductase in the saliva
- The test measures the rate at which an indicator dye, diazoresorcinol changes its color from blue to red to colorless on reduction by the mixed salivary flora.
- Saliva is collected by chewing a special flavored paraffin and expectorating directly into the collection tube upto the 5 ml calibration mark
- Sample is mixed with a fixed amount of diazoresorcinol and the change in color is noted after 30 seconds and 15 minutes.

Results

Color	Time	Score	Caries activity
Blue	15 min	1	Nonconducive
Orchid	15 min	2	Slightly conducive
Red	15 min	3	Moderately conducive
Red	30 sec	4	Highly conducive
Pink/white	30 sec	5	Extremely conducive

Saliva Tongue Blade Method[42]

- The test estimates the number of *S. mutans* in mixed paraffin stimulated saliva, when cultured on Mitis-Salivarius Bacitracin (MSB) agar medium.
- Patient chews paraffin wax for 1 min, thus displacing plaque microorganisms into the saliva
- The subjects are then given a sterile tongue blade which they rotate in their mouth ten times, so that both the sides of the tongue blades are thoroughly coated. Excess saliva is removed by withdrawing the tongue blade through closed lips.
- Both sides of the tongue blade are then pressed on to an MSB agar medium in a petridish. It is then incubated at 37°C for 48 hours.

- Counts of > 100 colony forming units (CFU by this method is proportional to greater than 10^6 CFU of *S. mutans* per ml of saliva by conventional methods.

Rapid Caries Activity Test by Resazurin Disk[43]

- This method of caries activity test has a characteristic color reaction developing with in 15 minutes at 32–37°C.
- The color of the disk changes form blue to bluish violet, reddish violet and then to red or colorless with saliva of the individuals
- The resazurin disk is highly sensitive to gram +ve microorganisms such as *S. mutans, S. mitis,* Lactobacilli and Actinomyces series.
- The color change was due to a chemical reaction (oxidation-reduction reaction) and not a pH effect.

HEALTH EDUCATION[44-46]

It derives form a Latin word 'educare' meaning to bring out and to lead.

Dental health education is an integral part of general health education. Therefore, the achievement of dental health goals will require the application of principles and processes that are effective in other aspects of health education.

The degree to which dental health education goals can be achieved is determined by a series of interrelated factors, which include:

1. The accessibility of dental health services and of advice in which individuals have confidence.
2. The economic feasibility of putting into practice the dental health measure advocated.
3. The acceptability of the proposed dental health practices in terms of the customs, traditions, and beliefs of individual families and groups
4. The extent to which people already have the kinds of learning experience needed to enable them to understand or to desire the benefits that arise from new or modified dental health behavior and such behavior may often require a considerable personal sacrifice of a financial, social or psychological nature.

Definition

Health education is defined "as a process that informs, motivates and helps people to adopt and maintain healthy practices and lifestyles, advocates environmental changes as needed to facilitate this goal and conducts professional training and research to the same end."

Objectives of Health Education

1. Informing people
   - Regarding scientific knowledge about prevention of disease and promotion of health
   - This will melt away the barriers of ignorance, prejudice and misconceptions people have about health and disease.
2. Motivating people
   - Simply telling the truth is not sufficient
   - They must be motivated to change their lifestyle accordingly
3. Guiding them into action
   - Helping people to use judiciously and wisely the health services available to them
   - Health education acts as the cement to bind together the brick of health program.

Approaches to Public Health

1. Regulatory
   - Health promotion, achieved through the law enforcement
   - Less likely to change the habit on a long run
   - Requires vast administrative machinery
2. Service
   - Aims at providing all the needed health facilities
   - When 'felt needs' were not established they were a failure
3. Educational
   - It involves motivation, communication and decision making
   - Slow but permanent results can be obtained.

Steps in the Adoption of New Ideas and Practices

1. *Unawareness:* Person lacks the knowledge
2. *Awareness:* Comes to know about the disease and its prevention
3. *Interest:* Seeks more detailed information
4. *Evaluation:* Weighs the pros and cons
5. *Trial:* Decision is put into practice
6. *Adoption:* Decides the new practice is good and adopts it.

Communication in Health Education

The purpose of communication is to transmit information from one person to another with a view to bring about behavioral changes.

Key Element in Communication

1. *Communicator:* The person who educates
2. *Message:* The knowledge or information
3. *Audience:* People to be educated

4. *Channel for communication or aides used for communication:* It can be auditory aids (tape recorder, microphone, etc.), visual aids (not requiring projection such as chalk board, posters, etc. or those requiring projection like slides, movie, etc.) or combined.

> Considerable information about the individual, his family background, social and cultural values, belief, perceptions, and aspirations should be done first. One of the main drawbacks in many dental health education programs has been the failure to make adequate educational diagnosis before prescribing program activities.

DIET ASSESSMENT,[36,47] ANALYZING AND COUNSELING

These form the steps involved in evaluating patients' diet and implementing a modified diet habit.

Diet Habit Assessment

The collection of information about food consumption and dietary habits is essential when relating diet to caries prevalence or incidence.

Various Methods Employed for Collection

A. Food balance sheets
B. Food accounts and estimated food records
C. Weighing methods and duplicate portion technique
D. Interview methods
E. Questionnaires

The choice of method is greatly affected by the purpose of study. Diet assessment can be made for individual patients or for a large group of people.

Food balance sheets (Used only for assessment of dietary habit of a given population): It is an indirect estimate of the amounts of foods consumed by a population at a certain time, expressed as per capita consumption per year. It is obtained by dividing the total amount of food with the total amount of population of the country and correlating it with the caries frequency and sugar consumption.

Advantage: It gives a total view of the country, effective while formulating a national food program.

Disadvantage: Reliability of data differs from one country to other and these data shows only the amount of food available and not consumed as food wastage is not considered. It is not useful for individual assessment.

Food accounts and estimated food records: In this method the accounts of food consumed are recorded (Table 7.3) over a certain period of time (3-7 days including weekends).

Table: 7.3: Diet chart (Sample of one day)				
Time	Food eaten	Method of preparation	Quantity	Sugar
7.00 am	Milk Chapathi Jam	Boiled With Ghee –	1 Glass 2 1 tsp	✓
10.00 am	Lassi with Sugar Gulab Jamoon	– Fried	1Glass+ 2tsp 2	✓
11.30 am	Burfi	Cooked in ghee	Small bite piece	✓
1.00 pm	Rice Vegetable curry	Boiled Fried in little oil	1 Medium Bowl 1 Small Bowl	—
4.30 pm	Water Melon Juice with sugar Glucose Biscuits	— Baked	1 Glass+ 2tsp 4	✓
8.30 pm	Rice Vegetable curry	Boiled Fried in little oil	1 Medium Bowl 1 Small Bowl	—
Total Sugar Exposures = 4 per day				

It can be used by a group of people living in institutions, families or on individual basis. A person has to keep record of the amount of food taken over 3-7 days which also includes a weekend. The amount of sugar containing foods can also be written specifically.

Advantage: Large sample can be obtained by it and it is cheap as there is no need for trained persons.

Disadvantage: May not represent a typical week, bias by the individual, just the fact that the person is maintaining the record may result in change in eating habits and accuracy depends on the reliability of the data.

Weighing methods/duplicate portion technique

It is also called as recipe method or double portion method. Portion similar to those consumed are collected by the subjects and then analyzed by the investigators. Meals eaten outside the home, must also be taken into account. They are then weighed.

Advantage: It is more accurate.

Disadvantage: Limited sample size, much work is involved and high cost.

Interview methods

There are two variations:

a. Diet recall—food consumed by people during 1-2 days is recalled (1 day or 24 hours recall).

b. Diet history—questions are made on the general food patterns and habits over a longer period of time, even 1 year or more.

Advantage: Large sample can be utilized as less time is consumed, cheap and direct communication is possible

Disadvantage: Attitude of the interviewer is important in decision making and one day history does not give correct data.

Questionnaires

It is similar to interview, but there is no interviewer. The individual is given questionnaires that has to be completed by tick marking the correct answer. But this requires marking only those items in the questions and other items may not be entered.

Dietary Goal at Modification

1. Restriction of the frequency of in between meal snacking
2. Reduce consumption of sugar to a maximum of 10% of the total energy intake, and increase the intake of starch and fiber containing food stuffs
3. Avoid products that contain high concentration of sugar and which are retained for long periods of times in the oral cavity such as candies and sweets or at least restrict them once a week
4. Use of sugar substitutes
5. IDA national workshop on 'oral health goals for India and strategies to achieve them by 2000 AD had suggested sugar consumption should be not more than 10 kg/person/year.

Diet Counseling

In some patients a single dietary habit may explain the high levels of caries activity, such as frequent eating of sweets or snacking at night and this can be easily corrected. In others a complex eating situation is found. The eating pattern may be characterized by snacking with virtually no ordinary satiety giving meal or a proper nutrient intake. In such cases change in basic behavior is necessary.

A change in behavior is affected by the fact that humans are neophobic. Therefore changes should be brought on slowly and gradually. The advice given should be compatible with the home environment, religion, financial status, patients medications, metabolic disorders, etc.

Three Basic Stages of Behavior Change

1. Contemplation stage—patient gains insight of the fact that his/her eating habits may be associated with a disease and it has to be changed.

2. Stage of behavioral change
3. Maintenance stage.

Areas of Influence for Promoting Dietary Behavior Modifications

* Laws and regulation
* Cultural norms and values—use of famous personalities and value of an attractive smile
* Education, to create awareness
* Food production—reduction in the cariogenic food production and sale
* Availability of food—making healthier choice the easier choice
* Improving socioeconomic status
* Media—through advertisements
* Diet assessment and counseling.

Dietary modification is synonymous with restricted intake of sugars. But such approach attracted few followers and is not practical on a public health scale. More pragmatic approach would be to encourage sugar substitution by the use of hypoacidogenic and nonacidogenic sweetners.

Xylitol, as discussed is one of the promising dietary approach on the current scene. Xylitol chewing gum has been shown to reduce levels of *S. mutans* by altering their metabolic pathway.[48-49] It also enhances remineralization and arrests dentin caries. A number of potentially effective strategies have been implemented such as use of preservatives with enhanced antibacterial activity increased use of natural inhibitors of demineralization such as various phosphates, components like polyphenols (found in chocolates) oat and pecan hulls and cheese and other bovine milk products.

Food with Low Cariogenic Potential

* Relative high protein content
* Moderate fat content to facilitate oral clearance
* A minimal concentration of fermentable carbohydrates
* Strong buffering capacity
* High mineral content
* pH > 6.0
* Ability to stimulate salivary flow.

Remineralizing Agents

1. Fluorides: This is explained in detail in the next chapter
2. Casein phosphopeptides
3. Novamin
4. Hydroxyapatite
5. LASER

Casein Phosphopeptides (CPP)[50-54]

Casein phosphopeptides are used alone or as CPP-ACP (Casein phosphopeptides with amorphous calcium phosphate) or CPP-ACFP (Casein phosphopeptides with amorphous calcium fluoride phosphate). They are derived from casein which is a milk protein. CPP-ACP has shown to reduce demineralization and enhance remineralization of the enamel subsurface carious lesions. The main function of casein phosphopeptides is to modulate bioavailability of calcium phosphate levels by maintaining ionic phosphate and calcium supersaturation to increase re-mineralization. The role of ACP is also said to control the precipitation of CPP with calcium and phosphate ions. The advantage of CPP-ACFP is the availability of calcium and phosphate in one product. Each molecule of CPP can bind to 25 calcium ions, 15 phosphate ions and 5 fluoride ions. CPP also is believed to possess antibacterial and buffering effect on plaque and also interfere in the growth and adherence of *S. mutans* and *S. sobrinus*. Combined with fluoride CPP-ACP has an additive effect on caries activity. It has also been observed that adding CPP-ACP to soft drinks with tendency for demineralization may actually reduce the erosion capacity of the soft drinks. CPP-ACP has also been added to dentifrices, mouthrinses, chewing gums, lozenges.

NovaMin[55]

NovaMin® (Calcium Sodium Phosphosilicate) is the trademark product of NovaMin Technology Inc (NTI). It is a bioactive glass composed of minerals that naturally occur in body and react when it comes into contact with water, saliva or other body fluids. This reaction releases calcium, phosphorus, sodium, and silicon ions in a way that results in the formation of new HydroxyCarbonateApatite (HCA) crystals.

Hydroxyapatite[56,57]

Carbonated hydroxyapatite nanocrystals, with size, morphology, chemical composition and crystallinity comparable with that of dentine, is said to remineralize enamel, thus proving beneficial in the management of dental caries. A concentration of 10% nano-hydroxyapatite is optimal for remineralization of early enamel caries. It has been used in tooth pastes (as fillers) and pit and fissure sealants. Hydroxyapatite crystals can effectively penetrate in the dentin tubules and obturate them. They can cause closure of the tubular openings of the dentin with plugs within 10 minutes and a regeneration of a surface mineral layer.

Lasers[58-62]

The ability of the laser to alter the surface of enamel and increase its resistance to acid challenge is utilized. The CO_2 laser is efficiently absorbed by the tooth minerals and is transformed rapidly into heat and forms a ceramic like surface that is highly resistant to acid attack. Laser treatment appears to be particularly useful for treatment of pit and fissure surfaces. Nd:YAG lasers have also been used for etching the enamel without any risk of pulpal irritation.

Ozone Therapy[63,64]

Ozone is a chemical compound consisting of three oxygen atoms (O_3—triatomic oxygen). Ozone therapy has proven to be effective in preventive treatment of dental caries. It is usually advocated in dentistry for sterilization of cavities, root canals, periodontal pockets, and herpetic lesions. It interferes with the metabolism of bacterial cell, most likely by inhibiting and blocking the operation of the enzymatic control system. A sufficient amount of triatomic oxygen breaks through the cell membrane and this leads to the destruction of the bacteria. Ozone therapy canals stimulate remineralization of incipient caries following treatment for a period of about six to eight weeks.

PIT AND FISSURE SEALANTS[65-82]

The anatomical pits and fissures of the teeth have long been recognized as susceptible areas for initiation of dental caries. Robertson wrote in 1835 that the caries potential was directly related to the shape and depth of the pits and fissures. GV Black noted that 43-45% of all caries occurred on the occlusal surfaces. Debris remained in the fissure sites regardless of the means of prophylaxis.

The National Health and Nutrition Examination Survey (NHANES III) conducted in 1988-1991 demonstrates that occlusal caries accounted for 56% of the caries in children and adolescents, compared to the 32% of buccal caries or 12% of proximal caries.

Caries reduction of about 92% is achieved if the sealant remains intact over the pits and fissures for a period of 5 years. Fluorides benefit the smooth surface whereas sealants prevent fissure caries, thus providing an overall protection. This is because on smooth surface at least 1 mm of enamel is found superficial to the dentinoenamel junction. In contrast to the base of the fissure, which may lie close to or actually within the dentin. Since enamel caries can be remineralized by fluoride, benefits of fluoride is more to the smooth surface caries and also fluoride may not be able to reach the deeper pits and fissures.

History

Hyatt, 1924 first advocated the term 'Prophylactic Odontotomy' and published the same in 1923. He advocated filling the fissures of teeth with silver or copper oxyphosphate cement as soon as the teeth erupted and then later, when they completely erupted into the oral cavity a small occlusal cavity is prepared and filled with silver amalgam.

Bodecker, 1929 suggested widening the fissures mechanically so that they would be less retentive to food particles and called it as 'Fissure Eradication.'

Gore, 1939 used polymers as sealants. He used solutions of cellulose nitrate in organic solvents to fill surface enamel made porous by action of acids in saliva.

Buonocore, 1955 observed that attachment of acrylic resin to tooth surface was greatly increased after treatment of enamel with concentrated phosphoric acid solution.

Bowen, 1962 used BISGMA, but it was too viscous and required dilution with other monomers.

Roydhouse, 1968 used BISGMA monomer using MMA as a diluent together with peroxide amine poly-merization system. He found 30% reduction of caries over a period 3 years.

Buonocore, 1970 utilized same system but employed an ultraviolet sensitive polymerization inititator (benzoin methyl ether).

Requirements of the Materials Used as Pit and Fissure Sealant

- Reduced water sorption and solubility
- Increased hardness and abrasion resistance after curing
- Sufficient strength, surface hardness, dimensional stability, etc
- Good flow
- Suitable short setting time and adequate working time
- Same thermal conductivity as tooth
- Good bond strength with enamel
- Chemically inert, anticariogenic, etc
- Low volatility
- Reduced polymerization shrinkage.

The deeper parts of fissures contain organic debris and bacteria. Prophylaxis removes debris from only the surface, but does not penetrate below the visible orifice of the fissure. Although the sealant may fill deep fissures under the best conditions, bonding to the clean enamel surface is usually confined to the inclined planes of the fissure and the contents of the fissure within the body of the tooth are sealed in.

Materials Used as Sealant

1. Cyanoacrylates:
   - Discovered in late 1950's
   - Used as surgical adhesive and tooth sealants
   - In presence of traces of moisture they polymerize rapidly to hard and brittle polymers on etched tooth surface.

   Mechanical durability is not satisfactory and they are not biodegradable. Hydrolysis to potentially toxic materials occurred, as initially methyl cyanoacrylate was used. This was later replaced by butyl and isobutyl ester which was found to be more stable.
2. Polyurethanes:
   - For example, epoxylite (contain 10% sodium monofluoro phosphate with liquid polyurethane and utilizes citric acid as etchant),
   - Not regularly used due to poor mechanical properties and oral durability and toxicity
3. Dimethacrylates:
   - MMA is highly volatile and lack penetration
   - Enamite, a new sealant utilizes MMA-PMMA system initiated by butyl boron. It binds better and is less affected by immersion in water
   - BISGMA is a viscous amber liquid of low volatility diluted with MMA (Ratio of 3 : 1) for use as sealant.
4. Glass ionomer:
   - Developed by McLean and Wilson
   - Hydrophilic, good adhesion, biocompatible, flu-oride release. This is an added advantage over the routinely used BIG GMA resin. The fluoride that is released improve caries resistance, remineralize enamel caries and also alters the bacterial adhesion
   - Used for fissure whose orifice exceeds 100 μm.
   - Long-term retention rate, wear resistance of glass ionomer cements is questionable.
   - Since it is less technique sensitive than resins, they are recommended as transient sealants in incompletely erupted teeth and in children whom isolation is difficult to achieve.
5. Fluoride releasing resin sealants:
   - With recent advent of fluoride releasing sealants, it is easier for the fluoride to reach the deeper enamel.
   - They increase the fluoride levels to 3500 ppm in deep enamel layers.
   - Modified urethane—BIS-GMA resin is used as fluoride releasing sealants.
   - Incorporating fluoride does not alter the properties of the resin.

Classification of BIS GMA Sealants

1. Based on curing method
   First generation: Polymerized with ultraviolet light of 350 nm wavelength. Absorbed UV light excessively and prevented complete polymerization of the sealant. Light intensity varied from lamp to lamp
   Second generation: Self cured or chemically cured. Most of them are unfilled. Can be transparent, opaque or tinted. Filled resin increased wear and abrasion resistance than unfilled resin
   Third generation: Visible light cured of 430-490 nm wavelength. May be unfilled (usually white) or filled (usually clear)
   Fourth generation: With addition of fluoride for added benefit
2. Based on Presence of Filler
   Unfilled—better flow
   Semifilled—strong and resistant to wear
3. Based on color
   Tinted—for easy identification
   Clear—difficult to detect
   Opaque—for easy identification
   Pink (Fuji VII, GC Company)—better fluoride release.
   Newer resins are available that change color following polymerization. Clinpro™ sealant (3M ESPE) is one such pit and fissure sealant that is pink in color and changes to natural white upon polymerization.

Properties of BIS-GMA

Biocompatibility

- Nonirritating to tissue
- Allergic reactions must be kept in mind
- Abraded surface may promote plaque accumulation and encourage caries and staining.

Ease of Manipulation

- Good results depend on manipulation characteristics like proportioning, mixing, working time, method of placement, polymerization technique and setting time. If these are not well controlled it may contribute to poor interfacial bonding and low resin strength. Curing time of self-cure—90-180 seconds and working time is 2/3rd of curing time.

Viscosity and Penetration

- Usually used to fill wide shallow fissure but not narrow deep fissures, hence low viscosity is preferred. But the disadvantage is that the material flows off from the surface especially in the maxilla.
- It was found that even narrow fissures can be completely filled with a sealant having a high

coefficient of penetration so long as it is applied at the proximal edge of an occlusal surface and allowed to flow to the other edge.

Dimensional Stability

- Volatility, polymerization shrinkage and thermal contraction affect the placement and stress developed which in turn influence the mechanical properties and durability of bonding
- Extent of curing shrinkage is affected by the degree of conversion of monomer to polymer.
- Combination of thermal and polymerization shrink-age may produce high internal stresses. Cracks may develop in thin marginal layers of such sealants on hardening.
- Inhibition of polymerization by atmospheric oxygen producing an unpolymerized layer of monomer on the surface of a resin material and around the interior surface of air bubbles within the body of the material.

Physical and Mechanical Properties

- Thermal expansion and contraction as a result of hot and cold foods affect stresses generated at the interface with enamel.
- It is also affected by water absorption.
- Coefficient of thermal expansion of sealants is 7-10 times more than tooth.

Microleakage and Bacterial Survival

- Interface show minimal penetration.
- Studies have shown negligible microleakage after 6 months.
- Caries preventive effectiveness of fissure sealant is attributed to a combination of a decreased number of viable bacteria and lack of sufficient fermentable carbohydrate for the remaining bacteria to accumul-ate acid in cariogenic concentration.
- Also found a negative bacteriological result after 5 years in a fissure under the sealant.

Steps in the Placement of Sealant (Figs 7.17A to G)

1. *Thorough prophylaxis:* Polished with paste free of fluoride and glycerine. Application of fluoride makes the enamel surface difficult to etch and glycerine forms an impervious coating on the surface. The tooth should be thoroughly washed to remove the pumice from the fissures.
2. *Acid etch:* Removes organic material and debris from the surface and produces micro pores into which the monomer can penetrate. Degree of etching depends on nature and concentration of acid, duration of exposure, composition and site of enamel. 30-50%

orthophosphoric acid is used in liquid form for 30-60 seconds using sable hair brush. Liquid must be replenished if it flows from the surface. Etching permits the sealant to penetrate about 50 μm of enamel depth. Liquid etchant is preferred as they penetrate deep grooves better compared to the gel.

3. *Rinsing:* Tooth surface is rinsed thoroughly for 30 seconds with oil free air and water.
4. *Placement of material:* Some authors recommend placement of bonding agent prior to placement of sealant material. But care should be taken not to fill the fissure and pits with bonding agent. Fissure sealant is applied using sable hair brush and polymerized.
5. *Finish:* Feel gently with blunt explorer or small ball ended burnisher for the edges.

Indications and contraindications of sealant			
Surface diagnosis	*Clinical considera-tion*	*Pits and fissures that are sealed*	*Pits and fissures that are not sealed*
Carious	Occlusal anatomy Status of proximal surface General caries ac-tivity	If pits and fissures are separated by transverse ridge, a sound pit or fissure may be sealed Sound	Carious pits and fissure Carious
Questionable	Occlusal morphol-ogy Tooth age Status of proximal surface	Many occlusal le-sion, few proximal lesion Deep, narrow pit and fissure Recently erupted teeth Sound	Many proximal lesion Broad, well coalesced pit and fis-sure Teeth car-ies free for 4 years or more Caries
Sound			

Some of the commercially available pit and fissure sealants	
Sealant material	*Manufacturing company*
Helioseal	Ivoclar-Vivadent Inc
Helioseal F (with fluoride)	Ivoclar-Vivadent Inc
Seal–Rite	Pulpdent Corporation
Clinpro Sealant	3M-ESPE
Teethmate F	J Morita USA
Prisma Shield VLC	Dentsply Ltd

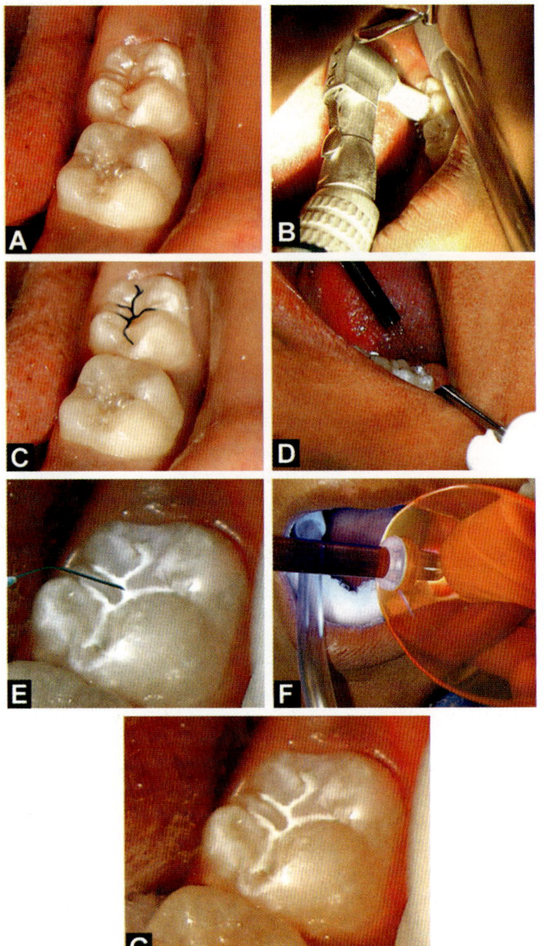

Figs 7.17A to G: Steps in the placement of sealant: (A) First permanent molar with deep grooves; (B) Oral prophylaxis; (C) Liquid etchant placed in the grooves; (D) Acid etch is washed with water and surface is dried; (E) Sealant is placed in the grooves with the help of the syringe. It can also be applied with a single tufted brush and varies as per the manufactures method of dispensing; (F) Sealant is cured using visible light; (G) Sealant is finished and checked for premature contacts

Sealant rention: Retention rates for sealants placed on permanent teeth were initially reported to be higher than those for deciduous teeth. 76% of retention was observed in primary molars upto a period of 2.8 years after placement. Permanent first molars exhibited varied retention rate from 92% after 1 year to 28% after 15 years. Although the retention rate was low, there was no significant increase in caries rate.

The reason for the difference was attributed initially to the prismless enamel in the deciduous teeth. Prismless enamel is the product of reduced functional activity during the terminal stages of amelogenesis, which resulted in the lack of enamel rod formation during the last 25 µm of enamel formation. Later it was found that since the prismless enamel occurred in only about 17% of the primary teeth, it may not be the sole reason for the difference in the reduced sealant retention and may be due to lower mineral content and higher internal prism volume.

> **Placement of pit and fissure sealant over carious fissure**[76,77]
>
> - Acid etching procedure itself removes 75% of the viable microorganisms
> - 4.5% of microorganisms were viable after 2 weeks
> - A total reduction of 99.9% of microorganisms were found after 2 years
> - Sealants act as a barrier that isolates the microorganisms from their source of nutrition and prevent colonization by new microorganisms.

ATRAUMATIC RESTORATIVE TECHNIQUE (ART)[44,82]

The atraumatic restorative technique (ART) is a procedure based on removing carious tooth structure using hand instruments alone and restoring the cavity with an adhesive restorative material. At present the restorative material of choice is glassionomer cement.

History

- Atraumatic restorative treatment was pioneered in the mid 1980s in Tanzania.
- In 1991, a community field trial started in Thailand, comparing ART with traditional treatment using dental drilling equipment and amalgam.
- Another community field trial was set up in Zimbabwe in 1993.
- The results of the study has shown that through the careful application of ART, about 85% of one-surface restorations in the permanent dentition will be in a good to acceptable condition upto about 3 years.
- The studies in Thailand and Zimbabwe, and also another community field trial, which started in 1995 in Pakistan, have clearly shown that pain is rarely experienced with this approach. In fact, if applied correctly ART is well received by the vast majority of patients.
- In conclusion, ART is quality treatment applicable to all communities.

Advantages of Atraumatic Restorative Technique

1. ART provides care for decayed teeth, which is nonthreatening, low cost, and can prevent extractions in most cases.

2. ART is based on modern knowledge about minimal intervention techniques thereby requires minimal tooth removal.
3. Because it is a noninvasive procedure, there are great potentials for its use in children as well as in fearful adults.
4. It also provides a restorative option for special groups in the community, such as the physically or mentally handicapped people living in nursing homes and the home-bound elderly.

Indication of Atraumatic Restorative Technique

1. Done where there is no power supply to run the motors required for cavity preparation such as in very remote villages.
2. When many people have to be treated such as in refugee camps.
3. Areas where it is difficult to take heavy equipments due to natural constraints. The equipments required for ART are few.

Contraindications of Atraumatic Restorative Technique

1. Presence of abscess or fistula associated with the tooth to be restored.
2. Presence of clinical pulp exposure.
3. Teeth that have been painful for a long time and may be associated with chronic inflammation of the pulp.
4. There is an obvious carious cavity but is not inaccessible to hand instruments.

Principles of Atraumatic Restorative Technique

The two main principles of ART are:
1. Removing carious tooth material using hand instruments only.
2. Restoring the cavity with a restorative material that adheres to the tooth surface.

Steps in Preparing the Cavity for Atraumatic Restorative Technique

1. Cotton rolls are placed alongside the tooth to be treated. This will absorb saliva and keep the tooth dry.
2. Plaque and other deposits are removed from the tooth surface with a wet cotton pellet, and then the surface is dried with a dry cotton pellet.
3. The extent of the caries is judged.
4. The access to the caries is widened by placing the blade of the dental hatchet into the cavity and turning the instrument forward and backward like turning a key in a lock. This movement chips off small pieces of carious enamel.

5. Carious dentin is then removed with the excavators by making circular scooping movements around the long axes of the instrument.
6. The unsupported enamel that may be present is very weak and is removed with the blade of the hatchet.
7. Restoring the cavity with glass ionomer cement using finger press technique as explained in glass ionomer section.

PREVENTIVE RESIN RESTORATIONS (PRR)/ CONSERVATIVE ADHESIVE RESIN RESTORATION[69,83,84]

There may be deep pits and fissures present on tooth surface that require sealant therapy. In such situations if caries is present in one area or part of the pits or fissures then that particular caries is restored and remaining pits and fissures are protected with sealants. This was introduced by Simonsen in 1978 and was termed as preventive resin restoration. It is presently referred to as 'conservative adhesive resin restoration' due to confusion of the original term with pit and fissure sealant (Fig. 7.18).

Types of Preventive Resin Restoration

There are three types of preventive resin restorations based on the extent and depth of the carious lesion. They are:
1. Type A
2. Type B
3. Type C

Armamentarium required for preventive resin restorations
1. Local anesthesia (optional)
2. Rubber dam or cotton rolls
3. Cotton pellets
4. Burs: No. 114, 112 round (slow speed), No. 330 (high speed)
5. White finishing stone and carbide fluted finishing bur
6. Etching gel (tooth conditioner)
7. Sealant (filled)
8. Applicator
9. Bonding agent (unfilled)
10. Calcium hydroxide liner
11. Polymerization unit (visible light)
12. Composite resin (filled)
13. Plastic (Teflon) instrument
14. Marking paper

Type A Preventive Resin Restoration (Fig 7.19)

Type A comprises of suspicious pits and fissures where caries is limited to enamel. A slowspeed round bur is used to remove any decalcified enamel.

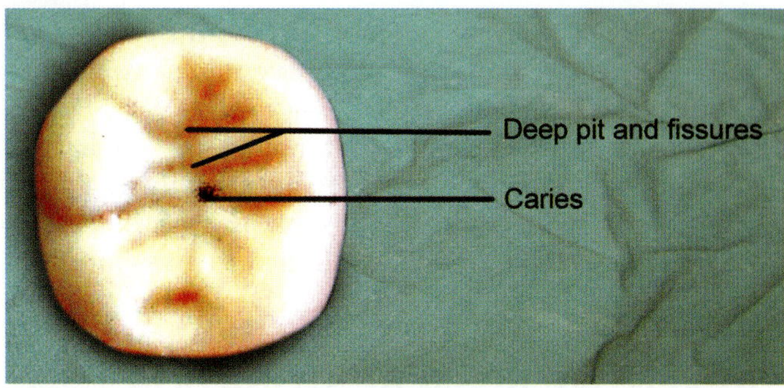

Fig. 7.18: PRR is indicated in cases where caries is present in some parts of the deep pits and fissures

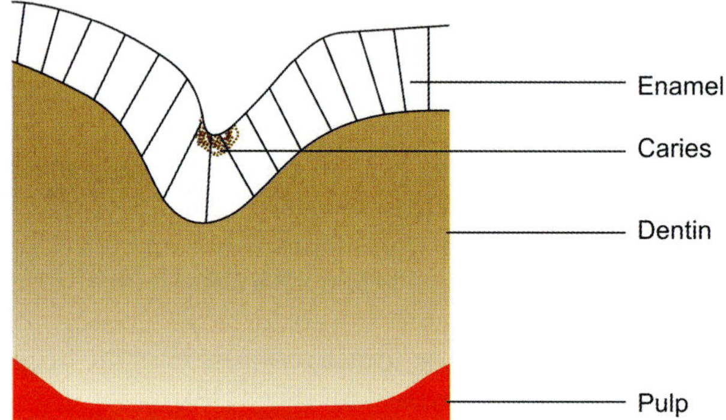

Fig. 7.19: PRR Type A: Suspicious pits and fissures where caries is limited to enamel

Steps involved are:
1. The surface is cleaned.
2. Cotton rolls or, preferably, a rubber dam is used for isolation.
3. Decalcified pits and fissures are removed with a slow-speed round bur.
4. Acid etching gel is placed over the entire occlusal surface for 60 seconds.
5. It is then washed for 20 seconds and dried for 10 seconds
6. The sealant is applied carefully, avoiding air entrapment in the preparation site.
7. It is polymerized with the visible light for 20 seconds.
8. The occlusion is adjusted, if needed, with finishing bur.

Type B Preventive Resin Restoration (Fig. 7.20)

Type B comprises of incipient lesion extending into dentin that is small and confined.
Steps involved are:
1. Thorough prophylaxis of the surface.
2. Placement of a rubber dam.
3. Carious pits and fissures are removed with a slow-speed round bur.
4. Fast setting calcium hydroxide is placed over the exposed dentin.
5. Acid etching gel is placed over the entire occlusal surface for 60 seconds.

6. It is then washed for 20 seconds and dried for 10 seconds.
7. A coat of bonding agent is applied on the walls of the preparation.
8. The preparation is then filled with composite resin material.
9. The filled sealant material is applied over the entire occlusal surface and all layers are simultaneously light cured.
10. Occlusion is adjusted and the surface is finished and polished.

Type C Preventive Resin Restoration (Fig. 7.21)

Type C is characterized by the presence of deep caries and need for greater exploratory preparation in dentin.
1. Thorough prophylaxis of the surface
2. Placement of a rubber dam
3. Carious pits and fissures are removed with a slow-speed round bur. Since it involves deep caries, local anesthesia may be required.
4. A bevel is placed on the enamel cavosurface margin of the preparation
5. Fast setting calcium hydroxide is placed over the exposed dentin.

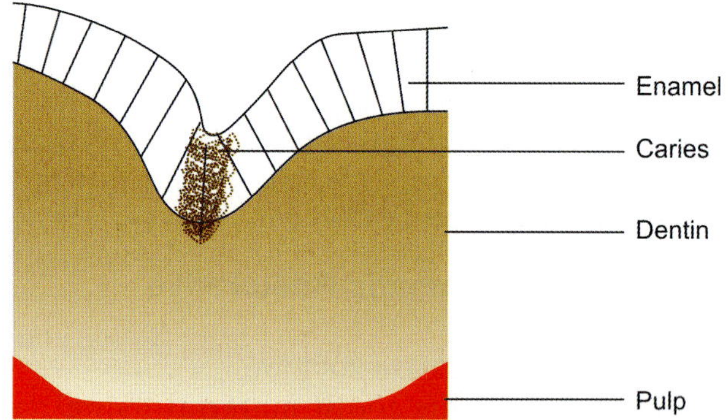

Fig. 7.20: PRR Type B: Incipient lesion extending into dentin that is small and confined

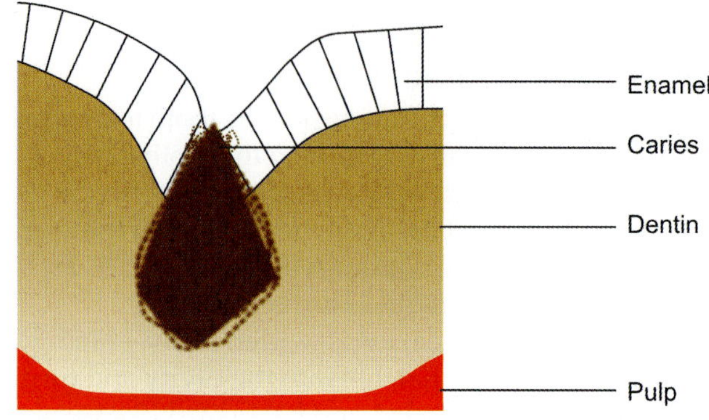

Fig. 7.21: PRR Type C: Deep caries extending deep into dentin

6. Acid etching gel is placed over the entire occlusal surface for 60 seconds.
7. It is then washed for 20 seconds and dried for 10 seconds
8. A coat of bonding agent is applied on the walls of the preparation
9. The preparation is then filled with composite resin material
10. The filled sealant material is applied over the entire occlusal surface and all layers are simultaneously light cured
11. Occlusion is adjusted and the surface is finished and polished.

CHEMOMECHANICAL CARIES REMOVAL CONCEPTS[85,86]

Chemomechanical caries removal (CMCR) is a non-invasive technique of removing infected dentine using a chemical agent. The method of caries removal is based on dissolution followed by scooping or excavating the softened dentin. It was introduced to dentistry as an alternative method of caries removal and is mainly indicated to overcome the discomfort of burs. Various agents have been used such as Carisolv, which is the most successful and commonly used agent. Carisolv gel is a 2-component mixture. Equal parts of the two are mixed to form the active gel substance. One of the components primarily contained three amino acids (glutamic acid, leucine and lysine) and sodium hydroxide. The other fluid contained the reactive hypochlorite component (NaOCl).

Other agents used are papacarie. Papacarie is composed basically of papain, chloramines and toluidine blue. Papain interacts with exposed collagen by the dissolution of dentin minerals through bacteria, making the infected dentin softer, and allowing its removal with noncutting instruments.

ORAL HYGIENE MAINTENANCE

Oral Hygiene Aids

Types of oral hygiene aids that are used to maintain oral hygiene are:
1. Toothbrush
2. Dentifrices/toothpaste
3. Dental floss
4. Oral rinses
5. Disclosing agents

Toothbrushes[87-89]

The overall objectives of toothbrushing are to remove plaque and food debris as well as to atraumatically stimulate gingival tissues.

Components of a Brush (Fig. 7.22)

A tooth brush consists of head and a handle connected by a neck. The head portion contains bristles, made of nylon.

Head

Correct head size of a brush should be selected for attaining maximum maneuverability in the oral cavity. The length of the head should not be >2.5 cm for children. The width should be 6-7 mm for children such that it is sufficient enough to cover 3 adjacent teeth.

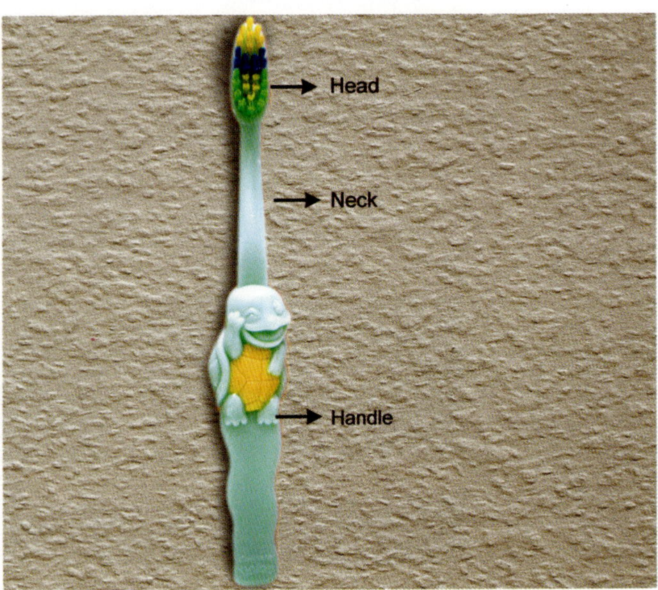

Fig. 7.22: Components of a toothbrush

Bristles (Fig. 7.23)

Texture of the bristles are characterized by:
1. Diameter of the filament
2. Length of the exposed bristle. It is about 11 mm
3. Size of the hole into which the filaments comprising a tuft are inserted
4. Number of tufts in a given area
5. Number of bristle filament in each tufts.

Arrangement of the tufts, and their basic designs

1. *Straight:* All the tufts are of same height (Fig. 7.24A)
2. *Curved or concave:* Tufts at the sides are longer and they gradually reduce in height towards the center giving a curved down or concave shape (Fig. 7.24B).
3. *Convex:* Tufts at the center are longer and they gradually reduce in height towards the center giving a curved up or convex shape (Fig. 7.24C).
4. *Serrated:* Tufts are of different height alternately giving a serrated appearance (Fig. 7.24D).

Nylon bristles loose up to 27% of its stiffness when saturated with water.

Diametre of the bristle denoting the brush type:
Soft brush—0.16–0.22 mm,
Med—0.23–0.29 mm
Extrahard—> 0.30 mm

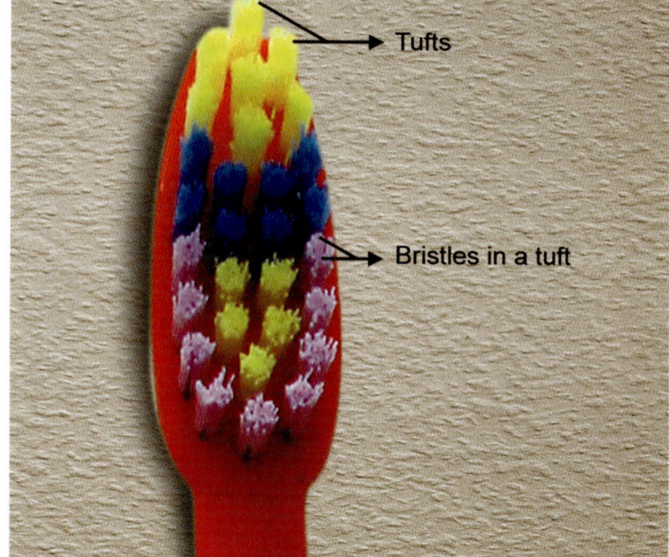

Fig. 7.23: Bristles are grouped to form tufts

Ideal Pedodontic Brush

- Diameter of each nylon filament—0.16–0.22 mm
- Tufts—24–33
- Long handle
- Small head size

Modifications in Brushes

1. *Finger brushes (Fig. 7.25):* These brushes are used when few teeth have erupted and will also help to accustom the child to normal bristle brushes.

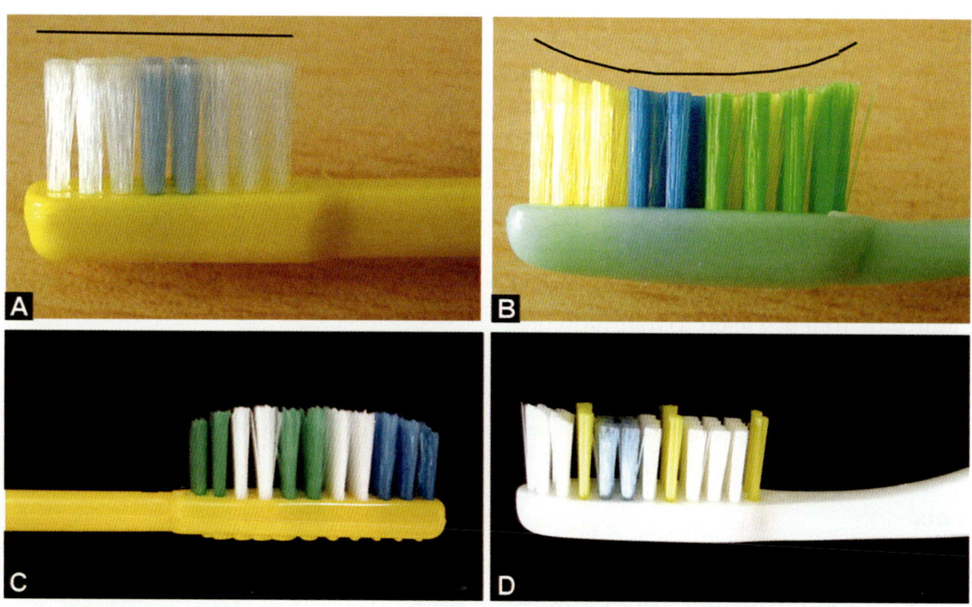

Figs 7.24A to D: Different types of arrangement of tufts: (A) Straight; (B) Concave; (C) Convex; (D) Serrated

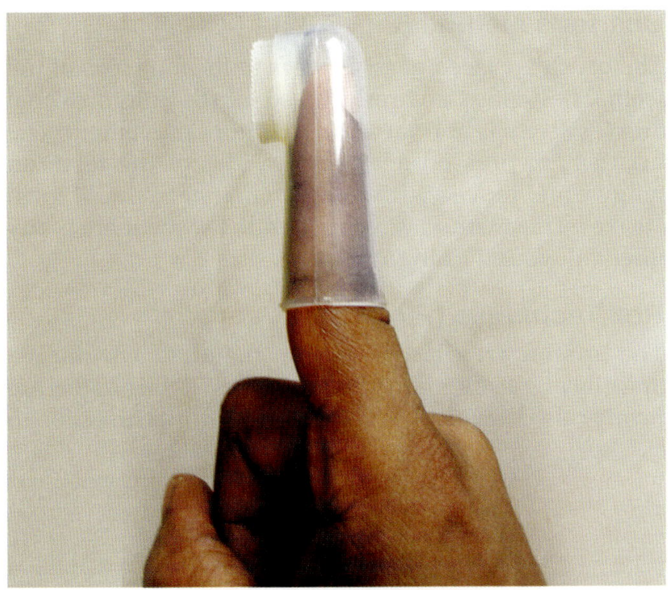

Fig. 7.25: Finger brush

2. *Orthodontic brushes (Fig. 7.26):* It consists of outer rows of longer bristles and inner rows of shorter and stiffer bristles.
3. *Special sulcular cleansing brushes:* Used for periodontal pockets and is not regularly used in pediatric practise.
4. *Pacemaker 45:* Bristles are automatically placed at 45° angle to the tooth surface.
5. *Interdental or proximal brushes (Figs 7.27A and B):* It consists of a holder to which brushes of different shape and size can be fixed as per the need of the patient. Single tufted brushes can also be used to clean the interproximal areas.
6. *Travelling brushes:* The brush can be folded and placed inside a box.
7. *Toothette (Fig. 7.28):* It consists of cotton rolled over a stick. It is used to clean the teeth or gumpads of very small children after wetting it with water. Tooth paste is not used along with toothette.
8. *Brush for the disabled children:* with elastic strap, bicycle handle, etc
9. *Electric or battery operated toothbrushes (Fig. 7.29):* It requires no manual dexterity since the bristles move by battery power. Three types of movements may be present. They are:
   i. Rotation in an arc of about 60°, so that the bristles sweep the tooth similar to roll method
   ii. Back to fourth horizontal action as in horizontal scrub
   iii. An elliptic movement combining oscillating with back and forth movements.

It is especially useful in preschool children when used by parents or children with extensive prosthetic or orthodontic appliance and in handicapped children.

TOOTHBRUSHING PROGRAM FOR CHILDREN

Techniques used are:[90-96]
1. Bass/modified Bass technique
2. Scrub technique
3. Modified Stillman technique

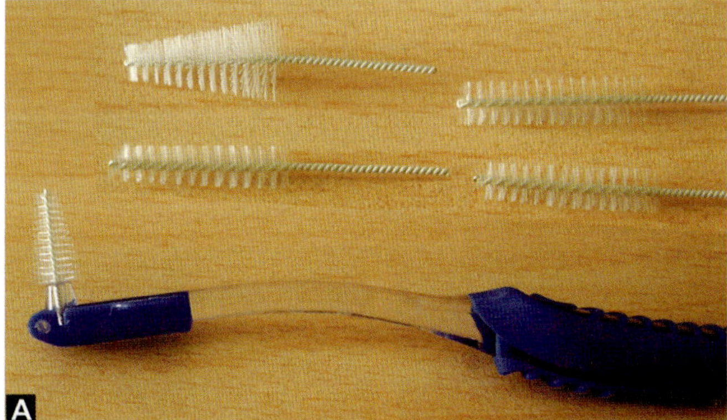

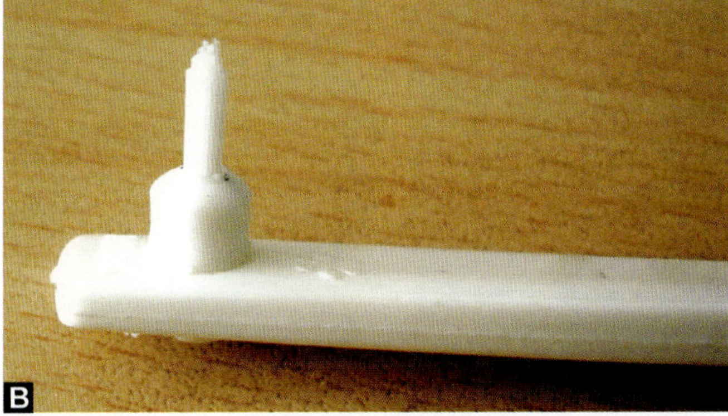

Figs 7.27A and B: Interdental and proximal brushes: (A) Interdental brushes of different shape with holder; (B) Single tufted brush

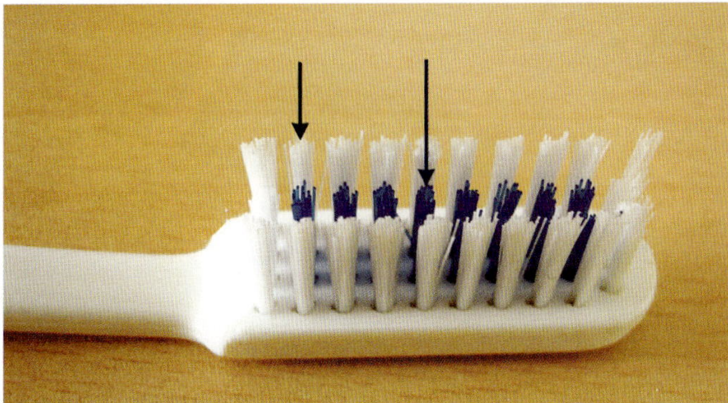

Fig. 7.26: Orthodontic brushes. Note the outer longer bristles (Black arrow) and inner shorter bristles (Blue arrow)

4. Charter's method
5. Roll technique
6. Physiologic method
7. Fones technique

Bass/Modified Bass Technique (Fig. 7.30)

The brush is placed at 45 degrees angle to the long axis of the teeth and the bristles are gently forced into the gingival sulcus and the interproximal area. It is then moved in short back and forth strokes with a vibratory action for 1 to 15 seconds for each area. The occlusal surfaces are brushed with anteroposterior short strokes. In a modified bass method, after the vibratory motion is applied, the brush is rolled towards the occlusal surface.

Modified Stillman Technique (Fig. 7.31)

The bristles are placed at 45 degrees to the apices of the teeth on the gingival margin so that they rest partly on the gingiva. The brush is then moved mesiodistally with a gradual movement towards the occlusal plane. This cleans the interproximal area and vigorously massages the gingival tissues.

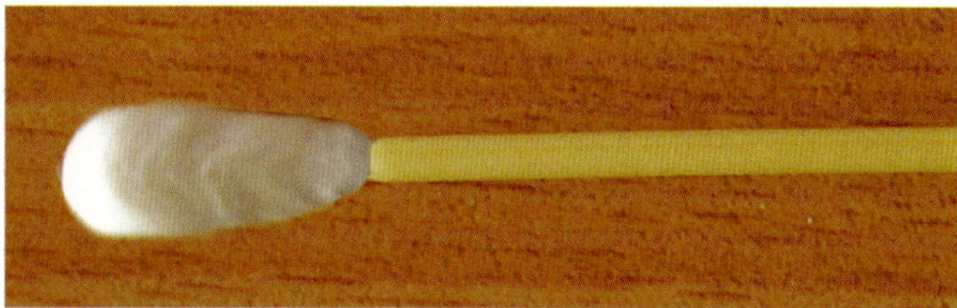

Fig. 7.28: Toothette

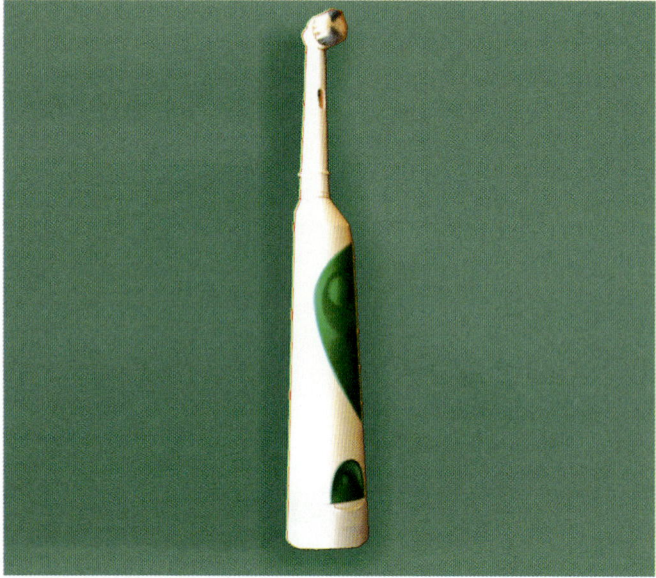

Fig. 7.29: Battery operated toothbrushes

Charter's Method (Fig. 7.32)

The brush is placed at 45 degrees to the long axis of the teeth. The bristles are firmly forced into the interproximal areas with a slight rotary and vibratory movement. The bristles are pressed against the sides of the teeth an gingiva and moved with short circular or back and forth strokes. This method is recommended when there is any gingival wound or injury.

Roll Technique (Fig. 7.33)

The bristles are placed high on the attached gingiva apically at a 45 degree angle. The sides of the bristles are firmly rolled against the gingiva in a coronal direction to

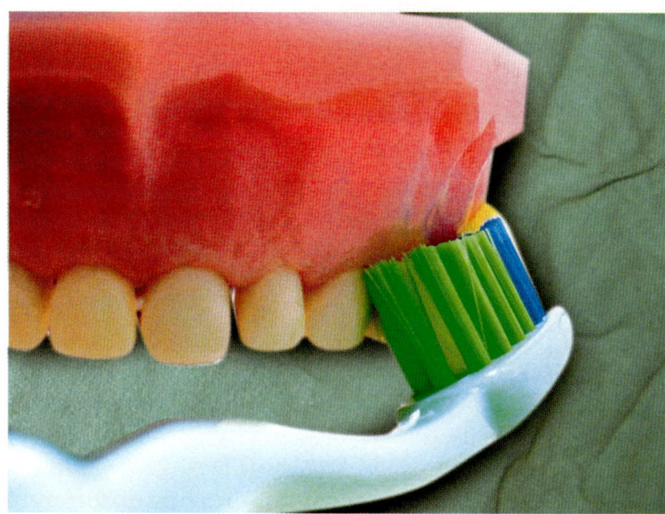

Fig. 7.30: Position of the brush for bass technique

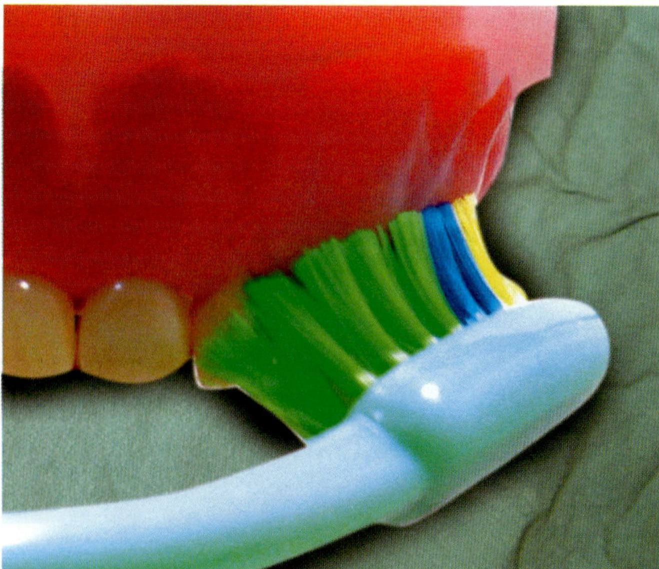

Fig. 7.31: Position of the brush for stillman technique

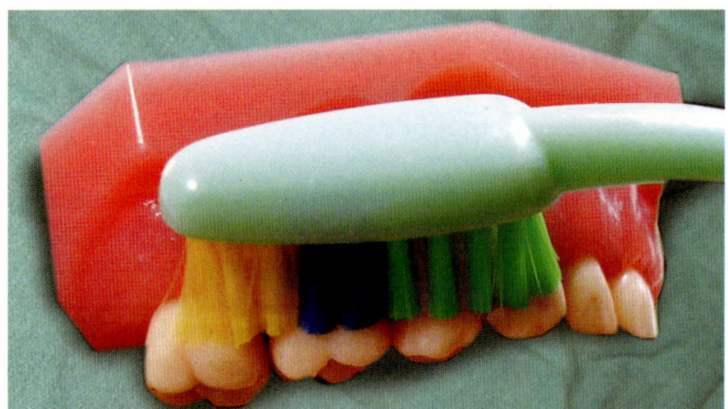

Fig. 7.32: Position of the brush for charter method

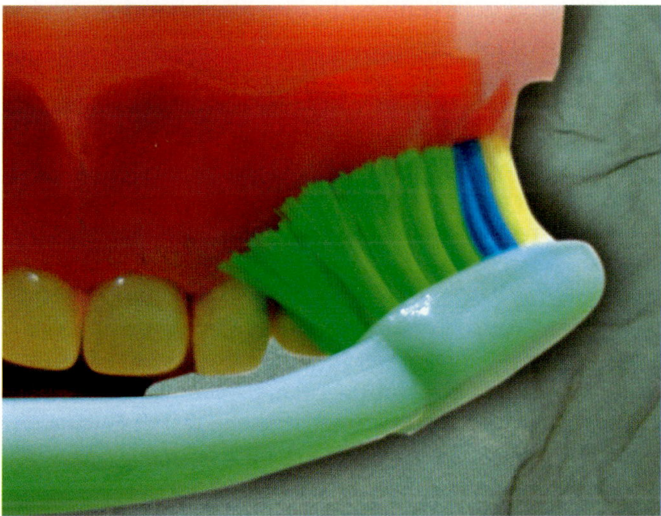

Fig. 7.33: Position of the brush for roll technique

blanch the tissues momentarily and the brush is rubbed against the tooth surface in occlusal direction. It can easily be performed and is used by many people. It is more appropriate when the patient is in normal health.

Scrub Technique (Fig. 7.34)

It is the most commonly used technique. The bristles are placed at 90 degrees to the tooth surface and the brush is moved back and forth as in scrubbing a floor. It just cleans the surface and is not a very good technique to remove plaque from the interproximal areas. This technique may also result in tooth abrasion and gingival recession. Since this method does not require extensive techniques it is ideal for use in children.

Physiologic Method (Fig. 7.35)

This method is based on the belief that the action of brushing the teeth should simulate the passage of food over the crown towards the gingiva. It requires a soft brush and the brushing is done by sweeping from a coronal portion apically towards the gingival margin and the gingiva.

Fone's Technique (Fig. 7.36)

The brush is firmly pressed against the teeth and gingiva with the bristles at right angles to the buccal surfaces and the handle parallel with the occlusal plane. The patient occludes the teeth and the brush is moved in a rotary action with as large a radius as possible. This technique is effective for young children with minimal manual dexterity.

Recommended Brushing Techniques for Children

- Most children find horizontal scrub technique easier to perform.
- Scrub or circular scrub are best for young children with little manual dexterity and it is more effective than roll technique.
- Incisal and occlusal areas and facial and lingual two thirds are frequently not brushed. So these areas should be double checked by parents (Figs 7.37A to E).
- Soft to medium brushes are more efficient
- Time taken is at least 2½ to 3 minutes to cover the entire surface
- Removing plaque thoroughly once every day is sufficient to maintain healthy gingiva, thoroughness of brushing is important than frequency
- Parents brush their children's teeth until the later have achieved manual dexterity, i.e. 5-6 years of age.

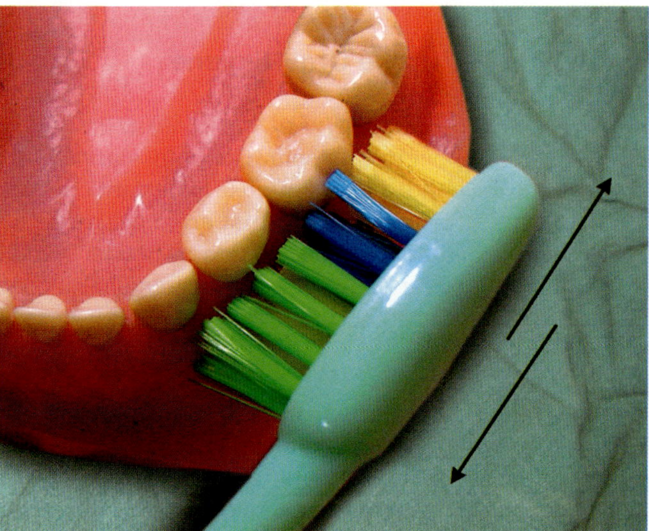

Fig. 7.34: Position of the brush for scrub technique

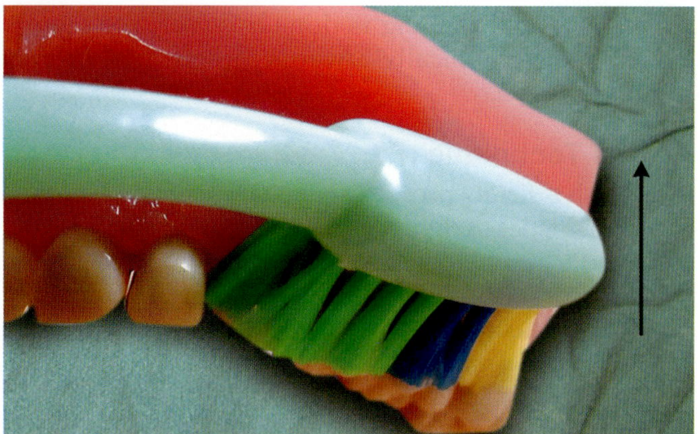

Fig. 7.35: Position of the brush for physiologic method

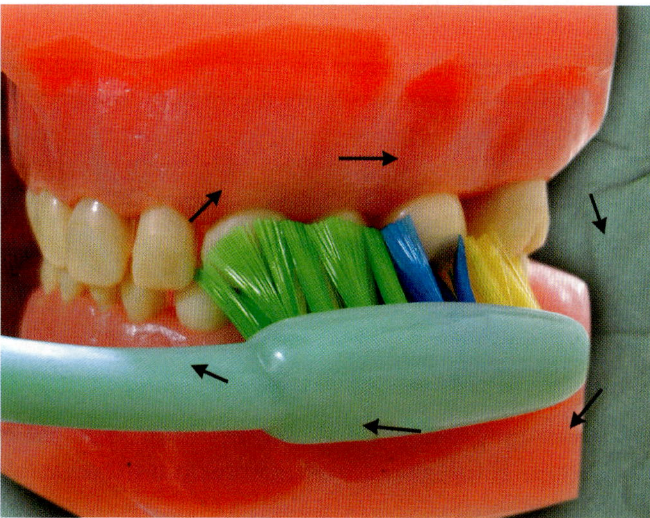

Fig. 7.36: Position of the brush for Fone's technique

Guidelines for Home Oral Hygiene
Prenatal Counseling

The best time to begin counseling actually starts before the birth of the child. This is because expectant couples, particularly if the child is their first are most receptive to preventive health recommendations. They have to be counseled regarding their own oral hygiene habits and the role they shall play as models to their children.

Infant (0 to 1 Year Old) (Fig. 7.38)

The child should be cradled with one arm while the gum pads are massaged with the other hand. This position will provide a sense of security to the child.

The gum pads are cleaned with damp cloth or guaze. As teeth erupt small soft bristled tooth brush is used and there is no need of using any kind of paste.

Toddler (1 to 3 Years Old) (Figs 7.39A to C)

Routine brushing is done by the parent. Plane tooth brush and water is used while brushing.

Positioning of the child and parent is important. Three positions can be used.

1. This position requires two persons. They sit on a chair facing each other, their knees touching each other. The child lies with head towards the person who will be brushing and legs towards the other adult. This position requires two people and may not be possible always (Fig. 7.39A).
2. This position also requires single person. He/she sits on the floor with his or her legs stretched out and the child is made to lie on the leg. The child's leg can be locked in between his/her leg. Left hand is used to retract the cheek and the right hand is used to brush (Fig. 7.39B).
3. This position requires single person. He/she sits on the floor with his or her legs stretched out in front and the child is positioned on the lap. The Childs head is supported by the parent's left hand or the child's head can be rested against the mother's body (Fig. 7.39C).

Preschooler (3 to 6 Years Old) (Fig. 7.40)

The parent stands behind the child and both face the same direction. The child rests his or her head back into the parent's left arm and right hand is used for brushing. This hand can be used also to retract the cheek, while the other hand is used to brush. This is also appropriate for flossing.

Fluoride tooth paste can be used that is pea sized if the child has learned to expectorate. It is also during this stage that fluoride gels and rinses for home use may be introduced in small quantities and limited to those patients demonstrating a moderate to high risk of caries. The use of other chemotherapeutic plaque control agents is generally not recommended.

Parents must continue to take the responsibility of the child's oral hygiene.

School Age (6 to 12 Years Old)

This stage is marked by acceptance of increasing responsibilities by the children. Parental involvement is still needed. However, instead of performing the oral hygiene, they can switch to active supervision. By the second half of this stage, most children can brush and floss themselves. Parents may need to brush or floss their child's teeth in certain difficult to reach areas of the mouth or if there is a compliance problem. One useful adjunct, the disclosing agent may be beneficial at this stage. Children at this age can be motivated quickly and can be explained the importance of keeping their teeth clean and healthy.

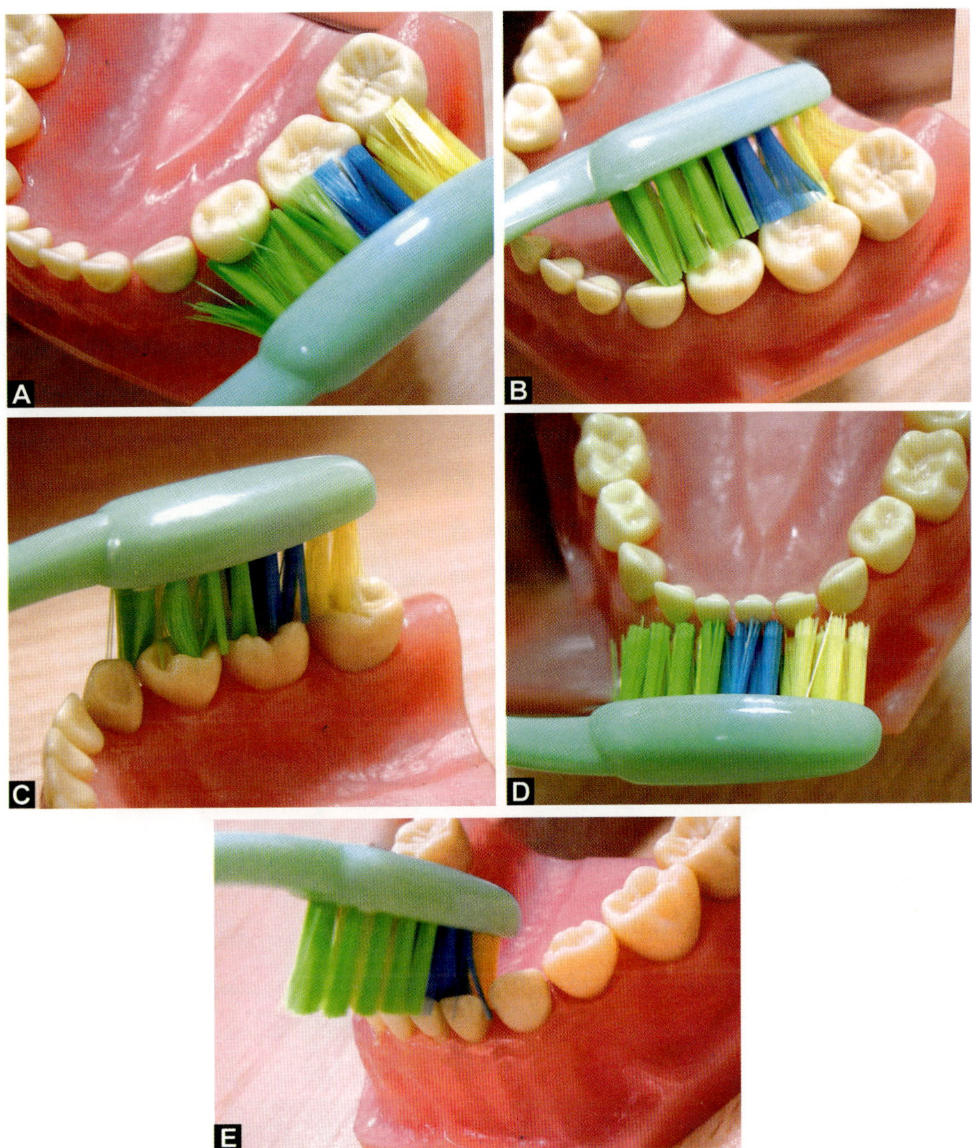

Figs 7.37A to E: All the areas of the tooth should be adequately brushed. This should be demonstrated to the patient: (A) Buccal surface of posterior teeth; (B) Lingual or palatal surface of posterior teeth; (C) Occlusal surface of posterior teeth; (D) Labial surface of anterior teeth; (E) Lingual or palatal surface of anterior teeth

In addition, the use of chlorhexidine or listerine can be introduced to those at risk for periodontal disease and caries.

Adolescents (12 to 19 Years Old)

Although the adolescent patient usually has developed the skills for adequate oral hygiene procedures, compliance is a major problem during this age period. Motivating an adolescent to assume responsibility for personal oral hygiene may be complicated by reactions of rebellion against external authority and some incapacity to appreciate long-term consequences. In addition, poor dietary habits and pubertal hormonal changes increase the adolescents' risk for caries and gingival inflammation. They should be constantly motivated.

Common extrinsic stains:[97,98]

1. Green stain:
   - Boys are more affected
   - Color varies from dark green to light yellow
   - Seen on the labial surface of maxillary anterior teeth at the gingival third
   - Fungi and fluorescent bacteria may be responsible

Contd...

Contd...

2. Orange stain:
   - Occurs less frequently
   - Chromogenic bacterial are responsible
   - Seen in the gingival third of the tooth and is associated with poor oral hygiene
3. Black stain:
   - Seen as dots or thin line of black along the gingival contour. Also seen on tooth irregularities.
   - More difficult to remove
   - May be seen in spite of good oral hygiene
   - Actinomyces is said to be responsible

Dentifrices[87]

The word meaning is derived from latin, dens = tooth and fricare = to rub

The primary purpose of a dentifrice is to clean and polish the accessible surfaces of the teeth when used in conjunction with a tooth brush. It must provide maximum cleaning with minimum abrasion, prevent accumulation of stains, and retard the development of objectionable mouth odors.

Composition

Abrasives (20-50%)
Abrasion that occurs during the use of dentifrice is a function of:
- Inherent hardness of the abrasive material
- Particle size and shape of the milled product
- Properties of the abrasive slurry like pH, viscosity, heat conductivity, etc.

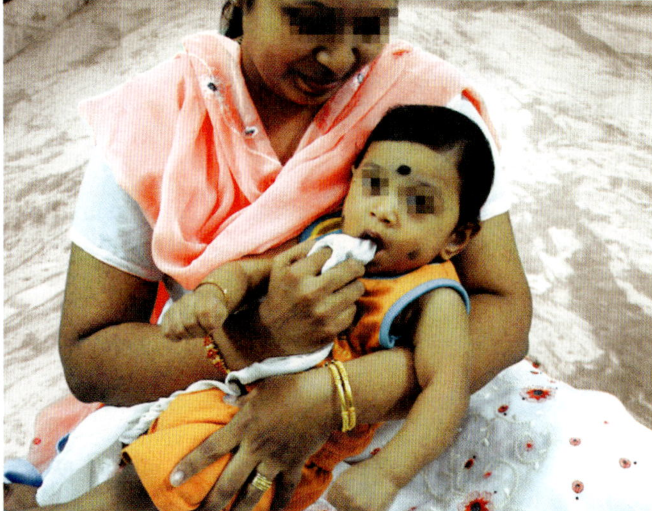

Fig. 7.38: The child is cradled on the left arm and right hand is used for cleaning the gum pads

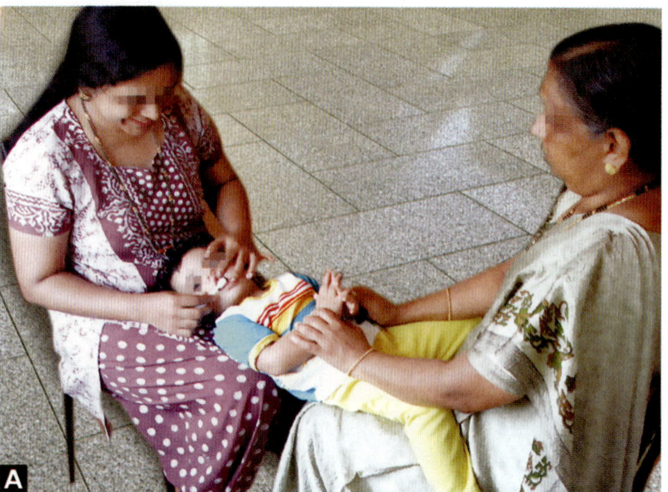

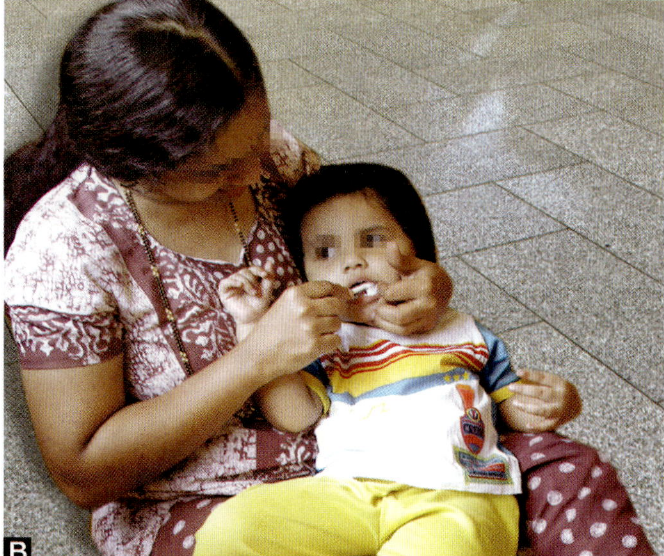

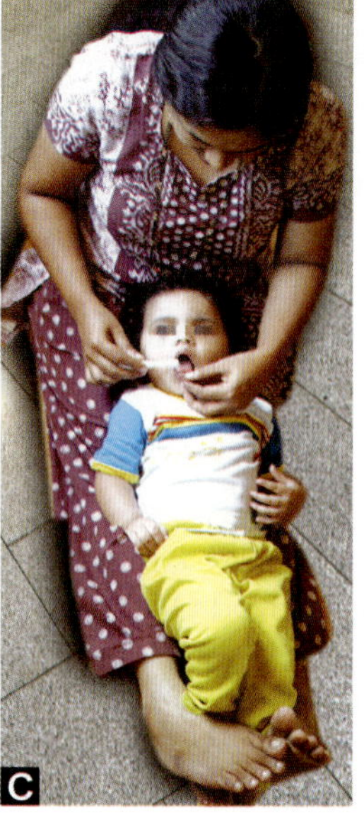

Figs 7.39A to C: Positions used for brushing the teeth of a toddler: (A) Requiring two persons facing each other; (B) Single person and child in a sitting position; (C) Single person and child in a sleeping position

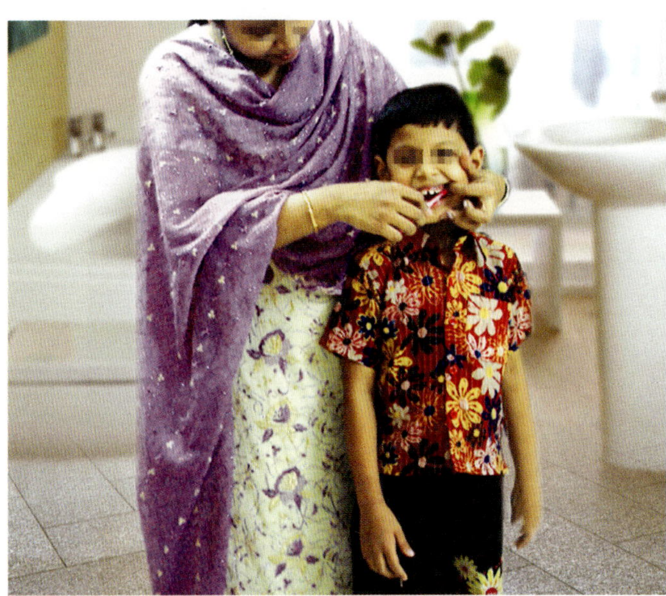

Fig. 7.40: Brushing position for a preschooler

- Hardness of the bristle
- Stress applied during brushing
- Properties of the abraded surface

Increased wear is associated with—harder abrasive, sharper particles, low pH, injudicious brushing with hard bristles, excessive pressure.

Commonly used abrasives

- Silica gel
- Phosphate salts—DCP
- Insoluble sodium metaphosphate
- Calcium and magnesium carbonates
- Aluminium oxide

Abrasion = wearing off
Polish = implies the placing of successively finer scratches until a smooth clean surface is attained.

Humectants: It prevent loss of water and subsequent hardening of the paste when exposed to water. Material used as humectants are glycerol, sorbitol, propylene glycol

Binders: They are hydrophilic colloids that stabilize the formulation and prevent separation of the solid and liquid phases during storage. Gum Arabic, gum karaya, gum tragacanth, alginates, Irish moss extract, etc. are used as binders. They disperse or swell to form a viscous material.

Surface active detergents: They lower the surface tension, penetrates and loosens surface deposits and emulsify or suspend the debris. Sodium lauryl sulfate is commonly used. It is soluble in water and functions in acid or alkali solution and do not form precipitate in hard water or saliva, provide foaming action and a pleasant sensation. Other substances used are sodium coconut monoglyceride sulfonate, sodium n-lauryl sarcosinate, poloxalene.

Flavoring agent: Principle agents are – mint, essential oils of anise, clove, eucalyptus, citrus, menthol, cinnamon and tutti-frutti. It may also contain synthetic sweetener like saccharin.

Preservatives: dichlorophene, benzoates, p-hydroxybenzo-ates, formaldehyde, methyl/ethyl or propyl paraben are used as preservatives.

Other ingredients

Coloring agents: Green, erythrocin, tartrazine, tin oxide
Therapeutic agents: Ammonia and urea, chlorophyll, antibiotics like penicillin, bacitracin, erythromycin, chlorhexidine, hydrogen peroxide, fluoride, desen-sitizing agents-formaldehyde, potassium or silver nitrate, zinc chloride, sodium citrate, sodium fluoride, strontium chloride or triclosan.
Anti calculus agents: 3.3% pyrophosphate, tetrasodium pyrophosphate, disodium pyrophosphate.

Nasadent—dentifrice used in space shuttle, and does not contain detergents, so does not require expectoration.

Dental Floss[99-102]

Parmly first published the paper on the use of dental floss for cleansing the interproximal area of teeth.

1882—First floss was made commercially by Codman and Shurtleff

1948—Bass gave specifications for manufacturing dental floss, as follows

Material—should be of high tenacity bright nylon yarn, 2 denier/filament

Construction—twisting 5 threads of 70 denier, 34 filament yarn

Twists—3 s' twist, steam set
Size—350 denier

Denier (D) defined on the basis of the weight of a 500 denier floss. The denier of any yarn is its weight in a 9000 mts length. Thus 9000 mts of a 500D yarn should weigh 500 gm.

Classification of Dental Floss

According to American National Standard Committee, floss can be of three types:

Type I: unbounded dental floss comprised of yarn having no other additives.

Type II: bonded dental floss comprised of yarn having no additives other than binding agents or having additives that contribute only to cosmetic performance of floss, such as wax.

Type III: bonded or unbounded containing a drug additive intended to give a therapeutic prophylactic, such as fluorides.

Unwaxed floss: It is associated with ease of passing through tight interproximal areas and splaying action may tend to cover a larger area.

Waxed floss: Commonly used in clinics for ligating rubber dam and checking interproximal contact. The problem encountered is that some wax from the floss may remain on the tooth surface and aid in plaque adhesion.

Taflon floss: They are made of polytetrafluoroethylene fibers manufactured by WL Gore and Associates exclusively for Procter and Gambler. Teflon flosses do not tear or wear easily.

Effectiveness of Dental Floss

- Remove efficiently interproximal plaque and reduce plaque scores, gingival inflammation and bleeding.
- Tooth brushing combined with flossing was the most efficient.

Usage of Dental Floss (Figs 7.41A and B)

Flossing is recommended in children with closed proximal contacts. Initially parents should take the resposibility of flossing upto the age of about 9 years.

It may be difficult for younger children to expertise the art of flossing or a parent might find it difficult to floss her child's teeth. This can be made easier by the use of floss holders. They are available in different shapes that enable younger children or parents to floss. Commonly used folders are 'Y' shaped (Fig. 7.42A). Floss of required dimensions are cut and tied across the short arms and the remaining material is tied around the wheel that is used as reservoir. Ready made floss with holders (Fig. 7.42B) is also available. But the floss material available is limited and there is no provision for reservoir, hence the same floss has to be used for the entire mouth.

Disclosing Agents[45,103]

It is difficult to visualize thin plaque in unstained vision. For efficient plaque control it becomes necessary to visualize plaque, which also helps in patient education. Disclosing agents are chemical substances that stain the plaque which makes them clear on the enamel.

Uses of Disclosing Agents

1. Estimating the patients oral hygiene status
2. In educating and motivating patient and parents regarding proper brushing habits

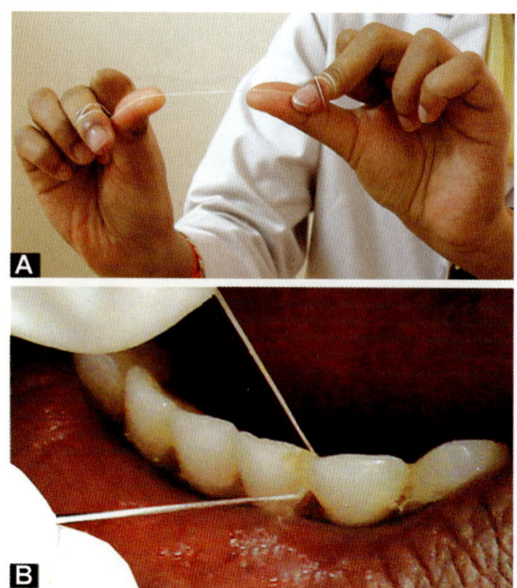

Figs 7.41A and B: (A) Method of holding dental floss; (B) Positioning of floss in between the teeth

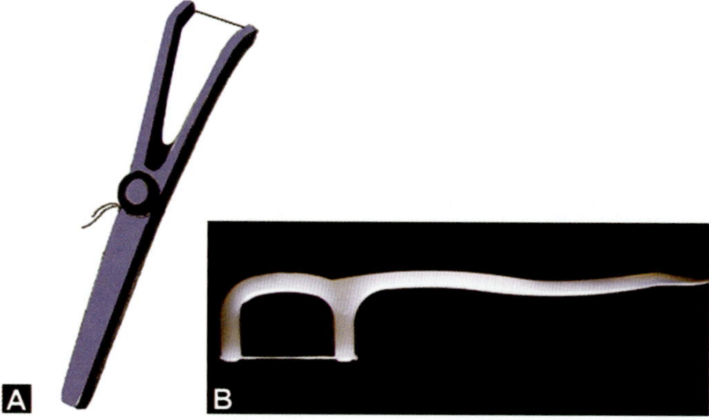

Figs 7.42A and B: Different types of floss holders: (A) 'Y' shaped floss holder; (B) Ready made floss holder with floss attached to it

3. Evaluation of the patient in recall appointments
4. At homes, patients can themselves evaluate the oral hygiene procedure.

Disclosing agents can be dispensed as solutions, wafers, capsules or tablets. During routine use by the patient it is advisable to use disclosing solutions after brushing and flossing to evaluate the efficiency of their brushing.

Materials Used as Disclosing Agents

The common agents used as disclosing agents are:
1. Two tone
2. Erythrocin
3. Bismark brown
4. Basic fuchsin

5. Fast green
6. Mercurochrome
7. Displaque
8. Fluorescent dyes

Some agents stain the older plaque in one color and new plaque with another. For example, two tone disclosing solution is a dye that differentiates plaque by staining older plaque in blue tones and more recent thin deposits in red or pink tones.

Fluorescent dyes are used in conjunction with a special mirror (Plak lite) with absorbency range of 200-540 nm wavelength. It utilizes tungsten light and filters or utilizes standard operatory light and optical filters or UV light. The patient examines his/her image in the mirror and the stained teeth has brilliant yellow-green color. The dye is not visible to naked eye and does not discolor the gingiva and mucosa. But the disadvantage is that of additional cost of the filters and light and also detection of plaque necessitates a darkened room.

Use of Disclosing Agent (Figs 7.43A to C)

A good disclosing agent stains the plaque deeply and may also stain pellicle faintly, but should not discolor the lips and gingiva. To avoid this, the lips, gingiva, tongue, etc may be covered with layer of vaseline or the agent carefully applied only onto the tooth surface.

They are easy to use. Few drops are dropped into the mouth and swished with few drops of water or can also be swabbed directly on the tooth surface with cotton. They should not irritate the soft and hard tissues.

SUGAR SUBSTITUTES[104-108]

It is a known fact that human beings have a weakness for sweets and also sucrose is known to be one of the etiological agents in the formation of caries. Advising people to refrain from eating sucrose is practically not possible. Hence replacements for sugar were introduced.

Sugar substitutes can be of two types:
A. Noncaloric sweetners/intense sweetners
B. Caloric sweetners/nutritive sugar/sugar substitutes.

Noncaloric Sweetners

They are substances of synthetic or natural origin that tastes much sweeter than sugar weight by weight. They yield little or no energy, provide no bulk and are to be used in very small quantities in drinks or blended with sugar substitutes in foods and snacks. Their main commercial success is based on weight control and diabetic products.

Example: Saccharin, cyclamates, aspartame, etc.

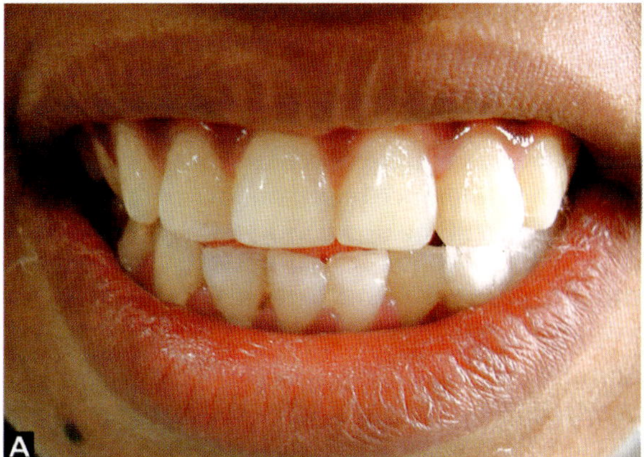

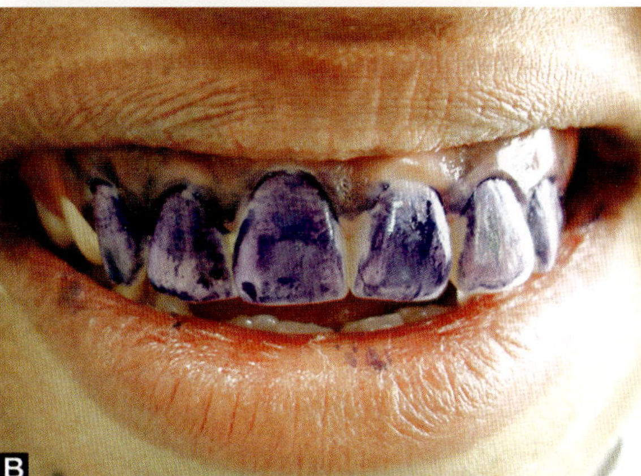

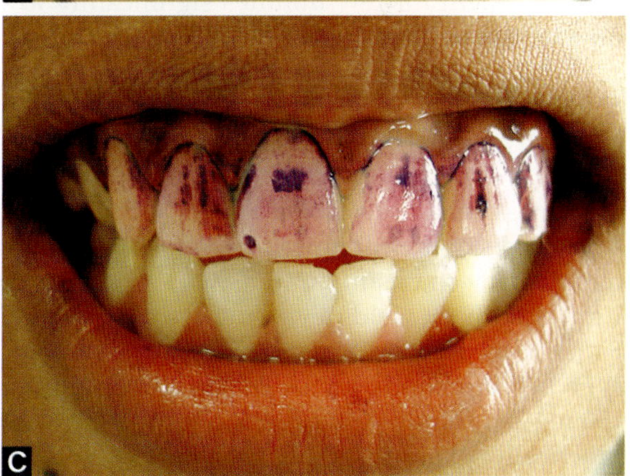

Figs 7.43A to C: Steps in disclosing plaque with two tone disclosing agent: (A) Pretreatment picture, where plaque is not visible clinically; (B) Disclosing agent is applied on the teeth for about one minute; (C) After rinsing the mouth, Old plaque appears as blue in color and new plaque appears pink

Sugar Substitutes/Caloric Sweetners

They are usually carbohydrates or carbohydrate substitutes. They can be metabolized to yield energy and they add bulk to the food products.

They are equally or less sweet tasting than sucrose and require blending with intense sweetners. Their main commercial value lies in products for the diabetics and in "safe for teeth" sweets.

Example: Sorbitol, xylitol, fructose, glucose.

Ideal sweetner selection is based on:

- Consumer acceptance
- Consumer tolerance based on metabolic capacity
- Product should be non cariogenic

Commonly Used Substitutes

1. Xylitol
2. Sorbitol
3. Saccharine
4. Cyclamates
5. Aspartame

Xylitol

- Naturally occurring in raspberries, strawberries, plums, lettuce, cauliflower, mushrooms, etc.
- Sweetness is similar to sucrose
- Slowly absorbed from the gastrointestinal tract
- Side effects: Diarrhea due to osmotic action, predisposes to renal calculi formation, epithelial hyperplasia and neoplasia of bladder.
- Majority of the bacteria including *S. mutans* and *lactobacilli* do not metabolize xylitol
- Most of the chewing gums contain xylitol, and chewing them for few minutes significantly lowers the salivary and plaque level of *S. mutans.*

Sorbitol

- Naturally occurring in cherries, plums, pears, apples, berries and algae
- Sweetness is half of sucrose
- Absorbed slowly from the small intestine by passive transport mechanism.
- 1 gm of sorbitol yields 4 cal energy
- Side effects: Gastric upset and acts as laxative.
- WHO recommends intake of sorbitol be limited to 150 mg/kg/day
- Practically all strains of bacteria ferment sorbitol to produce acids but the rate is very slow.
- Compared to sucrose and other carbohydrates it causes less caries, and also associated with reduced plaque accumulation
- May be added to the dentrifices due its sweetening properties and as humectant.

Saccharin

- Used widely as sugar substitute
- It is 200 times sweeter than sucrose. More than 0.1% tends to become bitter and may induce vomiting

- Side effects are rare, few cases of photosensitization and allergic reactions such as urticaria have been reported.
- Excreted in urine
- Available as tablet, liquid or in powder form
- Interferes with the growth and metabolism of *S. mutans*
- Maximum allowed dose is 1 gm/day for 155 lb person.

Cyclamates

- Used as sodium cyclamate
- It is 30 times sweeter than sucrose
- Side effects: Minimal laxative effect. Long-term use may cause growth retardation.
- It is not fermentable by oral microorganisms.

Aspartame

- 180 times more sweeter than sucrose
- Loss of sweetness on storing and cooking is the main drawback
- Should be avoided in patients with phenylketonuria, during pregnancy
- Unstable in extreme of pH changes.

For a substitute to be accepted commercially it should:

- Have sufficient sweetening power
- Be nontoxic
- Be reasonably inexpensive
- Be thermostable
- Have long shelf time
- Should not react with other components of food.

LEVELS OF PREVENTION, CARIES POINT OF VIEW[45,109]

According to WHO (1970) levels in the prevention of caries can be mainly divided into primary, secondary and tertiary levels.

Primary Prevention Level

Primary level of prevention involves the action taken prior to the onset of disease, which removes the possibility that a disease will ever occur.

It is aimed at reducing the occurrence of new cases of disease in a population. This is accomplished by introduction of fluoride in communal water supplies or the avoidance of sucrose containing in between meal snacks. Primary level of prevention can be sub divided into sub levels, health promotion and specific protection (The actions taken are summarized in table given below).

Level of prevention	Primary prevention		Secondary prevention	Tertiary prevention	
Preventive services	*Health promotion*	*Specific protection*	*Early diagnosis and prompt treatment*	*Disability limitation*	*Rehabilitation*
Services provided by the individual	Diet planning Demand for preventive services Periodic visits to dental clinic	Appropriate use of fluoride Injestion of fluoride Use of fluoridated toothpaste Oral hygiene practises	Self examination and referral Utilization of dental services	Utilization of dental services	Utilization of dental services
Services provided by the community	Dental health education programs	Community and school water fluoridation School mouth rinse program	Periodic screening and referral Provision of dental services	Provision of dental services	Provision of dental services
Services provided by dental professional	Patient education Plaque control program Diet counseling Caries activity tests	Topical fluoride application Pit and fissure sealant	Complete examination Prompt treatment of incipient lesions Preventive resin restoration Pulp capping	Complex restoration Pulpotomy Pulpectomy Rct Extraction	Removable and fixed prosthesis Minor tooth movements Implants

Secondary Prevention Level

Secondary level of prevention involves action which halts the progress of a disease at its incipient stage and prevents complications.

It aims at reducing the prevalence of caries by early diagnosis and prompt treatment. The use of radiographs to detect initial carious lesions leads to prevention at the secondary level. (The actions taken are summarized in table given above).

Tertiary Level

Tertiary level of prevention involves actions which limits the disability progress of a disease helps in rehabilitation.

SCHOOL DENTAL HEALTH PROGRAM[45,110-112]

Objectives of School Dental Service

The objectives according to the American Dental Association are:
1. To help every school child appreciate the importance of a healthy mouth.
2. To help every school child appreciate the relationship of dental health to general health and appearance.
3. To encourage the observances of dental health practices, including personal care, professional care, proper diet, and oral habits.
4. To enlist the aid of all groups and agencies interested in the promotion of school health.
5. To correlate dental health activities with the total school health activities.
6. To stimulate the development of resources to make dental care available to all children.
7. To stimulate dentists to perform adequate health services for children.

Advantages of a School Based Program
1. The children of different age groups are available for preventive or treatment procedures.
2. School atmosphere is less threatening than private offices.
3. Collective education can also be provided along with individual treatment.
4. The dental service supplements the nursing services by helping to provide total health care for school children.

Disadvantages of a School Based Program
1. Performing dental treatment in a school is difficult due to certain limitations such as insufficient dental chairs, etc.
2. Short school hours and long vacations may hinder the program.

Elements of School Based Programs
1. Improving school—community relations
2. Conducting dental inspections

3. Conducting health education
4. Performing specific programs
   - Tooth brushing program
   - Mouth rinse program
     - Fluoride tablet program
     - School water fluoridation
     - Sealant placements
5. Referral to dental care
6. Follow-up of dental inspection

Treatment protocol for early childhood caries

1. Preventive Care

Professional Care
- Educating parents regarding importance of deciduous teeth
- Diet counseling
- Dental health education to parents regarding gum pads cleaning, tooth brushing, frequent mouth rinsing
- Advocating fluoride supplementation if needed
- Advocating fluoride containing dentifrices once a day only after four years of age
- Applying fluoride varnish topically
- Application of fissure sealants in first and second primary molars
- Regular recalls for routine monitoring for dental health
- Reinforcing and motivating parents to continue supervised home care

Home Care:
- Elimination of cariogenic food items from the diet
- Substitution with tooth friendly food
- Discouraging bottle feeding at night
- Falling asleep with pacifiers should be stopped

- Cleaning of gum pads during infancy period is encouraged
- Digital or baby tooth brushing as the teeth erupts
- Initiating mouth rinsing habit after consuming any solid or drinks
- Regular visit to dental clinic once in six months

2. Restorative

Incipient or White Spot Carious Lesions
- Professional topical fluoride application and observation of the lesion for reversal
- Fissure sealant application

Carious Lesions in Enamel and Dentin
- Preventive resin restoration
- Glass ionomer fillings
- Composite restoration in anterior teeth
- Posterior composite restoration
- Amalgam restoration in posterior teeth
- Nickel chrome stainless steel crowns
- Anterior and posterior crown restorations

Carious Lesions with Pulp Involvement
- Pulp therapy with full coverage caronal restoration
- Extraction with space management

FLUORIDES

INTRODUCTION

Fluoride is one of the essential agents used in preventive dentistry effective against dental caries. It has also been described as an essential nutrient in the Federal Register of United States Food and Drug Administration (1973) and also by WHO expert committee.

Fluoride is derived from a Latin word fluor, meaning to flow, since it was used as a flux. It is most electronegative with atomic weight 19 and atomic number 9.

HISTORICAL EVOLUTION OF FLUORIDES AS CARIES PREVENTIVE AGENT[113-120]

1901: Dr Frederick McKay of Colorado, USA discovered permanent stain on the teeth of his patients which was referred to as "Colorado brown stain." McKay named the stain as mottled enamel.

1902: Dr JM Eager, a US marine hospital surgeon, stationed in Italy reported a high proportion of Italian residents in Naples who had ugly brown stains on their teeth known as 'denti di chiaie.'

1916: McKay and Black examined 6873 individuals in USA and reported that an unknown causative factor of mottled enamel was possibly present in domestic water during the period of tooth calcification.

1930: Kemp and McKay observed that no mottling occurred in people who grew up in bauxite prior to 1909, the year in which bauxite had changed its supply from shallow wells to deep drilled wells.

1931: New methods of spectrographic analysis led to the identification of fluoride in the drinking water, Churchill HV (Bauxite)
Similar discoveries were also made independently by Smith MC, Lantz EM, Smith HV (Arizona) Velu H, Balozet L (France) at about the same time.

1931: Shoe leather survey: Trendley H Dean carried out a survey in the US, which was a continuation of McKay's work, to find out the extent of geographical distribution of mottled enamel.

1935: Dean gave his mottling index
1 ppm—no stain
2.5-3 ppm—dull chalky appearance
4 ppm—discrete pitting

1941: "21 city" study, carried out by Dean et al. The objective was to define the water fluoride levels which represented the best compromise between low caries experience and a level of fluorosis which could be considered acceptable. The first part consisted of clinical data from children 12-14 years old with life-time residence in 8 suburban Chicago communities with stable mean fluoride levels. The project later added 13 additional communities in 4 other American states. This was a land mark epidemiologic survey which led to the adoption of 0.7-1 mg fl/ liter of water as optimum amount of fluoride in drinking water.

1945: World's first artificial fluoridation was started at Grand Rapids, USA

1969: Fluoridation was endorsed by the WHO.

Fluoride is found in abundance in the nature and is distributed in the lithosphere, biosphere, hydrosphere and the atmosphere.[121-124]

Fluoride in the Lithosphere

Fluoride though is considered as a trace element from the biologic point of view is present in abundance in the earth's crust and presents as 13th among them.

In the lithosphere, the fluoride is present as inorganic fluoride in:
- Siliceous igneous rocks
- Alkalic rocks
- Geothermal waters and hot springs
- Volcanic gases and fumaroles

Some of the fluoride containing minerals are[124]
Apatite, 34% of fluoride $Ca_5(PO_4)_3(OH,F,Cl)$
Cryolite, 54% of fluoride Na_3AlF_6
Fluorite 49% of fluoride CaF_2

In the Biosphere

Some plants accumulate more fluoride and hence are the rich source of this mineral. Few plants like tea plants actively accumulate fluoride and the fluoride concentrations reach between 0.03–25.7 ppm fluoride. The fluoride level in the soil directly influences the fluoride concentration of the plants grown in such a soil.

In the Hydrosphere

River contains fluoride in the free form but complex fluoride increases with increasing salinity, in sea water. Sea water contains 1.2–1.4 ppm fluoride 47% of which are present as MgF. Sardines, salmon, mackerel and other fish contain about 20 ppm of fluoride on a dry weight basis.

In the Atmosphere

Fluoride in the atmosphere is maximum near industrial area who by product is fluoride as seen around the aluminium factory. Fluoride emissions are heaviest in the vicinity of industries involved in the production of aluminium from cryolite, phosphate fertilizers, fluorinated hydrocarbons, plastics, uranium and other heavy metals and hydrogen fluoride.

FLUORIDE IN INDIA

In India, areas with high fluoride minerals are extensive (Fig. 7.44). The main fluoride bearing areas are Gujarat, Rajasthan and Andhra Pradesh where about 70-100% of the districts are affected. Only about 10-40% districts are affected in the states of Jammu & Kashmir, Kerala, Chhatisgarh and eastern India. The remaining states have about 40-70% of the districts affected by increased fluoride in their water.

Besides these areas, fluoride is also found in some areas of Karnataka, Bihar, West Bengal, Punjab and North West Himalayas.

Whatever may be the primary source of fluorine, the element is ultimately dispersed in the environment and is found in air, atmosphere, soil and water.

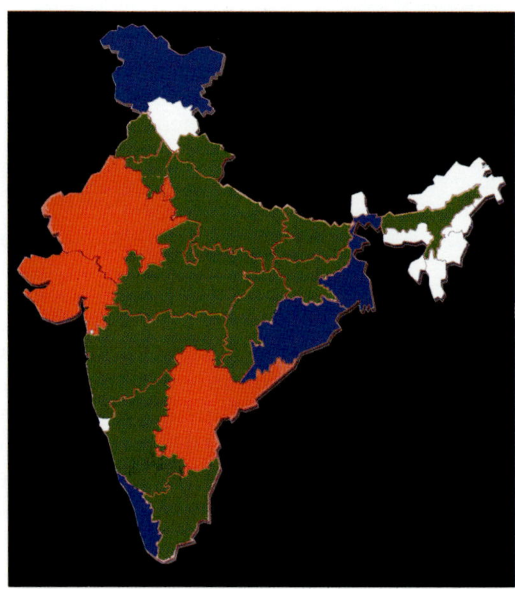

Fig. 7.44: Areas of increased fluoride distribution in India
Red—States having 70-100% of districts affected
Green—States having 40-70% of the districts affected
Blue—States having 10-40% of districts affected

Accordingly, the fluorides reach the living organisms through these elements.

ABSORPTION OF FLUORIDE[125,126]

The rate and amount of fluoride absorption are determined by many factors:
- Physical form of the dose: Fluoride in the liquid form is better and quickly absorbed than in the solid form.
- Presence of food in the stomach: Fluoride absorption is slow in the presence of food.
- Composition of gastric contents: Certain items such as milk combine with fluoride and delay or prevent its absorption.
- Gastric pH: Reducing the pH enhances the fluoride absorption. Ionic fluoride is converted to hydrogen fluoride, which is a weak acid and an uncharged molecule that freely passes through gastric membrane.
- Gastrointestinal motility: Fluoride absorption is reduced with increased motility as seen in case of diarrhea.
- Concurrent oral administration of cations like Ca, Mg, Al: They bind with fluoride thus making it unavailable for absorption.

Fluoride is absorbed from the entire gastrointestinal tract. About 90% of the dietary fluoride is absorbed and the maximum 10% is exereted through faces.

Fluoride is poorly absorbed with milk because:

- Of formation of low soluble calcium fluoride
- Binding of Fl to casein and colloidal $CaPO_4$
- Clotting of milk due to gastric acidity, acts as physical barrier for further access of fluoride to mucosal surface of the GI tract.

DISTRIBUTION OF FLUORIDE IN THE BODY[126,127]

Fluoride in Plasma

The plasma concentration fluoride is about twice to that of the cells.

It exists in 2 general forms
1. Ionic (also called as inorganic or free fluoride)
2. Nonionic (bound fluoride)

Together they form the total plasma fluoride and are about 12 µm/L. Plasma half-life for fluoride is about 4-10 hours. The rate of elimination of fluoride is proportional to the plasma concentration. That is, higher the plasma concentration the faster is the elimination and vice versa.

Fluorides in Soft Tissues

It mainly depends upon the blood flow to the tissue. The brain tissue and the adipose tissue accumulate the least amount while the kidney, heart and lungs accumulate the maximum amount of fluoride.

Fluorides in Teeth and Bone

Teeth

Fluoride concentration in enamel is not uniform. Outer enamel concentrates more fluoride than the inner layers. In dentin the concentration of fluoride is more at the pulpal end. Cementum accumulates the maximum amount of fluoride.

Bone

More than 95% of the fluoride in the body is retained in the bones and this retention is irreversible. When the intake falls, fluoride from the bones are released into the plasma and later excreted.

Accumulation in bones depends on:

- *The fluoride intake:* Amount of fluoride accumulated is directly related to the amount of fluoride intake.
- *Type of bone:* Cancellous bone retains more fluoride than compact bone.
- *Age:* Fluoride accumulation is maximum in growing bones.
- *Duration of fluoride exposures:* Amount of fluoride accumulated is directly proportional to the duration of exposure to fluoride.

> Amount of fluoride in the tooth
> Outer enamel—2,200-3,200 ppm
> Dentin—200-300 ppm
> Cementum—4,500 ppm
> Pulp—100-650 ppm

> Fluorides are deposited in dental tissues in successive stages during the life of the tooth. The initial deposition occurs while the organic and mineral phases are being laid down. Next it is deposited from the tissue fluids during the pre-eruptive maturation phase. Finally fluoride is acquired topically during posteruptive maturation and aging period.

EXCRETION OF FLUORIDE[128]

Excretion through the kidneys forms the major route for the elimination of fluoride. Renal clearance of fluoride is about 30-50 ml/min. About 30% is excreted within 3 hours and remaining 40-60% is excreted within 24 hours. Increase in urine pH increases the fluoride excretion. Remaining fluoride is excreted through the feces (10%), Breast milk (0.001-0.005 ppm), Sweat (10-25%) and saliva (0.01-0.05 ppm).

MECHANISM OF ACTION OF FLUORIDE[129-137]

Hypothesis regarding fluoride anticaries mechanism of action:

1. Effect on hydroxyapatite crystals
   a. Decreasing its solubility
   b. Improving its crystallinity
   c. Remineralization
2. Effect on bacteria
   a. Inhibiting enzymes
   b. Suppressing cariogenic flora
3. Effect on the enamel surface
   a. Desorbing protein/bacteria
   b. Lowering the free surface energy
4. Alteration of the tooth morphology.

Decreasing the Solubility of Hydroxyapatite Crystals

Fluoride reduces the solubility of hydroxyapatite crystals during acid attack. Two theories are used to explain this.

  i. Void theory: Voids are normally present in any crystal which decreases the stability and increases the chemical reactivity. In hydroxyapatite crystal, fluoride fills up these voids and makes the crystal stable, by formation of additional as well as stronger hydrogen bonds leading to lower solubility and greater resistance to dissolution in acids.
  ii. FAP vs HAP: It is said that fluorapatite is less soluble than hydroxyapatite.
  $Ca_{10}(PO_4)6OH_2 + Fl = Ca_{10}(PO_4)6Fl_2$

Improving the Crystallinity of Hydroxyapatite

Fluorides increase the crystal size and produce less strain in the crystal lattice. This takes place by conversion of amorphous calcium phosphate to crystalline hydroxy-phosphate.

Various calcium phosphate phases are:

- Dicalcium phosphate dihydrate (DCPD)
- Dicalcium phosphate anhydrate (DCP)
- Tricalcium phosphate (TCP)
- Octa calcium phosphate (OCP).

Remineralization

It is a process of deposition of apatite or like material in enamel and dentin tissues after partial loss of normal mineral.

Fluoride stimulates apatite precipitation. Frequent application of low level fluoride will effectively inhibit demineralization and enhance remineralization.

Therefore the best strategy for caries management would be to focus on the methods of improving the remineralizing process. Various commercial products are available that contain fluorides that aid in remineralization.

Enzyme Inhibition

Fluoride has enolase inhibition effects and inhibits glucose transport also. Enolase is a metalloenzyme that requires divalent cation for its activity (Mg++). Fluoride due to its increased reactivity forms complexes with divalent cations. Thus it inhibits the metalloenzyme.

It also has shown to inhibit nonmetalloenzymes like phosphatases, acetylcholinesterase, etc. All the above effects are interrelated through PEP (Phospho Enol Pyruvate) phospho transferase system that is found in *S. salivarius, S. mutans, S. sanguis.* This leads to reduced acid production and reduced glucose transport into the cell.

Suppressing the Flora

Fluoride suppresses the growth of bacteria. Stannous fluoride is more potent. Stannous ion oxidizes the thiol group present in the bacteria required for its metabolism.

Desorption of Protein and Bacteria

Hydroxyapatite crystals are amphoteric with both positive and negative receptor site. Acidic protein group binds at calcium site and basic protein groups bind at phosphate site. Fluoride inhibits the binding of acidic protein to hydroxyapatite.

Lowering the Free Surface Energy

Fluoride by reducing the free surface energy prevents accumulation of plaque.

Alteration of Tooth Morphology

Dentition in fluoridated communities show a tendency towards rounded cusps, shallow fissures, wider tooth and improved alignment. All these make the tooth at less risk for development of caries.

DIFFERENT MODES OF FLUORIDE ADMINISTRATION

1. *Systemic:* In this mode fluoride is taken in a dietary form. Fluoride is absorbed into the circulation and reaches the developing teeth. Fluoride is also secreted into the saliva and gingival crevicular fluid.

2. *Topical:* They are moderate to high concentration fluoride applied topically on the tooth surface.

SYSTEMIC FLUORIDES

1. Water fluoridation
2. Salt fluoridation
3. Milk fluoridation
4. Fluoride tablets.

Water Fluoridation

Definition

"Controlled adjustment of the concentration of fluoride in a community water supply so as to achieve a maximum caries reduction and a clinically insignificant level of fluorosis."

Important Studies[138-140]

In US and Canada, studies on fluoridation of water began in 1945.

January 1945—studies were done at Grand Rapids (Experimental city) and Muskegon (Control city).

May 1945—studies were done at Newburgh (Experimental city) and Kingston (Control city)

1946—Studies were done at Evanston (Experimental city) and Oak Park (Control city).

The results of all these studies were as follows

- Fluoride is the etiological factor for the observed low caries levels in areas with naturally fluoridated drinking water
- There is no difference between the effect of naturally and artificially fluoridated water
- Controlled addition of fluoride to water is technically possible within narrow limits.
- When fluoridation was discontinued in a community, there was a dramatic increase in the dental caries incidence.

> Caries reduction benefits to primary teeth was 40-50% and to the permanent teeth was 50-60%.

> Fluoride benefit is not uniform and varies depending on tooth surfaces:
> Buccal and lingual—85%
> Inter proximal—75%
> Pit and fissures—35%

Optimum concentration of fluoride in the drinking water to produce maximum anticaries benefit and minimum toxicity.

This varies according to the climatic condition. In the tropical climates, water consumption is more than in cold climates and hence the amount of fluoride added to drinking water must be less than in cold climatic region.

A formula given by Galagan and Vermillion is used to decide the amount of fluoride that should be added to the drinking water and is as follows:

Galagan and Vermillion formula:[141] Amount of fluoride in ppm = 0.34/E

Where E = – 0.038+0.0062 × temperature in °F.

Recommended= 0.7 to 1.2 ppm (0.7 ppm in tropical climate and 1.2 ppm in cold climate).

Advantages of Water Fluoridation

- As people drink water daily, fluoride is consumed along with it
- Large number of people can benefit
- Cheap and effective.

Disadvantages of Water Fluoridation

- Interfere with human rights and fundamental liberties that every individual whether one likes it or not should consume fluoridated water.
- Other modes of fluoride intake should be considered. There is increased risk of overdosage of fluoride in individuals consuming other fluoride supplements.
- The entire population should consume water from one source. Fluoridation is not possible in area where people drink water from their individual well or rivers.

School Water Fluoridation[142]

It is a suitable alternative, where community water fluoridation is not feasible. Children can benefit by drinking fluoridated water when fluoride is added to the school water tank. The amount of fluoride added to the school water is more as they spend only 20-25% of their total working hours in school. The recommended level of fluoride is 4.5 times that of the optimum level.

Disadvantages

- Children are already 5-6 years when they attend the school. Benefits of systemic fluoride are maximum during the developing stages of fluoride. Most of the tooth crowns would have already formed by then they are relatively less beneficial.
- Continued monitoring of water is required. School authorities should hire a person who is well informed regarding the risk associated with adding excess fluoride to the water. He should monitor the total activity regularly.

Different Fluoride Compounds Used for Water Fluoridation

1. Sodium fluoride was used initially and is expensive. Sodium silicofluoride is preferred alternatively due its low cost.
2. Fluorosilicic acid (hydrofluorosilicic acid)—it is corrosive and requires careful supervision.
3. Fluorspar (calcium fluoride)—it costs 1/3 as much as sodium silicofluoride, but difficult to dissolve.
4. Ammonium fluosilicate.
5. Sodium silicofluoride.

Salt Fluoridation[142]

Introduced in Switzerland (1955) by Wespi. Initially 90 mg fl/kg salt was used, later it was increased to 200-350 mg fl/kg of salt. Clinical trials in Switzerland, showed 20-25% reduction of caries with 90 mg of fluoride. It was then decided that to obtain the same amount of fluoride benefit as water fluoridation, the amount in salt has to be increased to 300 mg/kg yielding 1.5 mg fl/5 gm of salt.

Method of Production of Fluoridated Salt

In Switzerland and Hungary fluoride is added by spraying concentrated solution of sodium fluoride or potassium fluoride to salt on a conveyer belt.

In USA sodium fluoride and calcium fluoride are first mixed with a suitable phosphate carrier salt and these premixed granules are added to the salt.

Advantages

- Individualized monitoring is not required, as the levels are adjusted to provide optimum levels of fluoride, keeping in account that a person consumes 5-8 gm of salt per day
- Everyone consumes salt, irrespective of ethnic or regional variation
- Readily acceptable, as the addition of fluoride to salt does not change the color, odor, consistency or taste.

Disadvantages

- Special plant has to be set up for fluoridation of the salt
- Consumption of fluoridated salt in areas with increased fluoride concentration in drinking water may lead to overdose.

Milk Fluoridation[142]

It was first mentioned by Zeigler in 1956. 36.3% caries reduction was observed with 2.5 mg of sodium fluoride added to milk daily in school meals.

There was a controversy concerning the binding and complexing of fluoride with calcium and milk protein thus reducing its anti caries effect.

Erickson (1958) using radioactive isotope technique proved the availability of fluoride from milk. But the release of fluoride from milk is mild and slow compared to that from water.

Disadvantages

- Fluoride is available to only those who drink milk. In India children living in low socioeconomic areas may not drink milk daily
- In most of the rural areas there is no central milk supply, hence fluoridation is not possible.

Fluoride Tablets[142]

It was introduced in the late 1940's intended to be used as a substitute for fluoridated water. Fluoride tablet is prescribed by a dental practitioner for individual patients keeping in account the fluoride concentration in the drinking water and other fluoride supplements consumed.

Availability

- Tablets or drops to be swallowed, chewed or sucked
- Tablets available as 0.25 mg, 0.5 mg, 1.0 mg
- Sodium fluoride, acidulated phosphate fluoride, potassium fluoride or calcium fluoride.

Dosage: It is calculated keeping in mind the water fluoride level of the community (Table 7.4). Less amount of fluoride in tablet form is recommended for children residing in areas having increased level of fluoride in drinking water. Therefore for children residing in areas where the drinking water level of fluoride is more than 0.6 ppm, fluoride supplement is not required.

TOPICAL FLUORIDES

1. Solution/thixotropic gels/foam
2. Dentifrice
3. Rinse
4. Varnish
5. Slow release system

Systemic fluoride has many disadvantages and the associated risks has definitely outnumbered its beneficial effects.

Efficient methods of fluoride therapy at the individual level surfaced in 1941, when the first clinical study of NaF was carried out by Bibby.

Topically applied fluorides are deposited onto the surface of the tooth and they tend to provide local protection at or near the tooth surface. Plaque, saliva and oral mucosa also serves as a reservoir for fluoride

Table 7.4: Amount of fluoride supplementation, based on the age and amount of fluoride in drinking water according to ADA February 1994

	Fluoride concentration of drinking water (ppm)		
Age	< 0.3	> 0.3 < 0.6	>0.6
0-6 months	–	–	–
6 month-3 years	0.25 mg	–	–
3-6 years	0.5 mg	0.25 mg	–
6-16 years	1.00 mg	0.5 mg	–

ions. During a cariogenic challenge, fluoride from these sources is mobilized to assist remineralization.

Topical fluorides can be used at home or applied by professional in the clinics. Topical fluorides advocated for home use contain comparatively less amount of fluoride and are used daily or regularly. Professionally applied fluoride agents contain very high amount of fluoride and are applied less frequently, majority being biannually.

SOLUTION/THIXOTROPIC GELS/FOAM

They may be in the form of sodium fluoride, stannous fluoride or APF. Thixotropic gels are better than solution due their high viscosity and inherent property to flow under pressure. They contain methyl cellulose that is responsible for their viscosity. Use of foam reduces the risk of overdosage.

Sodium Fluoride[143]

- 2% NaF is used
- Neutral pH
- 9,200 ppm of available fluoride
- 29% effective in caries reduction
- Milestone studies were done by Bibby and Knutson in 1941, 1942, 1947, 1948, using varied fluoride concentration and number of appointments.

Knutson's Technique

It is the technique recommended by Knutson for the application of 2% neutral sodium fluoride.

It consists of 4 applications at weekly intervals in a year at age group of 3, 7, 11, and 13 years. This age group was selected depending on the eruption of deciduous dentition, first permanent molar and incisors, premolar and canines and second molars respectively.

Oral prophylaxis was done on the first day of each series. The teeth were isolated and dried. The solution is applied on the teeth with cotton applicators or trays can be used for gels. Once applied the solution is allowed to dry on the tooth without reapplication for 4 minutes.

The patient is asked not to swallow the gel or solution but should be expectorated, and not to eat or drink for 30 min and not to eat for the next 1 hour.

Disadvantage of Knutson's Technique

- Patient has to make 4 visits within short time
- Interval of upto 4 years between series may be too long for maximal cariostatic protection.

Method of preparation of 1 liter of neutral NaF: 20 gm of NaF is dissolved in 1 liter of distilled water. It is stored in plastic bottles as fluoride reacts with silica of glass to form SiF_2, reducing the available fluoride.

Mechanism of action: When sodium fluoride is applied on the tooth surface there is rapid influx of fluoride leading to the formation of calcium fluoride. The calcium fluoride forms a layer on the tooth surface blocking further entry of fluoride ions. This sudden stop of the entry of fluoride is termed as "Chocking off effect". Fluoride then slowly leaches from the calcium fluoride. Thus calcium fluoride acts as a reservoir for fluoride release and that is the reason why sodium fluoride is kept untouched on the tooth for 4 minutes.

Stannous Fluoride[144-146]

- 8% SnF_2 is used
- 2.4-2.8 pH
- 19,500 ppm of available fluoride and 32% effective in caries reduction
- Dudding and Muhler in 1962 described the use of stannous fluoride and 8-10% was tested and found to be effective.

Method of preparation: It has to be freshly prepared as it is unstable. The stannous ion gets oxidised to stannic ion which is not effective. 0.8 gm of SnF_2 is dissolved in 10 ml of water to obtain 8% SnF_2.

Application (Muhler's Technique)

- Annual application
- Thorough prophylaxis and isolation is followed by quadrant wise application.
- Applied continuously for 4 minutes. Reapplication is done every 15-30 seconds.

Mechanism of action: SnF_2 reacts with hydroxyapatite with the formation of 4 products

1. Stannous trifluorophosphate (main product)
2. Stannous hydroxy phosphate (formed in low concentrations of SnF_2 and is responsible for the metallic after taste
3. Calcium trifluorostannate (formed in high concentrations of SnF_2)
4. Calcium fluoride.

Disadvantages

- Undergoes rapid oxidation and is unstable
- Should be freshly prepared
- Taste is disagreeable
- Gingival tissue irritation
- Staining of teeth.

Acidulated Phosphate Fluoride (APF)[147-149]

- 1.23% is used
- 12,300 ppm of available fluoride
- 3.0 pH
- 28% effective in caries reduction
- 1963—Brudevold and Weelock did a study to find optimum acid concentration to provide maximal fluoride deposition and minimal demineralization and also found adding phosphate provided maximum benefit.

Preparation of 1.23% APF: 20 gm of NaF is dissolved in 1 liter of 0.1m phosphoric acid. To this 50% hydrofluoric acid is added to adjust the pH to 3.0 and fluoride concentration to 1.23%.

Application (Brudevold's Technique)

- Prophylaxis and isolation is done first. Fluoride is applied with cotton applicators and kept wet for 4 minutes.
- Biannual application.

Mechanism of action: Initially it leads to dehydration and shrinkage in volume of hydroxyapattite crystals and formation of dicalcium phosphate dehydrate (DCPD). The DCPD formed is highly reactive with fluoride, leading to formation of fluorapatite (FAP). The amount and depth of fluoride deposited as FAP depends on the amount and depth at which DCPD gets formed. Since for the conversion of whole of DCPD formed into FAP, continuous supply of fluoride is required, APF has to be applied every 30 seconds and the teeth are kept wet for 4 minutes.

Disadvantages

- Acidic
- When stored in glass container, etches the glass
- Prolonged exposure to composite or porcelain, results in loss of surface material and unaesthetic appearance.

Characteristics	Sodium fluoride	Stannous fluoride	APF
Percentage	2%	8%	1.23%
ppm of fluoride	9,200	19,500	12,300
pH	Neutral	2.4-2.8	3.0
Frequency of application	4 at weekly interval at 3,7,11 and 13 years	Biannually	Biannually
Tooth pigmentation	No	Yes	No
Gingival irritation	No	Yes	No
Caries reduction	29%	32%	28%

Fluoride Gel[150,151]

- Easier to work permits application in trays—entire dentition can be treated at one time
- NaF and APF gels—contain the same concentration of fluoride and pH as their respective aqueous solutions. They are as effective as the solutions in caries reduction.
- Gels contain—cellulose compound for viscosity
- Thixotrophic gels—gels that flow under pressure penetrate better interproximally and do not drip.

Fluoride Foam[150]

- pH is 6.0
- It is marketed only in some countries
- Much lighter and requires application of little amount of the material
- Risk of over dosage is reduced.

Others

Ammonium fluoride, titanium fluoride, amine fluoride—hold fluoride in contact with tooth surfaces for longer periods. Used in toothpaste, rinses and gels and is under study.

Professional application of APF (Figs 7.45A to C)

1. Patient and the parents should be explained regarding the benefits and risks of topical fluorides
2. Patient is made to sit upright on the dental chair so that the saliva and excess fluoride is not accidentally swallowed
3. Saliva ejector is held in place to remove excess fluoride and saliva
4. Trays are filled to 1/3 to 1/2 its height. The tray is then placed in the mouth and the flanges are pressed against the tooth surface.
5. Excess fluoride is removed with saliva ejector
6. Lower arch is done first followed by the upper. If upper is done first the saliva that has been pooled in the floor

Contd...

Contd...

of the mouth will make it difficult to place the lower tray.

7. The trays are placed in contact with the tooth for 4 minutes. It is then removed and discarded. Fluoride on the tooth surface is removed by saliva ejector or asking the patient to spit the excess.
8. Patient is not allowed to wash his mouth. Rubbing with cotton is avoided for removal of excess fluoride from the tooth surface.
9. Instruction are given to the patient which includes-
   - Not to drink any liquid food for at least half and hour
   - Not to eat any solid food for one hour at least
   - To report immediately if any symptoms of acute toxicity is noticed.

Methods of Increasing the Fluoride Uptake by the Enamel

1. Increasing the time of contact of fluoride with the enamel
2. Pretreating the enamel with 0.05M phosphoric acid
3. Addition of casein phosphate to fluoride preparation.

FLUORIDE DENTIFRICES[142,152-154]

It is a simplest and rational way of combating caries. It combines the mechanical effect of tooth brushing with fluoride benefit. It was first introduced by Bibby in 1945 and Muhler in 1955.

Amount of Fluoride Present in the Dentifrice

Ideally 1000 ppm of fluoride should be present but dentifrices containing less or more than 1000 ppm of fluoride are also available. Two-three years old children usually ingest majority of the dentifrice during brushing. Hence dentifrice containing less amount of fluoride should be prescribed to a preschooler. On an average 0.5 gm of paste is used twice daily.

Fluoride toothpaste that contain 1000 ppm fluoride, contain 500-600 ppm of free fluoride in 50 gm of tooth paste. Therefore a 200 gm tube of tooth paste contains 140 mg of free fluoride.

Sodium fluoride and sodium monofluorophosphate are preferred as fluoride agents, due to their compatibility with abrasives and absence of brown staining and metallic taste unlike stannous fluoride.

Abrasive Compatibility

Basic problem with fluoride dentifrice is the incompatibility of the fluoride agent (Sodium fluoride) with

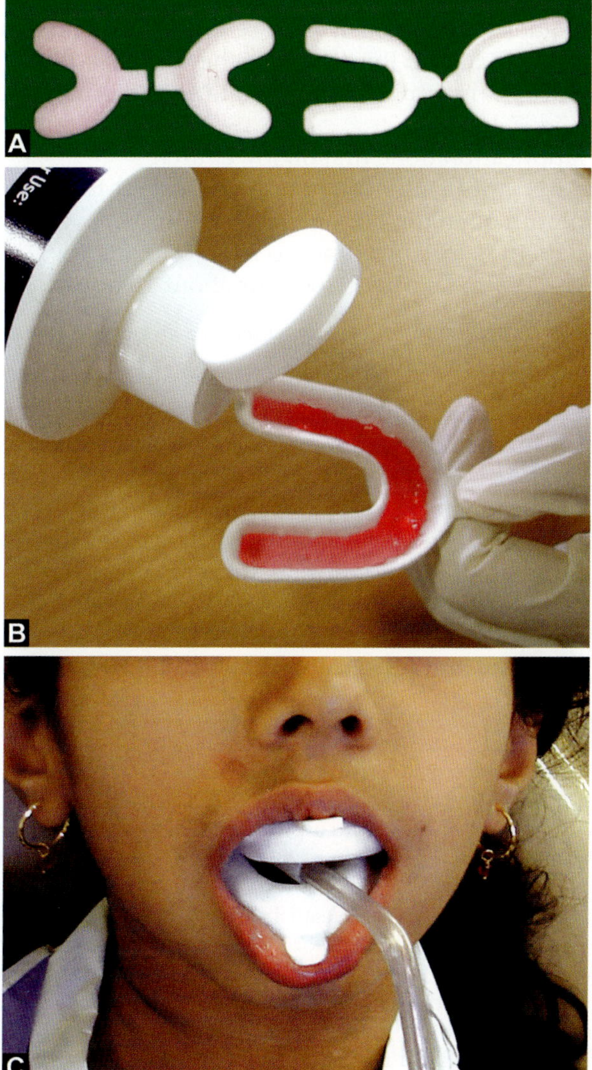

Figs 7.45A to C: Steps in the application of fluoride: (A) Trays used for fluoride application; (B) The trays are loaded with fluoride; (C) The tray is kept in the mouth for 4 minutes, with saliva ejector in place to remove excess material and saliva

calcium containing abrasives. These abrasives combine with fluoride to form calcium fluoride thus reducing the freely available fluoride making it inactive. This has been overcome by the introduction of monofluorophosphate.

Abrasives that are compatible with monofluorophosphate and sodium fluoride are:
- Calcium pyrophosphate
- Hydrated silica
- Sodium bicarbonate
- Acrylic polymer
- Insoluble sodium metaphosphate

Abrasives that are compatible with Monofluorophosphate are:

- Alumina trihydrate
- Anhydrous dicalcium phosphate
- Dicalcium phosphate dihydrate
- Calcium carbonate.

FLUORIDE RINSES[150,155]

- Sodium fluoride, stannous fluoride and acidulated phosphate fluoride are used as rinse
- 20 and 40% reduction in caries was seen when 0.2% and 0.05% Sodium fluoride was used respectively.
- Most frequently used is sodium fluoride rinse - 0.2% for fortnightly rinse (909 ppm) and 0.05% for daily rinse (227 ppm)
- Method of rinsing: 10 ml of the solution is swished vigorously for 1 minute and expectorated.
- Large scale or home method of rinse preparation: 200 mg NaF tablet + 5 tsp fresh clean water (25 ml).
- Commercially available rinse of 200 mg NaF contains – 10 mg of sodium fluoride + lactose (filler).

School Rinse Programs[142,150]

- 2 gm of sodium fluoride powder is mixed with 1000 ml of water to make 0.2% solution of sodium fluoride. As the powder is readily available and inexpensive and also teachers can master the art of mixing and dispensing, it proves to be the best method of topical fluorides for the school children.
- Children in large group is made to stand in a line. Each is given a small cup with the measured amount of rinse. They are asked to put the solution into the mouth and swish it for one minute. Then all of them are told to expectorate the solution. Children in a school can be grouped based on their class and fortnightly rinse is effective.
- Mouth rinsing is not recommended for preschool children and less amount (5 ml) is to be used for kindergarten children.
- 10 ml of 0.05% NaF contains 2.3 mg fluoride.
- Weekly fluoride rinse program has become standard for organized school based programs in USA
- In India, fluoride rinse program on a large scale has not been implemented.

Advantage of School-based Rinse Programs

- Safe and effective
- Relatively inexpensive
- Easy to learn and do
- Non dental personnel can supervise
- Well accepted by participants
- Less time is required—5 minutes.

Disadvantage of School-based Rinse Programs

- School teaching hours are compromised
- Teachers and parents should be educated and motivated regarding the benefits
- During long school vacations rinse program cannot be done.

FLUORIDE VARNISHES[142,156-158]

Fluoride varnish was first developed in Europe (1964) by Schimdt. The main advantage of varnish is that it increases the time the fluoride is in contact with the tooth.

Indications

- Handicapped children
- Incipient caries lesion
- After restorative treatment is complete under general anesthesia
- Very young children who cannot expectorate the gel or foam.

Commonly Used Fluoride Varnishes

1. Duraphat
2. Fluorprotector
3. Carex.

Duraphat

- 5% sodium fluoride in organic lacquer
- 22,600 ppm fluoride
- Hardens into a yellowish brown coating in the presence of saliva.

Fluorprotector

- Contains difluorosilane in polyurethane lacquer
- 7,000 ppm of fluoride.

Carex

- Contains lower fluoride concentration than duraphat (1.8%) but anticaries effect is equivalent to duraphat.

  The amount of fluoride introduced into the enamel is more with fluor protector but duraphat is found to be more effective in caries solution. This is because the silane fluoride of fluorprotector reacts with water to produce hydrofluoric acid, which penetrates into enamel readily and forms tags 0.5-1.0 μm long, leading to increased fluoride concentration. But these tags prevents further fluoride penetration thus reducing the anticaries effect.

Steps Involved in the Application of Varnish

- Prophylaxis
- Isolation required is very minimum. It is sufficient to just remove the thick mucous coat on the tooth surface. Isolation is not done with cotton as it tends to stick to the varnish and presence of mild moisture tends to hasten the setting of the varnish.
- Varnish is applied with single tufted small brush (Fig. 7.46)
- Application done first on lower arch
- After application, the patient is asked to keep the mouth open for 4 minutes.
- Patient is instructed not to rinse or drink for 1 hour and not to take solid food for about 18 hours.

Topical fluoride can be used routinely for any child. But some of the definite indications

- Caries active individuals
- Children shortly after periods of tooth eruption
- Individuals who are on salivary flow reducing medications
- Individuals with disease that decrease salivary flow
- Patients after periodontal surgery, when roots are exposed
- Individuals with eating disorder
- Mentally and physically challenged individuals.

Recent advances in fluoride research

Fluoride is the most effective preventive agent in dentistry and attempts have been made to utilize it in a variety of ways to reap systemic and topical benefits in the prevention of dental caries. The recent advances in fluoride research are:
Iontophoresis
Iontophoresis has been used in dentistry for the past 80 years. It is based on the theory that a small electric current will help drive fluoride ions further into dental enamel, producing the desired effect. Iontophoresis has been used most frequently to treat hypersensitive teeth, usually in conjunction with a topical fluoride agent. Consequently, it is difficult to prove conclusively that iontophoresis significantly helps penetration of fluoride into the enamel.
Fluoride—chlorhexidine preparations
Chlorhexidine is a powerful inhibitor of gingivitis and plaque formation and has been used with fluoride to prevent gingivitis and dental caries. They are compatible with each other.
Fluoride containing dental cements
Certain dental restorative materials increase the solubility of enamel. The solubility property of these materials was reduced when fluoride was incorporated in to them.
When stannous fluoride was incorporated into the liquid of zinc phosphate cement, it was found that enamel became less soluble, however the reductions diminished over time. Sodium monofluorophosphate was successfully incorporated into zinc oxide eugenol cement.
The matrix of glass ionomer cement consists of sheathed droplets of calcium fluoride. The slow leaching of fluoride from this matrix would impart anticaries action similar to that of silicate cement.

Fluoride treatment for children with rampant caries [0.3 -0.7 ppm water F level] [As per Council on Dental Therapeutics of ADA, 1986]				
Age	*0-2 Years*	*2-3 Years*	*3-13 Years*	*>13 Years*
Dietary supplement	Not required	0.25 mg daily	0.5 mg daily	Not indicated
Professionally applied Topical fluoride	APF solution or gel applied 4 times a year	APF solution or gel applied 4 times a year	APF solution or gel applied 4 times a year	APF solution or gel applied 4 times a year
Self applied fluoride	Not required	Not required	Self-application of gel in a tray daily for approximately 4 weeks thereafter continue with daily fluoride rinse (0.05% NaF)	

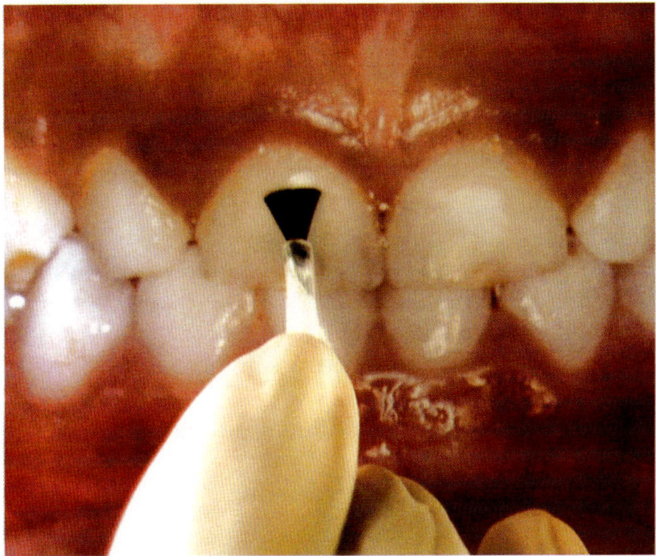

Fig. 7.46: Fluoride varnish is applied using single tufted brush

FLUORIDE TOXICITY

Toxicity is due to excessive ingestion of fluoride and can be acute or chronic. Acute toxicity is due to ingestion of large dose of fluoride in a short period of time while chronic toxicity is due to ingestion of excess fluoride in low doses over a prolonged period of time.

Acute Fluoride Toxicity[142,159]

Safely tolerated dose is 8-16 mg/kg body weight. When fluoride is consumed beyond this limit it can lead to symptoms of toxicity.

Lethal dose of fluoride is 32-64 mg/kg body weight. When fluoride is consumed beyond this limit it can lead to death.

Factors influencing acute toxicity

- *Form of administration:* Fluoride administered in liquid form is absorbed quickly, hence the symptoms of toxicity is rapidly seen.

- *Age:* Younger the age more severe and faster are the symptoms of toxicity.
- *Rate of absorption:* Rate of absorption depends on many factors already discussed initially in this chapter.

Signs and symptoms of acute fluoride toxicity

- Nausea, vomiting, abdominal pain, increased salivation, nasal discharge
- Generalized weakness, carpopedal spasm
- Reduced plasma calcium level, increased plasma potassium level
- Weak thready pulse, fall in blood pressure
- Depression of respiratory center
- Cardiac arrhythmia
- Coma and death.

Management of acute toxicity

Immediate management should be aimed at:
- Reducing the fluoride absorption by inducing vomiting through emetics
- Increasing fluoride excretion by increasing the alkalinity of the urine and fluid replacement
- Plasma calcium and potassium level monitoring

Management based on the amount of fluoride ions ingested	
< 5.0 mg/kg	Milk Induce vomiting
>5.0 mg/kg	Induce vomiting Milk, 5% calcium gluconate, Hospitalization
> 15.0 mg/kg	Induce vomiting Cardiac monitoring - peaking of T wave and prolonged QT interval in a ECG Slow administration of 10 ml of 10% calcium gluconate Maintain adequate urine output Supportive measures for shock

Possible ways to reduce the intake of excess fluorides especially at home:

1. Parental supervision
2. Small amount of tooth paste to be used
3. Products with low fluoride level to be used
4. Teaching children not to swallow paste or rinse
5. Strict adherence to professional advice

> Molecular conversion ratio
> NaF = 1/2 2
> SnF_2 = 1/ 4.1
> Na_2PO_3 = 1/ 7.6

Calculations of the percentage of fluoride ion in the total amount of fluoride agent swallowed

- Multiply the percentage of the fluoride agent with the molecular conversion ratio of that particular fluoride agent to obtain the percentage of fluoride ions present
  Example: For 2% sodium fluoride
  $2 \times 1/2.2 = 0.9\%$ fluoride ions
- To convert the percentage of fluoride ion to fluoride mg/gm, multiply the percentage of fluoride ions with 10
  $0.9 \times 10 = 9$ mg of fluoride ions in one gram of sodium fluoride
- To calculate the amount of fluoride ions swallowed, multiply the fluoride in mg/gm with the total amount of agent swallowed. This gives the total amount of fluoride ions present in the amount swallowed
  9 mg/gm × total amount of sodium fluoride swallowed = total amount of fluoride ions swallowed
- From this the toxic dose of fluoride can be calculated for a given child based on the body weight as total amount of fluoride ions swallowed/weight of the child in kg.

Chronic Toxicity[160-163]

It is caused due to ingestion of excess amount of fluoride over a prolonged period of time. It can cause dental and skeletal changes referred to as dental and skeletal fluorosis respectively.

Dental Fluorosis

Direct inhibitory effect on enzymatic action of ameloblasts by fluoride leads to defective matrix formation and subsequent hypomineralization in case of fluorosis.

Mild changes are seen when water fluoride level increases to more than 3 ppm.

Severe changes are seen when water fluoride level increases to more than 4-8 ppm.

Management of Dental Fluorosis

Dental fluorosis may range from mild to severe changes. The changes include discoloration, surface roughness, pitting or surface erosion. Treatment includes bleaching, composite restoration, veneers or complete crown restorations.

> Daily dose of >0.07 mg Fl/kg body weight/day for children with developing teeth may result in fluorosis.

Index used for Measuring Fluorosis

1. Dean's index
2. Thylstrup and Fejerskov scoring
3. Horowitz index

1. Dean's Index
Score Criteria
0 Normal
0.5 Questionable with few flecks to occasional white spots
1 Very mild, small, opaque, paper white areas scattered irregularly, involving < 25%
2 Mild, involving < 50 %
3 Moderate - all the surfaces are involved with attrition and brown stain
4 Severe - discrete or confluent pitting and corroded appearance.

2. Thylstrup and Fejerskov Scoring
Score Criteria
0 Normal translucency of enamel after prolonged drying
1 Narrow wide lines, corresponding to the perikymata
2 More pronounced lines, occasionally confluencing
3 Merging and irregular cloudy areas
4 Entire surface is chalky white
5 Entire surface is opaque with pits that are < 2 mm in diameter
6 Regularly arranged pits forming horizontal bands with <2 mm vertical extension
7 Loss of outer most enamel with irregular surface not covering more than ½ of the surface
8 Loss of outer most enamel covering more than ½ the surface
9 Loss of main part of enamel with change in anatomic appearance of the tooth.

3. Horowitz Index
Score Criteria
0 No evidence of fluorosis
1 Snow capped tooth with areas of white extending up to the 1/3rd of the incisal edge and cusp tips
2 Extending more than 1/3rd but less than 2/3rd

3 Extending more than 2/3rd
4 Stains and any of the above
5 Discrete pitting without stain
6 Discrete pitting with stain
7 Confluent pitting and loss of enamel.

Difference between fluorosis and hypoplasia		
Characteristics	*Fluorosis*	*Hypoplasia*
Area affected	Entire surface	Centered, smooth, Limited extent.
Lesion shape	Follow incremental lines	Round or oval
Demarcation, Color	Diffuse, Opaque white/brownish white	Clearly differentiated Opaque white, creat yellow, to dark reddish
Teeth affected	Homologous teeth Early erupting teeth are least affected. Premolar and second molar are severely affected	Common on the labial surface of single or homologous teeth. Any teeth can be affected

DEFLUORIDATION OF WATER[122]

The states having high fluoride levels (endemic fluoride belts with fluoride content in water more than 4.00 ppm) are:

- Punjab
- Haryana
- Rajasthan
- Gujarat
- Madhya Pradesh
- Andhra Pradesh
- Tamil Nadu
- Delhi

Several methods that have been implemented to defluoridate the community water are as follows. These may be divided into two basic types:

I. Based upon cation exchange process or adsorption,
II. Based upon addition of chemicals to water during treatment.

Ion Exchange Method

By addition of the following agents it is possible to reduce the fluoride content of water:

A. A sulphonated saw dust impregnated with 2% alum solution is used.
B. Dried and crushed bone
C. Activated carbon
D. Magnesia: It removes the excess fluoride but pH of treated water was beyond 10 and its correction by acidification or recarbonation was necessary.
E. Defluoron 1: Saw dust impregnated with 2% alum.
F. Defluoron 2: This was developed in 1968. It is a sulphonated coal and works on the aluminum cycles.
G. Carbion: It is a cation exchange resin of good durability and can be used on sodium and hydrogen cycles.

Nalgonda Technique of Defluoridation

The Nalgonda technique involves addition in sequence of sodium aluminate or lime, bleaching powder and filter alum to the fluoride water followed by flocculation, sedimentation and filtration. The technique is extremely useful both for domestic as well as for community water supplies. It is a technique in Andhra Pradesh, India for community water defluoridation in the 1970's.

Mechanism of Defluoridation by Nalgonda Technique

Rapid mix: Rapid mixing is an operation by which the coagulant is rapidly and uniformly dispersed through the single or multiple phase system. This helps in the formation of microflocs and results in proper utilization of chemical coagulant, preventing localization of concentration and premature formation of hydroxides which leads to less utilization of coagulants.

Flocculation: Flocculation is the second stage in the formation of settlable particles [FLOCS] from destabilized colloidal sized particles and is achieved by gentle and prolonged mixing.

Sedimentation: It is the separation from the water by gravitational setting of suspended particles that are heavier than water.

Filteration: This is the final step. The water is allowed to stand for about half an hour and the water collected at the top is utilized for drinking.

> **Global goals for oral health 2020 by WHO**
>
> The WHO goals 'Oral Health by 2000' had stimulated awareness of the importance of oral health amongst national and local governments and acted as a catalyst for securing resources for oral health in general. Therefore, even though not all countries had achieved the goals, they provided a key focus for the effort. Recently, the FDI, WHO and IADR have embarked on the activity of preparing goals for the new millennium, for the year 2020, and these are presented here.
>
> **Goals**
>
> 1. To minimize the impact of diseases of oral and craniofacial origin on health and psychosocial development, giving emphasis to promoting oral health and reducing oral disease amongst populations with the greatest burden of such conditions and diseases.

Contd...

Contd...

2. To minimize the impact of oral and craniofacial manifestations of systemic diseases on individuals and society, and to use these manifestations for early diagnosis, prevention and effective management of systemic diseases.

Objectives

1. To reduce mortality from oral and craniofacial diseases.
2. To reduce morbidity from oral and craniofacial diseases and thereby increase the quality of life.
3. To promote sustainable, priority-driven policies and programs in oral health systems that have been derived from systematic reviews of best practices (i.e. the policies are evidence-based).
4. To develop accessible costeffective oral health systems for the prevention and control of oral and craniofacial diseases.
5. To integrate oral health promotion and care with other sectors that influence health, using the common risk factor approach.
6. To develop oral health programs that will empower people to control determinants of health.
7. To strengthen systems and methods for oral health surveillance, both processes and outcomes.
8. To promote social responsibility and ethical practices of care givers.
9. To reduce disparities in oral health between different socioeconomic groups within a country and inequalities in oral health across countries.
10. To increase the number of health care providers who are trained in accurate epidemiological surveillance of oral diseases and disorders.

Targets

By the year 2020 the following will have been achieved over baseline:

Pain

1. A reduction in episodes of pain of oral and craniofacial origin.
2. A reduction in the number of days absent from school, employment and work resulting from pain of oral and craniofacial origin.
3. A reduction in the number of people affected by functional limitations (this covers a number of measurable factors such as pain and impairments, missing teeth, traumatized incisors and congenital dental and facial anomalies.
4. A reduction in the prevalence of moderate and severe social impacts on daily activities resulting from pain, impairments and aesthetics (this includes missing teeth, dental anomalies, enamel defects such as fluorosis, traumatized incisors, severe gingival recession and oral malodor.

Functional Disorders

A reduction in the numbers of individuals experiencing difficulties in chewing, swallowing and speaking/communicating. This covers a large number of measurable factors related to tooth loss and congenital and acquired facial/dental deformities.

Contd...

Infectious Diseases

To increase the numbers of health care providers competent to recognize and minimize the risks of transmission of infectious diseases in the oral health care environment.

Oropharyngeal Cancer

1. To reduce the prevalence of oropharyngeal cancer
2. To improve the survival (5-year survival rate) of treated cases
3. To increase early detection
4. To increase rapid referral
5. To reduce exposure to risk factors with special reference to tobacco, alcohol and improved nutrition
6. To increase the number of affected individuals receiving multidisciplinary specialist care.

Oral Manifestations of HIV Infection

1. To reduce the prevalence of opportunistic orofacial infections.
2. To increase the number of health providers who are competent to diagnose and manage the oral manifestations of HIV infection.
3. To increase the numbers of policy makers who are aware of the oral implications of HIV infection.

Noma

1. To increase data on Noma from populations at risk.
2. To increase early detection.
3. To increase rapid referral.
4. To reduce exposure to risk factors with special reference to immunization coverage or measles, improved nutrition and sanitation.
5. To increase the number of affected individuals receiving multidisciplinary specialist care.

Trauma

1. To increase early detection
2. To increase rapid referral
3. To increase the number of health care providers who are competent to diagnose and provide emergency care
4. To increase the number of affected individuals receiving multidisciplinary specialist care where necessary.

Craniofacial Anomalies

1. To reduce exposure to risk factors with special reference to tobacco, alcohol, teratogenic agents and improved nutrition
2. To increase access to genetic screening and counseling
3. To increase early detection
4. To increase rapid referral
5. To increase the number of affected individuals receiving multidisciplinary specialist care
6. To increase early detection of seriously handicapping malocclusions and their referral.

Dental Caries

1. To increase the proportion of caries free 6-year-old
2. To reduce the DMFT particularly the D component at age 12 years, with special attention to high-risk groups within populations, utilizing both distributions and means.

Contd...

Contd...

3. To reduce the number of teeth extracted due to dental caries at ages 18, 35–44 and 65–74 years.

Developmental Anomalies of Teeth
1. To reduce the prevalence of disfiguring dental fluorosis as measured by culturally sensitive measures and with special reference to the fluoride content of food, water and inappropriate supplementation.
2. To reduce the prevalence of acquired developmental anomalies of teeth, with special reference to infectious diseases and inappropriate medications.
3. To increase early detection for both hereditary and acquired anomalies.
4. To increase referral for both hereditary and acquired anomalies.

Periodontal Diseases
1. To reduce the number of teeth lost due to periodontal diseases at ages 18, 35–44 and 65–74 years with special reference to smoking, poor oral hygiene, stress and inter-current systemic diseases.
2. To reduce the prevalence of necrotizing forms of periodontal diseases by reducing exposure to risk factors such as poor nutrition, stress and immunosuppression.
3. To reduce the prevalence of active periodontal infection (with or without loss of attachment) in all ages.
4. To increase the proportion of people in all ages with healthy periodontium (gums and supporting bone structure).

Oral Mucosal Diseases
1. To increase the number of health care providers who are competent to diagnose and provide emergency care.
2. To increase early detection.
3. To increase rapid referral.

Salivary Gland Disorders
1. To increase the numbers of health care providers who are competent to diagnose and provide emergency care.
2. To increase early detection
3. To increase rapid referral.

Tooth Loss
1. To reduce the number of edentulous persons at ages 35–44 and 65–74 years.
2. To increase the number of natural teeth present at ages 18, 35–44 and 65–74 years.
3. To increase the number of individuals with functional dentitions (21 or more natural teeth) at ages 35–44 and 65–74 years.

Health Care Services
To establish evidence-based services.

REFERENCES

1. MI Compendium of systematic reviews, in www.mi-comendium.org.
2. Tyas MJ, Anusavice KJ, Frencken JE, Mount GJ. Minimal intervention dentistry—a review. FDI Commission Project 1-97. Int Dent J 2000;50:1-12.
3. Mount GJ, Ngo H. Minimal intervention dentistry—a new concept for operative dentistry. Quintessence Int 2000;31:527-33.
4. Young DA, Kutch VK, Whitehouse J. A clinician's guide to CAMBRA: A simple approach. Compendium 2009; 30:92-1-4.
5. Reich E, Lussi A, Newbrun E. Caries-risk assessment. Int Dent J 1999;49:15-26.
6. FDI POLICY STATEMENT Minimal Intervention in the Management of Dental Caries, Adopted by the FDI General Assembly:1– Vienna, Austria, October 2002.
7. Anderson MH. A review of the efficacy of chlorhexidine on dental caries and the caries infection. J Calif Dent Assoc 2003;31:211-4.
8. Afflitto J, Prencipe M, Zhang YP, Clipper D, Gaffar A. Antibacterial and anticaries efficacy of a dentifrice containing triclosan and xylitol. J Dent Res 1998.
9. Lang NP, Hase JC, Grassi M, Hämmerle CH, Weigel C, Kelty E, Frutig F. Plaque formation and gingivitis after supervised mouthrinsing with 0.2% delmopinol hydrochloride, 0.2% chlorhexidine digluconate and placebo for 6 months. Oral Dis 1998;4:105-13.
10. Litt MD, Reisine S, Tinanoff N. Multidimensional causal model of dental caries development in low-income preschool children. Public Health Reports 1995;110(4): 607-17.
11. Nicolau B, Marcenes W, Bartley M, Sheiham A. A life course approach to assessing causes of dental caries experience: The relationship between biological, behavioural, socioeconomic and psychological conditions and caries in adolescents. Caries Res 2003; 37(5):319-26.
12. Featherstone JD. The caries balance: Contributing factors and early detection. J Calif Dent Assoc 2003;31(2):129-33.
13. Featherstone JD. The caries balance: The basis for caries management by risk assessment. Oral Health Prev Dent. 2004;2(Suppl 1):259-64.
14. American Academy of Pediatric Dentistry, Council on clinical affairs. Policy on use of a caries risk assessment tool (CAT) for infants, children and adolescents. Pediatr Dent 2002;25:18.
15. Alaluvsua S, et al. Salivary caries related tests in prediction of future caries increments in teenagers, a three year longitudinal study. Oral Micro Immunol 1990; 5: 77-81.
16. Disney J, et al. The university of North Carolina caries risk assessment study, further developments in caries risk prediction. Community Dent Oral Epidemiol 1992; 20:64-75.
17. Messer LB. Assessing caries risk in children. Aust Dent J 2000;45:10-6.
18. American Academy of Pediatric Dentistry. Dental home resource center. Available at: http://www.aapd.org/dentalhome/", 2010.
19. American Academy of Pediatrics Committee on Children with Disabilities. Care coordination: Integrating health and related systems of care for children with special health care needs. Pediatrics 1999;104:978-81.

20. American Academy of Pediatrics. Committee on Pediatric Workforce. Culturally effective pediatric care: Education and training issues. Pediatrics 1999; 103(1):167-70.

21. American Academy of Pediatrics Committee on Pediatric Workforce. Pediatric primary health care. AAP News November 1993;11:7. Reaffirmed June 2001.

22. American Academy of Pediatrics. The medical home. Pediatrics 2002;110:184-6.

23. American Academy of Pediatrics. Policy on oral health risk assessment timing and establishment of the dental home. Pediatrics 2003;111:1113-6.

24. Lewis CW, Grossman DC, Domoto PK, et al. The role of the pediatrician in the oral health of children: A national survey. Pediatrics 2000;106(6):E84.

25. Harrison R. Oral health promotion for high-risk children: Case studies from British Columbia. J Can Dent Assoc 2003;69(5):292-6.

26. American academy of pediatrics, section on pediatric dentistry and oral health. A policy statement: Preventive intervention for pediatricians. Pediatrics 2008; 122(6): 1387-94.

27. Nowak AJ, Casamassimo PS. The dental home: A primary oral health concept. J Am Dent Assoc 2002; 133(1):93-8.

28. Nowak AJ. Rationale for the timing of the first oral evaluation. Pediatr Dent 1997;19(1):8-11.

29. US Dept of Health and Human Services. Healthy People 2010: Understanding and improving health. 2nd ed. Washington, DC. US Government Printing Office; November 2000.

30. Nowak AJ, Casamassimo PS. Using anticipatory guidance to provide early dental intervention. J Am Dent Assoc 1995;126(8):1156-63.

31. Paul S, Casamassimo, John JW. Examination, diagnosis and treatment planning of the infant and toddler. Pediatric Dentistry, Infancy through Adolescence 4th Edition Elsevier Saunders 2005;206-19.

32. Scottish Intercollegiate Guideline Network. Prevention and management of dental decay in the preschool child. A national guideline # 83. November, 2005.

33. Pang DT, Vann WF Jr. The use of fluoride-containing toothpastes in young children: The scientific evidence for recommending a small amount. PediatrDent 1992; 14(6):384-7.

34. Ramos-Gomez FJ, Crall JJ, Gansky SA, Slayton RL, Featherstone JD. Caries risk assessment appropriate for the age 1 visit (infants and toddlers). J Calif Dent Assoc 2007;35(10):687-702.

35. Krasse B, Newbrun E. Objective methods of evaluating caries activity and their application, Pediatric Dentistry, Scientific foundation and clinical practice, Stewart RE, Barber TK, Troutman KC, Wei SHY, The CV Mosby Co. 1982;610-6.

36. Newbrun E. Cariology, Baltimore, The Williams and Wilkins Co. 1978.

37. Krasse B. Caries risk, Chicago, Quintessence 1985.

38. Hadley FP. A quantitative method for estimating Bacillus acidophilus in saliva. Jour. Dent. Res 1933;13:415-28.

39. Mc Ghee JR, Michalek SM, Cassele GM. Editors Dental Microbiology Philadelphia, Harper & Row, 1982;74:688.

40. Snyder ML. A simple colorimetric method for the diagnosis of caries activity. JAm Dent Assoc 1941;28:44.

41. Rapp GW. Fifteen minute caries test. J. Int Dent 1962; 31:290-5.

42. Kohler B. Bratthall D. Practical Method to Facilitate Estimation of Streptococcus mutans Levels in Saliva, J Clin Microbiol 1979;9:584-8.

43. Maki Y, Yamamoto H, Takaesu Y, Shibuya M, Kinoshita Y, Asami K. A rapid caries activity test by Resazurin Disc. Bull Tokyo Dent Coll 1986;27(1):1-13.

44. Peter S. Essentials of Preventive and Community Dentistry 4th Ed. Arya (Medi) Publishing House, 2010.

45. Jong AW. Community Dental Health 3rd Ed. Mosby Co. 1988.

46. Park K. Park's text book for Preventive and Social Medicine. 20th Ed. M/s Banarsidas Bhanot Pub. 2009.

47. Schachtele CF. Changing perspective on the role of diet in dental caries information. Nutr News 1982;45:13-5.

48. Tanzer JM. Xylitol chewing gum and dental caries. Int Dent J 1995;45 (Suppl):65-76.

49. Edgar WM. Saliva and dental health, Clinical implications of saliva-report of a consensus meeting. Br Dent J 1990; 169:96-8.

50. Aimutis WR. Bioactive properties of milk proteins focus on anticariogenesis. J Nutr 2004;134:989S-95S.

51. Cross KJ, LailaHuq N, Palamara JE, Perich JW, Reynolds EC. Physicochemical characterization of casein phosphopeptide-amorphous calcium phosphate. Nanocomplexes J Biol Chem 2005;280:15362-9.

52. Cross KJ, Huq N L, Reynolds EC. Casein phosphopeptides in oral health-chemistry and clinical applications. Curr Pharm Des 2007;13:793-800.

53. Schüpbach P, Neeser JR, Golliard M, Rouvet M, Guggenheim B. Incorporation of caseinoglycomacropeptide and caseinophosphopeptide into the salivary pellicle inhibits adherence of mutans streptococci. J Dent Res 1996;75:1779-88.

54. Reynolds EC. Remineralization of enamel subsurface lesions by casein phosphopeptide-stabilized calcium phosphate solutions. J Dent Res 1997;76:1587-95.

55. Burwell AK, Muscle D. Sustained Calcium Ion and pH Release from Calcium Phosphate-Containing Dentifrices. IADR/AADR/CADR 87th General Session and Exhibition, Miami 2009;1-4.

56. Lia R, Barbara P, Michele I, Lorenza C, Federica D, Michela M, Norberto R. The remineralizing effect of carbonate-hydroxyapatite nanocrystals on dentine. Materials Science Forum 2007;539-543(1):602-5.

57. Huang S B, Gao S S, Yu H Y. Effect of nano-hydroxyapatite concentration on remineralization of initial enamel lesion *in vitro*. Biomed Mater 2009;4:34104.

58. Fowler BO. Infrared studies of apatites. I. Vibrational assignments for calcium, strontium, and barium hydroxyapatites utilizing isotopic substitution. Inorg Chem 1974;13(1):194-206.

59. Nelson DGA, Featherstone JDB. Preparation, analysis and characterization of carbonated apatites. Calcif Tissues Int 1982;34:S69-S81.

60. Meurman JH, Voegel JC, Rauhamaa-Makinen R, et al. Effects of carbon dioxide, Nd:YAG combination lasers at high energy densities in synthetic hydroxyapatite. Caries Res 1992;26:77-83.

61. Nelson DGA, Williamson BE. Low-temperature laser Raman spectroscopy of synthetic carbonated apatites and dental enamel. Aust J Chem 1982;35:715-27.

62. Tode CDM. Laser applications in conservative dentistry TMJ 2004;54:392-405.

63. Nogales CG, Ferrari PA, Kantorovich EO, Lage-Marques JL. Ozone Therapy in Medicine and Dentistry. J Contemp Dent Pract 2008;9:075-084.

64. Huth KC, Paschos E, Brand K, Hickel R. Effect of ozone on noncavitated fissure carious lesions in permanent molars. A controlled prospective clinical study. Am J Dent 2005;18:223-8.

65. Nogales CG, Ferrari PA, Kantorovich EO, Lage-Marques JL. Ozone Therapy in Medicine and Dentistry. J Contemp Dent Pract 2008; 9:075-084.

66. Huth KC, Paschos E, Brand K, Hickel R. Effect of ozone on non-cavitated fissure carious lesions in permanent molars. A controlled prospective clinical study. Am J Dent 2005;18:223-8.

67. Taylor CL and Gwinnett AJ. A study of the penetration of sealants into pits and fissures. J. Am. Dent. Assoc 1973;87:1181.

68. Brown LJ, Kaste LM, Selwitz RH, Furman LJ. Dental caries and sealants usage in US children, 1988-1991. Selected findings from the third national health and nutrition examination survey. JADA 1996;127:335.

69. Hicks J, Flaitz CM. Pit and Fissure Sealants and Conservative Adhesive Restorations: Scientific and Clinical Rationale. Pediatric Dentistry, Infancy through Adolescence, 4th Edition, Elsevier Saunders, 2005;520-76.

70. Hyatt TP. Occlusal fissures: their frequency and danger. How shall they be treated? Dent Items Interest 1924;46:493.

71. Bodecker CK. The eradication of enamel fissures. Dent Items Interest 1929;51:859.

72. Buonocore MG. Simple methods of increasing the adhesion of acrylic filling materials to enamel surfaces. J Dent Res 1955;34:849.

73. Bowen RL. Composite and sealant resins: past, present and future. Pediatr Dent 1982;4:10.

74. Hicks J, Garcia-Godoy F, Donly K, Flaitz C. Fluoride releasing restorative materials and secondary caries. Dent Clin North Am 2002;46:247.

75. Ripa LW. The current status of pit and fissure sealants. A review. J. Public Health Dent 1983;43:216.

76. Richardson BA, et al. A 5 years, clinical evaluation of the effectiveness of fissure sealant in mentally retarded Canadian children. Communtiy Dent Oral Epidemiol 1981;9:170.

77. Ripa LW, Gwinnett AI, Buonocore MB. The prismless outer layer of deciduous and permanent enamel. Arch Oral Biol 1966;11:41.

78. Silverstone LM. The histopathology of early approximal caries in the enamel of primary teeth. J Dent. Child. 1970;37:17.

79. Silverstone LM, Dogon IL. The effect of phosphoric acid on human deciduous enamel surface *in vitro.* J. Int. Assoc Dent Child 1976;7:11.

80. Garcia-Godoy F, Summitt JB, Donly KJ. Caries progression of white spot lesions sealed with an unfilled resin. J ClinPediatr Dent 1997;21:141.

81. Mertz-Fairhurst EJ, Smith CD, Eilliams JE, et al: Cariostatic and ultraconservative sealed restorations: six year results. Quintessence Int 1993;23:827.

82. Smales RJ, Yip HK. The atraumatic restorative treatment (ART) approach for the management of dental caries. Quintessence Int 33: 427-32, 2002.

83. Simonsen RJ. Preventive Resin Restorations (I.) Quintessence Int 1978;1:69.

84. Simonsen RJ. Preventive Resin Restorations (II.) Quintessence Int 1978;2:95.

85. Munshi AK, Hegde AM, Shetty PK. Clinical evaluation of Carisolv in the chemicomechanical removal of carious dentin. J Clin Pediatr Dent 2001;26:49-54.

86. Ganesh M, Parikh D. Chemomechanical caries removal (CMCR) agents: Review and clinical application in primary teeth, Jn Dentistry and Oral Hygiene, 2011;3(3): 34-45.

87. Wei SHY, Hyman RM. Use of tooth brush in plaque control for children, pediatric dentistry, Scientific foundation and clinical practice, Stewart RE, Barber TK, Troutman KC, Wei SHY, The CV Mosby Co. 1982;640-51.

88. Park KK, Matis BA, Christen AG. Choosing an effective toothbrush, ClinPrev Dent 1985;7(4):5-10.

89. Updyke JR. A new handle for a child's toothbrush, J Dent Child 1979;46:123-5.

90. Bass CC. An effective method of personal oral hygiene II, J La State Med Soc 1954;106:100.

91. Stillman PR. A philosophy of the treatment of periodontal disease. Dent Digest 1932;38:315.

92. Charters WJ. Eliminating mouth infections with the tooth brush and other stimulating instruments. Dent Digest 1932;38:130.

93. Gibson JA, Wade AB J. Plaque removal by the Bass and Roll brushing techniques. J Periodontol. 1977;48(8):456-9.

94. McClure DB. A Comparison of toothbrushing techniques for the preschool child. J Dent Child 1966;33:2.0.

95. Bell DG. Teaching home care to the patient. J Periodontol 1948;19:149.

96. Fones AC. Mouth Hygiene, Philadelphia, Lea and Febriger, 1934.

97. HattabfnQudeimat MA, Al-Rimawi HS. Dental discoloration: an overview, J Esthet Dent 1999;11:291-310.

98. Slots J. The microflora of black stain on primary teeth, Scand J Dent Res 1974;82:484-90.

99. Parmly SL. Practical guide to the management of the teeth, Philadelphia, Collins and Crofit, 1819.

100. Bass CC. The optimum characteristics of dental floss for personal oral hygiene. Dent Items Interest 1948;70:921.

101. Wei SHY, Vidra JD. Plaque control and the use of dental floss in children, Pediatric Dentistry, Scientific foundation and clinical practice, Stewart RE, Barber TK, Troutman KC, Wei SHY, The CV Mosby Co. 1982;652-9.

102. Wright CZ. The flossing technique: Can it be effective in reducing caries and gingivitis in children? Mc Donald R, et al. Current therapy in dentistry St Louis: CV Mosby Co. 1980.

103. Arnim SS. The use of disclosing agents for measuring tooth cleanliness. J Periodontol 1963;34,227.

104. Scheinin A. Sucrose substitutes. Pediatric Dentistry, Scientific foundation and clinical practice, Stewart RE, Barber TK, Troutman KC, Wei SHY, 1982;590-7.

105. Yoshihiko H, Tsunenori M, Iluminada VL. X-ray Microanalysis of Remineralized Enamel Lesions by Xylitol-containing Chewing Gums Having Different Types of Calcium Phosphate. Japanese J Cons Dent 2005;48:648-55.

106. Manton DJ, Glenn WD, Fan C, Nathan J, Peiyan S, Eric RC. Remineralization of enamel subsurface lesions *in situ* by the use of three commercially available sugar-free gums. Int J Paed Dent 2008;18:284-90.

107. Toshinari M. Remineralization promoting effect of chewing gum containing fluoride and xylitol. Japanese J Cons Dent 2005;43:1-11.

108. Manning RH, Edgar WM, Agalamanyi EA. Effects of chewing gums sweetened with sorbitol or a sorbitol/xylitol mixture on the remineralization of human enamel lesions *in situ*. Caries Res 1992;26:104-9.

109. Mandel I. What is preventive dentistry. J Prev Dent 1974;1:25.

110. Wright FA. Children's perception of vulnerability to illness and dental disease. Community Dent Oral Epidemiol 1982;10:29-32.

111. Rubinson L, Tappe M. An evaluation of a preschool dental health program ASDC J Dent Child 1987;54:186-92.

112. Jenkins SR, Geurink KV. A Rural School-Based Oral Health Program J Dent Hygiene 2006;80:26.

113. Mc Kay FS. An investigation of mottled teeth I, II Den. Cosmos 1916;58:477-484,781-2.

114. Eager JM. Abstract: Chiaic Teeth. Dent Cosmos 1902; 44:300-301.

115. Black GV, McKay FS. Mottled teeth-an endemic developmental imperfection of the teeth heretofore unknown in the literature of dentistry. Dent cosmos 1916;58:129-56.

116. Kemp GA, McKay FS. Mottled enamel in a segregated population. Public health rep 1930;45:2923-40.

117. Churchill HV. Occurence of fluorides in some waters of the united states. Ind. Eng. Chem 1931;23:996-8.

118. Dean HT. Distribution of mottled enamel in United States. Public health rep 1933;48:704-34.

119. Dean HT. Classification of mottled enamel diagnosis. J Am Dent Assoc 1934;21:1421-6.

120. Dean HT, Arnold FA, Elvove E. Domestic water and dental caries, additional studies of the relation of fluoride domestic waters to dental caries experience in 4,425 white children aged 12-14 years of 13 cities in 4 states. Public health rep 1942;57:1155-79.

121. Smith FA, Ekstrand J. The occurrence and the chemistry of fluoride In Fejerskov O, Ekstrand J, Burt BA. Fluorides in Dentistry, 2nd Ed Munksgaard pub,1996.

122. Szpir M. Food safety: A tea-time mystery. Environ. health perspect. 2005;113(8):A518.

123. Weinstein LH. Effects of fluorides on plants and plant communities; an overview, In: Shupe JL, Peterson HB, Leone NC, Fluorides – Effects on vegetation, animals and humans. Salt Lake City: Paragon Press 1983;53-9.

124. Fuge R. Sources of halogens in the environment, influences on human and animal health. Environ Geochem and health 1988;10:51-61.

125. Whitford GM, Pashley DH. Fluoride absorption: the influence of gastric acidity. Calcif tissue Int 1984;36:302-7.

126. Ekstrand J. Fluoride Metabolism. In: Fejerskov O, Ekstrand J, Burt BA. Fluorides in Dentistry, 2nd Ed Munksgaard pub, 1996.

127. Robinson C. Kirkham J, Weatherell JA. Fluoride in teeth and bone. In: Fejerskov O, Ekstrand J, Burt BA. Fluorides in Dentistry, 2nd Ed Munksgaard pub, 1996.

128. Ekstrand J, Spak CJ, Ehrnebo M. Renal clearance of fluoride in a steady state condition in man: influence of urinary flow and pH changes by diet. Acta Pharmacol Toxicol 1982;50:321-5.

129. Brown W, Konig K. Cariostatic mechanism of fluoride. Caries Res 1977;11(Suppl 1):1.

130. Moss S, Wei S. Fluorides: An update for dental practice. New York: Medcom, Inc. 1976.

131. Young RA. Biological apatite vs hydroxyapatite at the atomic level. ClinOrthop 1975;113:249-62.

132. Frazier PD. X-ray diffraction analysis of human enamel containing different amounts of fluoride. Arch Oral Biol 1967;12:35-42.

133. Brown WE, Gregory TM, Chow LC. Effects fo fluoride on enamel solubility and cariostasis. Caries Res 1977; 11:118-41.

134. Bibby BG, Van Kesteren M. The effect of fluoride in mouth bacteria. J Dent Res 1940;39:117.

135. Wright DE, Jenkin GN. The effect of fluoride on acid production of saliva-glucose mixtures. Br Dent J 1954; 96:30-4.

136. Erricsson TH, Ericsson Y. Effect of partial fluorine substitution on the phosphate exchange and protein adsorption of hydroxyapatite. Helvetica OdontActa 1967;11:10-4.

137. Aasenden R, Peebles TC. Effect of fluoride supplementation from birth on human deciduous and permanent teeth. Archives of Oral Biol 1974;19:321-6.

138. Arnold FA, Dean HT, Knutson JW. Effects of fluoridated public water supplies on dental caries prevalence. Result of the seventh year of study at Grand Rapids and Muskegon. Mich public health rep 1953;68:141-8.

139. Ast DB, Smith DJ, Wacks B, Cantwell DT. The Newburgh-Kingston caries fluorine study XIV. Comined clinical and roentgenographic dental finding after ten years of fluoride experience. J Am den Assoc 1956;52:314-25.

140. Blayney JR, Tucker WH. The Evanston dental caries study. J Dent Res 1948;27:279-86.

141. Galagan DJ, Vermillion JR. Determining the optimum fluoride concentrations. Publ Health Rep Wash 1957; 72:491.

142. Tiwari A. Fluorides and dental caries. J Ind Dent Assoc., Spl Issue, 1986.

143. Knutson JW. Sodium fluoride solution;techniques for applications to the teeth. J Am Dent Assoc 1948;36:37-9.

144. Dudding NJ, Muhler JC. Technique of application of stannous fluoride in a compatible prophylactic paste and as a topical agent. J Dent Child 1962;29:219-24.

145. Muhler JC. Control of dental caries. Current Therapy in Dentistry. Vol 3 pg 791 Mosby, St Louis, 1968.

146. Jordon, et al. $Sn_3F_3PO_4$ the product of the reaction between stannous fluoride and hydroxyapatite. Arch oral Biol 1971;16:241-6.

147. Brudevold F, Savory A, Gardner DE, et al. A study of acidulated fluoride solutions I *in vitro* effects of enamel. Arch Oral Biol 1963;8:167-77.

148. Aasenden R, Brudevold F. The response of intact and experimentally altered enamel to topical fluorides. Arch Oral Biol 1968;13:543-52.

149. Chow LC. Brown WE. The reaction of Dicalcium phosphate dihydrate with fluoride. Jn Dent Res 1973; 52:1220-7.

150. Horowitz HS, Ismail AI. Topical fluorides in caries prevention. In Fejerskov O, Ekstrand J, Burt BA. Fluorides in Dentistry, 2nd Ed Munksgaard pub,1996.

151. Horowitz HS, Doyle J. The effect on dental caries of topically applied acidulated phosphate-fluoride: results after three years. J Am Dent Assoc 1971;82:359-65.

152. Bibby BG. Test of the effect of fluoride containing dentifrices on dental caries. J Dent Res 1945;24:297-303.

153. Muhler JC, Radhike AW, Nebergall WH, Day HG. A comparison between the anticariogenic effect of dentifrices containing SnF_2. J Am Dent Assoc 1955;51: 556-9.

154. Richards A, Banting DW. Fluoride tooth pastes In. Fejerskov O, Ekstrand J, Burt BA. Fluorides in Dentistry, 2nd Ed Munksgaard pub,1996.

155. Centers for disease control and prevention: Recommendations for using fluoride to prevent and control dental caries in the United States. MMWR Morb Mortal Wkly Rep 2001;50(RR-14):26.

156. Richardson B. Fixation of topically applied fluoride in enamel. J Dent Res 1967;46:87-91.

157. Seppa L, Koskinen M, Luoma H. Relationship between caris and fluoride uptake by enamel from two fluoride varnishes in a community with fluoridated water. Caries Res 1982;16:404-12.

158. Arends J, Schuthof J. Fluoride content in human enamel after fluoride application and washing. An *in vitro* study. Caries Res 1975;9:363-72.

159. Stanley BH, Herschel SH. The amounts of fluoride in current fluoride therapies: safety considerations for children. J Dent Child 1984;5:257-69.

160. Dean HT. The investigation of physiological effects by the epidemiological methods. In Moulton FR. Fluorine and dental health. Washington DC. American Assoc for the Advancement of Science, 1942;23-31.

161. Fejerskov O, Richards A, DenBesten P. The effect of fluoride on tooth mineralization In. Fejerskov O, Ekstrand J, Burt BA. Fluorides in Dentistry, 2nd Ed Munksgaard pub, 1996.

162. Horowitz HS, Heifetz SB, Driscoll WS, Kingman A, Meyers RJ. A new method for assessing the prevalence of dental fluorosis- The tooth surface index of fluorosis. J Am Dent Assoc 1984;109:37-41.

163. Bhakuni TS, Sastry CA. Defluoridation of water using cation exchangers treated with aluminiumsulphate solution. Environmental Health 1964;6:246.
Defluoridation of water by Nalgonda Technique. Neeri Technical Digest 1974;46.

QUESTIONS

1. What is MID and what are its concepts ?
2. What is caries risk assessment tool ?
3. Dental home and anticipatory guidance.
4. What is the purpose of caries activity tests? Explain any two tests in detail.
5. Role of health education in clinical practice.
6. Name some remineralizing agents. Explain any two in detail.
7. Classify pit and fissure sealants. Describe the steps in the placement of a resin sealant.
8. ART
9. What is Carisolv?
10. Enumerate different oral hygiene aids. Describe in detail dentifrices.
11. What are the different brushing techniques advised for children?
12. Xylitol as sugar substitute.
13. Enumerate levels of prevention and describe each of them in detail.
14. Describe the mechanism of action of fluorides
15. Explain Galagan and Vermilion formula.
16. Describe Knutson's technique in detail.
17. Compare fluoride gels with varnishes.
18. School rinse programs.
19. Clinical features and management of acute fluoride toxicity.

PEDIATRIC OPERATIVE DENTISTRY

INTRODUCTION

The aim of pediatric operative dentistry is to maintain the tooth in the dental arch in a healthy state, so as to prevent its loss and the development of subsequent problems.

It is important to understand the difference in structure between the deciduous and permanent teeth before planning any procedure.

FEATURES OF DECIDUOUS TEETH COMPARED TO PERMANENT TEETH

1. *Shorter crown:* The total height of the clinical crown of the deciduous tooth is less and hence the depth of the cavity should be similarly less. The mesial pulp horns extend higher occlusally than on permanent teeth, and thus risk for accidental exposure increases during cavity preparation.
2. *Narrow occlusal table (Fig. 7.47):* The occlusal table width of deciduous molars are very narrow compared to the permanent molar as presented in the figure. Accordingly the width of the cavity should also be less in a deciduous tooth.
3. *Constricted cervical portion (Figs 7.48 and 7.49):* The deciduous teeth is characterized by a prominent cervical ridge more pronounced on the buccal aspect and a steep cervical constriction cervical to the ridge. Care must be taken while preparing the proximal box, as there is risk of pulp exposure at the site of constriction. Class II cavity should be restored with proper placement of wedges at the constricted area so that the matrix band is adapted well to the tooth surface.
4. *Thinner enamel and dentin layers:* Enamel and dentin is much thinner, thus dental caries penetrates deeper to reach the pulp earlier in primary teeth. Care must be taken during cavity preparation, not to extend very deep as there is increased chance of pulp exposure.
5. *Enamel rods extend in a slightly occlusal direction from the DEJ in the gingival third (Fig. 7.50):* So enamel beveling at the gingivocavo surface line angle is not required, as no enamel rods remain unsupported.
6. *Broad and flat contact areas (Fig. 7.51):* Caries may remain undetected. The proximal box preparation may have to be extended widely to break the contact free. Cl II cavity.
7. *Wider mesiodistally than cervico-occlusal height:* This is important during the selection of the stainless steel crown.
8. *Lighter color:* Deciduous teeth are generally lighter or whiter in color compared to the permanent teeth. This has to be kept in mind during shade selection for composite restoration or crown restorations.

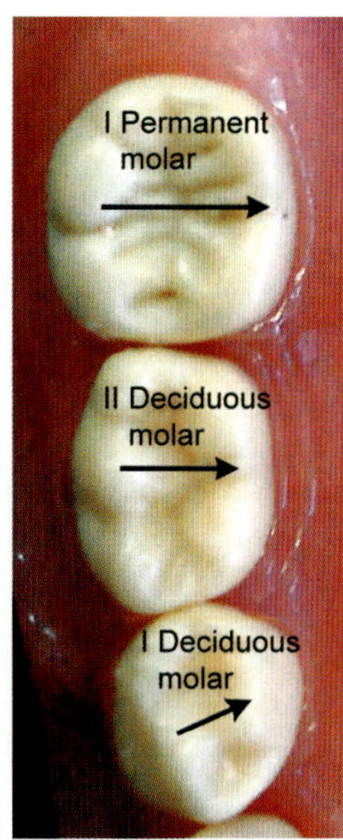

Fig. 7.47: The occlusal table of the deciduous molars is narrower compared to the permanent molar

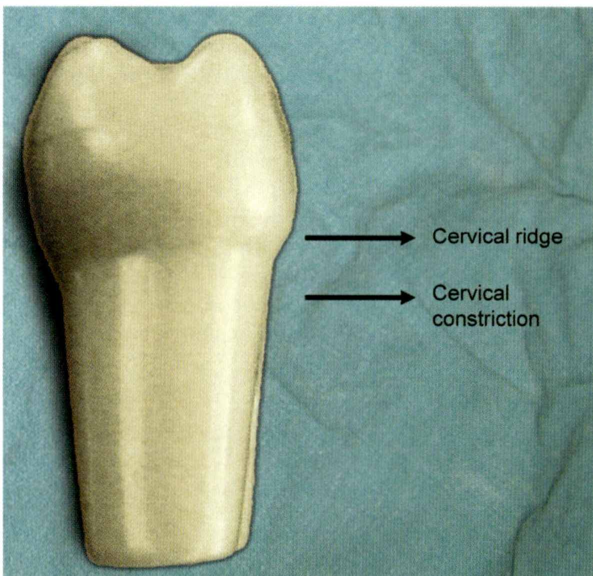

Fig. 7.48: Note the presence of cervical constriction apical to the cervical ridge

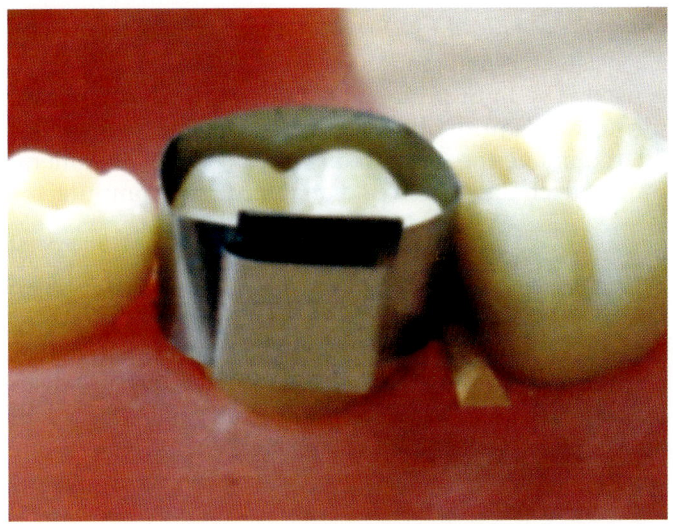

Fig. 7.49: Position of the wedge to hold the matrix band in close approximation to the tooth surface

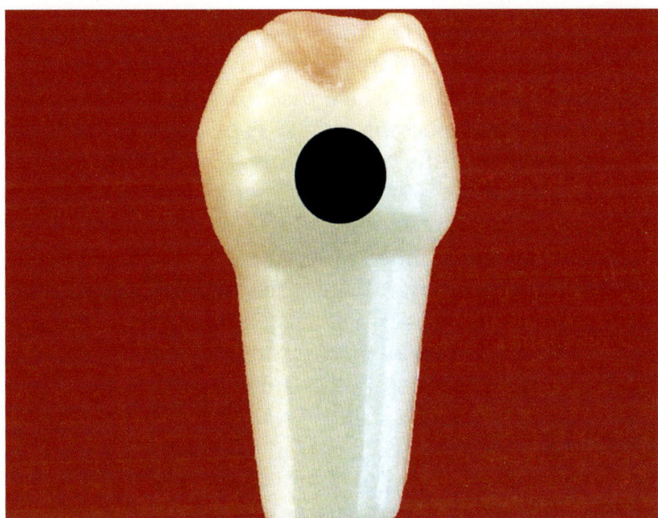

Fig. 7.51: Dark circle representing the broad and wide contact area in the deciduous tooth

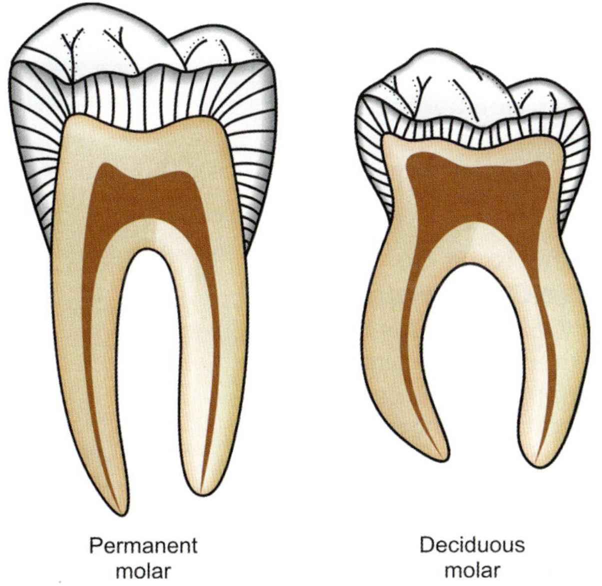

Fig. 7.50: Note the occlusal direction of the enamel rods at the cervical portion in deciduous tooth

Treatment decisions for pit and fissure caries and smooth surface caries

Caries unlikely	→	No treatment
Noncavitated	→	
Caries likely	→	Sealant and minimal intervention techniques
Cavitated	→	Restoration and topical fluoride therapy

DIAGNOSIS OF CARIES

Identifying caries at its early stage (preferably at the precavitation stage) is very essential to prevent significant tooth destruction.

A variety of diagnostic methods are available to detect caries activity at early stages.[1,2]

1. Identification of subsurface demineralization Inspection, radiographic and dye uptake, infrared laser fluorescence (Diagnodent), digital imaging, Fiberoptic transillumination, quantitative light fluorescence, etc.
2. Bacterial testing.
3. Assessments of environmental conditions like pH, salivary flow and salivary buffering.

Since no single test has been developed that is 100% predictive of later development of cavitated lesions, a concept of caries risk has been promoted. Once detected, patients at high-risk for caries can be treated with preventive methods that reduce their likelihood of developing cavitated lesions in the future.

Visual Evidence

Caries can be identified by the use of good illumination, tooth separators or transillumination for the presence of:

- *Opacification:* Due to demineralization in the subsurface of the enamel, initial caries appears as chalky white of opaque area without any loss of tooth structure. Care should be taken not to apply pressure with any instrument as there is risk of puncturing the surface enamel.

- *Surface roughness:* The rougness can be also confirmed by passing the explorer lightly over the surface.
- *Discoloration:* Subsurface discoloration without the presence of detectable cavity especially on the pits and fissures of the occlusal surface of the molars.
- *Cavitation:* Diagnosis of an obvious cavity does not require any extra armamentarium.

Differentiating initial caries from hypoplastic areas can be done by drying the surface. During drying, the water from the subsurface area is removed, leaving airfilled voids that make the area opaque and white. This can be reversed by wetting the surface with water.[3]

Tactile Evidence

By the use of sharp explorers, for the feel of:
- Roughness
- Softening

> Disadvantages of using sharp explorer are:
> Immature pits may break
> Spread of caries (inoculating loop)
> "Catch" may also depend upon:
> Shape of the fissure
> Sharpness of the explorer
> Force of application

Infrared Laser Fluorescence (Diagnodent)

It helps in the detection and quantification of occlusal and smooth surface caries. It uses a diode laser light source and a fiberoptic cable that transmits the light to a hand held probe with a fiberoptic eye at the tip. The light is absorbed and induces infrared fluorescence by organic and inorganic materials. The emitted fluorescence is collected at the probe tip and transmitted, processed and presented on a display window as an integer between 0 and 99. Increased fluorescence reflects carious tooth substance (numerical value higher than about 20).

The main disadvantage with this method is that, they have lower specificity value than visual examination leading to false identification of dentinal caries and unnecessary restoration. Therefore it cannot be used as primary diagnostic method.

Digital Imaging Fiberoptic Transillumination (DIFOTI)

It is similar to FOTI (Fiberoptic transillumination) that has been used for caries detection in dentistry since many years. The difference here in DIFOTI is that the images are visually observed using a digital charged coupled device (CCD) camera and computer.

Quantitative Light Fluorescence (QLF)

It consists of a small portable system in which laser source is used. The light illuminating the tooth is transported through a liquid-filled light guide. The fluorescent filtered images are captured using a color CCD camera. Data collected is stored and analyzed on a computer.

CAVITY PREPARATION

Definition

Cavity preparation is defined as the mechanical alteration of a defective, injured or diseased tooth in order to best receive a restorative material which will re-establish a healthy state of the tooth including esthetic corrections where indicated, along with normal form and function.

Objectives

1. All the defects must be removed and the pulp must be adequately protected.
2. The margins should be as conservatively located as possible.
3. The form of the cavity should be such that the restoration should not get displaced and the tooth or the restoration should not fracture under the force of mastication.
4. The restorative material that is used should be esthetic and functional.

Factors to be Considered before Cavity Preparation

1. Type of restorative material to be placed
2. Direction of the enamel rods
3. Support for the enamel rods
4. Location of the margins
5. Degree of smoothness desired

> General principles of cavity preparation for silver amalgam:[4]
> Initial cavity preparation stage:
> Step 1: Outline form and initial depth
> Step 2: Primary resistance form
> Step 3: Primary retention form
> Step 4: Convenience form
> Final cavity preparation stage:
> Step 5: Removal of any remaining enamel pit/fissure, and /or infected dentin, and/or old restorative material if indicated.
> Step 6: Pulp protection
> Step 7: Secondary resistance and retention forms
> Step 8: Procedures for finishing external walls
> Step 9: Final procedures: cleaning; inspecting; varnishing; conditioning.

CAVITY CLASSIFICATION

Black's Classification[4]

Class I (Figs 7.52A to C): Cavities on occlusal surface of premolars and molars: cavities on occlusal 2/3rd of the facial and lingual surfaces of molar: cavities on lingual surface of maxillary incisors.

Class II (Fig. 7.53): Cavities on the proximal surfaces of posterior teeth.

Class III (Fig. 7.54): Cavities on the proximal surfaces of anterior teeth that do not involve the incisal angle.

Class IV (Fig. 7.55): Cavities on the proximal surfaces of anterior teeth that do involve the incisal edge.

Class V (Fig. 7.56): Cavities on the gingival third of the facial or lingual surface of all teeth.

Class VI (Fig. 7.57): (Modified by Simon) Cavities on the incisal edge of anterior teeth or occlusal cusp heights of posterior teeth.

Finn's Modification of Black's Classification for Deciduous Teeth

Class I: Cavities on the pits and fissures of the molar teeth and the buccal and lingual pits of all teeth.

Class II: Cavities on the proximal surfaces of molar teeth with access established from the occlusal surface (Fig. 7.58).

Class III: Cavities on the proximal surfaces of anterior teeth that may or may not involve the labial or lingual surface (Fig. 7.59).

Class IV: Cavities on the proximal surfaces of anterior teeth that do involve the incisal edge.

Class V: Cavities on the cervical third of all the teeth including the proximal surface where the marginal ridge is not included.

Class VI: (Modified by Simon) Cavities on the incisal edge of anterior teeth or occlusal cusp heights of posterior teeth.

> General cavity preparation for glass ionomer restoration
> *Step 1:* Outline form
> *Step 2:* Convenience form to allow complete caries removal and placement of restorative material
> *Step 3:* Cavity extension and depth is limited to the extension of caries
> *Step 4:* Removal of unsupported enamel and deep caries
> *Step 5:* Pulp protection
> *Step 6:* Dentin conditioning
> *Step 7:* Restoration of the cavity with glass ionomer cement
> *Step 8:* Cleaning; inspecting; varnishing; conditioning.

Classification by Mount and Hume (1998)[5,6]

In this classification the cavity is defined based on the site of occurrence and the size of the cavity and numbers are allotted, as follows:

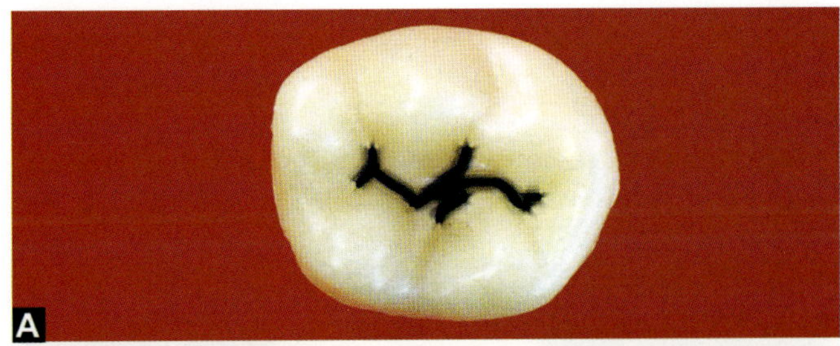

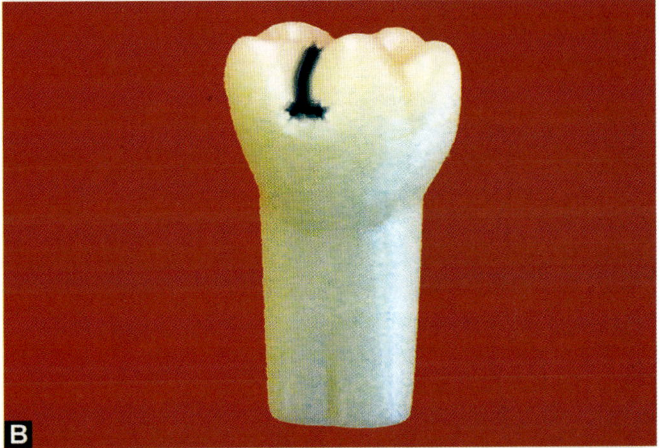

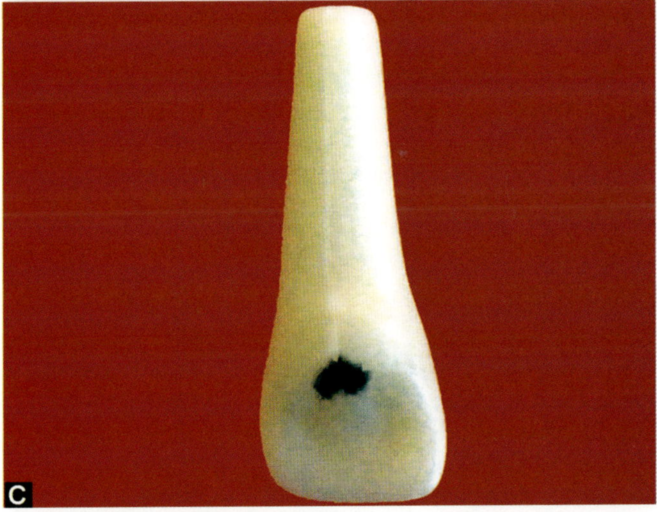

Figs 7.52A to C: Class I cavities involving the: (A) Occlusal surface of posterior teeth; (B) Occlusal 2/3rd of the facial and lingual surfaces of molar; (C) Lingual surface of maxillary incisors

Classification based on the Site of Occurrence of Carious Lesions

Site 1: Cavities seen in the pits, fissures and enamel defects of the occlusal surfaces of posterior teeth or other smooth surface that do not belong to site 2 or 3.

Site 2: Cavities seen on the proximal enamel immediately below areas in contact with adjacent teeth.

Site 3: Cavities seen on the cervical one-third of the crown or the root if they are exposed.

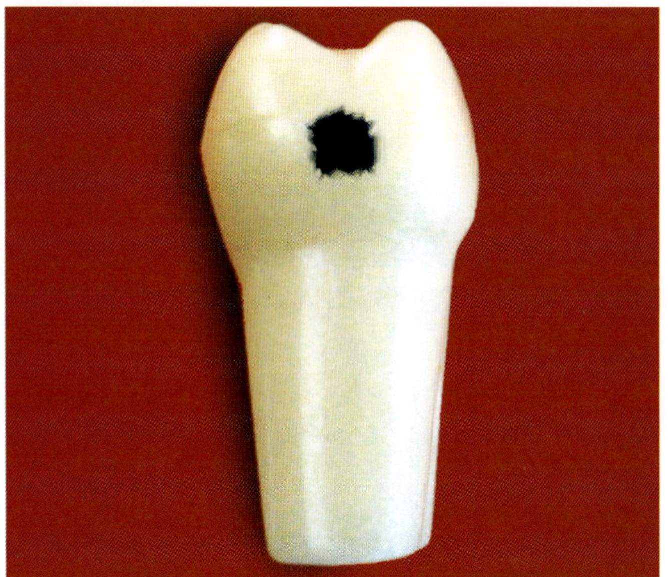

Fig. 7.53: Class II cavities involving the proximal surface of the posterior teeth

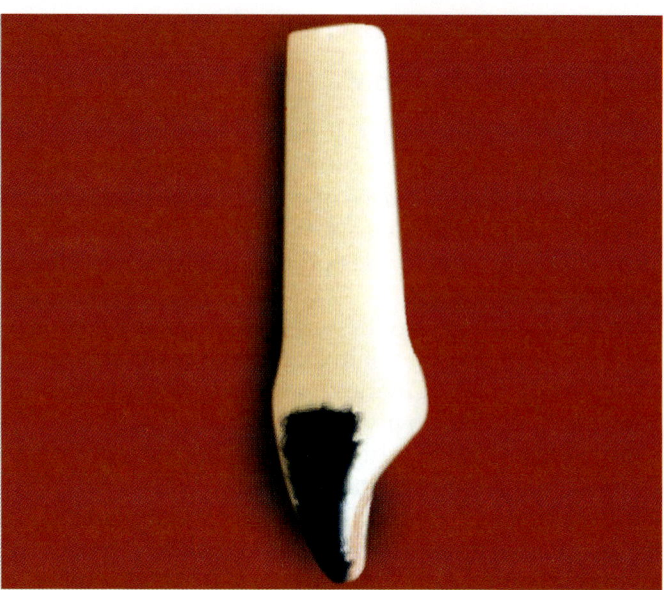

Fig. 7.55: Class IV cavities involving the proximal surface of the anterior teeth with the involvement of the incisal edge

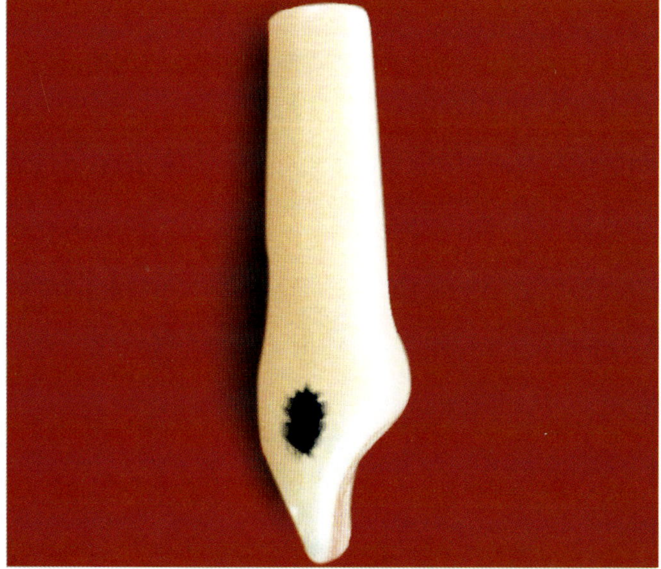

Fig. 7.54: Class III cavities involving the proximal surface of the anterior teeth without involving incisal edge

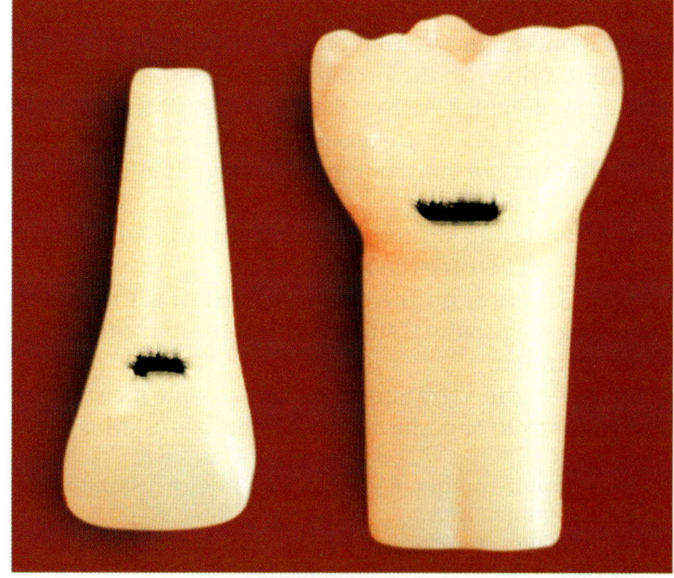

Fig. 7.56: Class V cavities involving the gingival third of the facial or lingual surface of all teeth

Classification based on the Size of Carious Lesions

Size 1: Minimal involvement of dentin that cannot be treated by remineralization alone.

Size 2: Moderate involvement of dentin. The amount of enamel remaining following cavity preparation is sound, well supported by dentin and not likely to fail under normal occlusal load. The remaining tooth structure is sufficiently strong to support the restoration.

Size 3: The cavity is enlarged beyond moderate. The remaining tooth structure is weakened extensively that cusps or incisal edges are split, or are likely to fail or left exposed to occlusal or incisal load. The cavity needs to be further enlarged so that the restoration can be designed to provide support and protection to the remaining tooth structure. Extensive caries with bulk loss of tooth structure has already occurred.

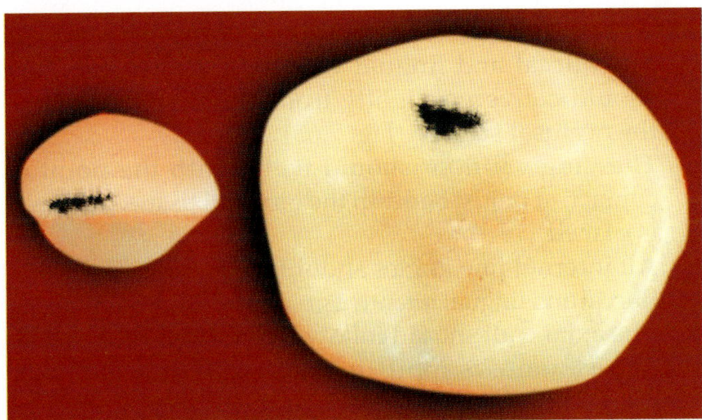

Fig. 7.57: Class VI cavities involving the incisal edge of anterior teeth or occlusal cusp heights of posterior teeth

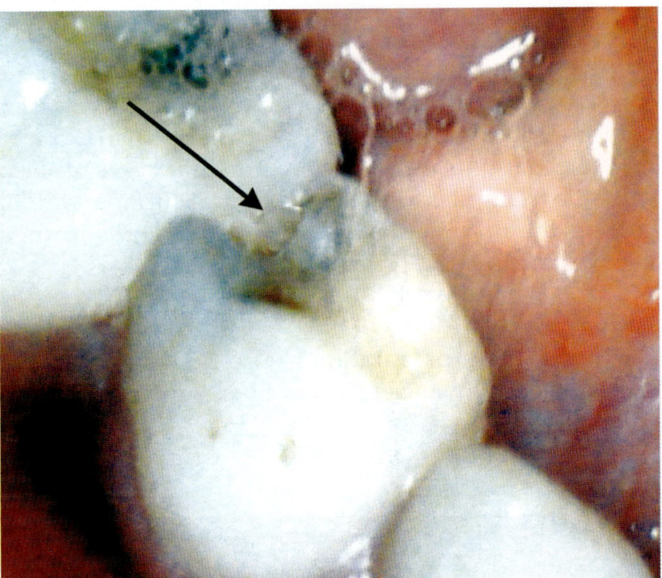

Fig. 7.58: Cavities on the proximal surfaces of molar teeth with access established from the occlusal surface

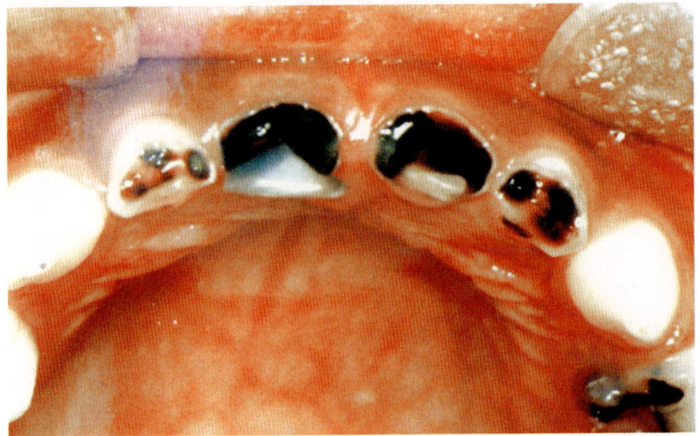

Fig. 7.59: Class III cavities on the proximal surfaces of anterior teeth that is extending to involve the labial and lingual surface

Site		Size		
	Minimal 1	Moderate 2	Enlarged 3	Extensive 4
1. Pit and fissure	1.1	1.2	1.3	1.4
2. Contact area	2.1	2.2	2.3	2.4
3. Cervical	3.1	3.2	3.3	3.4

AMALGAM RESTORATION FOR PRIMARY TEETH

Important points to be remembered while preparing a cavity for amalgam restoration are:

Occlusal (Fig. 7.60)

1. Outline form should include all fissures, areas of caries, pits and developmental grooves and should be dovetailed.
2. The extension of the occlusal portion of the cavity preparation depends on the primary molar involved:
   a. The occlusal portion usually is extended about one half the way across on the primary maxillary and mandibular first molars.
   b. For the primary mandibular second molar, extend the step completely across the occlusal surface.
   c. The primary maxillary second molar preparation includes only the nearest occlusal pit. The oblique ridge is not included unless undermined with carious lesions (Fig. 7.61).
3. The walls converge slightly with the greatest width at the pulpal floor (Fig. 7.62)
4. Cavosurface margins should be sharp
5. Angles of walls and floors should be slightly rounded

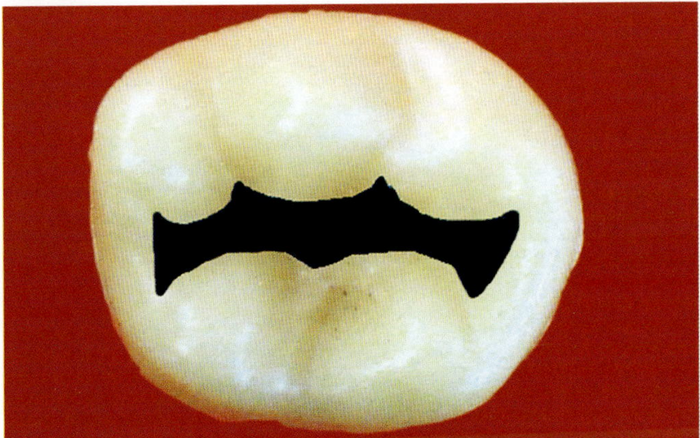

Fig. 7.60: Outline of the occlusal cavity should include all fissures, areas of caries, pits and should be dovetailed

6. Isthumus width should be one-third the width of the occlusal table
7. Depth of the cavity—0.2-0.8 mm into the dentin.

Proximal Box

1. The axiopulpal line angle should be gently rounded
2. The buccal and lingual walls should just extend into self-cleansing areas

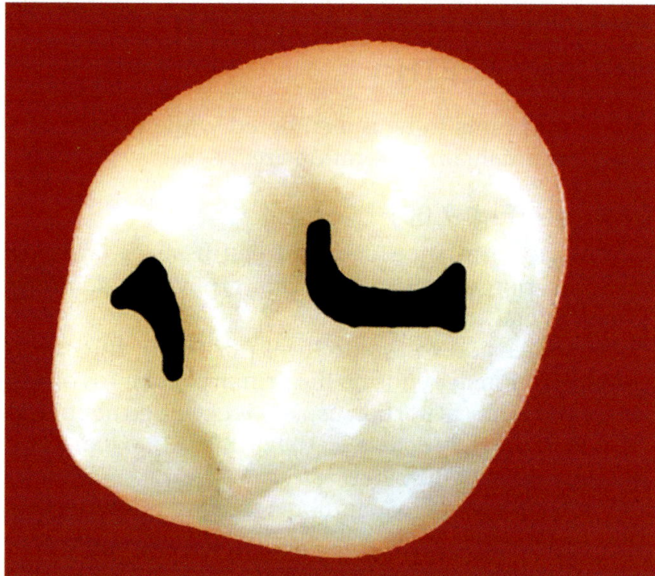

Fig. 7.61: Occlusal cavity preparation on a maxillary second molar does not cross the oblique ridge

3. A sharp 90° cavosurface angle is desirable
4. The buccal and lingual walls of the proximal box should converge slightly from the gingival floor to the occlusal surface (Fig. 7.63)
5. The gingival floor should be beneath the point of contact, at or just beneath the gingival tissue. No bevel is placed
6. All internal line angles should be gently rounded
7. Buccal and lingual retentive grooves are contraindicated
8. The axial wall should follow the contour of the tooth
9. The isthumus is approximately one-half to one-third the width of the occlusal surface.

CONSERVATIVE APPROACH FOR PROXIMAL CARIES IN DECIDUOUS TEETH

Tunnel Preparation

It is a type of cavity preparation made when the caries is located in the proximal surface, more than 2.5 mm from the marginal ridge. The proximal surface is reached from the triangular fossa in the occlusal surface without cutting the marginal ridge. Thus, a tunnel is formed keeping the marginal ridge intact.

Slot Preparation

This type cavity preparation is also done for proximal caries. The cavity outline is like a box with no step such as for gingival seat.

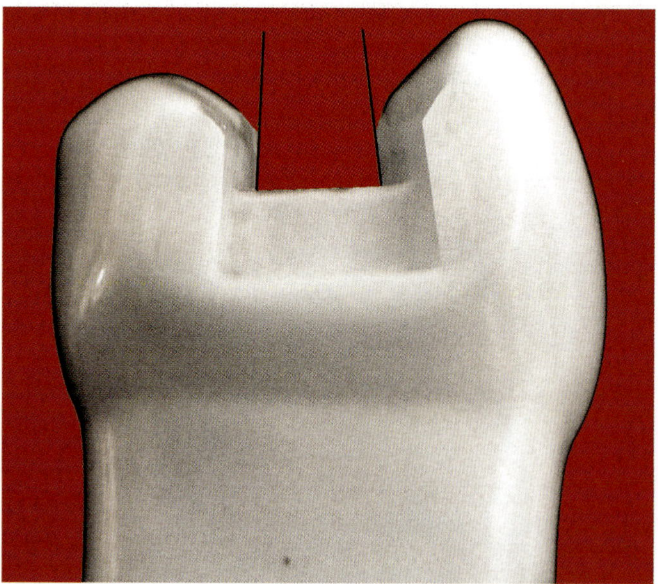

Fig. 7.62: The cavity wall should converge occlusally to provide retention to the restoration as seen from the proximal aspect

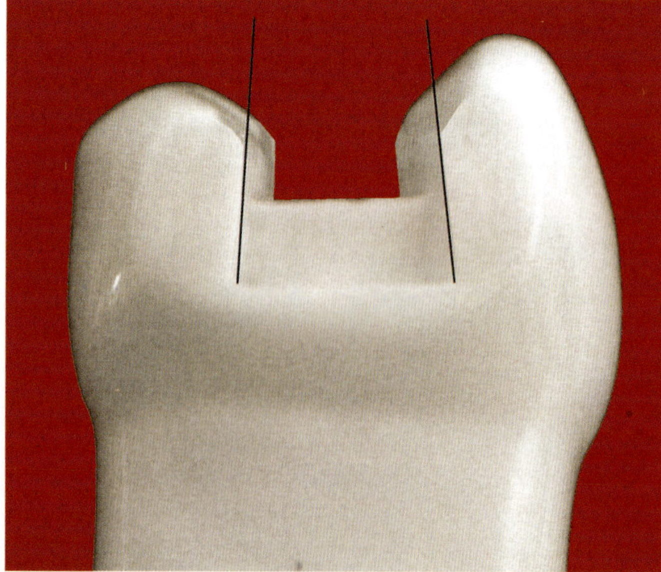

Fig. 7.63: The buccal and lingual walls of the proximal box should converge slightly from the gingival floor to the occlusal surface

Proximal Approach

This type cavity preparation is done when there is proximal caries and no adjacent teeth are present. So there is direct visualization of caries and also cavity preparation is directly done approaching from the proximal surface itself.

MATRIX BANDS, RETAINERS AND WEDGES

Matrix bands replaces the missing proximal surface of the tooth. Retainers are used to hold the bands in place. Wedges are used to adapt the matrix band closely to the tooth surface especially at the cervical constriction and thereby preventing any extension of material into the gingival tissue during condensation of the amalgam in a class II cavity preparation.

Classification of Matrix Band (Fig. 7.64)

The matrix band can be:
a. *Without retainers:* T-bands, spot welded
   With retainers: Tofflemire matrix retainers
b. *Metallic:* Spot welded, tofflemire matrix bands
   Nonmetallic: Mylar strip.

T-Band[7]

The T-band is available in several widths and thicknesses. This type of band is constructed at the time of the restoration. The disadvantage is that some difficulty may be experienced in placing this type of retainer as there is no retainer to hold the band in place.

Construction of T-band (Figs 7.65A to F)

1. Short and long arm are welded into a 'T'
2. The flanges of the short arm of 'T' are bent upwards

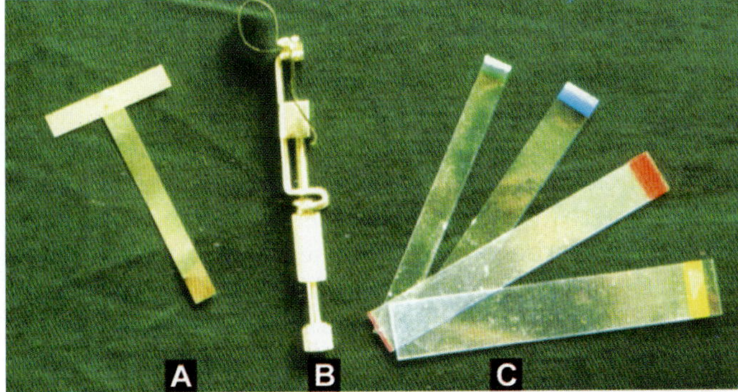

Fig. 7.64: Commonly used matrix band and retainers: (A) T-band; (B) Tofflemire; (C) Mylar strips

3. The long arm of the 'T' is bent into a circle
4. The short arm is folded over the circle formed. The wings should be loose enough for a sliding joint.
5. The matrix is placed on the tooth with the folded joint on the buccal side of the tooth.
6. The band is held with one finger and the tab is pulled tight around the tooth.
7. The tab is folded back over the joint distally.
8. The band is removed and flattened with the help of pliers.
9. The band is replaced on the tooth, the wedge placed and restoration completed.
10. When the restorative procedure is finished, the band is removed raising the tab over the joint and loosening the band.

Tofflemire (Fig. 7.66): Its use is restricted to a proximo-occlusal restoration done on a posterior tooth. It is available in straight and contra-angle types.

Mylar strips (Fig. 7.67): These are nonmetallic matrix band made of plastic used during glass ionomer and composite restorations.

Spot-Welded Matrix Band (Fig. 7.68)

The spot-welded matrix retainer lends itself to the philosophy of back-to-back amalgam restoration. It can be individually custom-made for each tooth.

The steps involved in fabrication are:
1. 5 cm length of band material is cut and the ends of the band are welded together in one spot to form a closed loop.
2. The loop is placed around the tooth and held firmly at the lingual surface with the index finger. With the No. 110 pliers, it is pinched together on the buccal portion until the band is drawn up snugly around the tooth.
3. The band is removed and welded together.
4. The excess band material is cut off 1 mm beyond the welded joint. The cut edges of the band are rounded and bent taking the excess back against the band.
5. The cervical and contact areas are contoured.
6. Holding the band with one finger, the wedge is inserted snugly at the cervical margin. A wedge can be inserted from either the buccal or lingual side to make sure the band is positioned snugly at the gingival margins and walls of the preparation.

Wedges

Different Types of Wedges

a. Based on the material used:
   – Plastic
   – Wooden

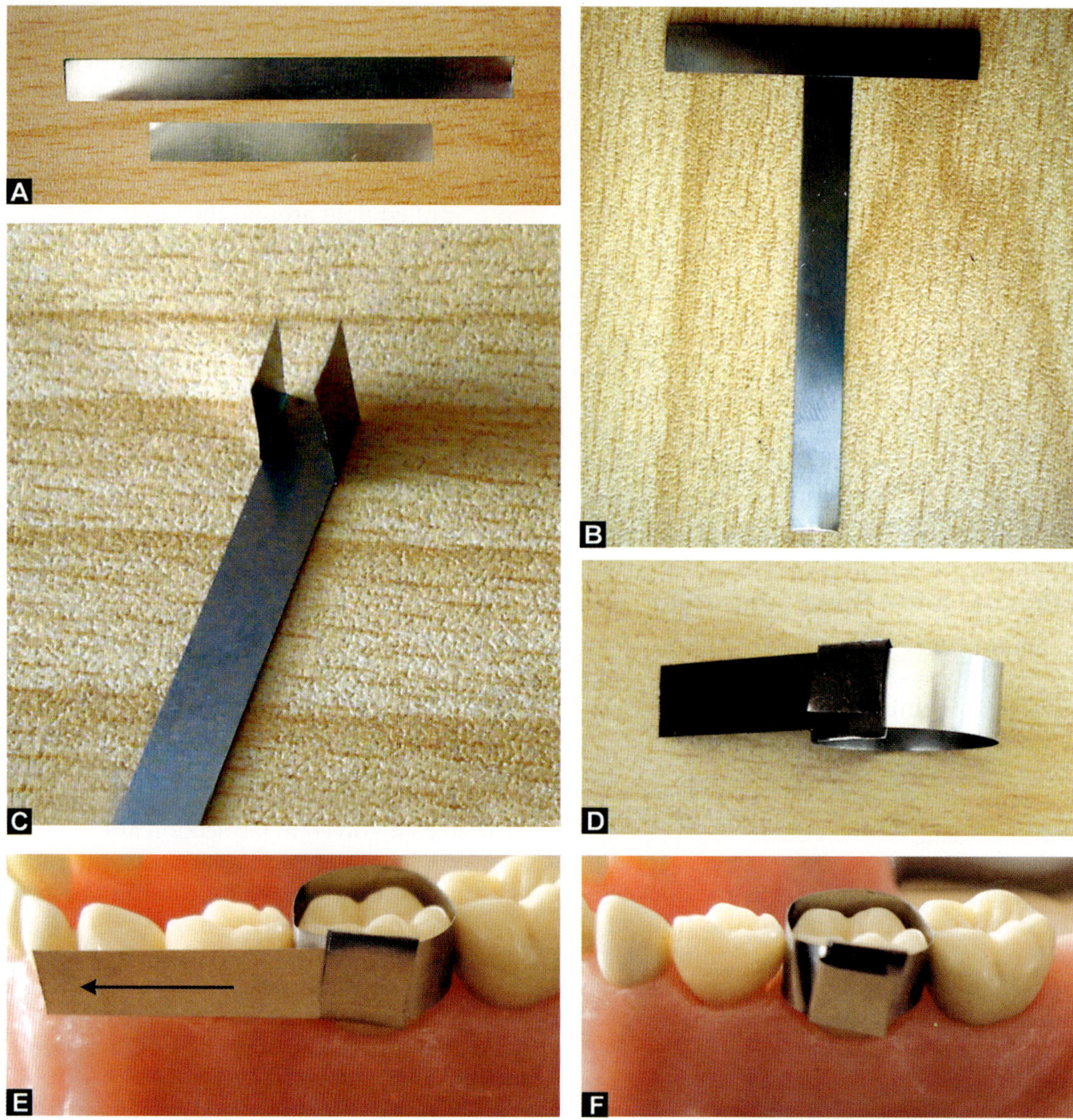

Figs 7.65 A to F: Steps in the constriction of T-band: (A) A matrix band is cut into a short and a long arm; (B) Short and long arm are welded into 'T'; (C) The flanges of the short arm of 'T' are bent upwards; (D) The long arm of the 'T' is bent into a circle. The short arm is folded over the circle; (E) The band is held with one finger and the tab is pulled tight around the tooth. The arrow indicates the direction of pull of the tab; (F) The tab is folded back over the joint

b. Based on the cross-sectional shape
   - Round
   - Triangular

Triangular wooden wedges are shown in Figure 7.69. Triangular wedges are preferred as they adapt well to the triangular embrasure space causing less trauma to gingiva.

Uses of Wedge

1. Adapts the matrix band close to the tooth
2. Protects the gingival papilla
3. Aides in mild tooth separation.

Results of Faulty Wedging

1. A concavity at the cervical portion of the proximal box can result if the rubber dam displaces the wedge or if too large a wedge is used. The purpose of the wedge in the primary dentition is to hold the matrix band at the cervical margins of the proximal box area.
2. An overextension of the restoration material may occur if the wedge is too loosely placed.
3. An open contact is caused by excessive wedging pressure, that to separates the approximating

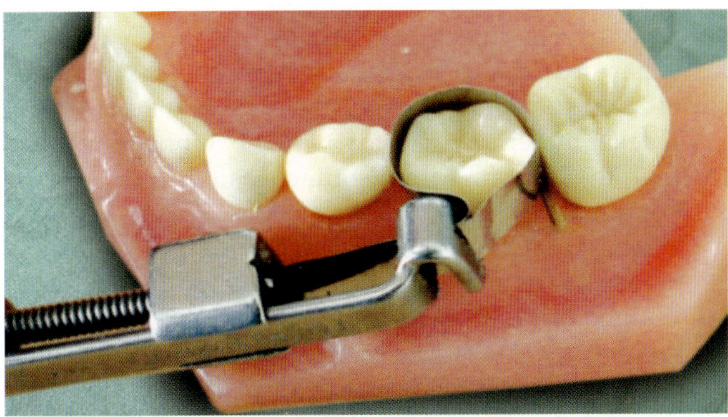

Fig. 7.66: Tofflemire retainer in position

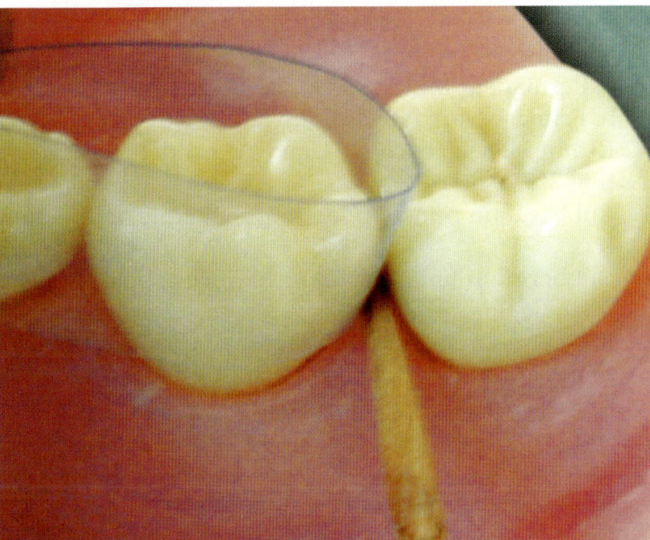

Fig. 7.67: Mylar strip in position

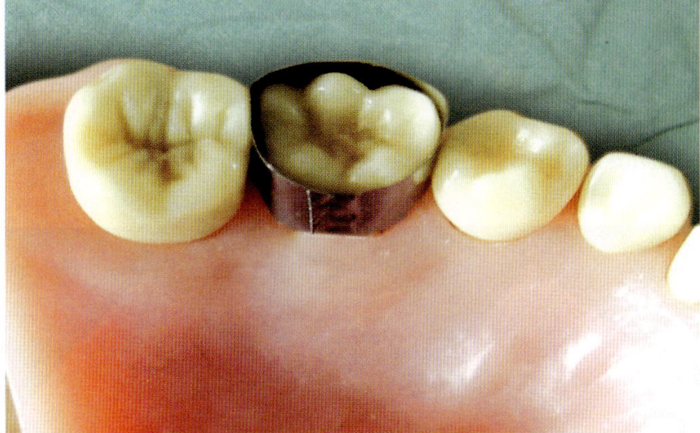

Fig. 7.68: Spot welded matrix band

contacts. If the child has primate spacing or space between the teeth, it is not necessary to restore the contact.

ISOLATION TECHNIQUES[8]

Objective of Isolation

- A dry, clean operating field
- Access and visibility
- Improved properties of dental materials
- Protection of the patient and operator
- Improved operating efficiency.

Isolation Involves Three Conceptual Elements

1. Moisture control—excludes saliva, sulcular fluid and gingival bleeding from the operating field.
2. Retraction and access—provides maximal exposure of the operating site. Involves maintaining mouth opening, depressing or retracting gingival tissue, tongue, lips and cheek.
3. Harm prevention—prevent aspiration or swallowing of small instruments, restorative debris or irrigation material and also prevents soft tissue injury.

Different Methods of Isolation

1. Rubber dam
2. High volume evacuator
3. Absorbents
4. Retraction cord
5. Mouth prop
6. Cotton rolls and holders
7. Medicines that reduce saliva—atropine, local anesthesia.

Rubber Dam[7,9-12]

It was introduced by SC Barnum in 1864. It is used to define the operating field by isolating one or more teeth from the oral environment. The dam eliminates saliva from the operating site and retracts the soft tissues.

Advantages of Rubber Dam

- It provides clean, dry operating field
- It provides clear access and visibility
- It improves properties of dental materials
- Protection of the patient and operator
- Improves operating efficiency
- Prevents aspiration of fluids used
- Prevents accidental ingestion of files/reamers
- Prevents injury to soft tissue such as tongue, cheek, gingiva
- Prevents patient from putting the tongue into the cavity
- Prevents the irrigating fluid coming in contact with oral soft tissues
- Reduced patient conversation
- Patient feels that the tooth is separated from the rest of the body and he will not feel the pain.

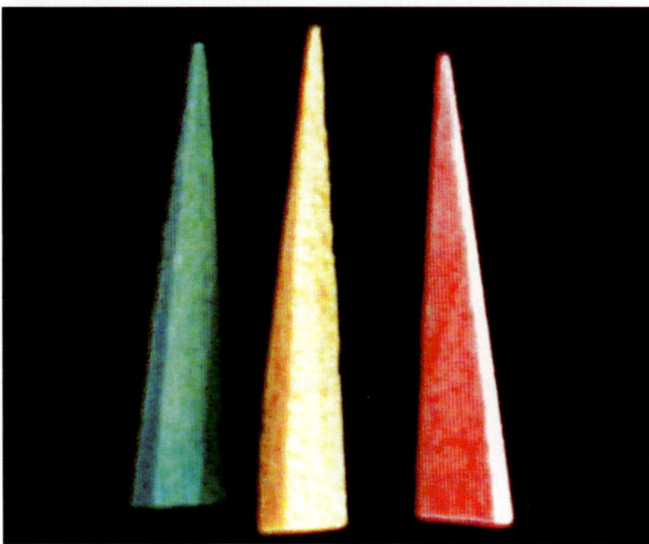

Fig. 7.69: Triangular wooden wedges

Disadvantages of Rubber Dam

- Time consumption
- Patient objection
- Certain conditions may preclude the use of rubber dam like:
  - Incompletely erupted teeth
  - Third molar isolation
  - Extremely malpositioned teeth
  - People suffering from asthma, mouth breathers.

Precautions to be Taken While Using Rubber Dam

- Patient must not be a mouth breather
- Clamps used must be tightly secured in place and a floss thread must be tied to the clamp, which helps retrieve the clamp if ingested or aspirated.
- The dam should be checked not to cover the nostril
- If patient is allergic to latex, rubber dam napkin should be used
- Lips should be lubricated to provide drying
- The clamp must not impinge on the gingiva nor traumatize the adjacent teeth.

Armamentarium Used for Rubber Dam Application

1. Rubber dam material (Fig. 7.70): It is made of latex material and is available as:
   Size 5 × 5 inches (Pediatric purpose) or 6 × 6 inches (Adult size)
   Thickness
   - Thin (0.006″)
   - Medium (0.008″)
   - Heavy (0.010″)
   - Extra-heavy (0.012″)
   - Special heavy (0.014″)

Color green, blue, black, brown.

It has a dull and bright surface. The dull surface should face the occlusal aspect as it reflects less light.

Thicker material resists tear and the thinner ones pass through the tight proximal contact easily.

2. Retainers:
   Wingless retainers (Fig. 7.71A)
   Retainers for anterior teeth (Fig. 7.71B)
   Winged retainers (Fig. 7.71C)
   Retainers are used to anchor the dam to the most posterior tooth to be isolated. Different sizes are available for different teeth.
   Parts of a retainer: It includes bow, jaws, prong (Fig. 7.72). The prongs contact the tooth at 4 regions, two on the buccal and two on the lingual.
   Clamps used for:
   a. Permanent Molars: Ivory 8A, 14A,14
   b. Primary Molars: SS White No. 27,26
3. Rubber dam forceps: Used to hold the retainer (Fig. 7.73).
4. Rubber dam punch: Used to punch hole on the dam (Fig. 7.74).
5. Rubber dam template: Guides during placement of the hole (Fig. 7.75)
6. Rubber dam holder/frame: It can be made of plastic (Fig. 7.76) or metal (Fig. 7.77). It is used to stretch the rubber dam sheet to gain clear access of the operating site.
7. Rubber dam napkin: Used to keep the dam away from the skin especially when the person is allergic to latex. It also absorbs moisture that may appear at the corner of the mouth (Fig. 7.78).

Placement of Rubber Dam[13,14]

Steps involved are:
1. Obtaining anesthesia
2. Evaluate the interproximal contact with dental floss
3. Mark the punch holes—using the template
4. Make punch holes using rubber dam punch

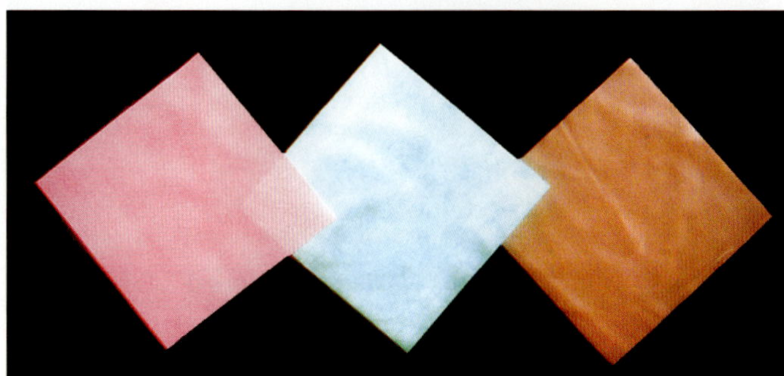

Fig. 7.70: Rubber dam material in pink, green and brown color

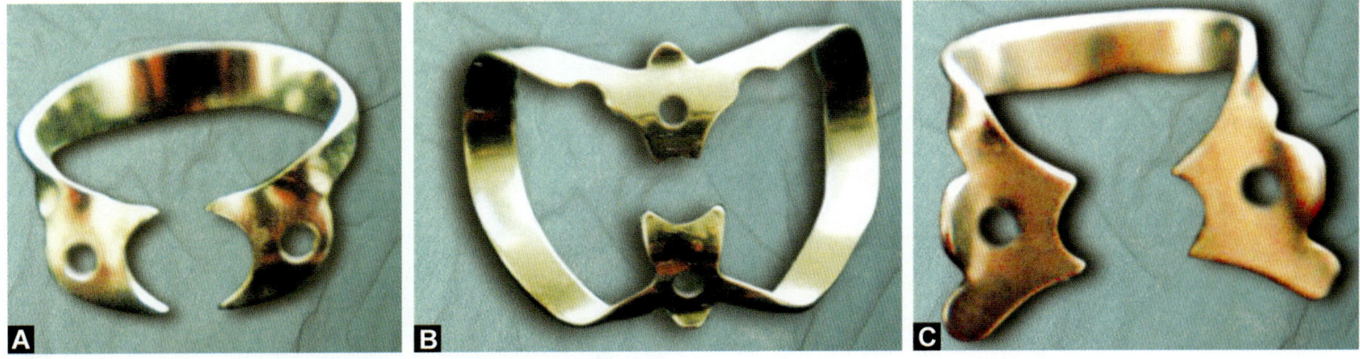

Figs 7.71A to C: Rubber dam clamps or retainers: (A) Wingless retainers; (B) Retainers for anterior teeth; (C) Winged retainers

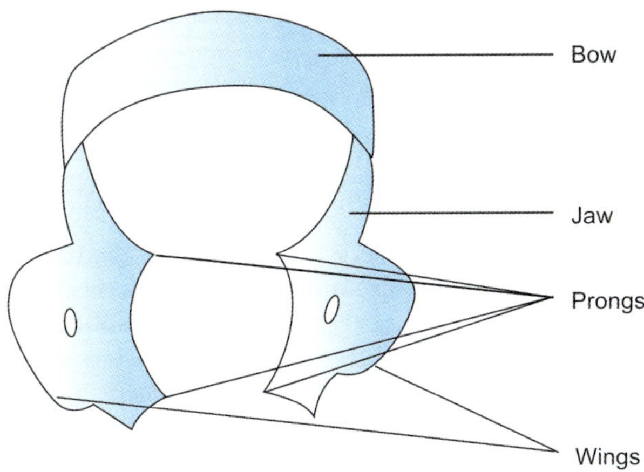

Fig. 7.72: Parts of a retainer

5. Lubricate the area of rubber dam around the punched hole with vaseline
6. Selection of the correct retainer
7. Rubber dam placement (one of the 3 methods)
   – Clamp is placed first on the tooth followed by the sheet
   – The sheet is placed first followed by the clamp
   – Both the clamp and the sheet are placed simultaneously; this is possible when winged clamp is being used.
   Areas where clamps cannot be placed, the sheet can be stabilized with dental floss tied around the neck of the teeth.
8. Placement of napkin and frame.

> Rubber dam clamp size preference:
> SS White No. 27 is preferred in primary teeth and Ivory No W14 in the young permanent teeth.

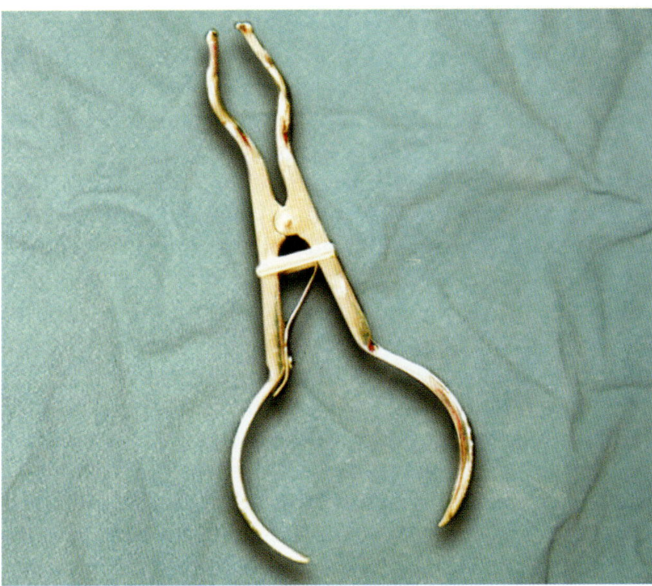

Fig. 7.73: Rubber dam clamp forceps

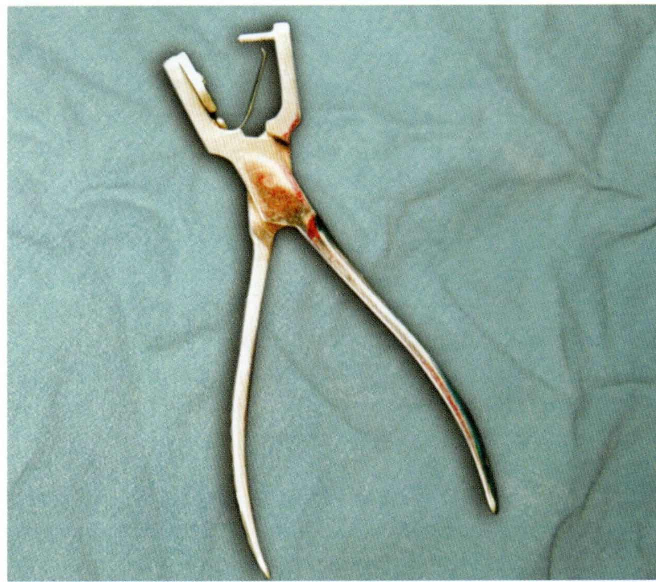

Fig. 7.74: Rubber dam punch

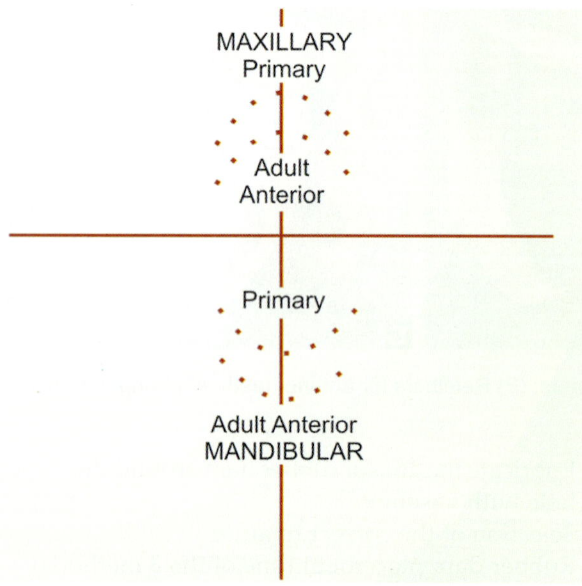

Fig. 7.75: Rubber dam template

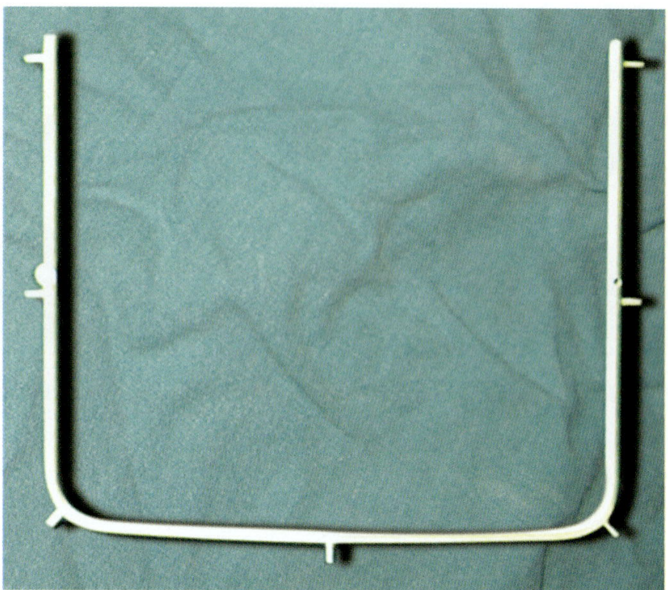

Fig. 7.77: Rubber dam frame (Metal)

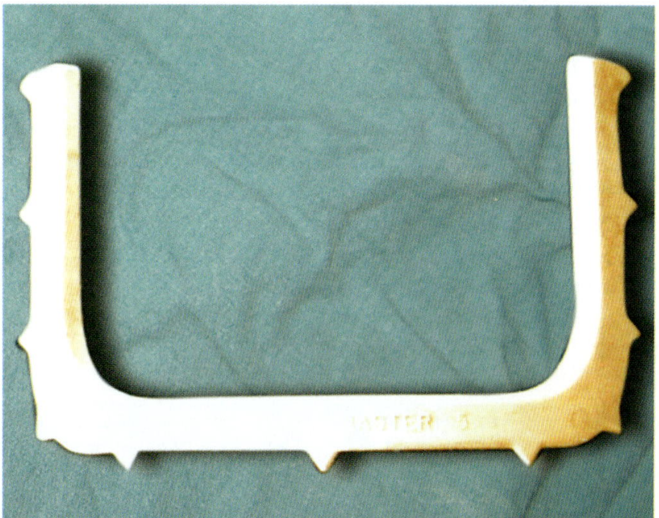

Fig. 7.76: Rubber dam frame (Plastic)

Errors in placement of rubber dam:

1. Off centered arch
2. Inappropriate distance between two holes
3. Incorrect arch form of holes
4. Inappropriate sized retainer
5. Retainer pinched tissue
6. Shredded or torn dam.

High Volume Evacuators and Saliva Ejectors

High volume evacuators (HVE) (Fig. 7.79) are used for suctioning water and debris from the mouth. The tip of the evacuator (Fig. 7.80) is placed near the operating area.

The saliva ejector (Fig. 7.81) removes saliva that collects on the floor of the mouth (Fig. 7.82). It is used in conjunction with sponges, cotton rolls and rubber dam. Saliva ejectors remove water slowly and are less efficient to pick debris (Fig. 7.83). It should be placed in an area least likely to interfere with the operator's movements usually in the floor of the mouth. The tip of the ejector must be smooth and made from a nonirritating material. Disposable and inexpensive plastic ejectors may be shaped by bending with the fingers and used.

Absorbents and Throat Shields

Absorbents such as cotton rolls (Figs 7.84A and B) and cellulose wafers are used for short periods of isolation and topical fluoride applications. They are alternatives when rubber dam application is impractical or impossible. Cotton rolls have to be positioned one each on the buccal and lingual vestibule adjacent to the working tooth and one in the upper buccal vestibule on the same side corresponding to the major salivary glands while operating in the lower quadrants. While operating on the upper quadrants, one cotton roll is positioned in the buccal vestibule adjacent to the working tooth.

Throat shields (Fig. 7.85) are indicated when small instruments are being used without rubber dam. A gauze piece (2 × 2 inch) that is spread over the tongue and the posterior part of the mouth acts as a shield. It helps to retrieve any instruments (Files or broaches) or restorations that would have accidentally slipped, which otherwise would have been aspirated or swallowed.

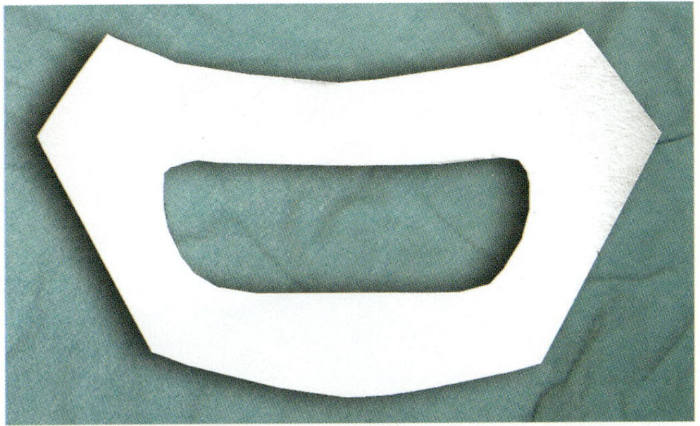

Fig. 7.78: Rubber dam napkin

- High copper alloy (Contains >6% < 30%)
- Admixed alloy (mixture of low and high copper alloy)

4. Zinc containing/Non-zinc containing
- Some alloys contain zinc. It acts as deoxidizer or scavenger (0-2%)

5. According to the method of dispensing
- As powder and liquid form
- As a capsule (Fig. 7.86)
- As pellets or pills of alloy powder
- As preamalgamated powder (3% of the Hg is mixed with the alloy powder and this facilitates faster reaction).

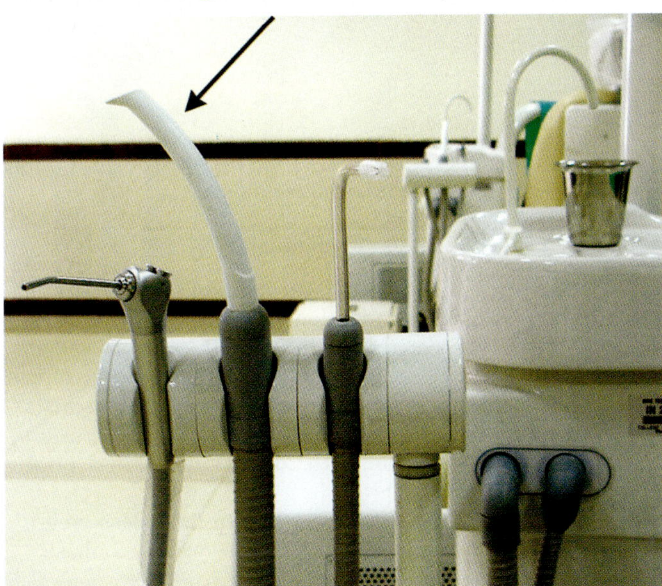

Fig. 7.79: High vacuum evacuators

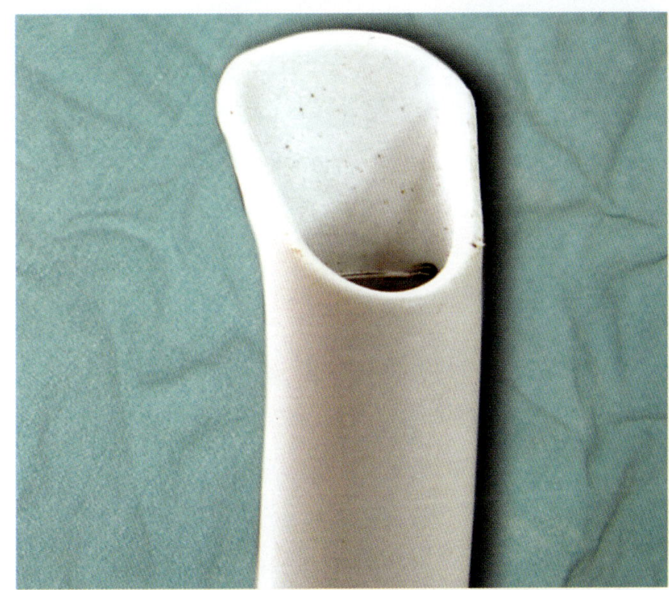

Fig. 7.80: The tip of HVE is wide enabling suctioning of debris

SILVER AMALGAM RESTORATIVE MATERIAL

Silver amalgam restorative material is obtained by the triturition of amalgam alloy with mercury.

Classification of amalgam alloy

1. According to the shape
- Lathe cut (Irregularly shaped)
- Spherical (Spherical in shape)
- Mixed (Contain mixture of lathe cut and spherical)

2. According to the size
- Fine cut (Partical size is 36 µ)
- Micro cut (Partical size is 26 µ)

3. According to the composition
- Low copper alloy (Contains <6%)

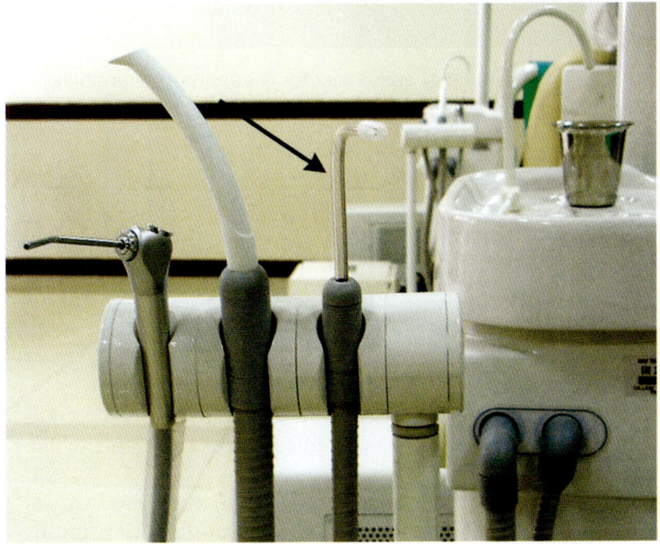

Fig. 7.81: Saliva ejector

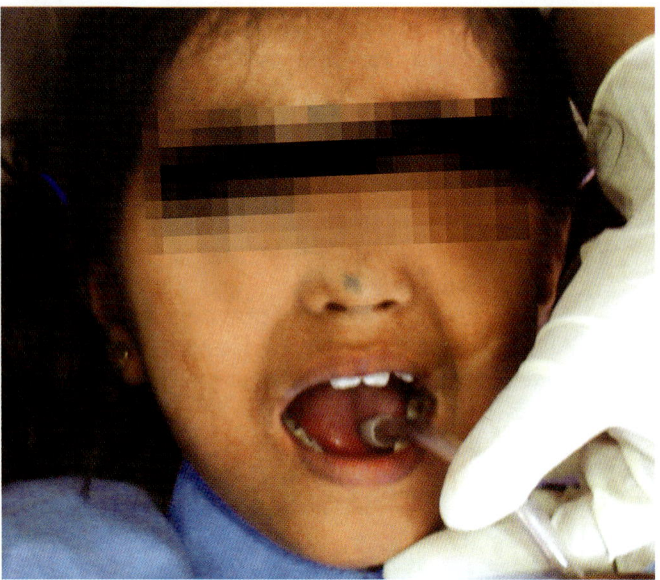

Fig. 7.82: The saliva ejector is placed in the floor of the mouth

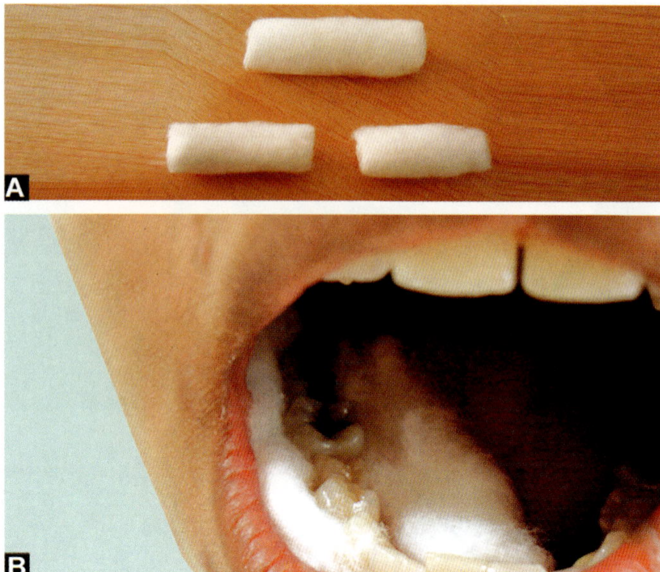

Figs 7.84A and B: (A) Cotton rolls used for isolation; (B) Cotton rolls position in the mouth

Criteria for selection of amalgam alloy

1. Small particles are selected: Better strength, good surface finish, good marginal adaption, poor corrosion resistance
2. Spherical is selected: Better strength, easy to carve, good finish, good marginal adaptation, good corrosion resistance and easy condensation. (Lathe cut resists condensation, may result in a porous, poor corrosion resistance restoration with rough surface and poor marginal adaptation)
3. High copper is preferred: Better strength, less creep, good corrosion resistance due to absence of γ-2 phase.

Drawbacks of silver amalgam

1. Good conduction of heat: Requires good insulation
2. Poor marginal adaptation: So varnish is applied
3. Poor esthetics
4. Poor modulus of elasticity, proportional limit and tensile strength
5. Electrolytic corrosion
6. Poor adhesion to tooth structure
7. Ditched amalgam.

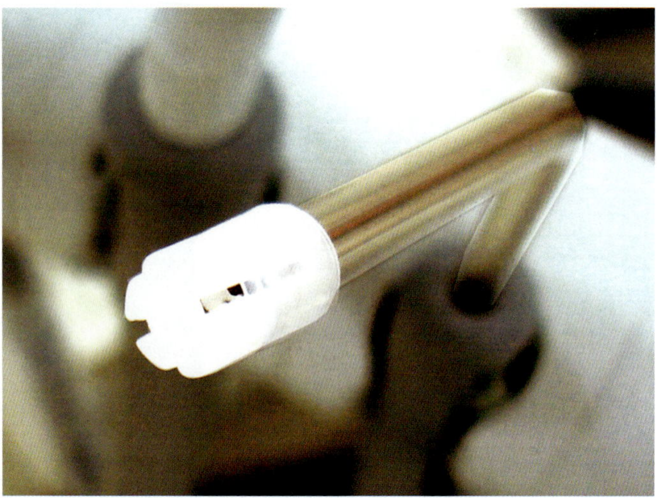

Fig. 7.83: The tip of saliva ejector is very narrow enabling suction of only liquids

Properties of amalgam

1. Increased mercury—leads to increased expansion, creep and corrosion
2. Compressive strength—Admixed is 430 Mpa after 7 days
3. Tensile strength—Admixed is 50 Mpa after 24 hours
4. Surface hardness—110 KHN
5. Working time—3-8 minutes
6. Setting time—5-10 minutes
7. Increased expansion is due to: increased mercury, short trituration, low condensation pressure and water contamination
8. Creep is associated with: increased or decreased trituration, time lag between trituration and condensation, increased mercury, less condensation force.

Condensation and Carving of Silver Amalgam

1. The amalgam alloy and mercury is dispensed and mixed as per the manufacturer's instructions (Fig. 7.87).
2. The material is loaded into the amalgam carrier (Fig. 7.88). Proximal box is first filled in a class II cavity. In other cavities it is started from one side slowly moving and filling the entire cavity.

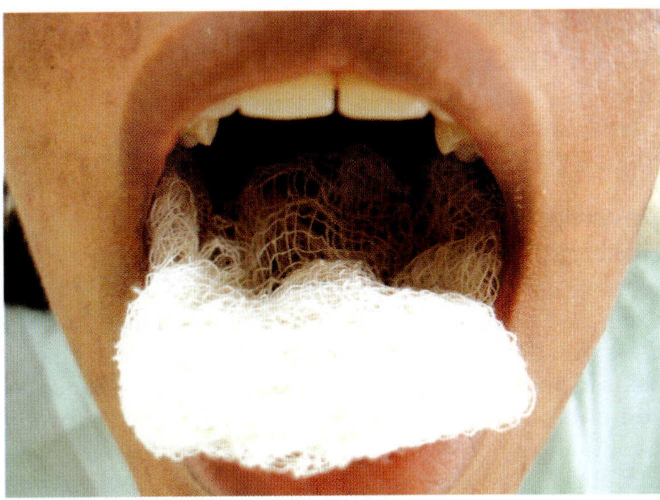

Fig. 7.85: Throat shield. It is especially useful when operating on the upper posterior tooth where the access is limited due to reduced mouth opening in children. While operating on the lower teeth, the tooth to be treated should be exposed and the shield can be placed on the tongue extending posterior to the operating tooth

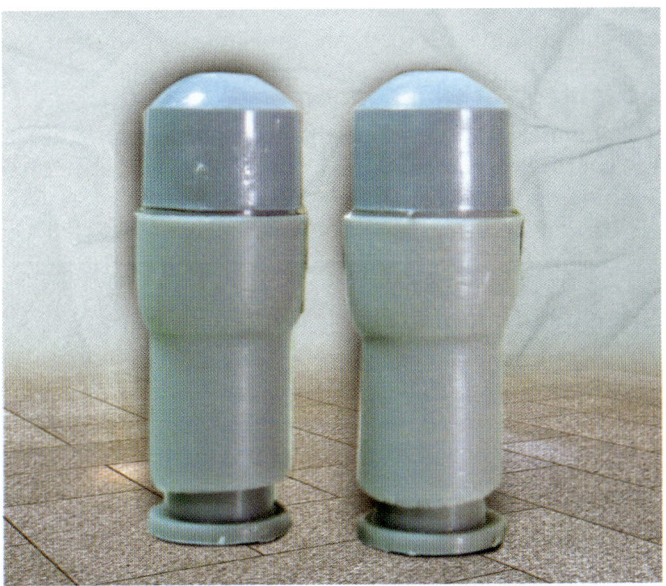

Fig. 7.86: Amalgam alloy and mercury in capsule form

3. The material is firmly condensed into the cavity. Amalgam is condensed using condensers. The initial condenser should be small (Fig. 7.89A) enough to condense the material into the line angles. Each condensing stroke should overlap the previous condensing stroke to ensure that the entire mass is well condensed. The cavity is overfilled and condensed with a large condenser (Fig. 7.89B). Parallelogram condenser (Fig. 7.89C) is used to condense narrow occlusal cavities.

4. This is followed by precarve burnishing of the amalgam. It is a form of condensation done with a large ball burnisher (Fig. 7.90A) using heavy strokes mesiodistally and faciolingually. This helps to remove all the excess amalgam and blends the restorative material with the cavity margins.
5. Initial gross carving of the restoration is done followed by fine carving of cuspal inclines, triangular fossa and the grooves. Hollenback, wards or diamond amalgam carvers are used for the purpose of carving amalgam (Fig. 7.91).
6. Wedges and the matrix band can be removed after initial carving.
7. Postcarve burnishing is done using ball burnisher (Fig. 7.90B): It involves the light rubbing of the carved surface to improve smoothness and produce a satin (not a shiny) appearance.
8. Finishing and polishing is done after 24 hours of insertion.

Armamentarium used for finishing and polishing of amalgam:

1. Pointed, white, fused alumina stone or a green carborundum stone is used to correct minor discrepancy
2. Green stone—is more abrasive than white stone and thus is used for correction of gross discrepancies
3. Finishing burs
4. Coarse rubber abrasive point at low speed
5. Medium and fine grit abrasive points in low speed
6. Final polishing—rubber cup with pumice and chalk.

Bonded Amalgam Restorations[15]

Retention of amalgam in a large cavity is very difficult. Dental adhesives are used as lining materials for amalgam to create bonded amalgam restoration. Amalgam is condensed over the uncured resin and this forms intermixing of resin and amalgam to form mechanical bond. The advantages of bonded amalgam restorations are amalgam retention, tooth reinforcement, and improved microleakage.

Amalgam bond, is the first one to be available commercially. It is a 4-META (4-methacryloxyethyl trimellitate anhydride) resin based adhesive. Other resin systems that are Panavia-F- Resin cement (dual cure, Kuraray Medical Inc. Japan), Dual cure (3M ESPE, USA).

Mercury Hygiene

Precautions that should be taken regarding the mercury exposure in dental office to protect the office staff and the patients are:

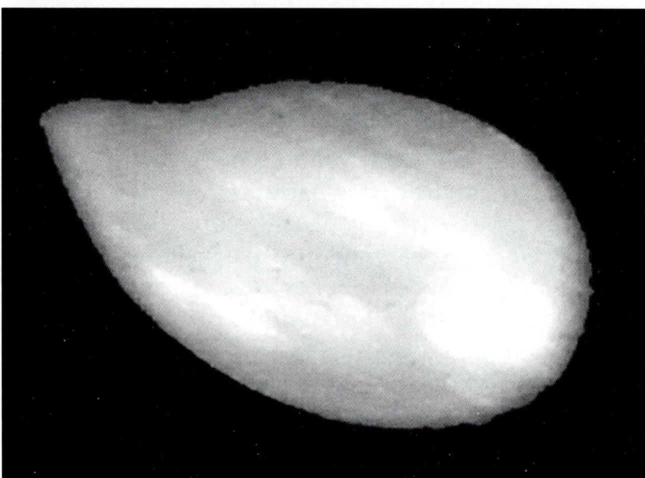

Fig. 7.87: Silver amalgam ready to use

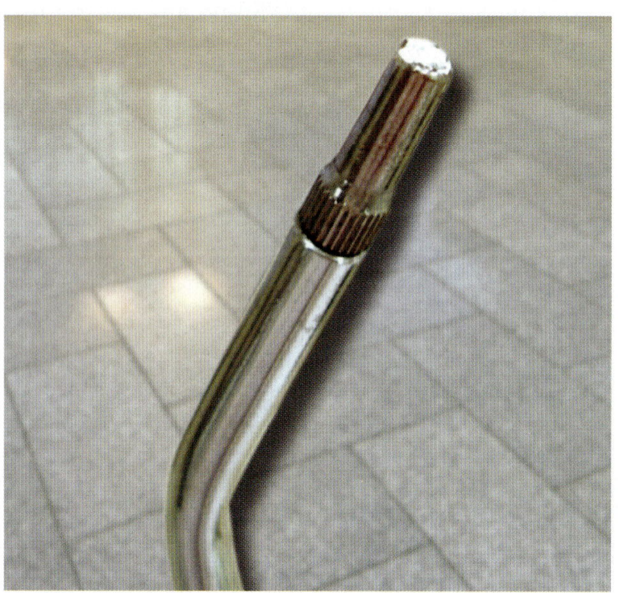

Fig. 7.88: Silver amalgam loaded into the amalgam carrier

- When removing an old amalgam restoration, rubber dam should be in place and high volume evacuation should be used. Glasses and disposable face masks should be worn.
- Amalgam capsules should be preferred to the conventional dispensing.
- Closed amalgamators should be used.
- Free mercury and amalgam scraps should be stored in an unbreakable, tightly closed container away from any source of heat preferably in water.
- Since mercury vaporizes at room temperatures, operatories should be well ventilated to minimize the mercury level in the air.

GLASS IONOMER (POLYALKENOATE) CEMENT[16-22]

Glass = formulation of glass powder
Ionomer = ionomeric acid with carboxyl group

Development of Glass Ionomer Restorative Material

During early studies in 1965 and 1966 AD, Wilson examined cements prepared by mixing dental silicate glass powder with aqueous solutions of various organic acids including polyacrylic acids. The first glass ionomer cements lacked workability and hardened slowly. Eventually Kent et al 1972, found a glass that was high in fluoride that gave usable cement, ASPA I which still had some drawbacks.

Later in 1972 Wilson and Crisp, found that adding tartaric acid, improving manipulation, extending working time and greatly sharpening the setting rate. This refinement of ASPA I was termed ASPA II and constituted the first practical glass ionomer cement. Over the years research workers have further improved glass ionomer cements in terms of setting rate, translucency and strength.

Advantage of Glass Ionomers

1. Chemical bonding to both enamel and dentin
2. Thermal expansion similar to that of tooth structure
3. Biocompatibility
4. Uptake and release of fluoride
5. Decreased moisture sensitivity when compared to resins.

Classification of Glass Ionomer Cement

Type I: Luting cement
Type II: Restorative cement
   Type II 1: Esthetic restorative cement
   Type II 2: Reinforced restorative cement
Type III: Lining or base cement

Dispensing of Glass Ionomer Cements[23]

1. *Powder (Liquid system):* The powder and liquid are dispensed and mixed manually. Appropriate sized scoop is used for accurate dispensing of the powder.
2. *Capsules:* The glass ionomer cement in the form of capsule system is a modern application method, which simplifies and allows procedures to be performed with greater ease and efficiency. These capsules contain pre-measured glass ionomer powder and liquid, which ensures correct ratio, consistency of mix and a predictable result. These capsules have angled nozzle that act as a syringe for accurate placement of the material in to a cavity or a crown for cementation.

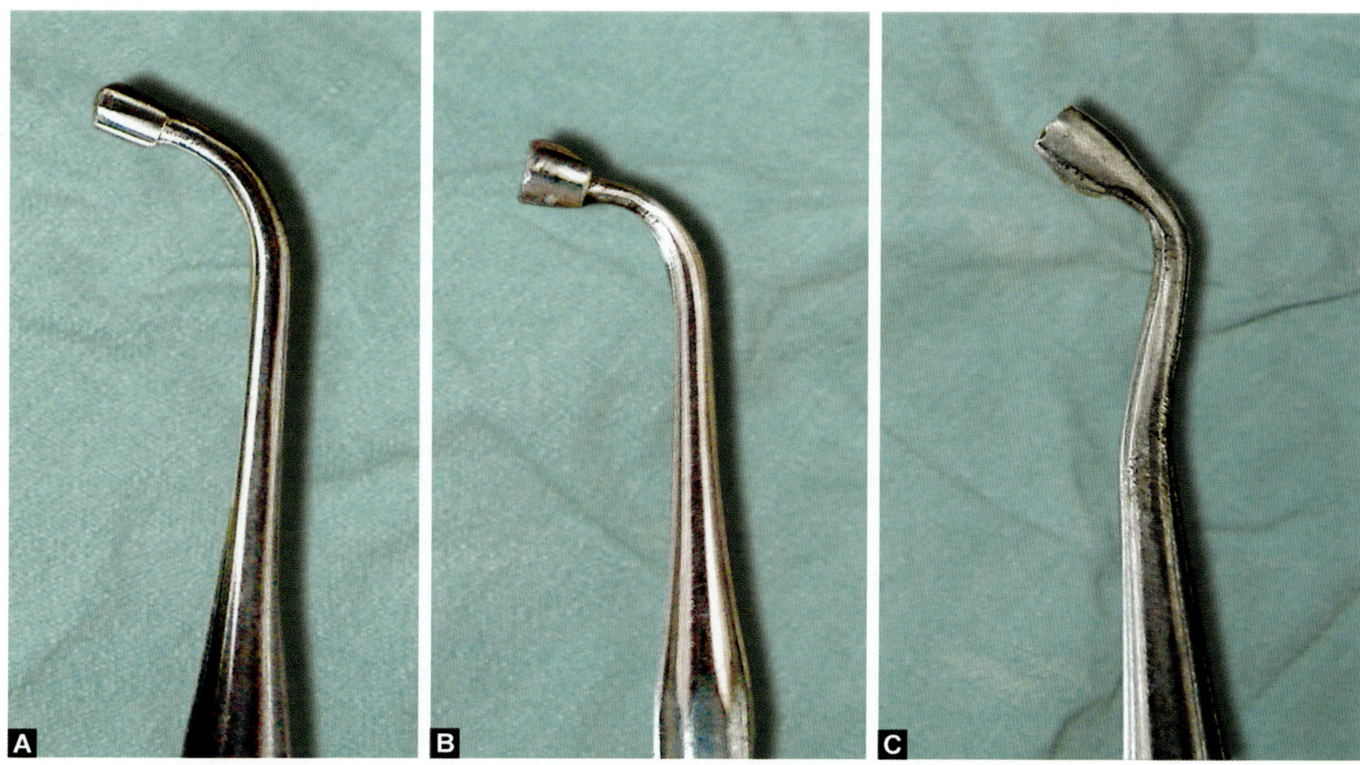

Figs 7.89A to C: Amalgam condensors: (A) Small round condenser; (B) Large round condenser;
(C) Parallelogram condenser

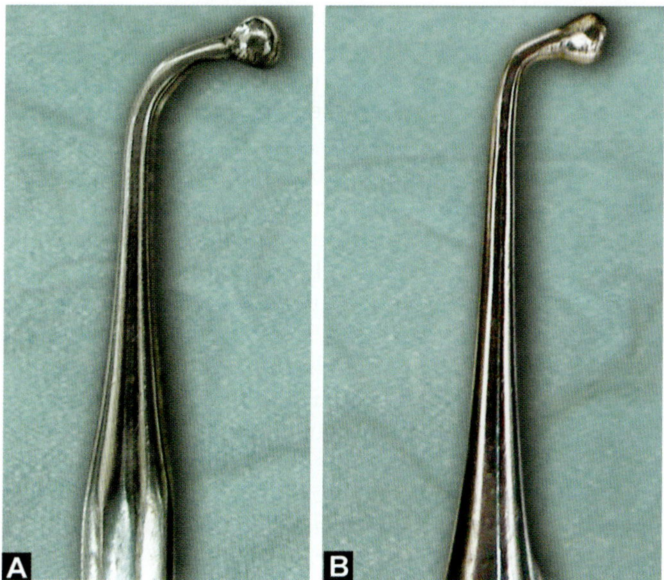

Figs 7.90A and B: Ball burnisher: (A) Large ball burnisher;
(B) Small ball burnisher

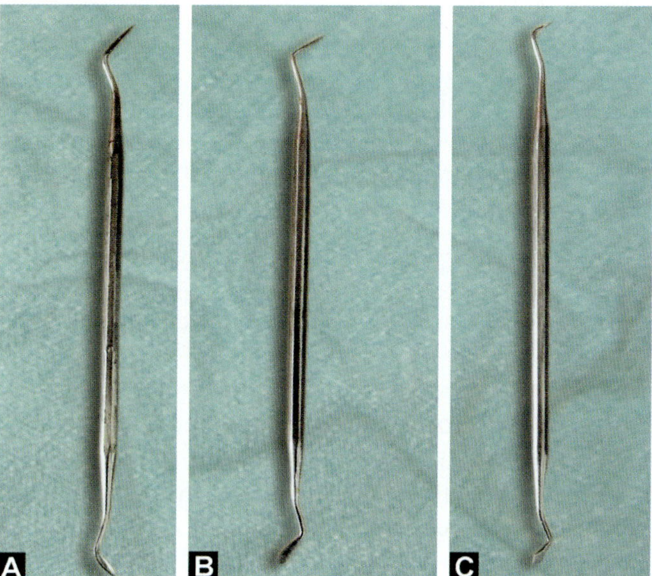

Fig. 7.91: Amalgam carvers: (A) Hollenback carver; (B) Wards
carver; (C) Diamond carver

3. *Paste (Paste dispensing system):* This is the latest development in the glass ionomer cement technology. This dispensing system was designed with the objectives of providing optimum ratio, easy mixing, easy placement, total reliability, using a specially designed cartridge and an easy-to-use material dispenser. In order to provide the material in a paste—paste consistency, an ultra fine glass powder was designed specifically. The low particle size provides the mixed cement with a thixotropic creamy consistency.

Composition of Glass Ionomer Cement

Glass ionomer cement is a product of an acid-base reaction. The basic component is a calcium aluminosilicate glass containing fluoride. The acid is a polyelectrolyte, which is a homopolmer or copolymer of unsaturated carboxylic acids known scientifically as alkenoic acids. Most commonly used is polyacrylic acid.

Powder

- Calcium fluoroaluminosilicate glass
- Lanthanum, strontium, barium or zinc oxide

Liquid

- Polyacrylic acid (50%)
- Itaconic acid (increases the reactivity and reduces the viscosity and tendency for gelation)
- Maleic acid, or tricarboxylic acid
- Tartaric acid—improves handling characteristics, increases viscosity and   working time and reduces setting time.

The three essential constituents of dental ionomer glasses are silica (SiO_2), alumina (Al_2O_3), and calcium fluoride or fluorite (CaF_2).

> The visual appearance of the glass depends on its chemical composition—glasses high in silica (>40%) are transparent, high in Al_2O_3 or CaF_2 are opaque.

> **Water settable GIC or anhydrous GIC**
>
> To extend the working time, the powder contains freeze dried acid powder. Water is used to mix the material.

> Glasses are prepared by fusing the components between 1100°C to 1500°C and then poured onto a metal plate. The glass is then ground to a fine powder depending whether it is a type I (30-50 µ), II (15-20 µ) or III(< 15 µ).

Setting Reaction of Glass Ionomer Cement[24,25]

When the glass ionomer cement powder and liquid are brought together to form a paste, the glass powder which is basic reacts with liquid that is acid, to form a salt hydrogel which is the binding matrix. Here water in the reaction medium forms a part of the hydrogel.

Different Stages in the Setting Reaction

- Initially the surface of the glass is attacked resulting in decomposition of the glass and release of Al and Ca ions
- These Al and Ca ions then migrate into the aqueous phase of the cement.

- As the reactions proceed the concentration of ions and the viscosity of the paste increases.
- Initially calcium ions forms part of the cross linkage with polyacrylic acid chains to form solid mass.
- Later within next 24 hours new phase is formed with aluminium ions becoming bound to cement matrix– leading to more rigid set cement.
- Gelation of the polyacids occurs by the metal ions leading to set cement.
- Calcium polyacrylate is responsible for the initial set and aluminium polyacrylate for the final hardening of the matrix.
- Sodium and fluoride do not participate in the cross linking of the cement. Some sodium ions may replace H+ of carboxylic group, but rest combine with fluoride to from NaFl which is uniformly dispersed within the cement.
- Unreacted glass particles are coated by silica gel (that forms during removal of the cations from the surface of the particles).
- Final set cement consists of agglomerated unreacted powder particles surrounded by a silica gel in an amorphous matrix of hydrated calcium and aluminium polysalts.

Role of Moisture Contamination and Dehydration

During the setting process the cement should be protected from two extremes—desiccation and aqueous environment. This can be achieved in an atmosphere of 80% relative humidity. The cement should be protected by varnish or petroleum jelly.

It is important to remember that after initial set but before the cement is fully hardened, a proportion of cement containing aluminium, calcium, fluoride and polyacrylate ions are in soluble form and so can be dissolved out of the cement by aqueous fluid leading to permanently weakened matrix.

If at this stage water is released out due to excessive drying, restoration will lose its aesthetic appeal, shrink and will become brittle. It may take 1 hour until the cement remains vulnerable to moisture. Hardening continues for 24 hours. Slow maturation continues over the period of months and becomes more rigid and gathers strength.

Factors Affecting Setting Characteristic of Glass Ionomer Cement

- *Role of fluorides:* Fluoride forms metal complexes that retards the binding of cations to anionic sites on the polyelectrolytic chain and thereby delaying gelation and prolonging working time. It also delays pH dependent gelation.

- *Role of tartaric acid:* It improves manipulation of the cement and increases the working time, it increases the viscosity and increase the strength of the set cement.

Factors Affecting Rate of Setting of Glass Ionomer Cement

1. Glass composition, especially the Al_2O_3/SiO_2 ratio and fluoride content. Increased ratio—faster is the set, shorter is the working time. Fluoride prolongs the working time.
2. Particle size—finer particle size-faster is the set and shorter is the working time.
3. Addition of tartaric acid sharpens the set without shortening the working time.
4. Relative proportion of constituents in the cement mix, i.e. glass/polyacid/tartaric acid/water. Greater proportion of glass and lower proportion of water, faster is the setting time and shorter is the working time.
5. Temperature of mixing—in higher temperature the faster is the set, shorter is the working time.

Properties of Glass Ionomer Cement[26-29]

Physical Properties

- Sets rapidly in the mouth.
- Initial compressive strength is low (24 hours)—150-200 Mpa but increases with time. After one year it can reach to 400 Mpa.
- Tensile strength (24 hours)—6.6 Mpa
- Hardness—70 KHN
- Solubility—0.7%
- Bioactive and possesses chemical bonding with the tooth.
- Coefficient of thermal expansion is close to that of the tooth causing less microleakage around the restoration.

Esthetics

- Translucent material.
- Color is much more stable. Resistance to stain is dependent on a good surface finish.

Adhesion

- Permanently adheres to the untreated enamel and dentin chemically.
- Principle barrier to adhesion is water.
- Mechanism of adhesion—chelation of carboxyl group of the polyacids with the calcium ions in the apatite of enamel and dentin forming strong ionic bonds. This ionic bonds are later replaced by hydrogen bonds

which increases the strength as the material sets. Surface conditioning also improves adhesion.

Biocompatibility

- Excellent marginal seal and fluoride release—reducing the risk of developing secondary caries
- Continuous fluoride release occurs around the restoration—tooth interface (3 mm) for a period of 18 months.
- The acid groups are attached to the polymer molecule which have limited diffusibility, hence the pulp effects are limited to areas immediately adjacent to the material. When fluid filled dentinal tubules are in direct contact with the unset material, 2 problems occur:
  1. High ionic concentration in the material cause dentinal fluid to rapidly diffuse outward into the cement producing a change in pulpal pressure, creating pain and sensitivity.
  2. Hydrogen ions may move into the tubules towards the pulp and cause chemical irritation. When the dentin thickness is less, there is less fluid to buffer the acid.
- Inflammatory response of pulpal tissue toward GIC is more than zinc oxide eugenol but less than zinc phosphate cement and resolves in 30 days without reparative dentin formation. It is said that a lining of calcium hydroxide or zinc oxide eugenol is required when less than 0.5-1 mm of sound dentin remains over the pulp.

> Initially citric acid was used as conditioner followed by 25% polyacrylic acid, tannic acid, ferric chloride, sodium or EDTA. The latest is the use of 10% polyacrylic acid for 15-20 seconds followed by rinsing for 20 seconds.

Steps Involved in Clinical Placement of Glass Ionomer Cement

1. Shade selection.
2. Isolation of the tooth, rubber dam is the material of choice.
3. Cavity preparation, the objective is to remove all caries and unsupported enamel. Minimal extension is the key word.
4. If the dentin thickness is 0.5-1 mm, lining of calcium hydroxide should be placed.
5. Surface preparation: The surface smear layer is removed by pumice wash. The tooth surface is conditioned with 10% polyacrylic acid application for 10-15 seconds followed by 30 seconds water rinse.
6. Cement is mixed according to the manufacturers instructions (Figs 7.92 A and B). It should be mixed

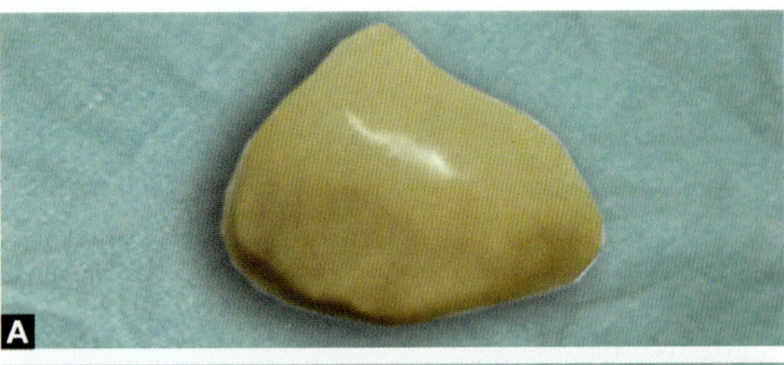

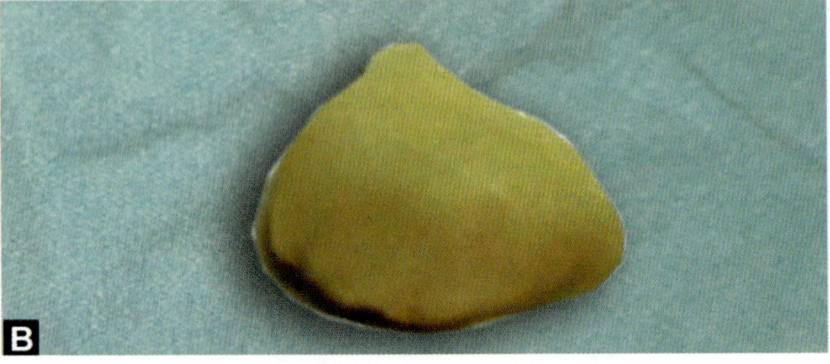

Figs 7.92A and B: (A) Glass Ionomer mix should have a glossy surface (Denoting the availability of free carboxyl group that is required for setting reaction) during placement into the cavity; (B) Set glass ionomer cement loosing its sheen

rapidly to gain working time and should not be more than 45-60 seconds. The tooth should be isolated all through.

7. Place a matrix wherever possible and fill the cavity with the GIC.
8. Remove the matrix and immediately protect it with waterproof material like varnish or vaseline.
9. Trim the excess with scalpel. Rotary cutting instruments should not be used.
10. After the removal of the excess material a layer of protective material is reapplied.
11. Finishing and polishing is done after 24 hours.
12. Reapply the protective material after finishing and polishing.

Critical Procedures for Glass Ionomer Restoration

1. Surface conditioning to remove the smear layer
2. P:L ratio must be maintained
3. Mixing time—not more than 45-60 seconds and surface should be glossy, due to the polyacid that has not participated in the reaction which helps in bonding.
4. Placement of material—with plastic instrument or injected. Mixed material should be used within 5 minutes and surface should be protected with varnish.
5. Surface finishing—delayed for 24 hours.

Modifications of Glass Ionomer Cement[23,30-32]

The chemistry is essentially the same for all three categories, but there are variations in powder/liquid ratio and powder particle size to accommodate the desired function.

Fiber reinforced glasses: The incorporation of alumina fibers and other fibers such as glass fiber, silica fiber, carbon fiber, etc to the existing glass powder at suitable filler/glass ratio was tried mainly to improve the flexural strength of the cement. Unfortunately, these composite materials are very difficult to mix if sufficient quantity of fiber is used to produce a significant increase in strength. In addition, resistance to abrasion decreases due to lack of bonding between fiber and matrix.

Metal reinforced glass ionomer cement: The addition of metal powders or fibers to glass—ionomer cements can improve strength; Metal fibers or amalgam alloy powders were used to improve the flexural strength. "Miracle mix" is the term used when amalgam alloy is mixed with glass ionomer and is used in core building. However, their aesthetics are poor and they are difficult to burnish. The metal/polyacrylate matrix interface was the weakest link.[33]

Cermet-ionomer cements: The solution to the problem of improving resistance to abrasion was the development of cermet-ionomer cements by McLean and Gasser. By sintering the metal and glass powders together, strong bonding of the metal to the glass was achieved. Ion leachable calcium aluminium fluorosilicate glasses were used in the preparation of the glass powder and a number of metal powders were tried, including alloys of silver and tin, pure silver, gold, titanium and palladium and gold and silver were found to be the most suitable materials.

Cermet-ionomer cements have greatly improved resistance to abrasion when compared with glass-ionomer cements and their flexural strength is also higher. However, their strength is still insufficient to replace amalgam alloys and their use should be confined to low stress-bearing cavity preparations.

Resin modified glass ionomers cement: This material was introduced to combat the problems of moisture sensitivity and lack of command cure. In their simplest form, these are GICs with the addition of a small quantity of a resin such as hydroxyethyl methacrylate (HEMA) or Bis-GMA in the liquid.[34] It was designed to produce favorable physical properties similar to those of resin composites while maintaining the basic features of the conventional glass ionomer cement.

In these materials the fundamental acid/base curing reaction is supplemented by a second curing process, which is initiated by light or chemical and are considered to be dual-cure cements if only one polymerization mechanism is used; if both mechanisms are used, they are considered to be tri-cure cements. These new materials are also called as hybrid ionomers.

It is done to improve the strength, fracture toughness and resistant to wear.

A. Silver alloy admix—mixing spherical silver amalgam alloy powder with Type II glass ionomer
B. Cermet—fusing glass powder to silver particles
C. Resin modified GIC—to overcome moisture sensitivity and low early strength. Also called as light cured, dual cure (LC and acid base reaction), tricure (dual cure and chemical cure), resin ionomer, compomers or hybrid ionomers.

Compomers are polyacid modified resin composites.[35]

Resin Modified Glass Ionomer Cement

Composition

Powder (Ion leachable glass)

- Initiator for light or chemical curing or both.

Liquid (Water)

- Polyacrylic acid/polyacrylic acid with carboxylic group modified with methacrylate and hydroxyethyl methacrylate monomers.

Setting reaction

Initial reaction is polymerization of methacrylate group, followed by acid base reaction.

Physical properties

- The difference is due to presence of polymerizable resins and less amount of water and carboxylic acid in liquid.
- Tensile strength is higher than that of conventional GIC
- Greater amount of plastic deformation
- Bonding similar to conventional glass ionomer cement
- Higher bond strength compared to composite resin
- Greater degree of shrinkage—due to polymerization, lower water and carboxylic acid content.
- Reduced water sensitivity
- Transient temperature increase during polymerization.

Advantages

- Extended working time
- Improved physical properties
- More resistant to dehydration and cracking.

COMPOSITE RESIN RESTORATIVE MATERIAL

"Composite materials" are formed from two constituents that are insoluble in each other." RL Bowen developed modern dental composite restorative materials in late 1950s and was introduced to dentistry in the early 1960s. He conducted experiments on reinforcing epoxy resins with filler particles.

Since epoxy resins have some disadvantages or shortcomings like slow cure and tendency to discolor, he combined the advantages of epoxy resin and acrylic resin leading to the development of BIS-GMA molecule. It is an aromatic ester of dimethacrylate, with epoxy resin as the backbone and acrylic as functional reactive group.

Composite restorative material is ideal for anterior tooth restoration due to its excellent color matching (Figs 7.93A and B).

Composition

1. *Resin matrix:* BIS-GMA is the most commonly used resin followed by urethane dimethacrylate. Diluent monomers like methyl methacrylate monomer or dimethacrylate monomers, such as TEGDMA

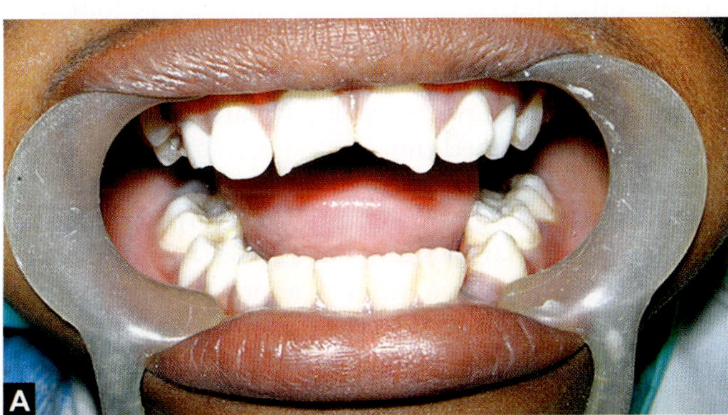
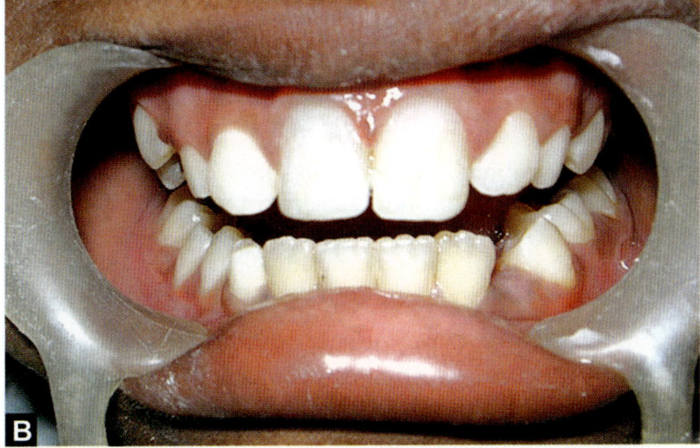

Figs 7.93A and B: Composite restoration of fractured central incisors: (A) Fractured teeth; (B) Restored with composite

(triethylene glycol dimethacrylate) are used to attain higher fillers levels and to produce pastes of clinically usable consistencies.

A blend of BISGMA + TEGDMA in 75: 25 wt% has a viscosity of 4300 centipoise, whereas that of 50: 50 blends is 200 centipoise.

TEGDMA allows extensive cross linking to occur between chains resulting in a matrix that is more resistant to solvents, but also increase the polymerization shrinkage.

2. *Filler particle:*
   - Improves the properties of the matrix material
   - Reduces polymerization shrinkage
   - Reduces water sorption and coefficient of thermal expansion
   - Improves tensile strength, compressive strength and modulus of elasticity and abrasion resistance.

Materials used as fillers are:
- Colloidal silica
- Quartz
- Barium
- Strontium
- Zirconium

Quartz has been used extensively as filler particularly in conventional composites. Advantage is that it is chemically inert but it is so very hard that it is difficult to polish and may abrade opposing teeth or restoration. Other materials are not as stable as quartz and may leach out into aqueous medium.

Translucency of the filler must be similar to that of tooth structure and its index of refraction must closely match that of resin. For BISGMA + TEGDMA combination refractive index is about 1.5. Most of the glass or quartz that are used as fillers have R. I. of 1.5.

> **Hardness**
> - Filler—600-1100 DPN
> - Matrix—80-130 DPN

> **Advantages of filled resin over unfilled resin**
>
> - Reduced polymerization shrinkage
> - Less water sorption and coefficient of thermal expansion
> - Improved mechanical properties—compressive strength, tensile strength, and modulus of elasticity.

3. *Coupling agent:* It provides a bond between the resin matrix and fillers, thus improving the physical and mechanical properties and providing hydrolytic stability by preventing water from penetrating along the resin – filler interface. For example, organosilanes are commonly used (e.g. 3-methoxy-propyl-trimethoxy silane). Others are titanates and zirconates.

4. *Inhibitors:*
   - Hydroquinone, butylated hydroxytoluene (<0.01%)
   - Minimizes or prevents spontaneous polymerization. It reacts with free radicals that are formed.
5. *UV Absorbers:* To improve color stability, e.g. 2 hydroxy-4 methoxy benzophenols.
6. *Activators:*
   - For self-cure—tertiary amine
   - Light cure—light
7. *Initiators:*
   - Self-cure—benzoyl peroxide,
   - Light cure—α-diketones like camphorquinone,
   - UV light benzoin methyl ether,
8. Pigments.

Classification of Composite Resins

Classification Based on Filler Particle Size

- Megafiller   – >100 µ (megafil)
- Macrofiller   – 10-100 µ (macrofil)
- Midifiller   – 1-10 µ (midifil)
- Minifiller   – 0.1-1 µ (minifil)
- Microfiller   – 0.01-0.1 µ (microfil)
- Nanofiller   – 0.005-0.01 µ (nanofil 10^{-9})
- Picofiller   – < 0.005 µ

> Heavily filled material contains inorganic filler about 75% wt. or more
> Lightly filled material contains inorganic filler about 66% wt. or less.

Based on the Mean Particle Size of the Major Filler

1. Conventional   – 8-12 µm
2. Small particle   – 1- 5 µm
3. Microfilled   – 0.04-0.4 µm
4. Hybrid   – 0.1-1.0 µ

Based on the Method of Polymerization

1. Self-cured
2. Light cured

Properties

A. Linear coefficient of thermal expansion is twice as much the value of amalgam and 3-4 times greater than that for tooth structures.
B. Most composites can be practically cured only to levels of 55-65% conversion of monomer sites, usually due to inadequate curing energy from visible light cure unit and is improved by post-curing.
C. Water absorption swells the polymer portion and promotes diffusion and desorption of any unbound

monomer. Water plasticizes the composite and chemically degrades the matrix into the monomer. Increased filler content, lower is the water absorption.

D. Microfill composites are the least wear resistant.

E. Composites with high matrix content and self cured have more tendency to undergo yellowing. Addition of UV light absorbers and antioxidants reduce this chance of yellowing.

F. Beveling tends to blend any color difference associated with margin and provides more surface area for bonding.

G. Good marginal integrity—Butt joints margin wear slowly but create a meniscus appearance against enamel. Beveling produces thinner ledges of material that are prone to fracture.

H. Biocompatible, but unpolymerized materials are potentially cytotoxic, they are very poorly soluble in water and are polymerized into a bound state before dissolution or diffusion.

I. Compared to unfilled resins, filled resins are more stronger, increased modulus of elasticity (increased modulus of elasticity—less is the flexibility and vice versa), good abrasion resistance and lower coefficient of thermal expansion.

Light Cured Composites

These materials are dispensed in a single paste form, thus requiring no mixing and so eliminating human variable.

- Working time is as chosen by the dentist. Cure is fast, deep and reliable compared to UV light cured composites.
- Increased color stability.
- Incremental technique is used for restoring the tooth with composite, as the depth of penetration is less, but this technique compensates for polymerization shrinkage.
- Wavelength of light used is 400-500 nm (peak intensity is 470 nm).
- Optimal polymerization is important for color stability, physical and biological properties.
- High intensity light should be used.
- Exposure time is 40-60 seconds.
- Resin thickness to be cured should not be more than 2-2.5 mm.
- Dark shades require longer exposure time, as they tend to absorb the light.
- Composites straight from the refrigerator takes longer to cure than those at room temperature.
- Light used cause retinal damage, so direct visualization of the light is avoided and protective shield should be used.

- Dual cured composites combine self curing and light curing.
- Unreacted monomer is capable of diffusing out of the polymer either into dentin or onto external tooth surfaces.
- Intensity of the light striking the composite is inversely proportional to the distance from the tip of the light source to the composite surface. Ideally tip should be within 2 mm and perpendicular to the surface.
- Output energy of light unit, should be 300 mw/cm^2 and is monitored with a radiometer.
- Degree of conversion of monomer to polymer is related to intensity and duration of exposure of light, i.e. about 20-60 seconds.
- The material can abrade steel, so use of steel instruments should be avoided during manipulation.
- The material should not be spatulated, as it may incorporate air.

> - Etching time of 15 seconds provide as strong a bond
> - Increased fluoride content of tooth is associated with longer etching time.

Acid Etch[36-43]

The purpose of acid etch is to form micropores for better resin-enamel micromechanical bond.

The technique of acid etching consists of applying ortho phosphoric acid (H_3PO_4) to enamel for 15-60 seconds, followed by rinsing and drying.

The recommended time for etching varied between 15-60 seconds but there seems to be not significant difference in sealant retention with variation in etching time. The currently recommended etching time for permanent teeth is 20 seconds and for deciduous teeth is 30 seconds.

The etched tooth exhibits porosity at three levels microscopically. First a narrow zone of enamel is removed by etching and is about 10 μm in depth. The second zone is the qualitative porous zone which is 20 μm in depth. It is characterized by large porosities and is easily distinguishable from the adjacent unetched enamel using polarized light microscopy. The third zone is the quantitative porosity with relatively small but large number of porosities and is about 20 μm.

The tooth to be etched is isolated from fluids by rubber dam, cotton roll or retraction cord. Liquid and gel etchants are available in the concentration of 37 or 50% H_3PO_4.

After acid etching, care should be taken that the area is kept free of saliva or sulcular weepage. If there is contamination the surface is re-etched for 10 seconds.

Etched enamel has a high surface energy, and allows resin to wet readily the surface and penetrate into microscopic porosity. Once the resin penetrates into the microporosity, it can be polymerized to form a mechanical bond to the enamel. These resin tags may penetrate 10-20 µm into enamel, but the length is dependent on the etching time.

Enamel should not be etched immediately after fluoride therapy as the microscopes created may not be adequate. So it is suggested that teeth be etched 2 weeks after APF treatment.

Liquid Etchant

They are used to etch large surface areas of enamel. Applicators include small cotton pellets, foam, sponge and brushes.

Acid is applied gently to the enamel surface keeping the extension to a maximum to 0.5 mm from the cavity margin past the extent of the restoration. Application is repeated every 10-15 seconds to keep the area moist for 30 seconds, care should be taken not to flood the area with acid or to rub the enamel. The area is rinsed with water for 10-15 seconds. The area is then dried with clean dry air. The enamel must appear as having a ground glass or lightly frosted appearance.

Gel Etchant

It is made by adding colloidal silica to acid. Thixotropic gels are most preferred, as controlled application is possible. Applied with a brush, paper point, instrument or syringe. Procedure is the similar to liquid etchant, but a long rinse is required to wash off the gel.

Three Basic Types of Surface Characteristics in Etched Enamel[44]

Type 1 Pattern: Most common pattern seen. Prism core material is preferentially removed, leaving the prism peripheries relatively intact.

Type 2 Pattern: Peripheral region of prism was removed leaving prism cores relatively unaffected.

Type 3 Pattern: There was a more random pattern, areas of which corresponds to type 1 and 2 pattern, together with regions in which the pattern of etching could not be related to prism morphology.

All three patterns were found in single samples of etched enamel, suggesting that there is no specific etching pattern produced in human dental enamel by the action of acid.

Type 4 Pattern: (Not described by Silverstone) Surface loss occurs without exposing the prism, usually seen in the cervical areas where prism do not extend upto the surface.

> Smear layer: Is 0.5-5 µm and consists of blood, saliva, bacteria, enamel and dentin particles. Some believe that smear layer acts as an effective, natural cavity liner that seals the dentinal tubules and reduces permeability making the smear layer a clinical asset, while others argue that smear layer interferes with adhesion of restorative material, serves as a focus for bacteria and its toxins.

Bonding Agent

These are unfilled resins that are applied on the etched tooth surface before the placement of the composite resin material. Composite material since it is more viscous does not penetrate the micropores created due to acid etching. The bonding agent is less viscous and flows into the micropores and bonds with the composite resin.

1. Enamel bonding system—unfilled or lightly filled liquid acrylic monomer mixture placed on the etched enamel surface resulting in tag formation.
2. Dentin enamel bonding system—it is also called as 'dentin bonding agents.' It includes ingredients that etch, prime and bond to dentin and also produce enamel bonding. Priming agent is 2 HEMA (Hydroxyethyl methacrylate). It is used to wet the dentin surface. They penetrate the remaining smear layer into the intertubular dentin and fill the space left by dissolved hydroxyl apatite crystals. Bonding agent is the same as discussed in enamel bonding system (unfilled or lightly filled liquid acrylic monomer mixture). It forms a network around the dentin collagen and when polymerized produces a hybrid zone.[45,46]

Individual Components of Bonding Agents

Dentin conditioner

Objective: To create a surface that is capable of micromechanical or chemical bonding with bonding agent.

Methods of conditioning

1. Chemical—acids, chelators
2. Thermal—lasers
3. Mechanical—abrasives such as aluminium oxide, creates a smear layer that might be used to enhance the bond strength of smear mediated dentin bonding agents.

Dentin primers

It forms thickness of 0.5-1 µ. Increases the wettability of bonding agent on the conditioned dentin.

Bonding agent

It forms resin tags into the tubules and more important is the penetration of bonding agents into intertubular dentin, to form a hybrid layer.

> Resin reinforced zone or Hybrid layer (Nakabayashi et al 1982):[47] The primer wets and penetrates the collagen network/meshwork, raising it almost to its original level. It also increases the surface energy of dentinal surface. Unfilled resin then penetrates the primed dentin, copolymerizing with the primer to form an intermingled layer of resin and collagen.

Critical Factors Affecting Adhesion

The surface of enamel over which the unfilled resin must flow should have surface energy higher than the resin. Instrumented surface release polar substances that form low energy surface layer.

A. Salivary and blood contamination—contamination after placement of a bonding agent and before curing is critical. If the bonding agent that utilizes the smear layer for bonding is used and is washed, the smear layer gets washed off. So in such cases following washing, the dentin is roughened, this allows the formation of a smear layer once again over which the bonding agent is placed. If the surface is contaminated, it is reconditioned with 37% phosphoric acid for 10 seconds followed by reapplication of bonding agent.

B. Oil contamination

C. Surface roughness of the tooth surface—mechanical retention may increase slightly.

D. Mechanical undercuts—they hold the restorative materials from bodily dislodgment from the preparation and may also resist microscopic movement of the restoration caused by thermal or polymerization influences.

E. Fluoride content of the tooth—etching time is doubled in tooth with increased fluoride.

F. Presence of plaque/calculus/stains/debris—they prevent etching and the surface becomes shiny when etched.

G. Presence of bases, liners or varnishes should not be applied.

H. Tooth dehydration—overdrying of dentin before the placement of the bonding agent is as damaging as placing bonding agent in a wet field.

I. Constituents of temporary cement—fresh eugenol could be a negative factor for resin polymerization. Eugenol is completely absorbed in ZnOE of >7 days old and rendered inert.

J. Intimate contact—>0.0007 between the tooth structure and the adhesive is ideal.

K. Clean tooth surface

L. Wettability of the adhesive—surface tension of the liquid must be less than the surface energy of the enamel and dentin. Freshly etched enamel has twice the surface energy than unetched surface.

M. Adhesion also depends on the amount of polymerization shrinkage of the resin.

> 4 META (4 methacryl oxyethyl trimellitate anhydride): It has both hydrophobic and hydrophilic groups. Improves the adhesion strength of resins to teeth by promoting intertubular penetration, impregnation and entanglement of the methyacrylate base monomer into dentinal substrates and their polymerization therein.

Steps in Composite Restoration

Oral Prophylaxis

- Done to remove plaque, debris and stain from the tooth surface for efficient bonding.
- Non-fluoride paste should be used, as the surface becomes more acid resistant with fluoride.
- Glycerin should not be used as it provides an impervious layer.

Shade Selection

- It is done prior to rubber dam application.
- Light source used- should be natural mid day light coming from the northern sky and slightly overcasted. If artificial light is used white fluorescent light is preferred.
- The eye of the operator and the tooth should be at the same level, and the operator should stand at a distance of not more than 3 feet.
- Hue—it is the main color, e.g. red, yellow, etc. CHROMA is the depth of the color – how far it is red, VALUE—darkness or whiteness of the color –shade
- Shade is also compared with the hair, pupil and skin color.

Beveling of the Cavity Border

- Bevel of 45° is given at the cavity border extending for 1-1.5 mm.
- It is done to increase the surface area available for bonding and to provide a gradual reduction in the material thickness and also helps in color blending with the tooth.

Acid Etching

- 37% (30-50%) orthophosphoric acid is commonly used for 15 secs. Others are 50% citric acid or 25% pyruvic acid.
- Available in gel and liquid form.
- Liquid—used for pit and fissure sealant and requires constant replenishing.

- Gel—is used in small areas, easy to control and rinsing time required is more.
- Etching cleans the tooth surface, increases the surface free energy by increasing the wettability, increases the surface area by formation of micropores, removes smear layer, opens dentinal tubules, increases dentinal permeability and decalcifies the inter and peritubular dentin.
- Problems encountered in deciduous teeth are- presence of outer prismless layer and increased organic content. Methods of improving bonding are- increased etching time, washing and re-etching, mechanical removal of the 0.1mm of prismless layer or use of coupling agent like butyl acrylate-acrylic acid copolymer in alcohol solution.
- Depth of decalcification is affected by—pH, concentration, viscosity and time of application.
- Changes seen—10 µ loss at the surface followed by 20 µ qualitative porous zone and the last zone is 20 µ quantitative porous zone.
- Pattern seen—type I honey comb appearance, type II cobble stone, type III combination and type IV seen on the cervical region where there is loss of surface layer without formation of micropores due to failure of the enamel rods to extend upto the surface. (prismless layer is seen on deciduous enamel, cervical portion and pit and fissure of permanent teeth).
- Applying bonding agent followed by curing.
- Incremental placement of composite materal followed by curing. Each increment of composite that is cured should be about 1.5–2 mm.

Finishing and Polishing of Composites

It should be kept to the minimum, aimed at providing the final contour and smooth finish. Care must be exercised with all rotary instruments to prevent damage to the tooth structure especially at the gingival marginal areas.

Finishing and Polishing

Carbide finishing bur is used to remove excess composite. Medium speed with light intermittent brush strokes and air coolant for contouring is used. Final polishing is achieved with rubber polishing paste. Sand paper disk can also be used with low speed and by constant shifting motion. Final polishing is done with a fine grit disk available in different sizes.

Wear of Composites

1. *Microfracture theory:* Filler particles are compressed onto the adjacent matrix during occlusal loading, creating microfractures in the weaker matrix. These microfractures may unite and lead to the loss of the surface layer of composite.
2. *Hydrolysis theory:* Debonding between the filler particle and matrix as the silane bond is hydrolytically unstable leading to loss of surface fillers.
3. *Chemical degradation theory:* Materials from food and saliva are absorbed into the matrix, causing matrix degradation and sloughing from the surface.
4. *Protection theory:* Weak matrix is eroded between particles.

Repair of Composites

Rebonding to Old Composite

Replacement of composite restorations becomes necessary following fracture of old restoration. The tooth should be cleaned with pumice and etched before placing the bonding agent and the material. Rebonding is achieved by a combination of new tag formation and chemical bond between the new composite and residual tags.

Repair of the Newly Placed Restoration

Addition can be made directly over the restoration that has been just cured and polished.

Properties of Composite Resins

1. Setting—commences immediately after mixing in selfcure with uniform rate of set through out the bulk and limited working time. The working time is longer with light cured. These materials tend to set slowly when exposed to light. Increased viscosity- retards diffusion of active free radicals from the surface layers to the lower unactivated layers, resulting in the material that is unset.
2. Polymerization reaction is exothermic. Heat liberated can irreversibly damage the pulp if not properly insulated. For an average sized restoration the temperature rise of chemical cure composites is about 5-10°C and that for light cure is 15-35°C.
3. Setting contraction—increased filler, and BIS-GMA causes less shrinkage. TEGDMA increases shrinkage. Shrinkage compromises marginal seal and places stress on tooth substance.
4. Thermal properties—this depends on inorganic filler content. Increased filler—decreased coefficient of thermal expansion (CTE). CTE is 6-7 times more than tooth substance.
5. Mechanical properties—depends upon filler content, type and efficiency of coupling.
   LC composite—compressive strength is 260 MPA.
6. Surface characteristics—initially surface layer is rich in resin then as wear occurs relatively soft resin matrix is worn preferentially leaving the filler particles protruding from the surface.

STAINLESS STEEL CROWNS

Selecting an ideal restorative material for restoration of a grossly decayed teeth is very challenging. Silver amalgam or cast crown restoration are the material of choice. Disadvantage of silver amalgam is that it requires additional reinforcement to give a truly satisfactory, long lasting results. Cast crown restoration, which avoids many of the difficulties encountered with amalgam, requires more tooth reduction and hence, cannot be used in deciduous and young permanent tooth because of the danger of pulp exposure. The advent of stainless steel crowns has been proved to be an ideal choice for such grossly decayed teeth. Introduced by Dr. William Humphrey,[48] (1950) stainless steel crown provides a fast yet effective means of restoring a tooth which in the past might have had to undergo either extraction or painstaking and laborious procedures for receiving a casting or extensive restoration of silver amalgam.

> Retention of a stainless steel crown depends primarily on a tight fit at the gingival margins and the shape of the preparation is relatively not important.

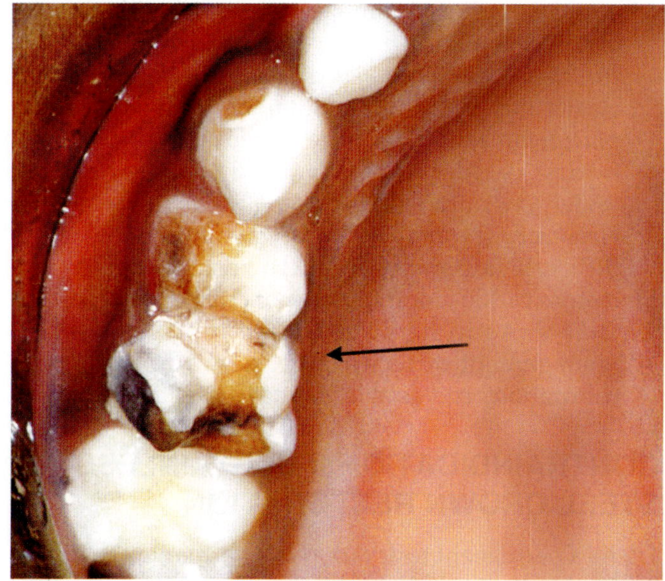

Fig. 7.94: Caries involving three or more surfaces indicated for stainless steel crown restoration

INDICATIONS OF STAINLESS STEEL CROWN RESTORATIONS[49,50]

1. *Extensive Caries (Fig. 7.94):*
   - Cl II cavity where one or more cusps are destroyed or weakend by caries.
   - Caries involving 3 or more surfaces
   - Rampant caries.
2. *Following pulp theropy:* The tooth becomes brittle and weakened following pulp therapy leading to fracture especially in mesiodistal direction leading to extraction. Thus a stainless steel crown should be routinely used following pulp therapy.
3. *Developmental defects (Fig. 7.95):* In amelogenesis imperfecta, dentinogenesis imperfecta or enamel hypoplasia, the enamel is chipped or worn off exposing the underlying dentin, which may also lead to reduction in vertical height of the crown. Cast crown is avoided, considering the pulpal morphology and reduced height of the tooth. Care must be taken while placing a stainless steel crown as enamel easily chips off. Usually when the patient reports for the first time, much of the tooth would have worn off, leading to reduced vertical height.

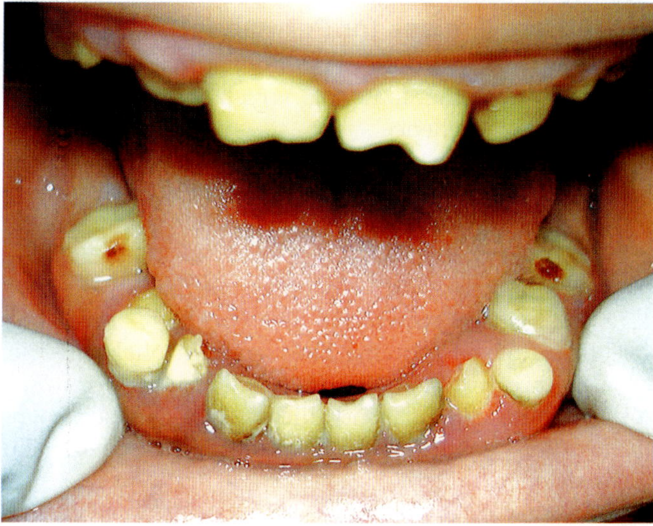

Fig. 7.95: Teeth with developmental defects indicated for stainless steel restoration

To restore the normal vertical dimensions, it may necessitate placement of the crown with increased occlusogingival dimensions. To prevent undue discomfort to the patient, crowns should be placed in pairs one on each side of the mouth, either in the same arch or the opposite arch.

4. *Bruxism:* Stainless steel crown can be given to compensate for the wear and to reduce the masticatory forces on the erupting permanent teeth.
5. *Fractured Incisors:* Stainless steel crown can be given as temporary restorative material which provides a means for retaining sedative dressing over the exposed dentin.
6. *Abutment for space maintainer (Fig. 7.96):* As in crown and loop space maintainer, used where band placement is difficult due to reduced undercut as in first deciduous molar or when the abutment undergoes pulp therapy.
7. *Handicapped children:* Oral hygiene maintenance is difficult, so stainless steel crowns are preferred to restore carious tooth than amalgam restorations.
8. *Others:* As in habit breaking appliance, in the management of recurrent caries around existing restorations and as abutment to a prosthesis.

CONTRAINDICATIONS TO STAINLESS STEEL CROWN RESTORATION

1. As a permanent restoration in a permanent dentition
2. Deciduous teeth that exhibits resorption of >½ of the root length.

Stainless Steel Crowns are Used as Temporary Crowns for Permanent Teeth

1. The margins of the crowns cannot be made as accurate as gold and other materials, which can be adapted for marginal excellence
2. They are not as durable for a long period as crowns made of precious metal.

COMPOSITION

1. Stainless steel crowns (18-8)
2. Nickel based crowns: They contain Nickel (72%), Chromium (14%), Fe (6-10%), Carbon (0.04%), Manganese (0.35%) and Silicon (0.2%). These crowns are very easy to adapt and have increased wear resistance.

Stainless steel	:	12-30% chromium is added to steel alloy (steel=carbon in iron)
	:	18-8 alloy contains 18% chromium and 8% nickel
	:	Strength: 211-1760 Mpa
	:	They resist tarnish and corrosion due to the formation of passivating layer of chromium oxide (Cr_2O_3)
	:	There are 3 types of steel: ferritic, martensitic and austenitic

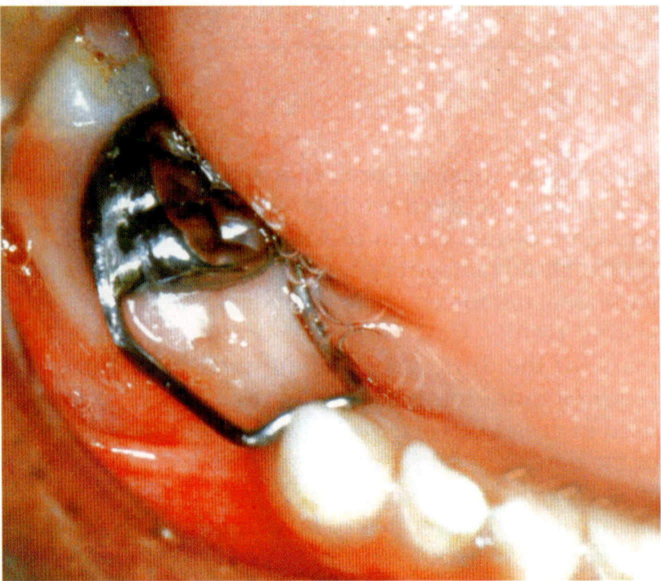

Fig. 7.96: Crown and loop space maintainer

Austenitic is preferred to ferretic because:
- Increased ductility and ability to be cold worked without fracturing
- Strengthening during cold working
- Greater ease of welding
- Ability to overcome sensitization (>650°C)
- Less critical grain growth, during annealing.

CLASSIFICATION OF STAINLESS STEEL CROWNS

Classification of Crown-based on Shape (Figs 7.97A to C)

1. *Untrimmed:* They are long and usually requires trimming, e.g. Sankim, Unitek crowns.
2. *Pretrimmed (prefestooned):* These crowns are short in length but are not contoured and so has a parallel sides, e.g. 3M stainless steel crowns, Denovo crowns.
3. *Precontoured:* These crowns are contoured and have a bell shape, e.g. 3M Ni–chromium ioncrowns, Unitek stainless steel crown.
4. *Prevented crowns:* They have resin-based composite bonded to the buccal and some part of occlusal surface, e.g. Nu Smile crowns.

Based on the Metal

1. Stainless steel crowns (Unitek, Rocky mountain)
2. Nickel Based crowns (Ion Ni-Chromium from 3M): It is made of nickel chromium alloy, containing

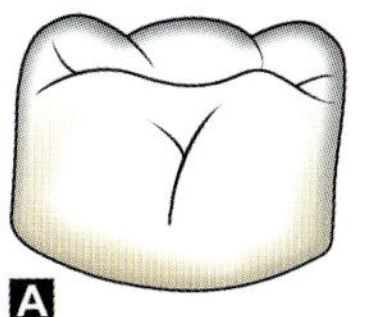 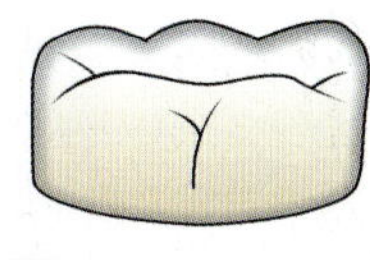 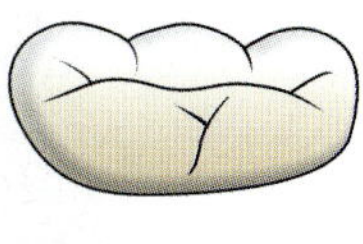

Figs 7.97A to C: Types of crown based on shape: (A) Untrimmed crown; (B) Pretrimmed crown; (C) Precontoured crown

nickel (70%), chromium (15%) and ferrous (10%). It is available as pretrimmed and precontoured crowns. They are easy to fit and require least amount of additional crimping, trimming and countouring.

EQUIPMENTS

Burs (Figs 7.98A to D)
- Round—for caries removal
- Flame shaped diamond bur—for occlusal reduction
- Long thin tapered diamond bur—for proximal, buccal and lingual reduction.
- Rubber wheel or point/green stone—for finishing and polishing.

Pliers (Figs 7.99A to C)
- Johnson No.114 (Rocky mountain)—for general contouring in the occlusal and middle region
- No. 417 (Unitek) crimping pliers—to produce marked curvature in cervical region.
- No. 112 (Dentarum)—to produce convexity and contact points.
- No. 137 Gordon—used for general contouring and shaping.

STEPS INVOLVED IN ADAPTATION OF THE PREFORMED STAINLESS STEEL CROWN[51-54]

Mink and Bernet in 1968 gave the basic principles for preparation of the tooth and adaptation of the crown.

1. Crown selection
2. Preoperative occlusal evaluation
3. LA administration
4. Rubberdam application
5. Placement of wedges
6. Tooth preparation
    - Occlusal reduction
    - Proximal reduction
    - Buccal and lingual reduction
    - Finishing
7. Trial fitting, trimming and contouring the crown
8. Finishing the crown

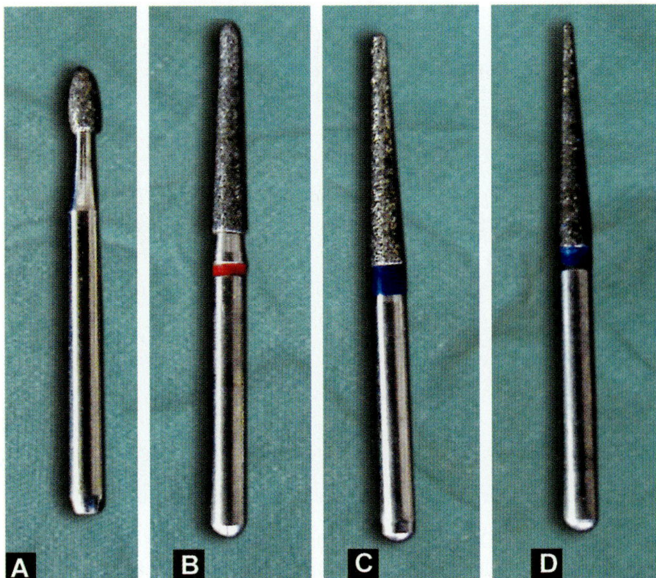

Figs 7.98A to D: Diamond burs used for tooth reduction for stainless steel crown restoration. Flame-shaped and long thin tapered bur are routinely used: (A) Flame-shaped bur; (B) Round end tapered bur; (C) Flat end tapered bur; (D) Long thin tapered bur

9. Cementation
10. Postcementation instruction.

Crown Selection

A correctly selected crown should cover all the tooth preparation and provide resistance to removal. Festooned crowns are superior because it most accurately reproduces the tooth morphology and requires least trimming and contouring. Primary molar with deep interproximal caries extending subgingivally may warrant the use of non-festooned crown to encompass the margins of the preparation. Two principles that should be kept in mind to obtain well-adapted crown are: (1) Establish correct occlusogingival crown length, and (2) crown margins should follow the natural contour of the tooth and the gingiva.

Factors to be Considered during Crown Selection

Mesiodistal width of the tooth: Preoperative mesiodistal width of the tooth to be crowned is measured with the callipers and matched with the stainless steel crown (Figs 7.100A and B). The crown selected should be of correct dimensions as a smaller crown will have no allowance for contouring and on the other hand it will be impossible to contour satisfactorily a grossly over sized crown. It should be also kept in mind that an over contoured or oversized crowns on 2nd deciduous molar can prevent normal eruption of the 1st permanent molars.

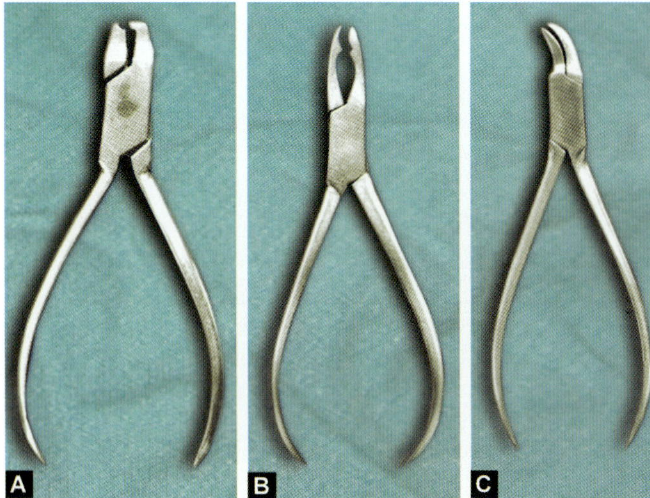

Figs 7.99A to C: Pliers used for fabrication of stainless steel crown: (A) Crimping pliers; (B) Johnson ball and socket plier, used to get a bell shaped contouring; (C) Gordon plier, used for general contouring and shaping

Occlusal anatomy (Figs 7.101A and B): Excessive occlusal anatomy may present with problems. Deep occlusal fissures and high cusps means that a greater reduction of the occlusal surface is required to avoid problems occurring when the crown is fitted. Such crowns without adequate reduction may not reach the correct gingival level and will rock.

Height of the crown (Figs 7.102A and B): The height of the crown should be same as that of the uncut tooth with cervical margin not more than 1mm below and parallel to the gingival margin.

Primate space: Preoperative assessment of the presence or absence of primate space should be done, when 1st deciduous molar is crowned. Impingement of this space may prevent early mesial shift of the 1st permanent molar.

Gingival marginal contour: The shape and contour of gingival margins differs from the 1st to 2nd molar as well from buccal to lingual to proximal aspect. Three forms of gingival margin contour has been described as 'Smile', 'Stretched S' and 'Frown' (Figs 7.103 and 7.104).

"Smile": The outline of the buccal gingiva of the second deciduous molar and the lingual gingiva of both the deciduous molars resemble a smile.

"Stretched S": Owing to the mesiobuccal cervical bulge, the gingival margin dips down in the buccal aspect of 1st deciduous molar as it continues from distal to mesial giving the configuration of a 'S' that has been stretched on one side.

"Frown": Due to short occlusocervical height at the mid point on the proximal aspect the gingiva dips down on either side of this midpoint giving a frown line.

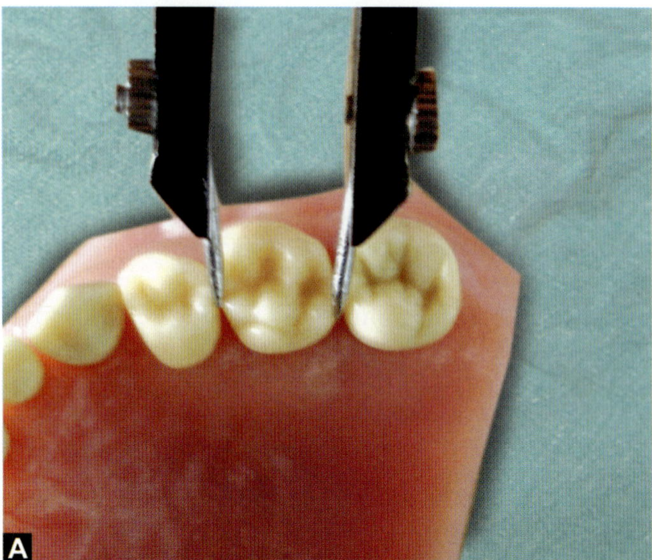

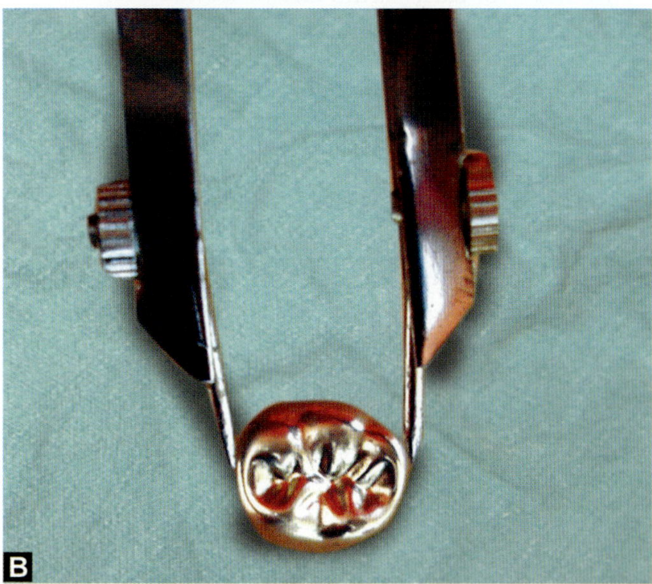

Figs 7.100A and B: Measurement of the mesiodistal width of the crown: (A) Mesiodistal width of the tooth is measured first with a divider; (B) The measurement is compared with the mesiodistal width of the crown

Preoperative Occlusal Evaluation

An instrument (probe) should be placed on the operating tooth so that the probe extends and touches the cusps of the two adjacent teeth (Fig. 7.105). This helps in later evaluation of the reduction and crown fit.

Local Anesthesia Administration

Local anesthesia reduces the discomfort to the patient during tooth reduction and crown manipulation.

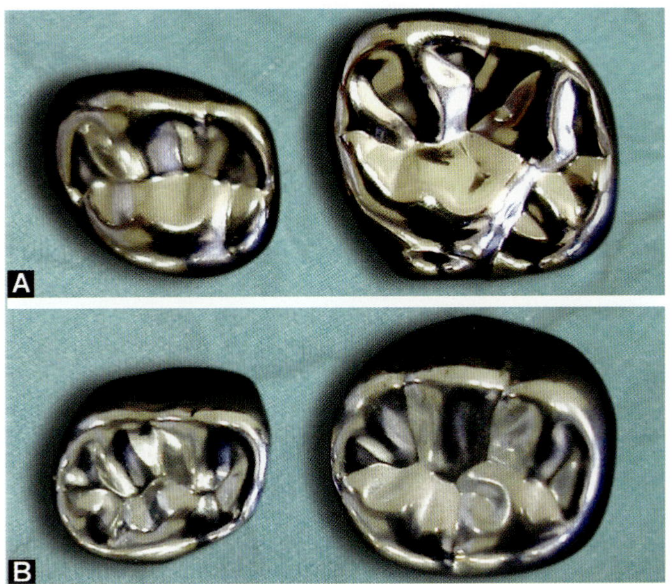

Figs 7.101A and B: Occlusal anatomy of the crowns: (A) Maxillary first and second deciduous molar crowns; (B) Mandibular first and second deciduous molar crowns

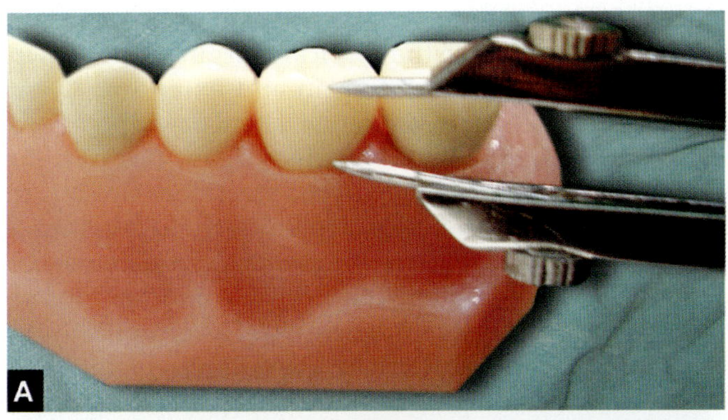

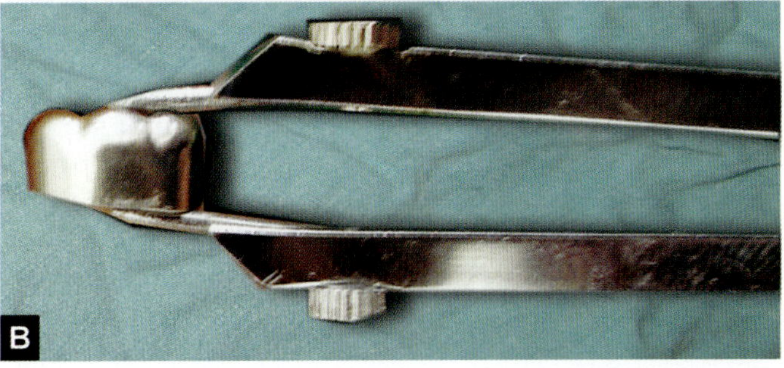

Figs 7.102A and B: Measurement of the height of the crown: (A) Height of the tooth is made first with a divider; (B) The measurement is compared with the height of the crown

Rubberdam Application

It prevents slipping of crown into the throat accidentally and also provides isolation if tooth has to undergo pulp therapy.

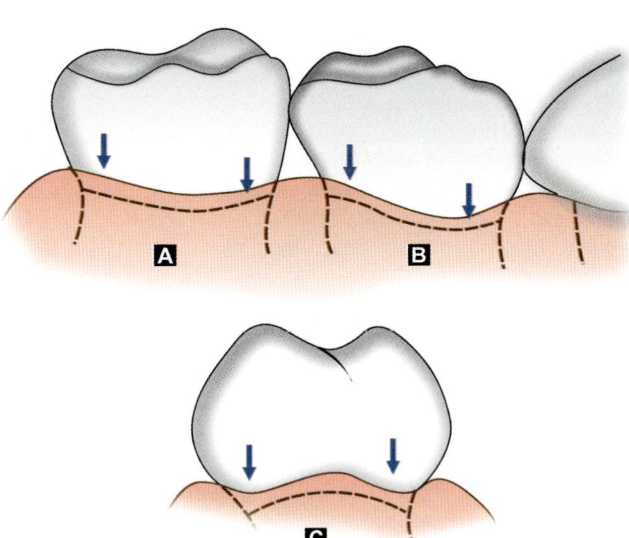

Figs 7.103A to C: Diagrammatic representation of the gingival contour line. Dotted line denotes cervical margin of the crown: (A) 'Smile'; (B) 'Stretched S'; (C) 'Frown'

Placement of Wedges

They are placed in the interproximal space which acts as tooth separators and also protects the underlying soft tissues.

Tooth Preparation (Figs 7.106A and B)
Occlusal Reduction

Large round bur, tapered fissure or flame shaped diamond can be used depending on the preference of the operator. The occlusal reduction of 1.5-2.0 mm follows the anatomy of the occlusal surface. Initial placement of 1 mm depth grooves in the occlusal surface followed by removal of remaining portion according to cuspal inclines makes the reduction easier and accurate. Sharp line angles should be rounded.

Proximal Reduction

The tappered fissure bur is used to reduce the trauma to soft tissues. The bur is moved in a buccolingual direction starting at the occlusal surface 1-2 mm away from the adjacent tooth, until the contact area clears gingivally and buccolingually. The gingivo proximal line angle should have a feather edge finish line. When finished one must be able to pass an explorer tip between the proximal surface and the adjacent tooth at the gingival margin.

Buccal and Lingual Reduction

Minimal but adequate buccal and lingual reduction is necessary. The buccal and lingual cervical bulges can

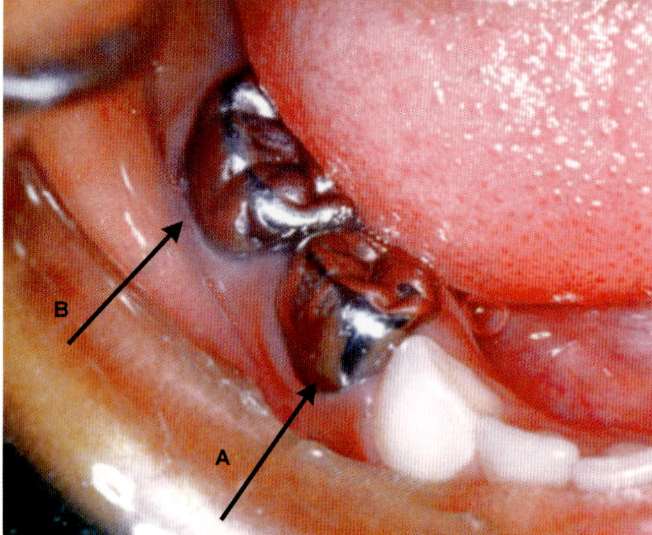

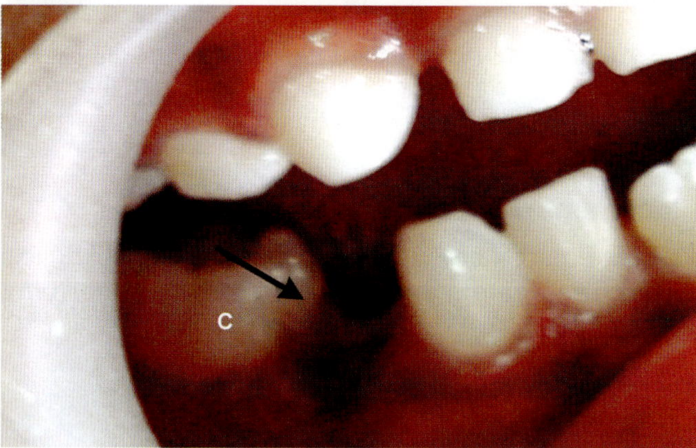

Fig. 7.104: Gingival contour line: (A) Stretched 'S' contour on the first molar; (B) 'Smile' contour on the second molar; (C) 'Frown contour on the proximal aspect

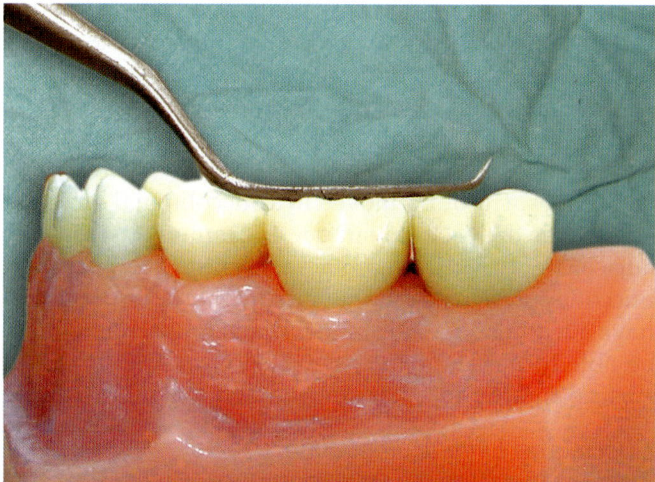

Fig. 7.105: Preoperative occlusal evaluation

be left uncut if they do not interfere in the placement of the crown.

Occlusal 1/3 of the buccal surface should be beveled to reduce the width of the occlusal table.

Finishing

All the line angles must be rounded. The occlusobuccal and occlusolingual line angles are rounded by holding the bur at a 30-45° angle to the occlusal surface and sweeping it in a mesiodistal direction.

Trial Fitting, Trimming and Contouring the Crown (Figs 7.107 to 7.109)

The purpose of crown trimming and contouring are respectively to leave the crown margins in the gingival sulcus and to reproduce the tooth's morphology. Retention of the stainless steel crown restoration is due to the firm contact between the tooth and the margins of the crown.

Seating of a crown on a mandibular molar is best done by first fitting the lingual side and then rotating it buccally. In the upper arch it is easier to fit the buccal side first. The position of the gingival margin is marked on the crown, to have the cervical margin of the crown parallel to the gingival margin and extending 1mm subgingivally. The excess material is cut with curved crown and bridge scissors away from the patient taking care that the slivers of the steel does not injure the patient. The margins are smoothened using a green stone. The crown is then contoured using a 114 plier and crimping plier resulting in a smooth flowing outline on the margin of the crown. The crown should snap into place when refitted. Care should be taken to see that there is no gingival blanching and no occlusal interference.

Finishing the Crown

It includes making of a bevel on the external surface of the crown margin around the entire periphery using a green stone held at 45° angle to the margin to reduce a feather edge margin. Final finishing is done with stone and rubber wheel to remove scratches and obtain shine.

Cementation

Cements used are ZnOE, $ZnPO_4$, polycarboxylate, glass ionomer cement. Glass ionomer is superior to all the above, while ZnOE is the least preferred.

Debris and hemorrhagic material are removed from the tooth surface by flushing with copious amounts of warm water. The tooth is isolated with cotton. All exposed dentin surface is protected with several layers

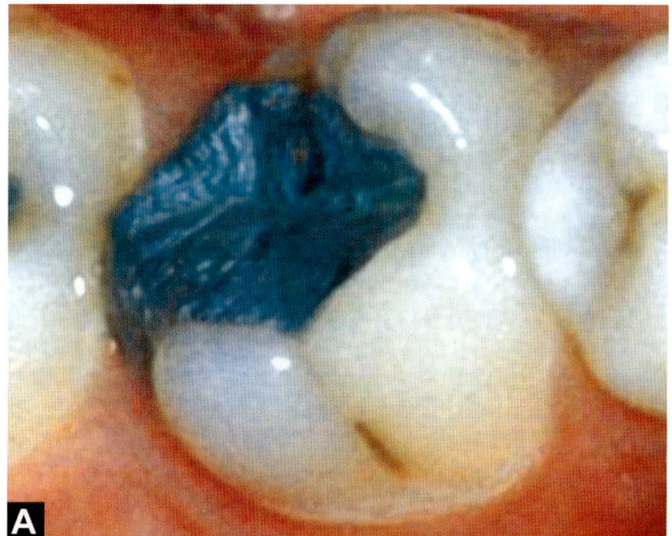

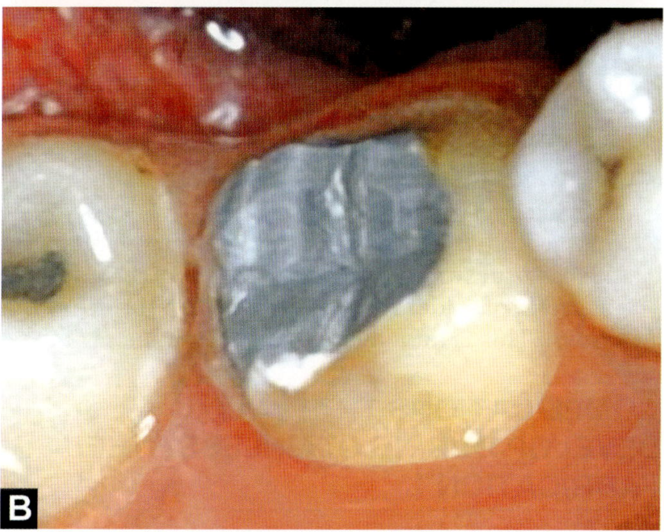

Figs 7.106A and B: Tooth preparation for stainless steel crown restoration: (A) Prereduction; (B) Postreduction

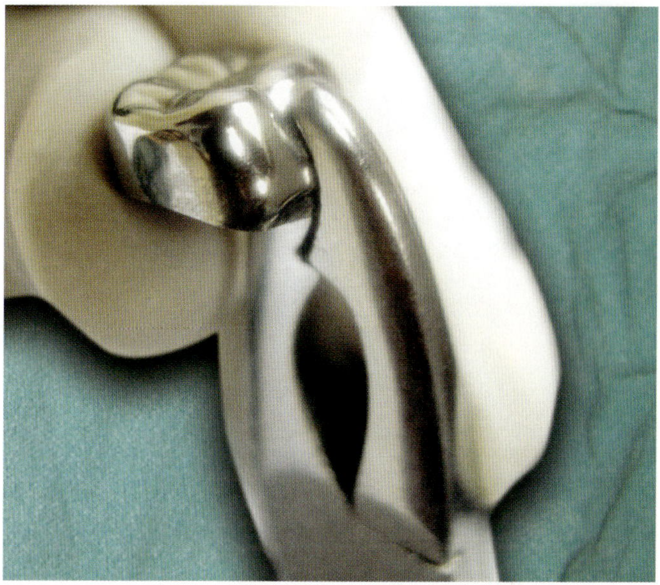

Fig. 7.107: Position of the plier during contouring

Luting Material	Film Thickness μm	Setting time Min.	Compressive Strength Mpa
ZnPO$_4$	18	5.5	103.5
ZnOE	25	4-10	27.6
Poly carboxylate	21	5.5	55.2
Glass ionomer	24	6.5	86.2

Postcementation Instruction

The patient should be instructed to avoid heavy chewing with the crown for 24 hours. Instructions should be given for maintaining oral hygiene and should be recalled once every 6 months for evaluation.

MODIFICATIONS OF STAINLESS STEEL CROWN[55-59]

A. When more than one stainless steel crown has to be prepared additional factors to be remembered are:
   a. Occlusal reduction of one tooth should be done completely before starting the second tooth. If done together there is a tendency to over reduce.
   b. Contact point between adjacent teeth should be broken producing 1.5 mm space at the gingival level.
   c. Both crowns should be trimmed, contoured and prepared for cementation simultaneously. Cementation of the distal tooth is done first and should be the same as during trial fitting.

of varnish. The crown is 1/2- 2/3 filled with cement that has been mixed to the luting consistency. The crown is seated on the tooth along the predetermined path of insertion. The cotton rolls are removed promptly and the patient requested to bite gently on the crown to ensure its being forced to place. The end of a tongue depressor, trimmed to the mesio distal size of the crown is placed between the crown and opposing tooth and the patient is asked to occlude gently. When the cement has been half set, the tongue depressor is removed, the occlusion is rechecked and excess cement is removed using scaler from the buccal and lingual aspects and floss can be used for proximal surface (Fig. 7.110).

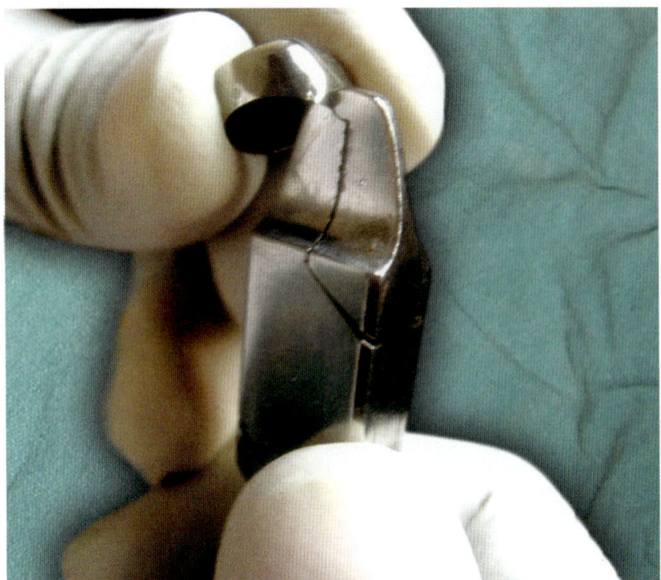

Fig. 7.108: Position of the plier during crimping

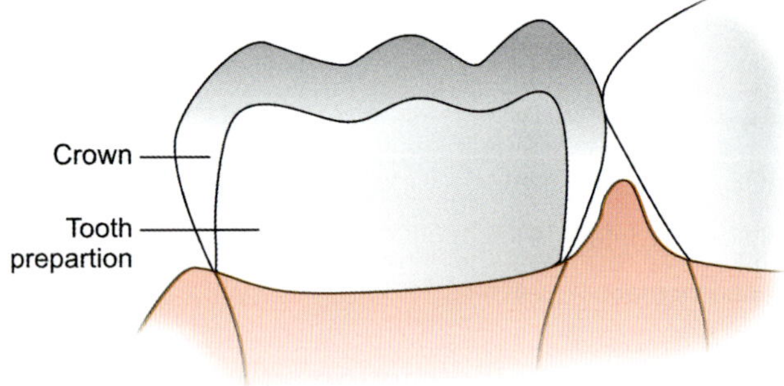

Fig. 7.109: Knife edge margin in the tooth preparation and fit of a stainless steel crown

B. Drifting of tooth and space loss: The crown required to fit a tilted tooth buccolingually will be too wide mesiodistally and crown selected to fit mesiodistally will be too small buccolingually. In such a case larger crown is taken and mesiodistal width is adjusted by using Howe utility plier. Alternate method when there is space loss is by using the crown of diagonally opposite arch.

C. Undersized crown (Fig. 7.111A): A vertical cut is made on the buccal surface of the crown. The margins are pulled apart and an additional piece of steel band material is spot welded to the buccal surface increasing the dimensions of the crown. After contouring, the crown is soldered, polished and cemented.

D. Over sized crown (Fig. 7.111B): The crown is cut vertically along the buccal wall. The free crown margin are approximated and overlapped over each other spot welded to reduce the crowns dimension. After contouring, the cut and relocated area is soldered and polished.

E. Deep subgingival caries in the interproximal surface (Fig. 7.112): This can be managed by 2 methods- use of unfestooned crown or a modified prefestooned crown. A normal prefestooned crown can be used by spot welding an additional band piece thus increasing the length of the crown wherever required.

F. Open contact (except the primate space): It can be corrected by using larger crown, taking care not to disturb the path of eruption of the erupting adjusting tooth. Contouring can also be done using 112 ball and socket plier if the gap is little. Localized addition of solder is also recommended.

G. Anterior teeth: Due to its strength and stability stainless steel crowns are preferred in grossly destroyed anterior teeth. Poor esthetics of stainless steel crowns can be improved by removing a portion of the labial surface of the crown or replacing it with a layer of composite resin. These crowns are also used in the correction of anterior cross bite, where the crown is cemented backwards to provide an inclined plane in the bite.

H. In bruxism: When there is greater risk of crown wear on the occlusal surface, the thickness of the metal on the occlusal surface can be increased by the addition of a layer of solder from the impression surface of the crown. This is known as Croll's technique.

COMPLICATIONS THAT MAY DEVELOP DURING STAINLESS STEEL FABRICATION

A. *Formation of interproximal ledge:* Leads to inability to seat the crown.

B. *Over extension of the crown:* This can be identified by the gingival blanching (Fig. 7.113) and can lead to loss of attachment and periodontal injury.

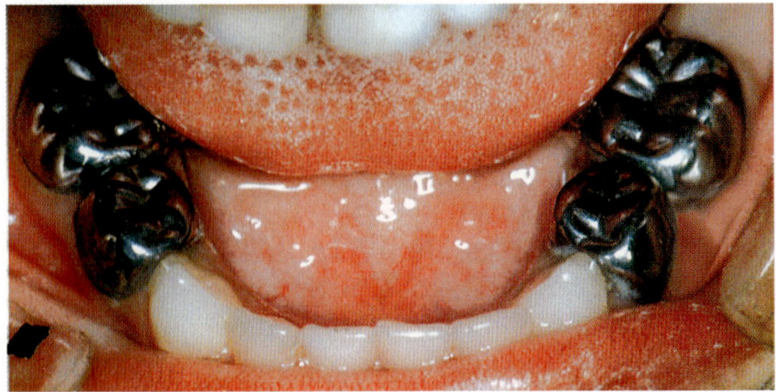

Fig. 7.110: Final placement of a stainless steel crown

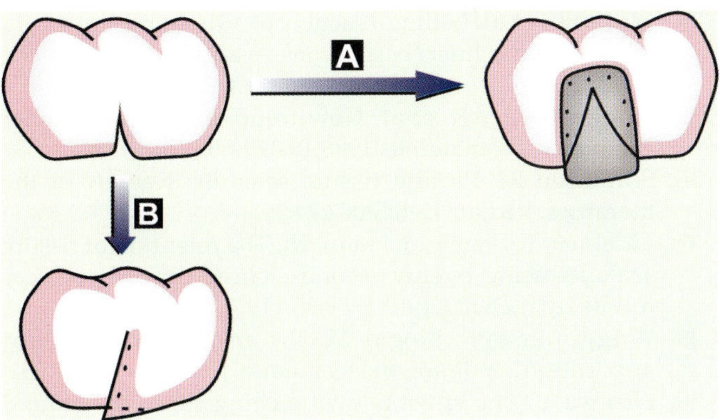

Figs 7.111A and B: Management of: (A) Undersized crown; (B) Over sized crown

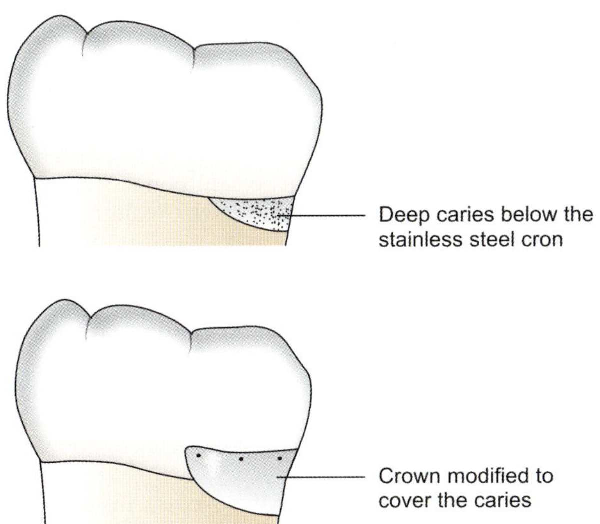

Fig. 7.112: Extension of stainless steel crown into the deep subgingival caries in the interproximal surface

C. *Under extension of the crown:* This will expose the tooth surface above the free gingival margin, making the area vulnerable for debris and plaque collection leading to caries formation and microleakage.

D. *Ingestion of crown:* Can be overcome by using a square piece of gauze as throat screen or by using rubberdam. Should this happen PA chest radiograph is mandatory and patient is referred to the physician. If the crown is not found in the radiograph it is assumed to pass uneventfully through the alimentary tract within 5-10 days and parents are adviced to keep a constant check. If not found abdominal X-ray is necessary to locate the crown.

E. Failure results from poor and inadequate preparation and improper gingival adaptation.

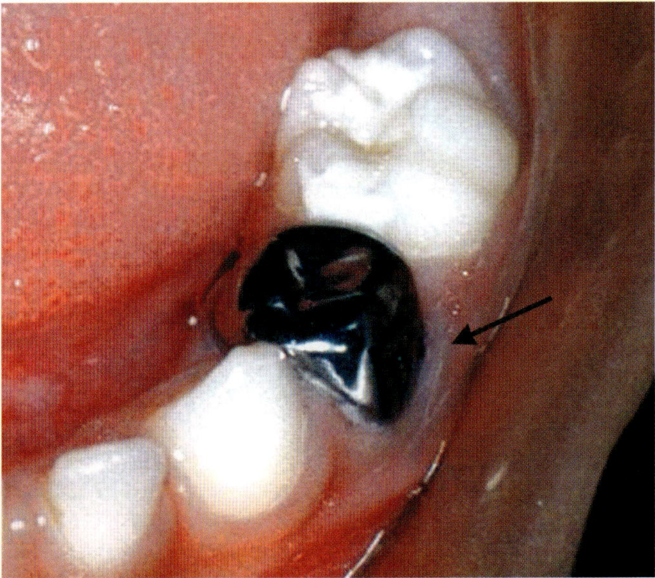

Fig. 7.113: Gingival blanching seen due to overextension of the crown (Arrow)

REFERENCES

1. Roberson TM. Cariology. The lesion, etiology, prevention and control in Roberson TM, Heymann HO, Swift EJ. Sturdevant's Art and Sciences of Operative Dentistry, 5th Ed. Mosby 2006;65-134.
2. Bader JD, Shugars DA. A systematic review of the performance of a laser fluorescence device for detecting caries. J Am Dent Assoc 2004;135:1413-26.
3. Roverson TM. Cariology, in Roberson TM, Heymann HO, Swift EJ. Sturdevant's Art and Sciences of Operative Dentistry, 5th Ed. Mosby 2006;65-134.
4. Black GV. Operative dentistry 8th Ed. Wood Stock Ill, Medico-Dental 1947-1948.
5. Mount GJ, Hume RW. A new classification for dentistry", Quintessence International 1997;28:301-3.
6. Mount GJ, Hume RW. Letter to Editor. Quint. Int 2000;31:375.
7. Curzon MEJ, Roberts F, Kennedy DB. Kennedy's Paediatric Operative Dentistry, 4th Ed. Wright Publishers, 1996.
8. Wilder AD. Preliminary considerations for operative dentistry, In, Roberson TM, Heymann HO, Swift EJ. Sturdevant's Art and Sciences of Operative Dentistry, 5th Ed. Mosby 2006;447-92.
9. Helpin ML, Michal BC. Improved moisture control with the rubber dam. A clinical technique. Pediatr Dent 1980; 2:59.
10. Jinks JM. Rubber dam technique in pedodontics. Dent Clin north Am 1966;327.
11. Smales RJ, Rubberdam usage related to restoration quality and survival. Br. Dent J 1993;174:330.
12. Mathewson RJ, Primosch RE. Fundamentals of Pediatric Dentistry, 3rd Ed. Quintessence Publishing Co.,Inc. 1995.

13. Cunningham PR, Ferguson GW. The instructions of rubber dam technique. J Am Acad Gold Foil Oper 1970; 13:5-12.

14. Medina JE. The rubber dam – an incentive for excellence. Dent Clin North Am 1967;255-64.

15. Setcos JC, Staninec M, Wilson NHF. Bonding of amalgam restorations: Existing knowledge and future prospects. Operative Dentistry 2000;25:121-9.

16. Wilson AD, Kent BE, Clinton D, Miller RP. The formation and microstructure of dental silicate cements. J Mater Sci 1972;7:220-38.

17. Wilson AD, McLean JW. Glass-ionomer cement. Berlin: Quintessence, 1988.

18. Mount CJ. Restoration with glass ionomer cement: requirement for clinical success. Oper Dent 1981;6:59-65.

19. Mount CJ. Glass ionomer cements: Clinical considerations. Clinical Dent. New York, Harper and Row 1984.

20. Forsten L. Fluoride release and uptake by glass-ionomers and related materials and its clinical effect. Biomaterials 1998;19:503-8.

21. Barry TI, Clinton DJ, Wilson AD. The structure of a glass ionomer cement and its relationship to the setting process. J Dent Res 1979;58:1072-9.

22. Wilson AD, Kent BE. A New Translucent Cement for Dentistry: the Glass Ionomer Cement, British. Dent. J 1972;132:133-5.

23. Upadhya PN, Kishore G. Glass Ionomer Cement – The Different Generation. Trends Biomater. Artif. Organs, 2005;18:158-65.

24. Hanting C, Hanxing L, Guoqing Z. The setting chemistry of glass ionomer cement, J Wuhan University of Technology—Materials Science Edition 2005;20:110-2.

25. Wilson AD. Secondary reactions in glass-ionomer cements J. Mat Science 1996;15:275-6.

26. Saito S, Tosaki S, Hirota K. Characteristics of glass-ionomer cements. In: Davidson CL, MjöR IA, editors. Advances in glassionomer cements. Berlin: Quintessence Publishing Co, 1999.

27. Mount GJ. Glass ionomers: a review on their current status. Oper Dent 1999;24:114-24.

28. Pelka M, Ebert J, Schneider H, Kramer N, Petschelt A. Comparision of two- and three-body wear of glass-ionomers and composites. Eur J Oral Sci 1996;104:132-7.

29. Xie D, Brantley WA, Culbertson BM, Wang G. Mechanical properties and microstructures of glass-ionomer cements. Dent Mater 2000;16:129-38.

30. Lohbauer U, Walker J, et al. Reactive fiber reinforced glass ionomer cements. Biomaterials 2003;24:2901-7.

31. Kawano F, Kon M, Kobayashi M, Miyai K. Reinforcement effect of short glass fibers with $CaO–P_2O_5–SiO_2–Al_2O_3$ glass on strength of glass ionomer cements. J Dent 2001;29:377-80.

32. Kobayashi M, Kon M, Miyai K, Asaoka K. Strengthening of glass-ionomer cement by compounding short bres with $CaO–P_2O_5–SiO_2–Al_2O_3$ glass. Biomaterials 2000; 21:2051-8.

33. Simmons JJ. The miracle mixture: Glass ionomer and alloyed powder. Text Dent J 1983;100:10-2.

34. Mitra SB, et al. Setting reaction of Vitrebond light cure glass ionomer liner/base. Trans Acad Dent Mater 1992; 5:1-22.

35. Guggenberger R, et al. New trends in Glass ionomer chemistry. Biomaterials 1998;19:479-83.

36. Simonsen RJ. Pit and fissure sealants: Review of the literature, Pediatr Dent 2002;24:393.

37. Eidelman E, Shapira J, Houpt M. The retention of fissure sealants using twenty-second etching time: three year follow up. J Dent Child 1988;55:119.

38. Waggoner WF, Siegal M. Pit and fissure sealant application: updating the technique. JADA 1996;127:351.

39. Hosoya Y. The effect of acid etching times on ground primary enamel. J Clin Pediatr Dent Spring; 1991; 15(3): 188-94.

40. Silverstone LM. Proceedings of the international symposium on the acid etch technique. St. Paul, North Central Publishing Co, 1975.

41. Hicks J, Flaitz CM. Pit and fissure sealants and conservative adhesive restorations: Scientific and Clinical Rationale. Pediatric Dentistry, Infancy through Adolescence, 4th Edition, Elsevier Saunders, 2005;520-76.

42. Redford DA, Clarkson BH, Jensen ME. The effect of different etching times on sealant bond strength, etch depth and pattern in primary teeth. Pediatr Dent 1986; 8:11.

43. Choi S, Rhee Y, Park JH, Lee GJ, Kim KS, Park JH, Park YG, Park HK. Effects of fluoride treatment on phosphoric acid-etching in primary teeth: an AFM observationMicron. Epub 2010;41(5):498-506.

44. Silverstone LM, Saxton CA, Dogon IL, Fejerskov O. Variation in the pattern of acid etching of human dental enamel examined by scanning electron microscopy. Caries Res 1975;9:373.

45. Van Meerbeek B, et al. Microscopy investigation: techniques, results and limitations. Am J Dent 2000;13: 3D-18D.

46. Nakabayashi N, et al. Identification of a resin-dentin hybrid layer in vital human dentin created *in vivo*: durable bonding to vital dentin. Quintessence Int 1992; 23:135-41.

47. Nakabayashi N, Takarada K. Effect of HEMA on bonding to dentin. Dent Mater 1992;8:125-30.

48. Humphrey WP. Uses of chrome steel in children's dentistry. Dent Surv 1950;26:945-9.

49. Randall RC. Preformed metal crowns for primary and permanent molar teeth: review of the literature, Pediatr Dent 2002;24:489-500.

50. Wei

51. Mink JR, Bennet IC. The stainless steel crown. J Dent Child 1968;35:186.

52. Spedding RH. Two principles for improving the adaptation of stainless steel crowns to primary molars, Dent Clin North Am 1984;28:157-75.

53. Kennedy DB. The stainless steel crown, Pediatric Operative Dentistry J Wright and Sons Ltd, Bristol 1976.

54. Rapp R. A simplified precise technique for the placement of stainless steel crowns on primary teeth J Dent Child 1966;33:101.

55. Mink JR, Hill CJ. Modification of the stainless steel crown for primary teeth, J Detn Child 1971;38:61-9.
56. Mc Donald RE, Avery DR. Restorative dentistry In. dentistry for the child and adolescent 6th Ed. St Louis Mosby 1994.
57. McEvoy SA. Approximating stainless steel crowns in space loss quadrants. J Dent Child 1977;44:105.
58. Croll, TP, Castaldi, CR. The preformed stainless steel crown for restoration of permanent posterior teeth in special case, JADA, 1978;97:644-9.
59. Croll TP. Increasing occlusal surface thickness of stainless steel crowns: A Clinical Technique. Pediatric Dentistry 1980;2:297-9.

QUESTIONS

1. Enumerate the differences between deciduous and permanent teeth.
2. What are the different methods of diagnosis of caries.
3. Principles of cavity preparation for amalgam restoration.
4. Properties of glass ionomer cement.
5. Modifications of glass ionomer cement.
6. Classify matrix and retainers. What is the use of matrix and retainers?
7. What are the different methods of isolation? Explain rubber dam in detail.
8. Components of composite resins.
9. Write in detail the steps involved in placement of composite restoration.
10. Give the indications and contraindications of stainless steel restorations.
11. Explain the steps involved in placement of stainless steel crowns.
12. What are the modifications of stainless steel crowns?

Pulp Therapy

INTRODUCTION

Pulp is a soft tissue that is surrounded by dentin. It is a tough fibrous tissue with not much elasticity which is attributed to collagen fibers present in them. The function of the pulp is summarized as being responsible for formation, nutrition, innervations and defence of dentin. It helps in the formation of secondary dentin, provides nutrition to dentin through odontoblasts, provides innervation through fluid and pheripheral receptors and defence is through the means of reparative dentin formation and blood cells. Dentin is formed around the pulp continuously in the form of secondary dentin and thus as age progresses the pulp regresses in size. Pulp in a deciduous tooth or young permanent tooth is, therefore, large in size compared to the tooth in adults. Anatomically, pulp can be divided based on its location into coronal and radicular pulp. Pulp is histologically made of two main zones—the peripheral and central. The peripheral zone is located just beneath the dentin. It is made of predentin, odontoblast cells, cell free zone of Weil (plexus of capillary and nerve fibers), cell rich zone (fibroblasts, undifferentiated mesenchymal cells and Korff's fibers). The central zone is surrounded by cell rich zone of the peripheral zone and consists of large vessels and nerves, ground substance (Hyaluronic acid, chondroitin sulfate and other glycoproteins) and collagen. Pulp consists of myelinated and nonmyelinated nerve fibers. The myelinated fibers are derived from trigeminal nerves. The nonmyelinated fibers form the majority types and are derived from the sympathetic division of the autonomous nervous system and are responsible for the regulation of blood flow in the pulp. Plexuses of Raschkow are myelinated nerve plexuses seen below cell rich zone in the central zone.[1-4]

Inflammatory Changes in the Pulp[4-10]

It was Seltzer et al in 1963 who gave a classic description of the histological changes seen in pulp following carious exposure.

Toxins reach the pulp through the dentinal tubules even before the bacteria can cause severe reaction in the pulp which may range from mild inflammation to abscess formation.

When the pulp is irritated, typical inflammatory changes are seen as observed in other parts of the body such as neutrophil chemotaxis, phagocytosis, release of lysosomal enzymes, vasodilatation. It is also important to realize that pulp tissue is located in an unyielding space within the chamber surrounded by dentin. When there is increased vasodilatation and increased permeability, fluid accumulates in the interstitial space leading to increase in pressure within the pulp and since there is no collateral circulation, it results in collapse of vessels and cell death. The healthy dental pulp has an interstitial pressure of 5 to 14 mm Hg and when it gets to 35 mm Hg, pulpal damage is irreversible.

Management of diseased pulp in a deciduous or young permanent tooth is a very challenging task due to the anatomy and reaction of the pulp which is further complicated by the age factor where it may be difficult to obtain accurate history and the fact that the tooth is constantly resorbing or developing.

DIFFERENCE BETWEEN PRIMARY AND PERMANENT PULP[11-16] (FIG. 8.1)

- Pulp chamber in a deciduous teeth is larger compared to the crown size
- The roots are thin and slender with narrow pulp canals
- Apical foramen is wider
- Mesial pulp horns extend closer towards outer surface. This increases the risk of pulp exposure during cavity preparation.
- Accessory canals extend from pulpal chamber to the interradicular area at the furcation. Therefore the radiographic changes (radiolucency that is caused due to widening of periodontal space and resorption of bone) is seen in the interradicular region rather than the periapical region.
- Deciduous pulp is highly vascularized. Thus it exhibits typical inflammatory response to any irritating stimulus, and is at high-risk for internal and external resorption. Localization of infection and inflammation is very poor for the same reason.

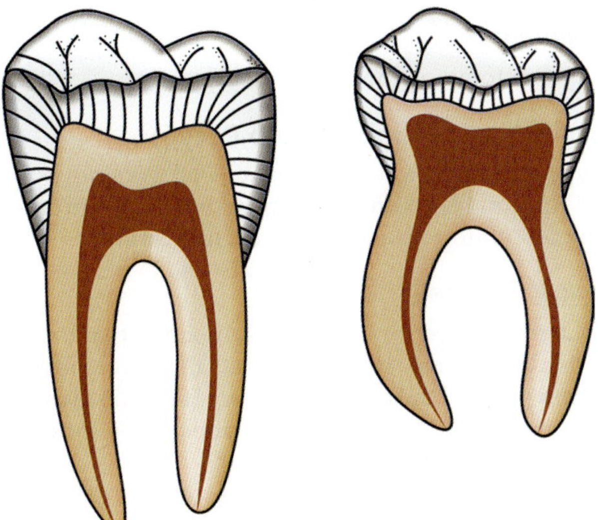

Fig. 8.1: Longitudinal section of permanent and deciduous molars

- Increased rate of reparative dentin formation is seen in deciduous teeth
- Root canals are ribbon shaped or have a hour glass appearance. The canals are narrower mesiodistally, which makes gross enlargement of the canal
- Multiple ramifications are common in deciduous pulp canal making complete debridement difficult if not impossible
- Histologically, there is not gross difference except for the presence of cap like zone of reticular and collagenous fibers in deciduous coronal pulp.
- Risk of pulp stones is less in deciduous teeth.
- Deciduous teeth are less sensitive to pain. This may be due to less number of nerve fibers in deciduous teeth. It is also noted that the nerve fibers extend up to predentin in permanent teeth but terminate in the odontoblastic area in deciduous teeth. The reason of reduced sensitivity is also said to be due to the fact that neural tissues are last to be formed during pulp development and first to degenerate when root resorption begins. Since the roots of the deciduous tooth begis resorbing as soon as completion the nerve fibers are never fully formed and this may be the reason for reduced sensitivity of deciduous teeth.

Type of nerve fibers in the pulp			
Type of fiber	Function	Diameter (μm)	Conduction Velocity(m/s)
Aα	Motor, proprioception	12-20	
Aβ	Pressure, touch	5-10	
Aγ	Motor	3-6	
Aδ	Pain, temperature, touch	2-5	
B	Preganglionic autonomic	<3	
C	Pain, Postganglionic sympathetic	0.5-1	

Etiology[17-26]

Physical (Mechanical) irritants: It is observed that slight elevation of temperature on the external surface of a tooth can raise the internal temperature of the pulp to the point that injury occurs. A temperature increase of 5.5° C above body temperature is said to be the threshold for damage to the pulp. Cutting a cavity without appropriate coolant can generate heat that may cause severe damage to the pulp. The heat produced during cutting is determined by factors such as the sharpness of the bur, the amount of pressure exerted on the bur and the length of time the cutting instrument contacts tooth structure. The temperature on the surface of a rotating dental bur in contact with dentin has been reported to be as high as 417° C. The ill-effect of heat on pulp is also dependent on the thickness of the dentin and is maximum when the thickness of dentin is less than 1 mm. Continuous blast of compressed air as during drying can damage to the pulp. During drying, the fluids from the dentinal tubules are sucked outwards and this will lead to displacement of odontoblasts. The damage is comparatively minimum compared to the damage that occurs due to overheating.

Chemical (Irritants such as acids, monomer, etc on pulp directly or through thin dentin): Dentin is capable of buffering and limiting the entry of hydrogen ions from reaching the pulp from the restorative materials.

Bacterial (Direct bacterial attack, toxins produced by the bacteria or may be anachoretic effect) insults: The mean dentin diameter is about 0.9 μm, whereas the diameter of the bacteria ranges from 0.2 to 0.7 μm. But the entry of bacteria is delayed in a vital tooth due to the outward movement of dentinal fluid and the presence of tubular contents. Conversely, bacterial invasion in a nonvital tooth is rapid. There are about 10 to 30 species of bacteria that form primary invaders and their count may range from 103 to 108 cells per canal. Endodontic bacteria mainly belong to Bacteroidetes, Spirochaetes, Fusobacteria, Actinobacteria, Proteobacteria, Synergistes or Firmicutes. Anachoresis is a process by which microorganisms are transported in the blood and lymph to an area of tissue damage, where they leave the vessel, enter the damaged tissue and establish an infection.

CLASSIFICATION OF PULPAL DISEASES[27]

Based on the extent of pulpal damage, disease of the pulp can be classified as:
1. Pulpitis
     i. Reversible pulpitis
    ii. Irreversible pulpitis
         – Hyperplastic pulpitis
         – Internal resorption
2. Pulp degeneration-pulp calcification
3. Necrosis

Reversible Pulpitis

Definition

"Mild to moderate inflammatory condition of the pulp caused by noxious stimuli, in which the pulp is capable of returning to the uninflamed state following removal of the stimuli." It is basically a clinical diagnosis made through subjective and objective findings.

Clinical Features

Reversible pulpitis may be due to direct or indirect injury to the pulp. It is related to recent restorations (lack of adequate insulation below a restoration), exposed thin dentin, trauma, etc. all of which resulting in inflammatory reaction within the pulp.

The typical features are the increased response to cold, hot or sweets. Pain that is associated with reversible pulpitis is sharp and transient in nature, lasting for a moment and subsides soon after removal of the stimuli.

Treatment

• A good restoration with adequate and effective insulation.

Irreversible Pulpitis

Definition

"Persistent inflammatory condition of the pulp, which is symptomatic or asymptomatic caused by a noxious stimulus." It is also basically a clinical diagnosis made through subjective and objective findings. It is normally continuation of reversible pulpitis resulting in progressive damage to pulp.

Clinical Features

Pain that is associated with irreversible pulpitis is sharp, piercing or shooting type. The typical feature is the presence of lingering pain (continuous in nature) that lasts for several minutes to hours after removal of the stimuli. Pain may also be aggravated by sudden changes in temperature, pressure or on lying down.

Treatment

• Pulpectomy or root canal therapy.

Hyperplastic Pulpitis (Pulp Polyp)

"Hyperplastic pulpitis is a form of irreversible pulpitis that originates from overgrowth of a chronically inflamed young pulp onto the occlusal surface."

Clinical Features

• Characterized by the development of granulation tissue, covered by epithelium, that protrudes as a polyp out of the pulpal chamber (Fig. 8.2) This is due to the ample vascularity and adequate exposure for drainage seen in young pulp.
• Occurs in tooth with extensive carious exposure of the pulp, associated with long standing, low grade irritation.

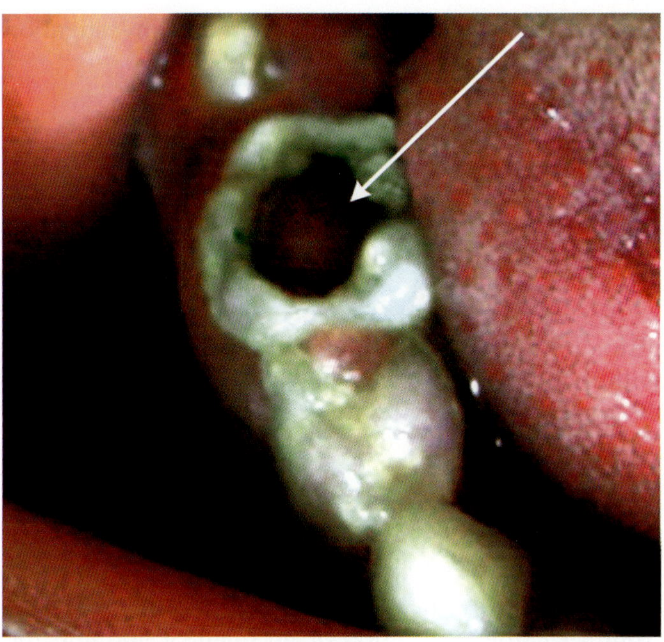

Fig. 8.2: Pulp polyp in the lower right second deciduous tooth

- Usually asymptomatic but pain may be present during mastication.

Treatment

Pulpectomy, root canal treatment or extraction.

Internal Resorption

Definition

"Idiopathic slow or fast progressive resorptive process occurring in the dentin of the pulp chamber or pulp canal of the teeth."

Clinical Features

Typically internal resorption exhibits no additional symptoms other than that of the existing pulpitis.
- Internal resorption may occur in pulp chamber or pulp canal.
- Crown may appear pink called as pink tooth when the internal resorption is present in the coronal portion. The enlarged inflamed pulp that occupies the resorbed area is seen through the thin dentin making the crown appear pink in color. Radiographically, no gross changes are seen except for widening of the pulpal chamber and thinning of the dentin.
- Internal resorption involving the root canal appears as round to oval radiolucent area that extends from the pulp canal.

- Internal resorption may proceed if left untreated to perforate the entire dentin thickness and communicate with the periodontal space. Prognosis becomes very poor when the tooth is associated with extensive resorption.

Treatment

- Pulp extirpation and routine endodontic procedure, if the resorption is mild to moderate. The process of resorption ceases after removal of the pulp.
- When the resorption is very extensive and prognosis is poor it is advisible to extract the involved tooth.

Necrosis of the Pulp

It is associated with the death of the pulp, and the tooth is termed is as being nonvital.

Clinical Features

- The involved tooth may be asymptomatic or associated with pain.
- It may also be associated with periapical abscess draining either intraorally or extraorally. The tooth may be then tender to biting or touch.
- The crown of the tooth may be discolored.

Treatment

- Pulpectomy or root canal therapy is the choice when the clinical crown is restorable.
- If the clinical crown is grossly destroyed due to caries, the treatment of choice is extraction following by suitable rehabilitation.

PERIRADICULAR DISEASES

As a consequence of pulpal necrosis, pathologic changes can occur in the periradicular tissues. Periradicular lesions have been classified based on their clinical and histologic findings.
1. Symptomatic (acute) apical periodontitis
2. Asymptomatic (chronic) apical periodontitis
3. Condensing osteitis
4. Apical abscess: Lesions associated with pain or swelling is referred to as acute and those with mild or no symptoms as chronic.

Apical Periodontitis

It may be symptomatic (acute) or asymptomatic (chronic). It indicates initial extension of pulpal inflammation into the periradicular region leading to inflammation of periodontal tissues. Symptomatic acute apical periodontitis is characterized by moderate to severe pain especially on biting and or percussion. Radiographic changes such as widening of periodontal ligament space may not be appreciable initially. In symptomatic apical periodontitis the involved tooth exhibits radiographic changes (root and bone resorption) with no clinical symptoms.

Treatment

- Pulpectomy, root canal treatment or extraction.

Condensing Osteitis

It may be symptomatic or asymptomatic and the tooth may or may not respond to electric or thermal stimuli. Radiographically, the presence of a diffuse concentric arrangement of radiopacity around the root of a tooth is pathognomonic. Treatment is root canal treatment.

Acute Alveolar Abscess

Definition

"Localized collection of pus in the alveolar bone at the root apex of the tooth, with extension of the infection through the apical foramen into the periradicular tissue."

Pulp in such a condition is necrotic most of the time.

Clinical Features

Initially the tooth that is affected is tender with soft tissue swelling. As it progresses, the swelling becomes more pronounced and the tooth becomes mobile and elevated from the socket. If left untreated, it may lead to osteitis, cellulitis and osteomyelitis. It can be also associated with slight rise in body temperature, chills, malaise and headache.

Radiographic changes are minimum—as the changes are confined to medullary bone only.

Treatment

- Establishment of drainage. An incision is given at the area where the abscess 'points'. Followed by root canal therapy or pulpectomy.

Chronic Abscess

It is seen in tooth associated with long standing, low grade infection of the periradicular tissues. It is most of the time associated with discharging sinus or fistula. Patients usually have no complaints except may be for occasional pain.

DIAGNOSIS OF PULP PATHOLOGY

The success of the treatment used depends mainly upon an accurate preoperative assessment of pulp status. Complete case history, examination and investigation forms the pre-requisite for correct diagnosis.

Diagnostic Features[4,27-30]

Pain

An accurate history must be obtained of the type of pain, including its duration, frequency, location and spread as well as aggravating and relieving factors.

The absence of toothache does not preclude a histologic pulpitis. The active lives of children, together with their short attention spans, may mean that minor discomfort passes without comment in a whirlwind of activities.

A positive history of toothache suggests definite pulp pathology. However it is difficult to correlate the type of pain with the degree of pathosis.

Sensitivity to thermal stimuli—indicates vital pulp.

Momentary pain—may be due to exposure of dentin from a leaking restoration or an open lesion and the pathosis is confined to coronal pulp.

Persistent pain—indicates widespread inflammation of the pulp, extending throughout the radicular filaments.

Pain may be radiated to other teeth, jaw, temple or sinuses. It then becomes difficult to identify the involved tooth.

Pain on percussion indicates that supporting periodontal fibers are inflamed. Depression of the tooth results in pain. The tooth may be slightly elevated from the socket and in premature occlusion. This increases the discomfort, especially during mastication.

Swelling

It may be present intraorally or extraorally.

Intraoral swelling (Figs 8.3 A and B)

It is usually apparent on the buccal aspect of the alveolus. There is less bone on the buccal aspect than on the lingual or palatal side, through which the inflammatory products from the periapical or inter radicular regions penetrate, taking the path of least resistance. The pressure of the swelling will eventually result in spontaneous drainage if treatment is not rendered.

The fine apical foramen precludes the drainage of the exudate through the open lesion and drainage occurs through the formation of fistula, usually seen at the junction of the attached gingiva and alveolar mucosa, corresponding to the site adjacent to the interradicular region.

The tissue adjacent to the fistula is inflamed. Once the fistula is formed, drainage is established and lesion is seldom acute and becomes a chronic lesion.

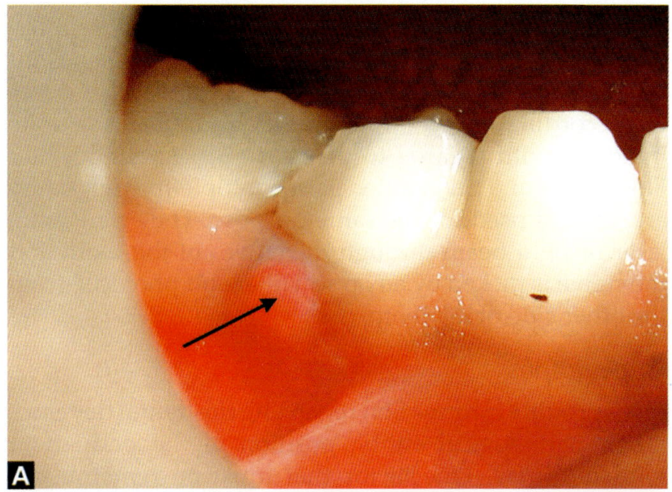

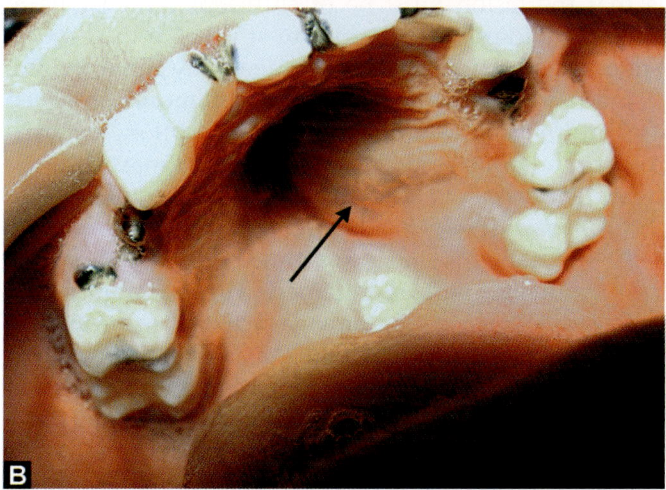

Figs 8.3A and B: (A) Intraoral swelling on the buccal aspect; (B) Intraoral swelling on the palatal aspect

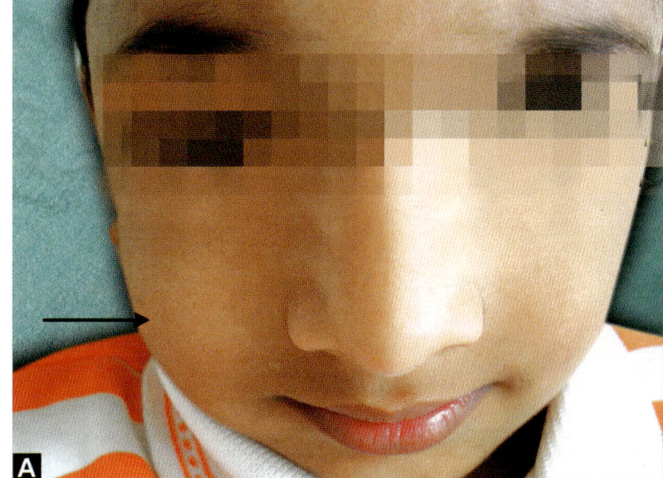

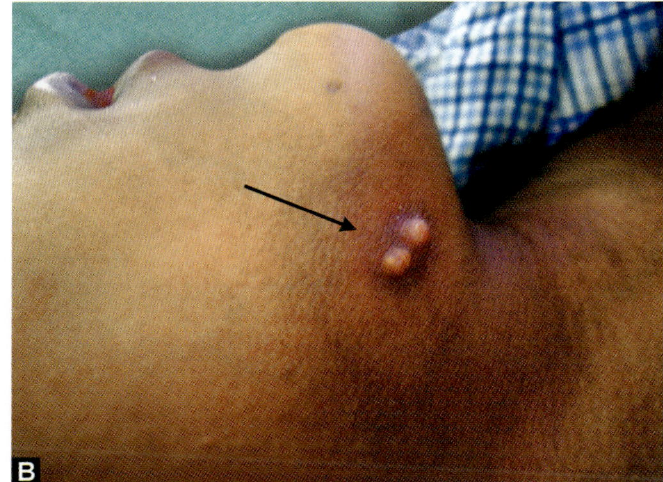

Figs 8.4A and B: (A) Extraoral swelling seen in a young boy due to an infected lower second right molar; (B) Extraoral sinus opening due to infection of lower right second deciduous molar

Extraoral swelling/cellulities (Figs 8.4A and B): It is due to the spread of exudate into various spaces along the fascial planes. In the mandibular arch, submandibular region is commonly involved and in the maxillary arch, the swelling may extend up to the infraorbital margin, may involve the upper eye lid or may be so severe as to close the child's eye. The drainage occurs through the path of least resistance, which is through the skin.

A tooth associated with swelling or fistula is usually nonvital. Sometimes one of the canals may contain inflamed but vital pulp. From the treatment point of view the tooth is considered nonvital.

Discoloration

Tooth that is nonvital tend to have a darker color (Fig. 8.5). Tooth associated with internal resorption at the pulp chamber tend to appear pink (Hence the name "Pink Tooth') (Fig. 8.6).

Mobility

Mobility associated with a deciduous tooth may be physiologic or may be due to any persisting pathology. Radiographic evaluation of the roots of deciduous tooth, the position of the developing tooth and amount of root completion of permanent tooth will determine the cause.

Pathological mobility is associated with pathologic root resorption/bone resorption.

Bone resorption is identified as radiolucency at the periapical or inter radicular region. It is not reliable to assess the degree of pathosis based on radiographic changes and mobility alone.

Vitality Tests

Pulp vitality tests, either thermal or electrical, are of little value in primary teeth. While they may sometimes give an indication of pulp vitality, the response does

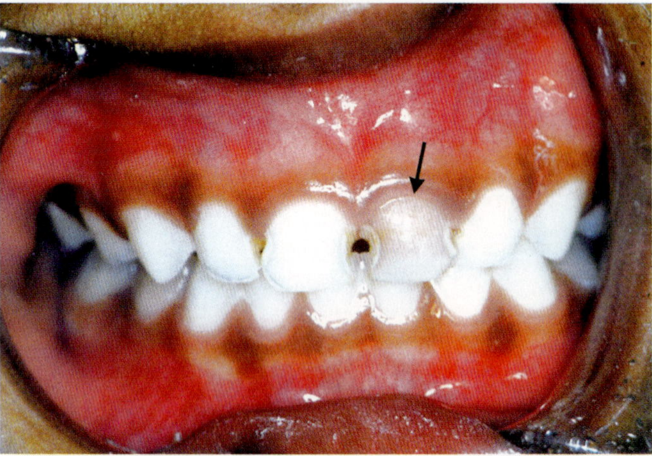

Fig. 8.5: Discolored nonvital upper deciduous central incisor

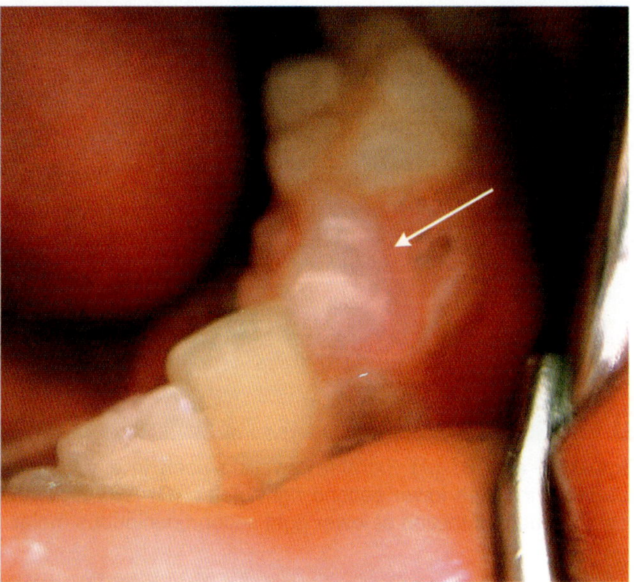

Fig. 8.6: Pink discoloration of the crown of the lower first deciduous molar due to internal resorption in the pulp chamber

not identify the degree of pathosis present. Fear of the unknown may make the child patient apprehensive of the electric vitalometer and he or she may then give the response they feel is correct rather than an accurate one, thus making it very unpredictable. More importantly a normal healthy primary teeth may not respond to vitality tests.

The real value of vitality tests, either thermal or electrical, is in the permanent teeth where comparison can be made with normal antimeres. The obvious example involves traumatized incisors, where serial testing may reveal the progress of the health of the pulp.

The pulp response may vary with recently erupted teeth, thickness of the tooth structure, presence of necrotic material, etc.

Recording the blood flow in the pulp is an accurate indicator with regards to the its status. Laser Doppler Flow meter and transmitted light photoplethysmography are devices used for the same purpose. They transmit a laser or light beam through the crown of the tooth and the signal is picked by an optical fiber and photocell from the other side of the tooth.

Radiographs

They provide information regarding the dental development, pathological entity, position of the permanent tooth bud, etc. One factor that must be remembered is that the lesion must be of sufficient dimensions to appear radiographically and must involve the cortical bone. Thus a lesion in its initial stages may go unnoticed.

Pathological entities that can be commonly observed are; pulp calcifications, internal resorption, external resorption, bone resorption all of which may alter the treatment plan.

I. *Internal resorption (Fig. 8.7):* It is associated with spontaneous pain at night and both the coronal and radicular pulp is inflamed. This contraindicates single visit pulpotomy and if the resorption is severe extraction may be the only choice.

II. *External resorption (Fig. 8.8):* Pathological resorption is invariably associated with nonvital pulp and extensive inflammation in the supporting tissues which may lead to external resorption. The only viable treatment is pulpectomy or extraction.

III. *Bone resorption (Fig. 8.9):* It is associated with a non vital pulp and may range from mild to severe bone loss depending on the presence of the persisting irritation. The involved tooth may be mobile and the extent of mobility is directly proportional to the amount of bone loss. If the resorption is minimum, pulpectomy is the treatment of choice but when the bone loss is extensive, extraction may be the only option. The radiolucency in primary molars is usually seen at the furcation and not at the apex. This is due to:
  – Exudate cannot penetrate the fine branching ramification of the molar root canals.
  – Presence of accessory canals in the furcation region.
  – Porous and permeable pulpal floor.

IV. Pulp calcification: Represents the pulp's response to a long-standing lesion and is associated with pulpal degeneration. This contraindicates single visit pulpotomy.

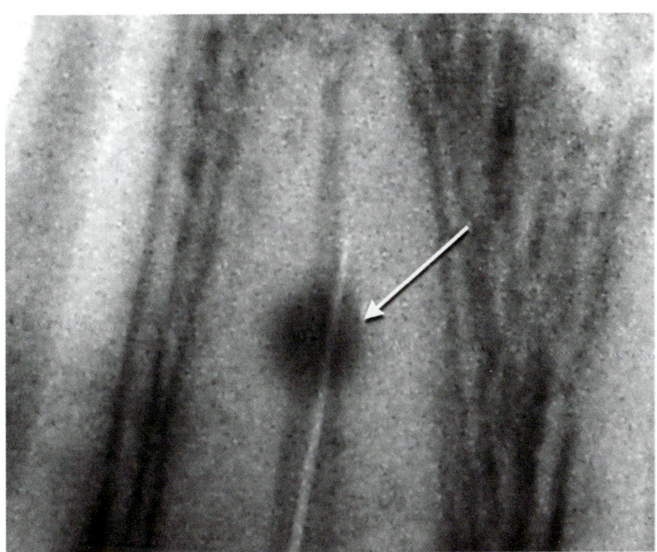

Fig. 8.7: Internal resorption seen with relation to upper central incisor

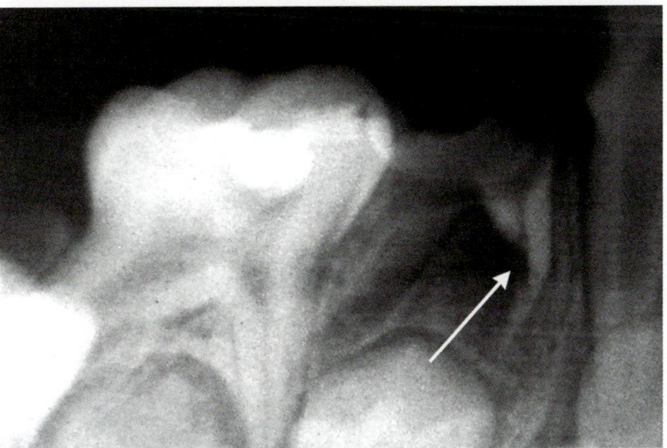

Fig. 8.8: External pathologic resorption seen with relation to distal roots of lower second deciduous molar

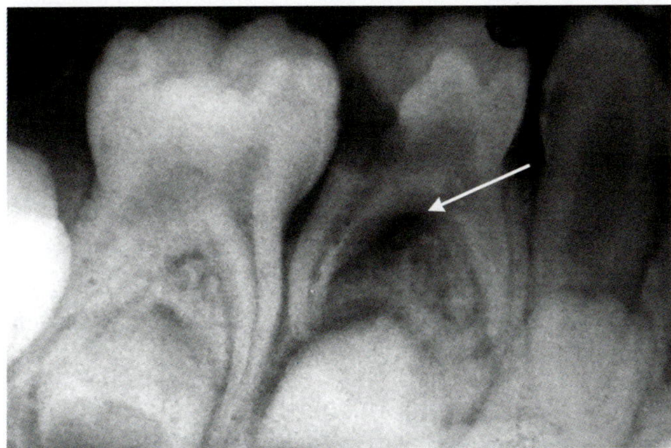

Fig. 8.9: Bone resorption in the deciduous molar is observed at the furcation whereas in permanent molars radiolucency is seen at the periapical region

INDIVIDUAL TOOTH ASSESSMENT

The following questions should be answered before planning a treatment:

1. Are there any prevailing medical factors that contraindicate endodontic therapy in deciduous teeth? (Example: congenital cardiac defects, immunosuppressed patients, diabetes, etc.)

2. Presence of medical or local conditions that contraindicate extractions such as bleeding or coagulation disorders, congenitally missing permanent successor, etc.

3. Can the tooth be restored back to function after pulp therapy is performed ? (Figs 8.10A and B)

4. Does the dental age of the child justify retention of the particular tooth? If the age of a child is above about 8 years it is very important to decide 'How long the tooth is going to stay in the oral cavity'. This depends on the dental age, amount of bone overlying the erupting permanent tooth.

5. Is the pulp status as such acquiescent to pulp therapy?

Objectives of pulp therapy[31-36]

According to AAPD guidelines, the primary objective of pulp therapy is to maintain the integrity and health of the teeth and their supporting tissues. The indications, objectives, and type of pulpal therapy depend on whether the pulp is vital or nonvital, based on the tooth's clinical diagnosis of normal pulp, reversible pulpitis, irreversible pulpitis, or necrotic pulp.

Teeth exhibiting signs and/or symptoms such as a history of spontaneous unprovoked toothache, a sinus tract, periodontal inflammation not resulting from gingivitis or periodontitis, excessive mobility not associated with trauma or exfoliation, furcation/apical radiolucency, or radiographic evidence of internal/external resorption have a clinical diagnosis of irreversible pulpitis or necrosis. These teeth are candidates for nonvital pulp treatment.

Teeth exhibiting provoked pain of short duration—which is relieved upon the removal of the stimulus, with analgesics, or by brushing—without signs or symptoms of irreversible pulpitis, have a clinical diagnosis of reversible pulpitis and are candidates for vital pulp therapy. Teeth with a normal pulp requiring pulp therapy are treated with vital pulp procedures. Vital pulp therapy is broadly defined as treatment initiated to preserve and maintain pulp tissue in a healthy state, tissue that has been compromised by caries, trauma, or restorative procedures. The objective is to stimulate the formation of reparative dentin to retain the tooth as a functional unit.

Different types of pulp therapy

Deciduous teeth	*Young permanent teeth*
1. Indirect pulp capping	1. Indirect pulp capping
2. Direct pulp capping	2. Direct pulp capping
3. Pulpotomy	3. Pulpotomy/Apexogenesis
4. Pulpectomy	4. Apexification

Pulpectomy and apexification are nonvital therapies. Remaining are vital therapies.

MANAGEMENT TECHNIQUES

Indirect Pulp Capping[4,27,37,38]

Indirect pulp capping is defined as "a procedure in which a material is placed on a thin partition of remaining carious dentin that, if removed, might expose the pulp in immature permanent teeth. This technique shows some success in teeth with the absence of symptomatology and with no radiographic evidence of pathosis.

Aim

To remove the infected dentin and leaving intact the affected dentin, so that the affected dentin will remineralize and act as a barrier above the healthy pulp.

Indications

- Deep caries in which the pulpal inflammation has been judged to be minimal and complete removal of caries would probably cause pulpal exposure.

Contraindications

- When there is wide spread inflammation or evidence of periapical pathosis.

Procedure (Figs 8.11A to E)

- Tooth is isolated with rubber dam.
- All the caries on the cavity walls and at the DEJ are removed, due to its closeness to the surface. Caries left in this area will likely cause failure due to the lateral spread.
- Large round bur or spoon excavator is used to remove the carious dentin. Round bur in slow speed is preferred, as there is more chance of removal of large segment of dentin with excavator
- Sedative dressing of calcium hydroxide is placed over the remaining dentin
- Tooth is then sealed with zinc oxide eugenol and amalgam

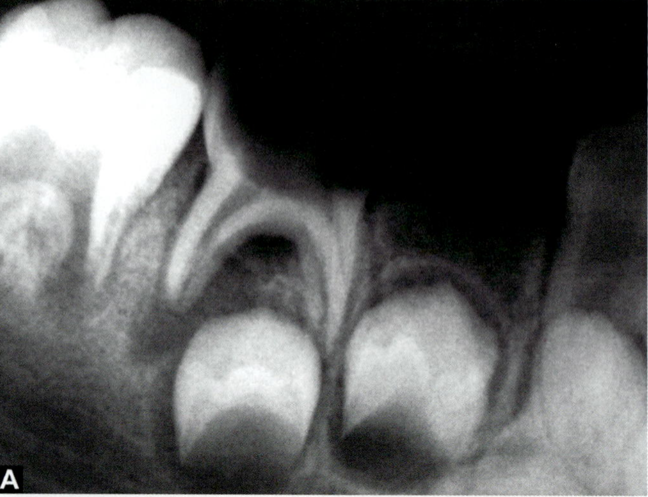

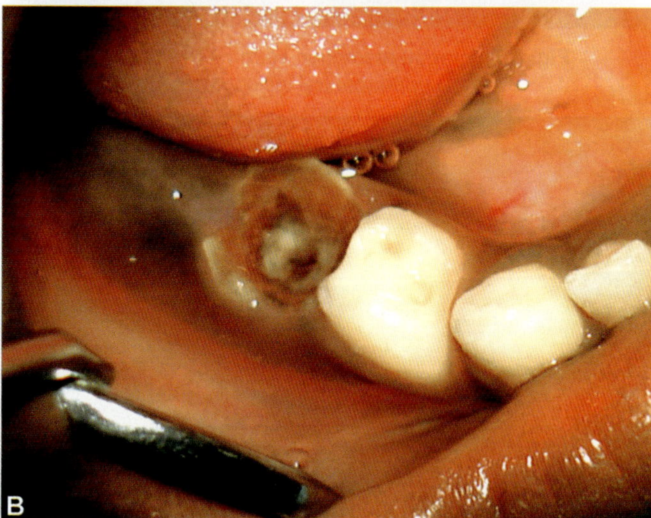

Figs 8.10A and B: Grossly decayed teeth which cannot be restored back to function is a contraindicated for any endodontic therapy; (A) Radiograph of a lower second deciduous molar; (B) Clinical picture of another case of a lower second deciduous molar with complete destruction of the clinical crown

- The treated tooth can be re-entered (if two step procedure is done) after 6-8 weeks and remaining caries is removed. The pulp is safe from exposure, due to the formation of reparative dentin
- The color would have changed from red rose to light gray or light brown. The texture changes from spongy and wet to hard
- Tooth is then permanently restored with stainless steel crown.

Affected Vs Infected Dentin[39,40]

- Carious dentin is characterized by the presence of affected and infected dentin. Affected dentin forms

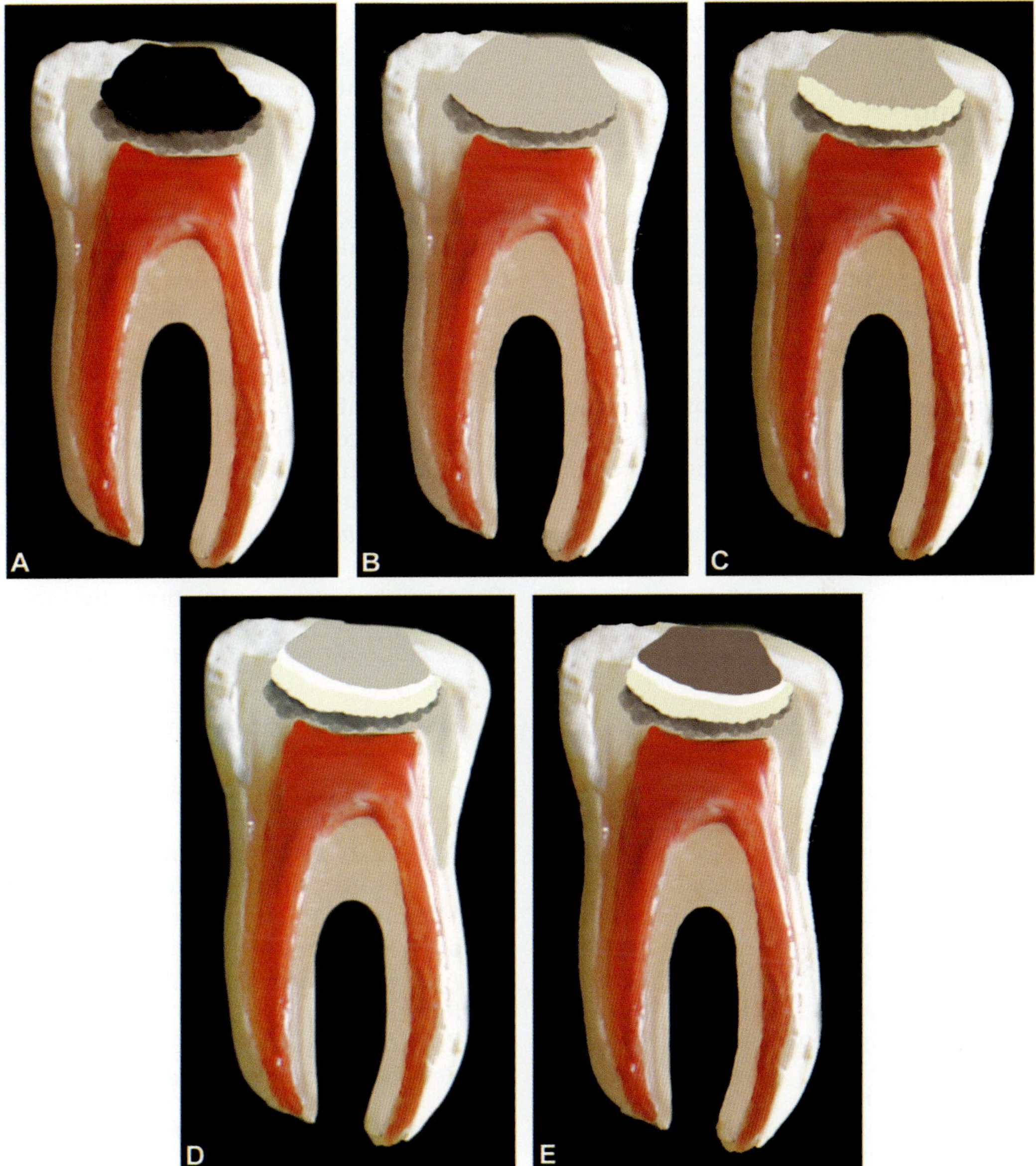

Figs 8.11A to E: Indirect pulp capping: (A) Deep caries close to the pulp; (B) Only infected dentin is removed leaving the affected dentin; (C) Calcium hydroxide is placed over the affected dentin; (D) Suitable base is placed over calcium hydroxide; (E) Tooth is sealed with amalgam restoration

the progressive front of the lesion preceded by the infected dentin. The infected dentin is characterized by the presence of microorganisms. The toxic products from these microorganisms demineralize the dentin to form the affected zone (Affected dentin do not contain microorganisms and hence are sterile). During cavity preparation, attempt is made to remove the infected dentin leaving intact the affected dentin, using the clinical criteria of softening and discoloration.

- But in most of the cases, it is very difficult to clinically differentiate between the infected and affected dentin. Dyes can be used to differentiate the infected dentin from the affected dentin.
- Dyes used to differentiate affected and infected dentin are:
  - 0.5% solution of basic fuchsin in propylene glycol: It is applied for 10 seconds. The outer or decomposed carious layer stains red. The inner or decalcified dentin does not take up the stain on short exposure
  - 1% acid red in propylene glycol: Carious dentin stains dark red and the noncarious dentin remains pink

– Mallory-Azan stain: Outer layer stains red and the inner layer stains blue.

Direct Pulp Capping[4,27,41]

Definition

"Placement of a medicament or a nonmedicated material on a pulp that has been exposed, in the course of excavating the caries, due to fracture or due to mechanical exposures during routine caries removal".

Indications

1. Mechanical exposures that occurs following trauma or during cavity preparation which is <1 sq mm, surrounded by clean dentin in an asymptomatic vital deciduous tooth
2. Mechanical or carious exposures <1 sq mm, in an asymptomatic vital young permanent tooth.

Contraindications

1. Cariously exposed deciduous teeth
2. Spontaneous pain
3. Swelling
4. Fistula
5. Tenderness to percussion
6. Pathologic mobility
7. Root resorption—external/internal
8. Periapical/interradicular radiolucency
9. Pulp calcifications
10. Profuse hemorrhage from the exposure site
11. Pus or exudate from exposure site.

> Clinical success of direct pulp capping depends upon the following salient features:
> - Maintenance of pulp vitality
> - Lack of undue sensitivity or pain
> - Minimum pulp inflammatory response
> - Ability of the pulp to maintain itself without progressive degeneration.

> Direct pulp capping is less preferred in primary teeth because:
> - Rapid spread of inflammation throughout the primary coronal pulp, due to increased blood supply. Therefore there is less chance that the infection will be limited to the exposed part of the pulp increasing the likelihood of rapid and widespread of bacteria.

Treatment Considerations

Debridement: During caries removal if there is a pulpal exposure, necrotic and infected dentin chips will be pushed into the exposed pulp, and this can impede healing, causing further pulpal inflammation. Therefore while excavating caries from a deep cavity, it should be remembered that peripheral carious dentin from the walls should be removed first followed by removal from the floor of the cavity.

Following a clinical exposure a nonirritating solution of normal saline or anesthetic solution should be used to cleanse the area and keep the pulp moist.

Hemorrhage and clotting: A blood clot formed after cessation of the bleeding, impedes the pulpal healing. Therefore care must be taken not to allow clot formation. The clot that is formed does not allow the capping material to contact the pulp tissue directly, or the clot material itself could breakdown, producing degradation products that act as substrate to the bacteria.

Bacterial contamination: Adequate seal following pulp capping is a must to prevent bacterial contamination. Stainless steel crown restoration is the most preferred one.

Ideal Requirements of Material Used for Direct Pulp Capping

- Stimulate reparative dentin formation
- Maintain pulpal vitality
- Bactericidal or bacteriostatic
- Adhere to dentin
- Adhere to restorative material
- Resist forces during restoration placement
- Must resist forces under restoration during lifetime of restoration
- Able to be sterilized
- Radio-opaque
- Provide bacterial seal
- Release fluoride to prevent secondary caries.

Materials Used for Direct Pulp Capping

1. Calcium Hydroxide
2. Zinc oxide eugenol: No calcific bridge formation occurs.
3. Mixture of corticosteroids and antibiotics (Ledermix): Made of powder and liquid components. Powder contains dimethyl chlortetracyline hydrochloride, triamcinolone acetonide, zinc oxide and calcium hydroxide. Liquid is made of eugenol and rectified oil of turpentine.
4. Polycarboxylate cements
5. Tricalcium phosphate cement
6. Cyanoacrylate
7. Collagen
8. 4 META (4-Methacryl oxyethyl trimellitate anhydride)—soaks into the pulp, polymerizes and forms a hybrid layer.
9. Mineral trioxide aggregate (MTA)

Since calcium hydroxide is one of the materials used traditionally in endodontics and minral trioxide aggregate is the latest and most recommended material, these materials will be discussed in detail.

Calcium Hydroxide[42-53]

Calcium hydroxide was originally introduced to the field of endodontics by Herman in 1930 as a pulp-capping agent. About 75% clinical success is observed when calcium hydroxide is used as a pulp capping agent. But its use today is wide-spread in endodontic therapy. It is the most commonly used dressing for treatment of the vital pulp. It also plays a major role as an inter-visit dressing in the disinfection of the root canal system. Calcium hydroxide possesses antibacterial property due to its high alkalinity (pH 11) and helps formation of a calcific barrier. But the calcium ions needed for the barrier formaon are derived from the blood stream and not from the calcium hydroxide material. The hydroxyl group is considered to be the most important component of calcium hydroxide as it provides an alkaline environment and activate alkaline phosphatases which play an important role in hard tissue formation. The calcified material which is produced appears to be the product of both odontoblasts and connective tissue cells and may be termed osteodentine.

Calcium hydroxide is supplied as powder or two-paste (hard setting) system. It is also supplied as light cured system. The powder form is mixed with sterile water (even locl anesthetic solution may be used) on a glass slab with a spatula to form a thick paste. Two-paste system (Dycal) that is used frequently is neutral in pH. Equal amount of both the pastes (catalyst and base pastes) are taken and mixed rapidly before placing it over the pulp. The setting time of this hard setting calcium hydroxide is very short and thus requires faster manipulation.

Procedure of Direct Pulp Capping with Calcium Hydroxide (Figs 8.12A to E)

- Adequate isolation
- Following pulp exposure, further manipulation of the pulp should be avoided
- Cavity is irrigated with saline and bleeding arrested with light pressure from sterile cotton pellet.
- Capping material is then placed over the exposure with minimum pressure and avoiding pushing the material into the pulp

A glass ionomer or reinforced zinc oxide eugenol material should be placed over it to provide a seal against microleakage since calcium hydroxide has a high solubility, poor seal, and low compressive strength. The use of glass ionomer cements or reinforced zinc oxide eugenol restorative materials has the additional advantage of inhibitory activity against cariogenic bacteria. Cement base is placed over the medicament followed by restoring the tooth with amalgam and stainless steel crown.

Histological changes

Following the use of alkaline calcium hydroxide as pulp capping agent (Fig. 8.13A):
- Pulp in direct contact with calcium hydroxide (alkaline pH) becomes necrotic after 24 hours.
- Necrotic layer is separated from healthy tissue by a deep staining basophilic material – calcium proteionate
- Partially calcified fibrous tissue lined by odontoblasts is seen below the calcium proteinate zone in 14 days.
- A zone of new dentin is observed within 28 days.

The reaction following the use of neutral calcium hydroxide (Dycal) as pulp capping agent is varied and is as follows (Fig. 8.13B):
- Pulp in direct contact with the material undergoes necrosis
- This necrosed tissue is removed by macrophages
- Granulation tissue are seen in the layer
- Odontoblasts are seen differentiating in the granulation tissue and form dentin.
- The dentin formed is in contact with the dycal. This makes it difficult to visualize the dentin bridge from the radio-opaque dycal material.

Drawbacks of Calcium Hydroxides

- Increased risk of resorption in deciduous teeth.
- It may degrade and dissolve beneath restorations.
- Interfacial failure during amalgam condensation.
- Dentin bridges beneath $Ca(OH)_2$ are associated with tunnel defects.
- Failure to provide a long-term seal against micro-leakage when used as a pulp capping agent and this may lead to penetration of microorganisms into pulpal tissue and induce pulpal irritation and potential pulpal death.

Mineral Trioxide Aggregate[54-65]

Mineral trioxide aggregate (MTA) is a new biocompatible pulp capping agent and excellent results have been reported with its use. MTA is a fine hydrophilic powder.

Commercially available MTA

ProRoot MTA (Dentsply),
White ProRoot MTA (Dentsply),
MTA- Angelus (Solucoes Odontologicas),
MTA- Angelus Blanco (Solucoes Odontologicas),
MTA Bio (Solucoes Odontologicas)

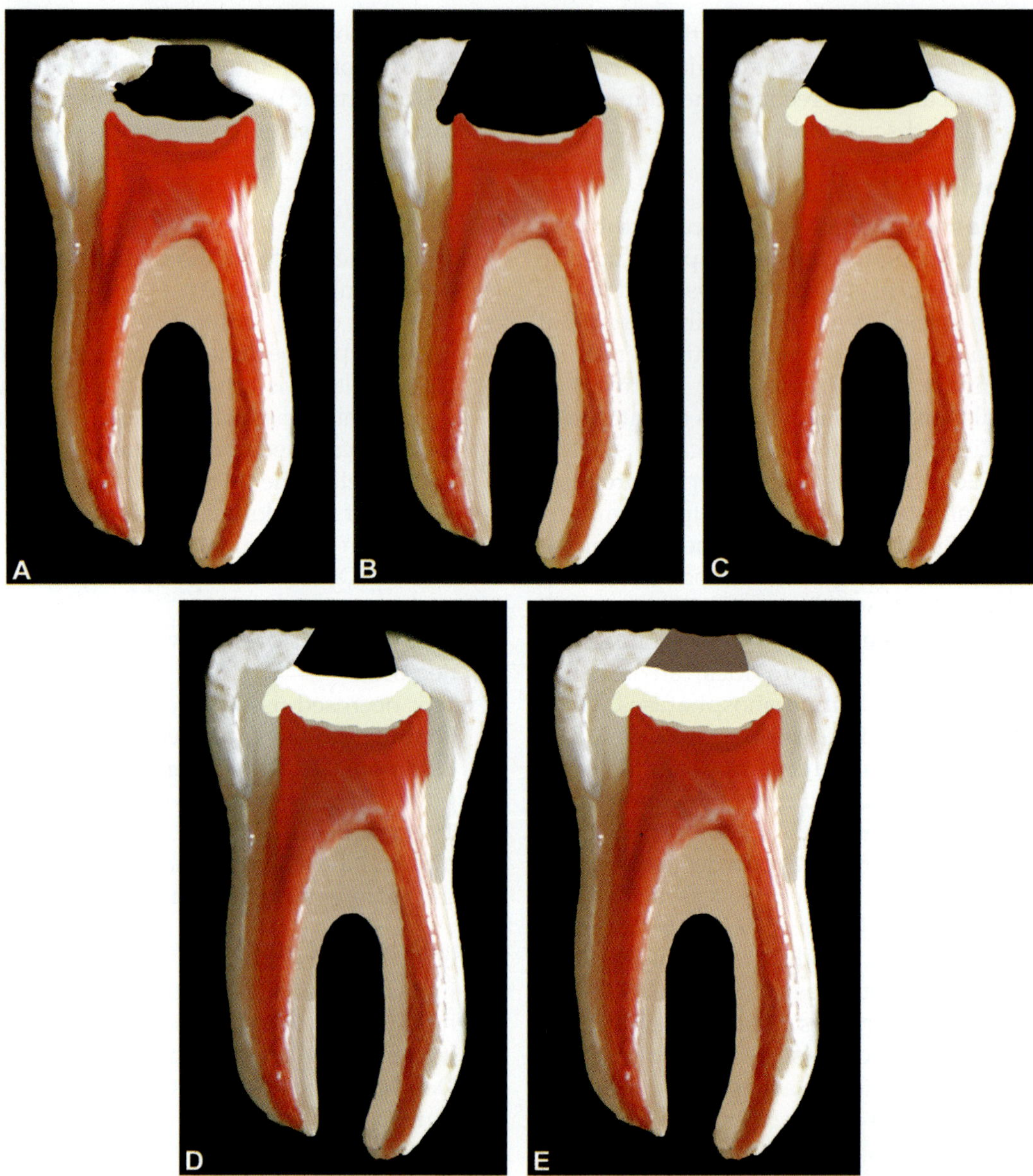

Figs 8.12A to E: Direct pulp capping: (A) Pulp horns are high; (B) Pulp horns exposed during cavity preparation; (C) Calcium hydroxide is placed over the exposed pulp; (D) Suitable base is placed over calcium hydroxide; (E) Tooth is sealed with amalgam restoration

MTA consists of tricalcium silicate, tricalcium aluminate, tricalcium oxide, silicate oxide and bismuth oxide. Bismuth oxide is added (17-18 wt%) to improve the properties and the radioopacity.

MTA are of two types—grey and white. The white and grey MTA differ mainly in their content of iron, aluminium and magnesium oxides. White MTA contains smaller particles with a narrower range of size distribution than grey MTA.[66,67]

Advantages of MTA

1. MTA produced significantly more dentinal bridge in a shorter period of time
2. Less pulpal inflammation seen
3. Ability to set in moist environment
4. It exhibits a superior marginal adaptation
5. Nonabsorble,
6. It forms a reactionary layer at the dentin interface resembling hydroxyapatite in structure.

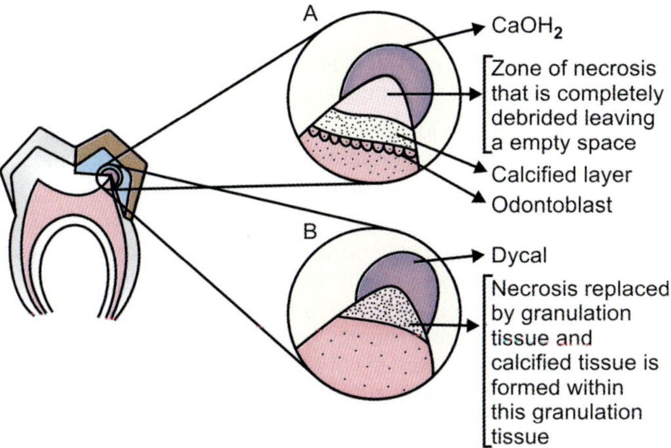

Figs 8.13A and B: Histological changes seen in pulp after placement of: (A) Calcium hydroxide; (B) Dycal

7. MTA stimulates cytokine release, induces pulpal cell proliferation, and promotes hard tissue formation.

Disadvantages of MTA

1. MTA takes longer time (about 2-3 hours) to set
2. Expensive
3. Difficult to store (hydrophilic)

Steps Involved in the Placement of MTA Over the Pulp

- Bleeding is controlled with a cotton moistened with Sodium Hypochlorite (NaOCl).
- Manipulation and setting reaction of mineral trioxide aggregate: The MTA paste is obtained by mixing 3 parts of powder with 1 part of water to obtain putty like consistency. Mixing can be done on paper or on a glass slab using a plastic or metal spatula. Mixing of MTA should be less than 4 minutes which, if prolonged, will result in dehydration. This mix is then placed in the desired location and condensed lightly with a moistened cotton pellet. MTA has a pH of 10.2 immediately after mixing and increases to 12.5 after 3 hours of setting which is almost similar to calcium hydroxide. MTA being hydrophilic requires moisture to set, making absolute dryness contraindicated. Presence of moisture (not excess water that makes the mix soupy) during setting improves the flexural strength of the set cement. Hydration of the powder results in a colloidal gel composed of calcium oxide crystals in an amorphous structure (33 percent calcium, 49 percent phosphate, 6 percent silica, 3 percent chloride and 2 percent carbon).

- MTA is placed over the exposed pulp using hand instruments or ultrasonic condensation. Hand condensation is done with the help of a plugger, paper point or messing gun. Ultrasonic condensation is done by first placing a hand instrument such as a condenser in direct contact with the MTA. Then an ultrasonic instrument is placed touching the shaft of the hand instrument and activated for several seconds.
- The material is padded into place with a moist cotton pellet
- The moist cotton pellet is placed on the MTA and the material is allowed to set. The rest of the cavity is filled with temporary filling material
- In the next visit the temporary material is removed along with the cotton pellet and the tooth is restored with a permanent restoration
- The entire cavity can also be filled with MTA, instead of temporary material. A wet piece of gauze is placed between the treated tooth and the opposing tooth for 3-4 hours. This can be done only in compliant patients. After 1 week, about 3-4 mm of the material from the occlusal surface is removed and final restoration placed over the set MTA.

Properties of MTA[68,79]		
Compressive strength	Within 24 hours of mixing was about 40.0 MPa and increases to 67.3 MPa after 21 days	Grey MTA exhibited greater compressive strength than white MTA
Radio-opacity	The mean radio-opacity of MTA is 7.17 mm of equivalent thickness of aluminium	MTA is less radio-opaque than IRM, super EBA, amalgam or gutta-percha and has similar radiodensity as Zinc Oxide Eugenol
Solubility	Set MTA shows no signs of solubility, the solubility might increase if more water is used during mixing	An acidic environment does not interfere with the setting of the MTA
Marginal adaptation and sealing ability	MTA superior to the other traditional root-end filling materials[37] MTA thickness of about 4 mm is sufficient to provide a good seal	MTA expands during setting which may be the reason for its excellent sealing ability

Contd...

Contd...

Antibacterial and antifungal property	By virtue of providing a good seal and preventing microleakage	Does not have direct antibacterial action against root canal bacteria
Reaction with other dental materials	MTA does not react or interfere with any other restorative material	Glass ionomer cements or composite resins, used as permanent filling material do not affect the setting of MTA when placed over it
Biocompatibility	That it is not mutagenic and is much less cytotoxic compared to super EBA and IRM.	Investigations by Koh et al revealed that MTA offers a biologically active substrate for bone cells and stimulates interleukin production. MTA is also said to stimulate cytokine production in human osteoblasts. This supports the superiority of MTA over formocresol as a pulpotomy medicament.
Tissue regeneration	MTA is capable of activation of cementoblasts and production of cementum	It consistently allows for the overgrowth of cementum and also facilitates regeneration of the periodontal ligament.
Mineralization	MTA induces dentin bridge formation	The tricalcium oxide in MTA reacts with tissue fluids to form calcium hydroxide, resulting in hard-tissue formation in a manner similar to that of calcium hydroxide. But the dentin bridge that is formed with MTA is faster, with good structural integrity and more complete than with calcium hydroxide.

Pulpotomy[39,80-88]

Definition

"Surgical removal of the entire coronal pulp, leaving intact the vital tissue in the canals, followed by placement of a medicament or dressing over the remaining pulp stump in an attempt to promote healing and retention of this vital tissue."

Objectives

- To remove the inflamed and infected pulp tissue and allowing the vital pulp in the root canals to heal, thus maintaining the vitality of the tooth.

Indications

- Carious or mechanical exposure of vital primary teeth and young permanent teeth, where inflammation is restricted to coronal pulp only.

Contraindications

- History of spontaneous pain
- Swelling
- Fistula
- Tenderness to percussion
- Pathological mobility
- External/internal root resorption
- Periapical or interradicular radiolucency
- Pulp calcifications
- Pus or exudate from exposures site
- Uncontrollable bleeding from the amputated pulp stump
- > half root length resorbed.

Types of Pulpotomy

A. Devitalization technique
B. Preservation technique
C. Regeneration technique

Devitalization technique

In this technique the pulp undergoes devitalization. *Materials used:* Electrocautery, laser and forma-cresol are commonly used.

Electrocautery: Carbonises and denatures pulp and eliminates bacterial contamination.

Laser: Creates a superficial zone of coagulative necrosis and this gets replaced by granulation tissue.

Formacresol: Buckley's formula or 20% formacresol is used. Formacresol fixes the tissue and renders it immune to bacterial attack.

Preservation technique

- In this technique minimum devitalization is present at the coronal portions of the pulp but not as severe and extensive as seen in devitalization technique. On the other hand it is noninductive as seen in regeneration technique.

- Gluteraldehyde, ferrous sulphate is used.

Regeneration technique

- This technique is inductive that is there is formation of calcific barrier or induces reparative dentin formation.
- Calcium hydroxide, BMP (bone morphogenic protien, has bone inducing property, so can be used to induce dentin also).

Partial Pulpotomy[89,90]

Partial pulpotomy (Cvek pulpotomy) is defined as "the surgical removal of a small portion of the coronal portion of a vital pulp as a means of preserving the remaining coronal and radicular pulp."

Cvek pulpotomy is indicated especially in the case of fractures involving the pulp. It involves removal of 2 mm of inflamed coronal pulp with a sterile bur in a high speed handpiece cooled with sterile solution. Calcium hydroxide dressing is placed over the residual tissue and sealed with zinc oxide eugenol cement or glass ionomer cement. When there is radiographic evidence of development of a hard tissue barrier (3-6 months), the tooth is restored with acid etch composite resin after removing the zinc oxide eugenol cement. Cvek reported 96% success rate with this technique regardless of the stage of root development, contamination by oral fluids (up to 7 days) or size of the original exposure (up to 4 mm). The procedure is similar to calcium hydroxide pulpotomy except that, only the pulp horns are surgically amputated, leaving behind considerable amount of healthy coronal pulp intact. High speed diamond burs are used with coolants for the amputation of the pulp.

Formocresol Pulpotomy

History[91-94]: It was Sweet in 1930's, who formulated the use of formocresol for pulpotomy in deciduous teeth and he recommended a multivisit technique. Multivisit technique was reduced to two visits by Doyle et al in 1962. The number of visits were subsequently reduced and in 1965 Spedding et al gave the presently used 5 minute technique. Garcia-Godoy and colleagues have recommended 1 minute application and found this to be adequate. But the 5 minute application time is the preferred one by the clinicians and is being routinely followed.

Mortal Pulpotomy

- It is a compromising treatment done on nonvital primary teeth, where pulpectomy is not practical
- Necrotic coronal pulp is removed
- Infected radicular pulp is treated with strong antiseptic solution (Beechwood Creosate) for 1-2 weeks.
- This is followed by replacement of antiseptic solution by an antiseptic paste.

Formocresol by its chemical structure is the combination

- Formaldehyde—19%
- Cresol—35%
- Glycerin—15%
- Water

Formaldehyde interacts with the protein portion of the cell and cresol enhances the action of formaldehyde.

Buckley's solution: The percentage of formocresol used is 20% (1/5 dilution) and was introduced by Buckley[95] in 1904.

Preparation of Buckley's solution

To prepare 150 ml. Buckley's solution (1/5th dilution) 120 ml of diluent is prepared first and added to 30 ml. of full concentration formocresol.

Diluent (120 ml) 3 parts glycerine (90 ml) + 1 part of distilled water (30 ml) = 120 ml.

Buckley's solution (150 ml)

4 parts of diluent (120 ml) + 1 part of formocresol (30 ml) = 150 ml.

= 150 ml formocresol of 1/5th strength is thus prepared.

Success following formocresol pulpotomy

Clinical success = 90-100%
Histological success = 70-80%
Success depends on accurate selection of the case.

Procedure for formocresol pulpotomy (Figs 8.14A to F)

1. Administration of local anesthesia and rubber dam isolation.
2. All caries should be removed.
3. Entire roof of the pulp chamber is cut with high-speed bur and water spray.
4. The coronal pulp is removed with the round bur or spoon excavator.
5. Pulp chamber is washed thoroughly, to remove all debris.

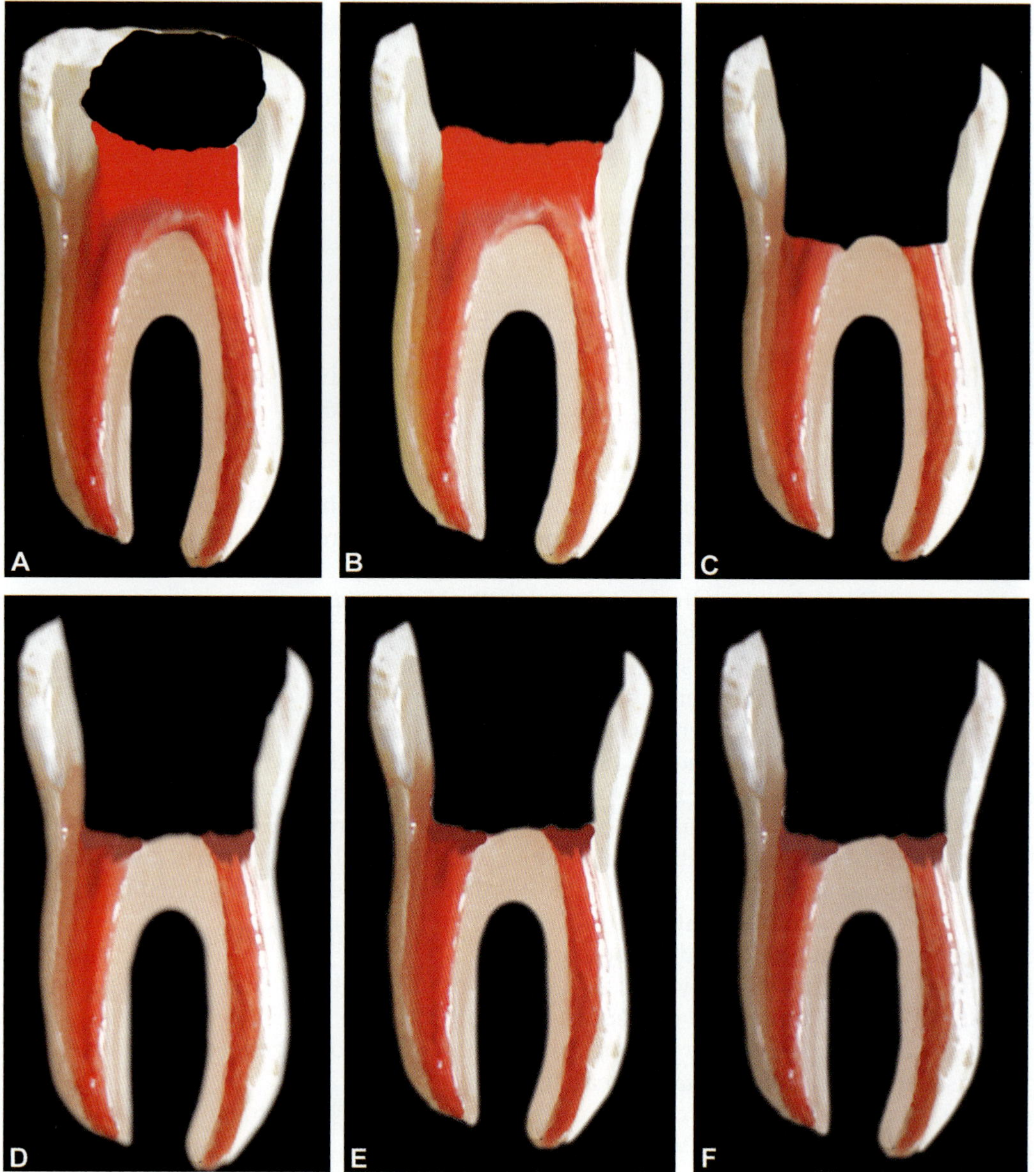

Figs 8.14A to F: Formocresol pulpotomy: (A) Caries extending up to the pulp; (B) Access opening made; (C) Coronal pulp removed; (D) Formocresol pellet placed on the amputated pulp stump for 5 minutes; (E) Zinc oxide eugenol mix is placed over the fixed pulp; (F)Tooth is sealed with amalgam restoration

6. Hemorrhage is controlled with cotton slightly moistened with saline, placed against the stumps of the pulp at the opening of the root canals. Bleeding should be controlled within 3-5 min.
7. Pulp status is assessed.
8. Cotton pellet moistened with 1/5th dilution formocresol is placed over the amputated pulp for 5 min.
9. When the cotton pellet is removed, the pulp stump must appear dark brown or even black, as a result of fixation.

10. Creamy mix of zinc oxide Eugenol is placed over the amputated pulp. Equal parts of formocresol can be added to eugeonl. The tooth is then restored with stainless steel crown restoration.

Histological changes following formocresol pulpotomy

As given by Massler and Mansokhani[96] in1959
Immediately following placement of the formocresol the pulp tissue became fibrous and acidophilic.
7-14 days later, 3 distinct zones appears. They are:
i. Broad acidophilic zone of fixation

ii. Broad pale staining zone of atrophy with few cells and fibers

iii. Broad zone of inflammatory cells extending apically from the border of the pale staining zone.

Progressive apical movement of these zones occur and at the end of one year the entire pulp will be comprised of only the acidophilic zone.

> Formocresol binds and renders tissue incapable of autolysis, but capable of replacement by granulation tissue.

Disadvantages of formocresol[97,98]

1. *Local toxicity:* There is no actual healing of the pulp and the tooth becomes devitalized.
2. *Systemic toxicity:* Studies have shown that full strength formocresol, is absorbed into the systemic circulation from the pulpotomy site. Excretion is via the kidney and lungs. Some amount of formocresol remains cell bound in the liver, kidney and lungs. Cytogenic and mutagenic effect is observed due to its ability to denature nucleic acids by forming methylol derivatives and methylene cross links. Formocresol is also said to produce irreversible damage to the protein portion of enzymes, genetic material, membranes, and connective tissue. It affects directly the protein biosynthesis and cell reproduction by interacting with DNA and RNA and destroys the lipid component of the cell membrane.
3. *Damage to succedaneous teeth:* It is seen that 1ml of formocresol diffuses through the apical foramen in 3 min. Thus there is high-risk for the formation of enamel defects in the permanent successor following the use of formocresol in a primary teeth.

Glutaraldehyde[99]

It has been widely tested, to replace formocresol. Studies have shown that application of 2-4% produces rapid surface fixation of the underlying pulp tissue.

Attributes of glutaraldehyde over formocresol

- Forms strong intra- and intermolecular protein bonds leading to superior fixation by cross linkage.
- Diffusability is limited, thus reducing the apical extension of the material
- Excellent antimicrobial property
- Less dystrophic calcification
- Produces initial zone of fixation that does not proceed apically
- Readily excreted from the body. About 90% is eliminated in 3 days

- 15-20 times less toxic than formocresol and have little potential for chromosomal interference or mutagenecity.

Pulpectomy[28,100-106]

Definition

"Removal of the entire pulp and subsequent filling of the canals of the primary teeth with a suitable resorbable material."

Indications

1. Primary teeth with pulp inflammation extending beyond the coronal pulp
2. Roots and alveolar bone with minimum pathologic resorption
3. Primary teeth with necrotic pulp and or periapical abscess
4. Pus at the clinical pulp exposure site.

Contraindications

1. Grossly destroyed tooth that is nonrestorable clinically
2. Periradicular involvement extending to the permanent tooth bud, where the risk of damage to the permanent tooth is high.
3. Root resorption—internal or external
4. Extensive mobility
5. Gross bone loss at the apex or at the furcation.

Types of Pulpectomy

Pulpectomy can be of two types, single visit or multi visit pulpectomy depending on the number of appointments required.

Single Visit Pulpectomy

Single visit pulpectomy is generally carried out as an extension of pulpotomy procedure, probably as an on the spot decision, when hemorrhage from the amputated radicular pulp stumps appear dark red (normal healthy bleeding is bright red in color) and is uncontrollable which is indicative of an inflamed tissue (Fig. 8.15). Other indication of single visit pulpectomy is a tooth with history of spontaneous pain without pulp necrosis, abscess or a fistula.

Procedure of Single Visit Pulpectomy (Figs 8.16 to 8.19)

- Done under local anesthesia and rubber dam isolation
- All caries should be removed.
- Entire roof of the pulp chamber is cut with high-speed bur and water spray.

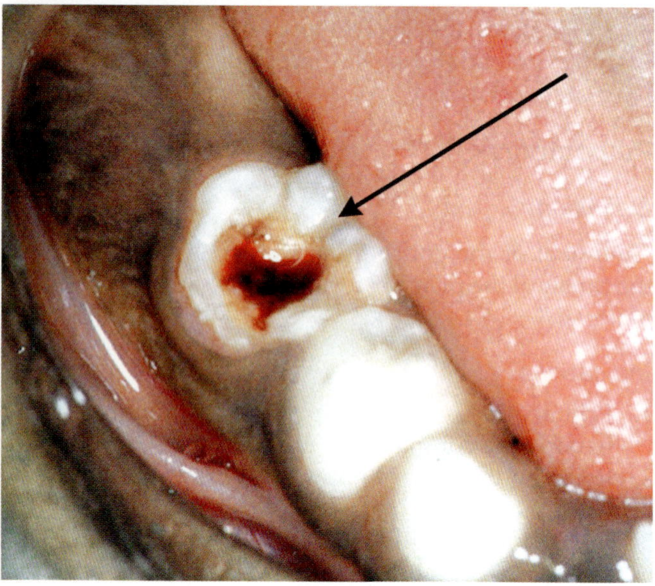

Fig. 8.15: Bleeding from inflamed vital pulp tissue

- The coronal pulp is removed with the round bur or spoon excavator.
- Pulp chamber is washed thoroughly, to remove all debris
- All accessible radicular pulp is removed with the broach. Care must be taken not to force the broach into the canal, as the barbs present in the broach can get caught to the canal wall and break inside the canal making it almost impossible to retrieve.
- Canals are enlarged with the aim of removing all the infected dentin and providing space for adequate obturation. No attempt is made to extend the instrument beyond the apex thus minimizing the risk of accidental injury to the permanent tooth bud.
- Hedstrom files are recommended since they remove hard tissue only on withdrawal, which prevents pushing infected material through the apices. The disadvantage of Hedstrom file is that it is weak and thus chances of breakage is high. K Flex files are stronger and hence are more resistant to fracture. Filing is done along with the use of lubricants. 5% sodium hypochlorite, hydrogen peroxide, saline, etc are used for irrigation. The canals should be instrumented to the resistance point, that usually corresponds to 2-3 mm from the radiographic apex. Each canal can be enlarged 3-4 instrument sizes greater than the first file
- Radiograph with the endodontic instrument need not be taken for working length determination.
- Canals are irrigated with saline and dried. Paper points are used for drying the canal walls.

- Canals are then obturated with suitable resorbable filling material.
- Zinc Oxide Eugenol mix is placed over the obturating material
- Tooth is sealed with amalgam restoration and finally restored with stainless steel crown restoration.

Multivisit Pulpectomy

- Used for nonvital primary teeth with or without associated abscess (Fig. 8.20)
- Clinical technique is similar to single visit pulpectomy but all the procedures are not done on the first visit. On the first visit pulp is extirpated, canals are irrigated, dried and the tooth is temporarily restored. On the second visit the canals are enlarged and if all the symptoms have subsided the tooth is obturated and permanently restored. Obturation is postponed untill the symptoms regresses.
- Between appointments, an antibacterial drug is sealed in the pulp chamber
- If pus is present, the canal can be left open to drain for 24 hours
- Systemic antibiotics are advised if cellulitis is present
- The number of appointments, timing and extent of instrumentation thus will be determined by the signs and symptoms at each visit.

Filling/Obturation of Deciduous Root Canals

Ideal requirements of material used

- Must be resorbable
- Should not interfere with eruption of permanent tooth
- Should be bactericidal
- Must be radio-opaque
- Must be nonirritant

Different materials used

- Zinc oxide eugenol
  - is used without catalyst. Lack of catalyst is used to allow adequate working time.
- Iodoform paste
  - Is also being used. It consists of zinc oxide and iodoform mixed into a paste. Its advantages over zinc oxide eugenol are
  - Potent bactericidal
  - Nonirritant
  - Radio-opaque
  - Chemically active until entirely resorbed
  - Good healing properties
  - Rate of resorption is faster

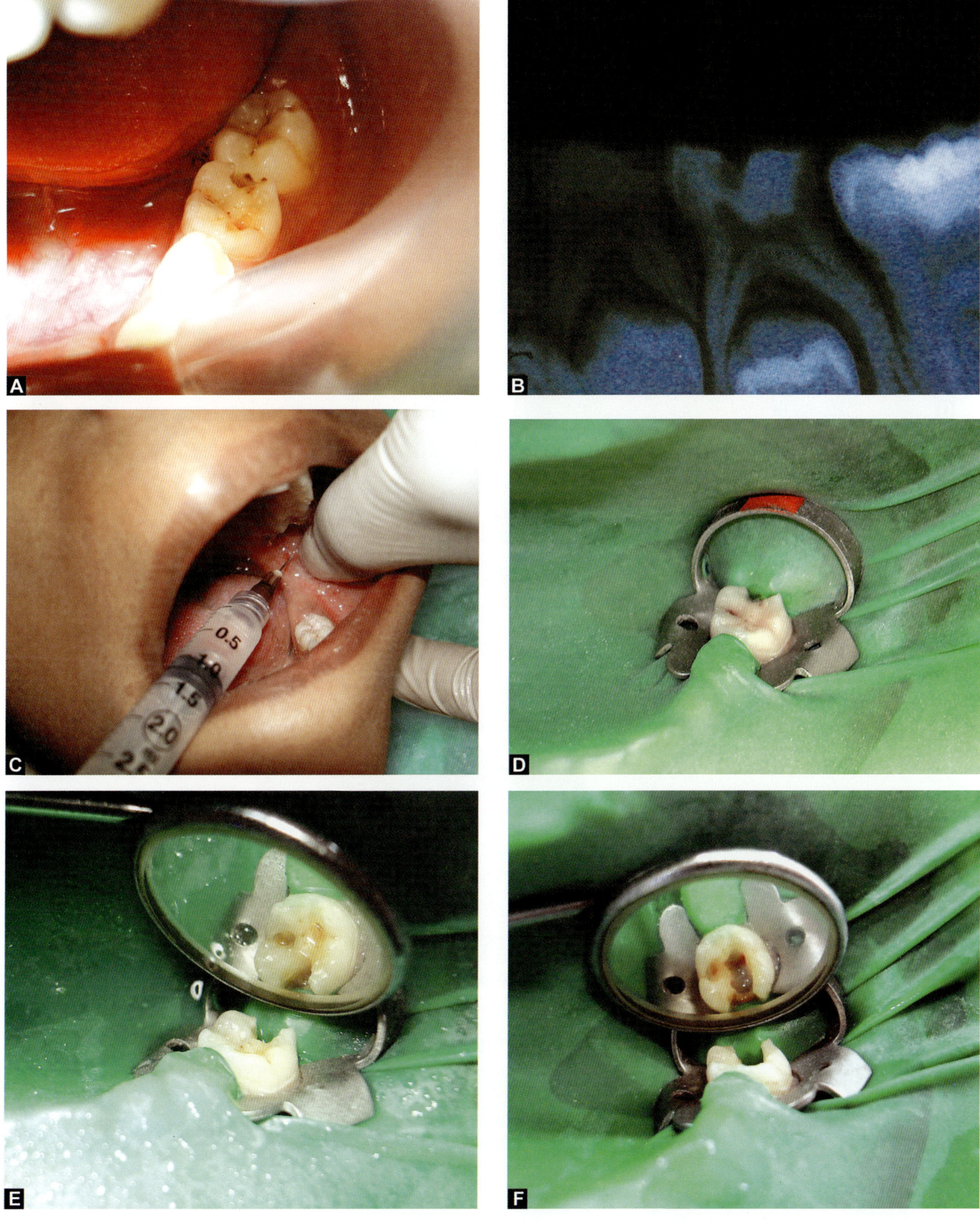

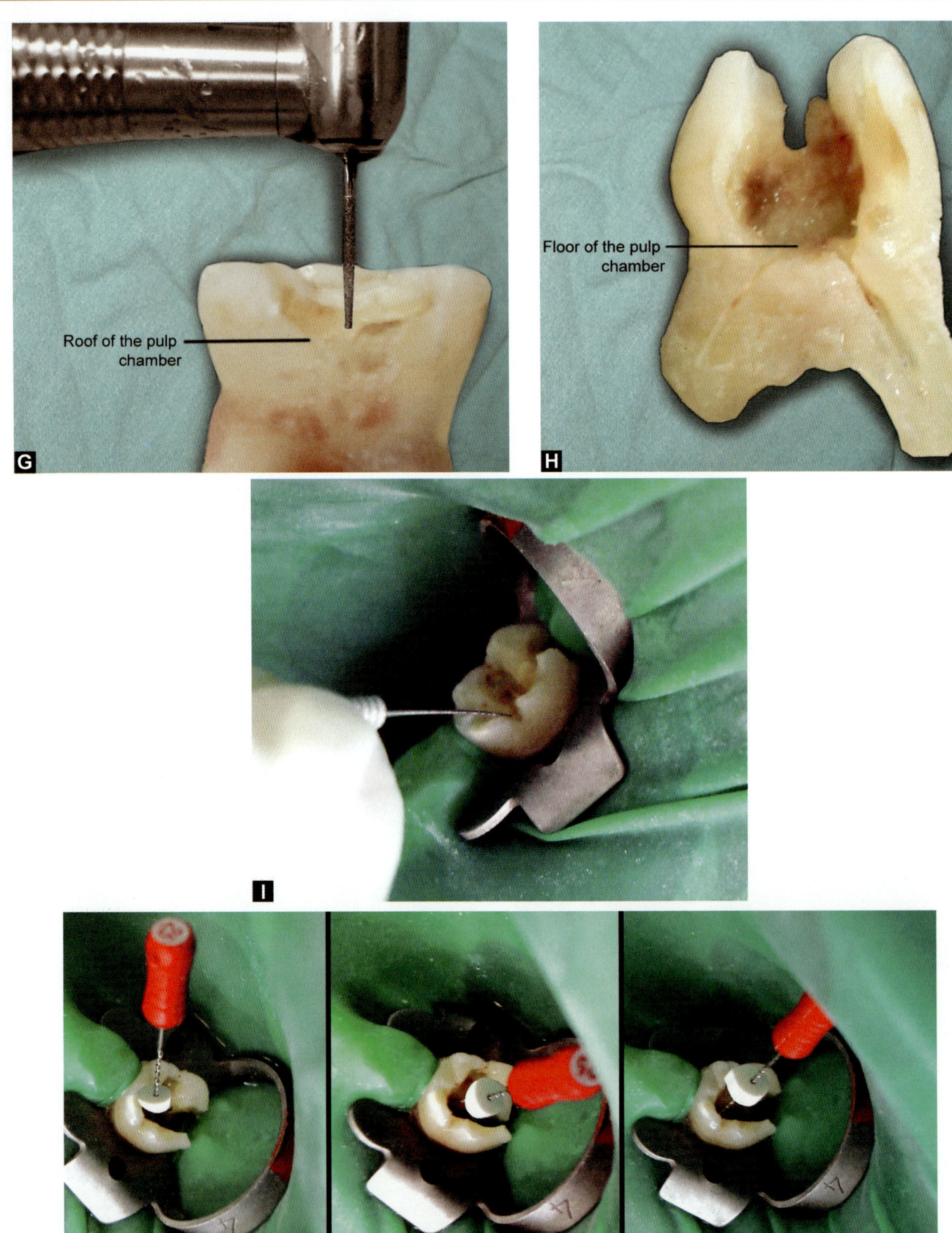
Roof of the pulp chamber
G
Floor of the pulp chamber
H
I
J

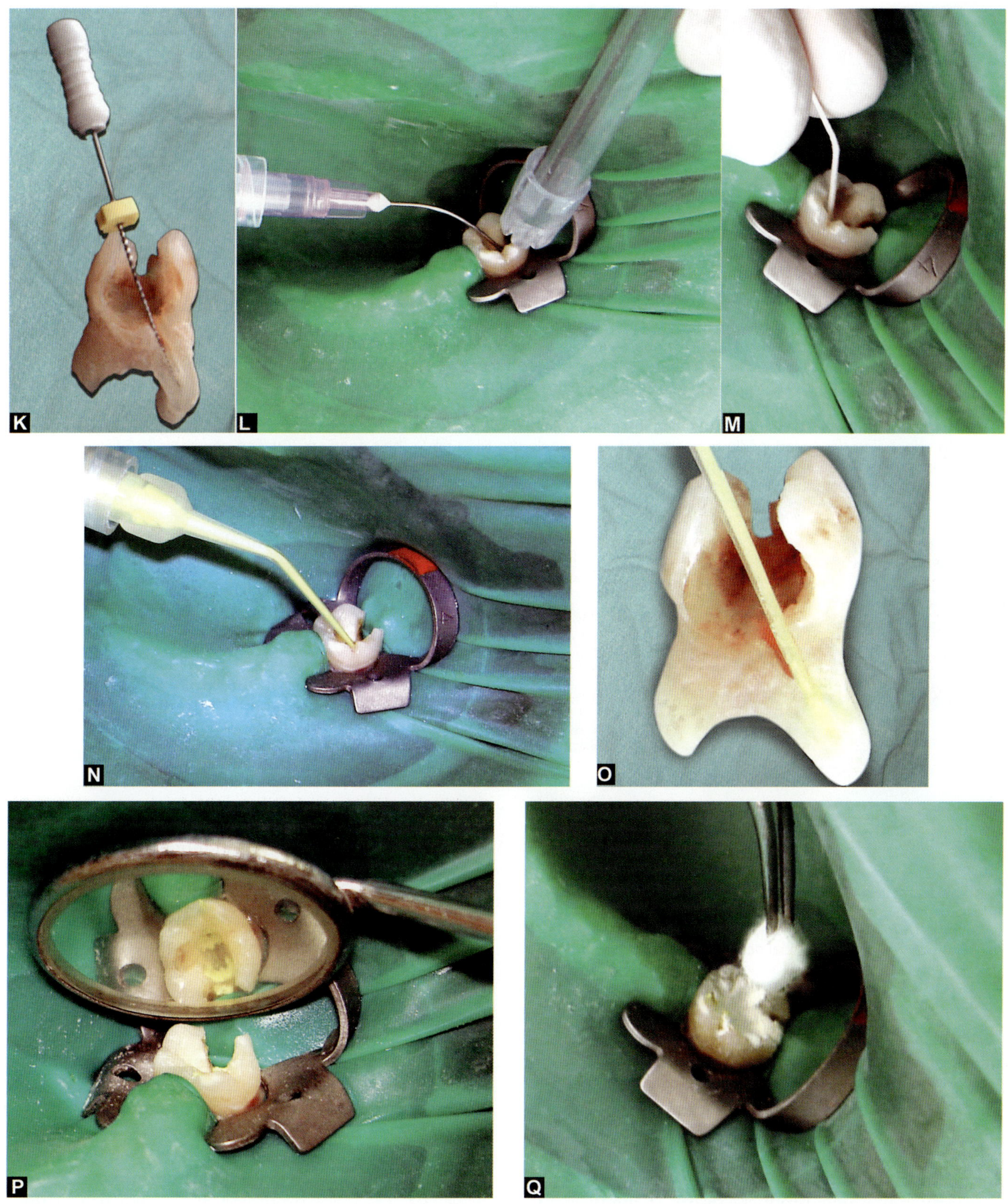

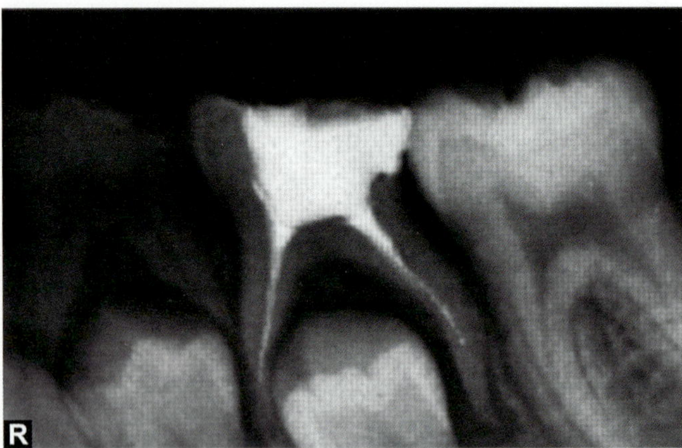

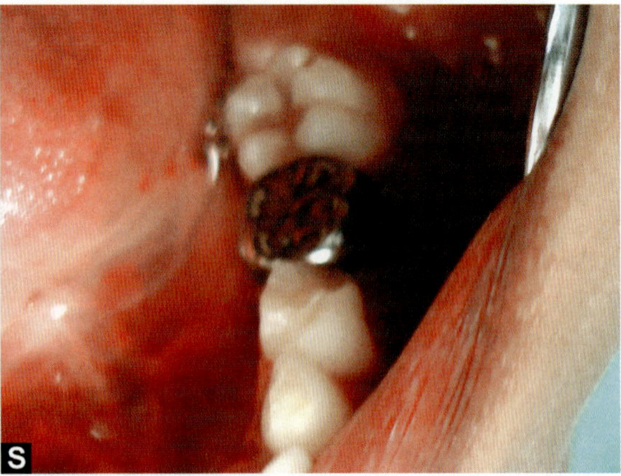

Figs 8.16A to S: Pulpectomy: (A) Preoperative clinical view; (B) Preoperative radiographic view; (C) Obtaining local anesthesia; (D) Application of rubber dam; (E) Removal of caries; (F) Access preparation; (G) Angulation of the bur; (H) Floor of the pulp chamber; (I) Removal of the pulp tissue with broach; (J) Endodontic files inside the canals; (K) Longitudinal section showing the instrument inside the canal; (L) Continuation irrigation is important during the procedure; (M) Drying the canal with paper point; (N) Obturating the canal with suitable material; (O) Longitudinal section showing the obturating material being deposited inside the canal; (P) The canals are filled up to their opening; (Q) The chambers are filled with temporary restoration material; (R) Radiographic view after obturation and temporary restoration; (S) Stainless steel crown as permanent restoration

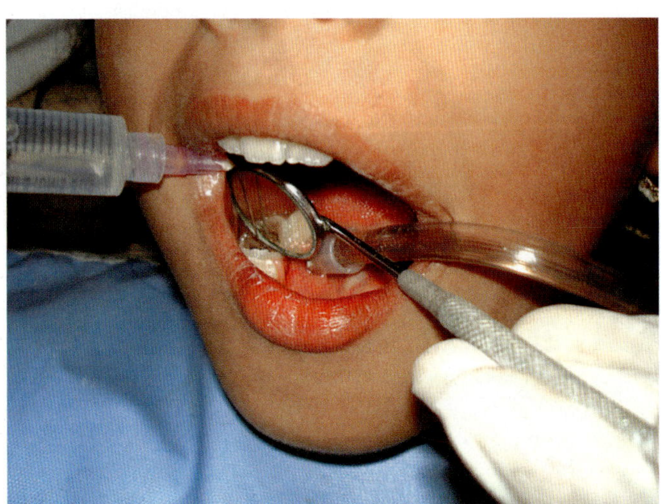

Fig. 8.17: Canals should be irrigated regularly during mechanical debridement

Iodoform paste is commercially available as KRI* and contains iodoform, camphor, para-chlorophenol, and menthol. Iodoform paste in combination with zinc oxide is available as Maisto's paste which, in addition to the above mentioned constituents, also contains thymol and lanolin. Iodoform paste in combination with calcium hydroxide has also been used; it is commercially available as Vitapex and Metapex. These iodoform-containing products resorb if inadvertently pushed beyond the apex, but the rate of resorption of the material from within the canals is faster than the rate of physiological root resorption. Another root canal filling material—a mixture of iodoform, calcium hydroxide, and zinc oxide—is commercially available as Endoflas; in addition, it has eugenol (triiodomethane, zinc oxide, calcium hydroxide, barium sulfate, and iodine di-stilo orthocresol, with the liquid consisting of eugenol and paramonochlorophenol. It is reported to resorb when extruded beyond the apex but resists resorption intraradicularly. Eugenol, one of its constituents, is known to cause periapical irritation.

Method of obturation

- The canals are dried thoroughly using paper points (Fig. 8.21)
- Lentulo spiral (Figs 8.22A and B), pressure syringe, Jiffy's syringe, amalgam condensor, local anesthetic syringe, tuberculin syringe, files, etc can be used to carry and deposit the material into the root canal.
- The material is mixed to the required consistency and is carried and deposited in the canal just short of the apex.
- Cotton held with cotton pliers can be used as piston to push the material into the canal
- Pressure syringe is one of the best devices used for obturation for the following reasons.
  - Avoidance of air trap
  - Even amount of material is deposited
  - 300 psi force produced allows the use of thick consistency.

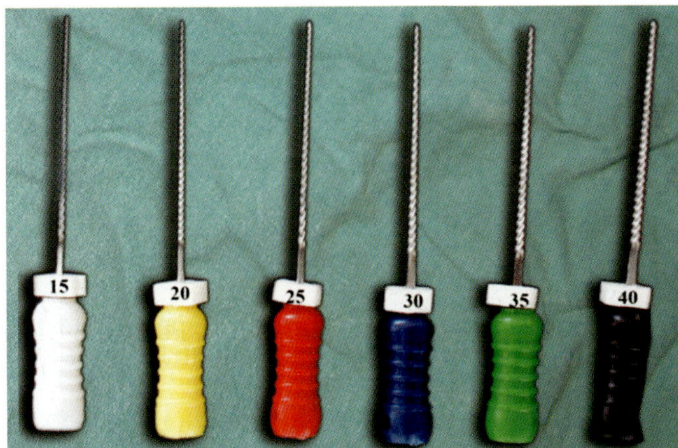

Fig. 8.18: Instruments are color coded based on the size No. 15 instrument: White; No. 20 instrument: Yellow; No. 25 instrument: Red; No. 30 instrument: Blue; No. 35 instrument: Green; No. 40 instrument: Black. The color repeats in the same sequence for further instrument size, e.g. No. 45 instrument is white

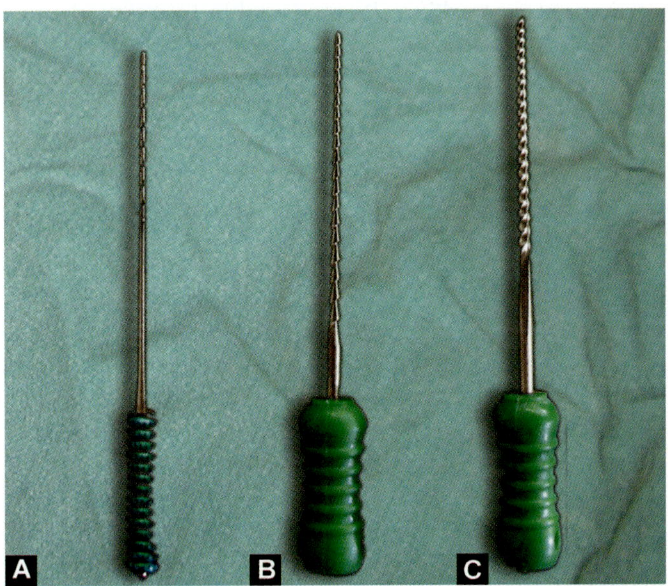

Figs 8.19A to C: Endodontic instruments used for canal debridement: (A) Barbed broach; (B) H-files; (C) K-files

Common Problems with Zinc Oxide Eugenol as Deciduous Tooth Obturation Material

- Zinc oxide eugenol material is harder and resorbs slowly compared to the root. Thus a small fraction of the material always extends beyond the root and may cause inflammatory changes in the adjoining tissues.
- As the resorption reaches the pulpal floor, the permanent tooth may get deflected from its normal path of eruption due to the presence and obstruction from the bulk of zinc oxide eugenol.

Problems Encountered in Deciduous Tooth Pulpectomy

- Multiple ramification—makes complete debridement impossible
- Ribbon shaped or hour glass shaped canals—discourages gross enlargement of the canal.

> In permanent teeth the objective of mechanical preparation is to provide an even circular apical 1/3rd. In primary teeth, attempt to prepare a circular apical 1/3rd mechanically may result in lateral perforation of the canal, due to its hour glass shape.

Evaluation of Success of Pulpectomy

- No purulent discharge from the gingival margin
- No abnormal mobility
- No postoperative pain
- No further resorption of root (except physiological)
- Resolution of sinus tract, by 6 months

Follow-up

- Monthly evaluation should be done preferably for six months period.
- Clinical and radiographic assessment should be made postoperatively to judge the outcome of the treatment.
- Following pulp therapy, it is advisable to place stainless steel crown to prevent fracture.

> If the succedaneous permanent tooth is missing, canals can be obturated with gutta percha.

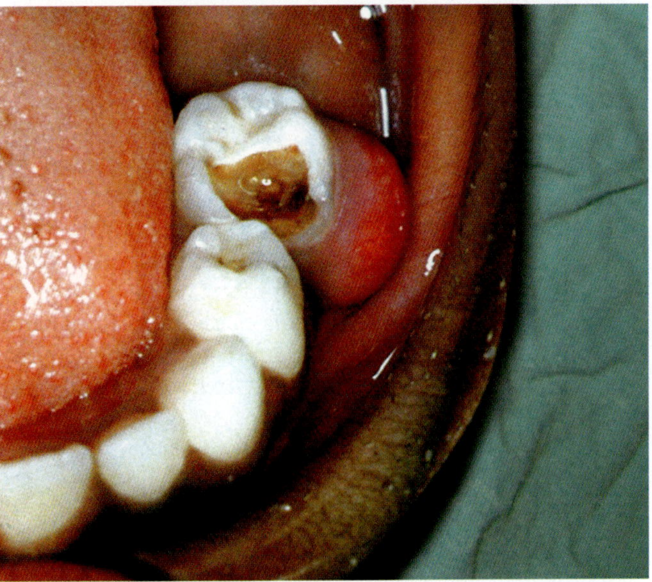

Fig. 8.20: Lack of bleeding from nonvital pulp tissue site

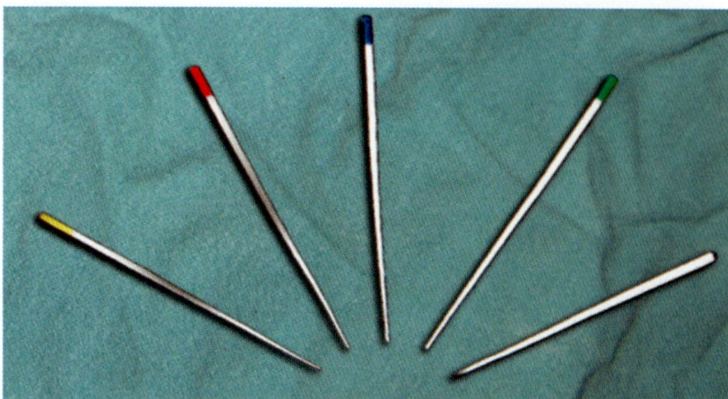

Fig. 8.21: Paper points are also color coded based on the size similar to the files/reamers/broaches

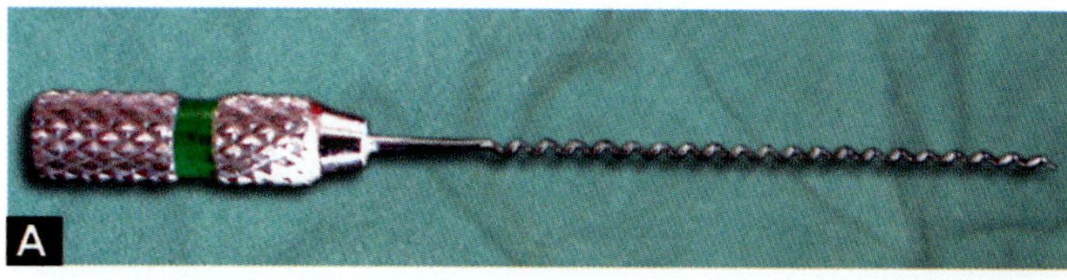

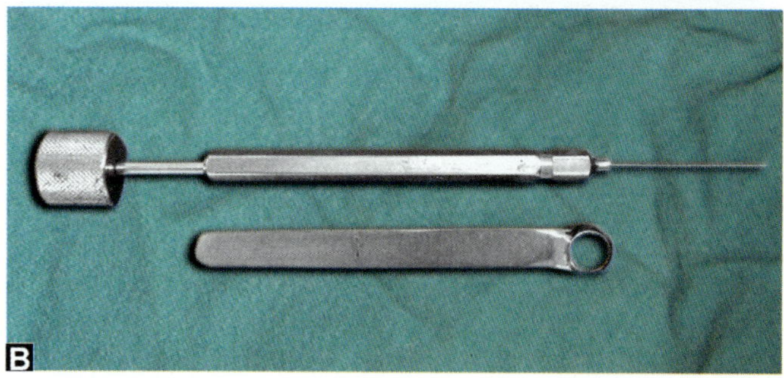

Figs 8.22A and B: (A) Lentulo spiral; (B) Pressure syringe

Treatment Modalities for a Permanent Tooth with Extensive Involvement of the Pulp

Treatment modalities depends on the stage of development of the root and the vitality of the pulp
Permanent tooth with vital pulp and open apex: Apexogenesis (Calcium hydroxide pulpotomy), followed by root canal treatment and permanent restoration.
Permanent tooth with vital pulp and closed apex: Root canal treatment followed by permanent restoration.
Permanent tooth with nonvital pulp and open apex: Three options of treatment are:
1. Apexification followed by root canal treatment and permanent restoration.
2. Apical plug with mineral trioxide aggregate.
3. Revascularization.
   Permanent tooth with nonvital pulp and closed apex: Root canal treatment followed by permanent restoration.

Apexogenesis/Calcium Hydroxide Pulpotomy/Cervical Pulpotomy (Figs 8.23A to C)

Indicated in vital permanent teeth with large pulp exposures and incompletely formed apices.

Aim

- To remove the infected coronal pulp and place calcium hydroxide over the healthy amputated radicular stumps
- A calcific barrier should form in response and the radicular pulp should retain its vitality so that root closure can occur.
- To achieve normal growth of the root to assume its normal length and apical closure.

Calcium hydroxide pulpotomy is considered as the first stage of treatment for vital cariously or traumatically exposed permanent teeth with incompletely formed apices.

The second phase of treatment following closure of the root apex is conventional root canal filling and permanent restoration. It is advisable to proceed with root canal treatment in permanent tooth as the second phase of treatment because; often there are linear calcifications along the length of the root canal after formation of a calcific bridge. This will progress until the canal appears to be completely calcified radiographically. Microscopic evaluation reveals pulp remnants in between the calcifications that have become strangulated and nonvital. Bacteria may migrate within these spaces to reach the periapical region resulting in periapical pathology. Once the canal has calcified to this extent, it may be impossible to negotiate it with instruments or EDTA and the choice of treatment is apical surgery or extraction. Thus to avoid similar postapexogenesis complications, root canal treatment is performed.

Care should be taken to remove the blood clot before placing calcium hydroxide over the amputated pulp. Leaving the clot has been attributed as one of the causes for dystrophic calcification and internal resorption.[107]

Apexification[4,28,108,109] (Figs 8.24A to E)

- Indicated in a nonvital pulp with incompletely formed or open apices (blunderbuss canal). The toxic products from the necrotic pulp causes death of the cells (Hertwig's epithelial rooth sheath) responsible for root growth, which reduces the chance of further root development and apical closure. It is almost impossible to get an accurate seal at the apex during obturation of a canal with wide open apex. Apexification is a procedure where a suitable material is placed in the root canal which aids in the formation of a calcific barrier at the apical end of the root canal acting as a natural seal. Calcific material that is formed may either be osteoid, cementoid or osteodentin.

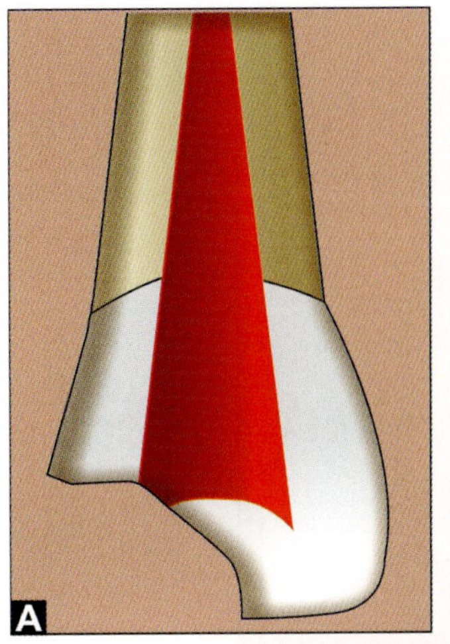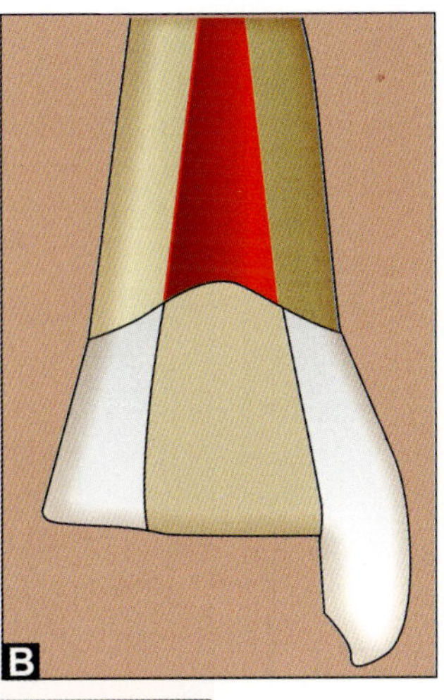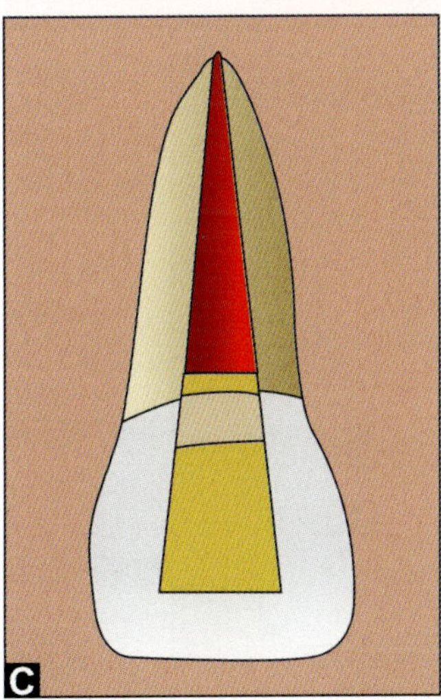

Figs 8.23A to C: Calcium hydroxide pulpotomy (Apexogenesis) procedure: (A) Fracture of the tooth exposing the pulp in an immature tooth; (B) Pulpotomy done using calcium hydroxide as the medicament; (C) Root formation completed. Calcific bridge seen at the coronal end

Alternative to apexification is apical surgery preceeded by root canal therapy. But this is not recommended in children because:
- Surgical techniques should be avoided
- Thin apical wall, may make apical surgery difficult
- Already short root may be further reduced by apical surgery.

Material

1. Calcium hydroxide—most preferred and first reported by Kaiser (1964) and popularized by Frank. It is mixed either with CMCP (camphorated parachlorophenol), saline, Ringer's solution, distilled water, anesthetic solution, etc.
2. Zinc oxide paste
3. Antibiotic paste
4. Tricalcium phosphate
5. Collagen—calcium phosphate gel
6. Mineral trioxide aggregate.

Procedure

- The tooth is anesthetized and isolated.
- Access opening is similar to conventional root canal treatment
- Barbed broach is used to remove the pulp and necrotic debris
- Diagnostic X-ray helps in assessing the root length (working length is approximately 2 mm from the apex)
- Hedstrom file is used along with constant irrigation to cleanse the canal off the debris
- Canal is dried and filled with calcium hydroxide or any other desired material
- Chances of success are greatly improved when the canal is filled in the absence of inflammation
- If acute signs are present, canal is debrided, irrigated and filled temporarily with antibacterial medicament like formacresol, beechwood creosote, CMCP or polyantibiotic paste.

Follow-up

- Evaluation of signs and symptoms are made regularly. IOPA is taken once in 2-3 months, to evaluate the amount of root closure
- Root appearance can be compared with that of the antimere
- Calcific repair may be complete in 6 months to 2-3 years
- If there is failure to see any radiographic change after 1 year, the tooth has to be re-zentered and calcium hydroxide must be replaced and X-ray taken to check the extent of calcium hydroxide in the canal
- Once the repair is complete, calcium hydroxide should be removed, canal irrigated and a root canal filling material placed
- Placement of posts within the canal should be avoided, as it weakens the remaining tooth structure
- Acid etched composite resin strengthens the tooth.

Apical Plug with Mineral Trioxide Aggregate[54,60]

Steps Involved in MTA as Apical Plug Placement

- Access opening is done under local anesthesia and rubber dam
- The root canal is cleaned with intracanal irrigants
- Calcium hydroxide paste can be placed in the canal to disinfect for about 1 week
- Calcium hydroxide is removed by rinsing. Excess moisture is removed from the canal

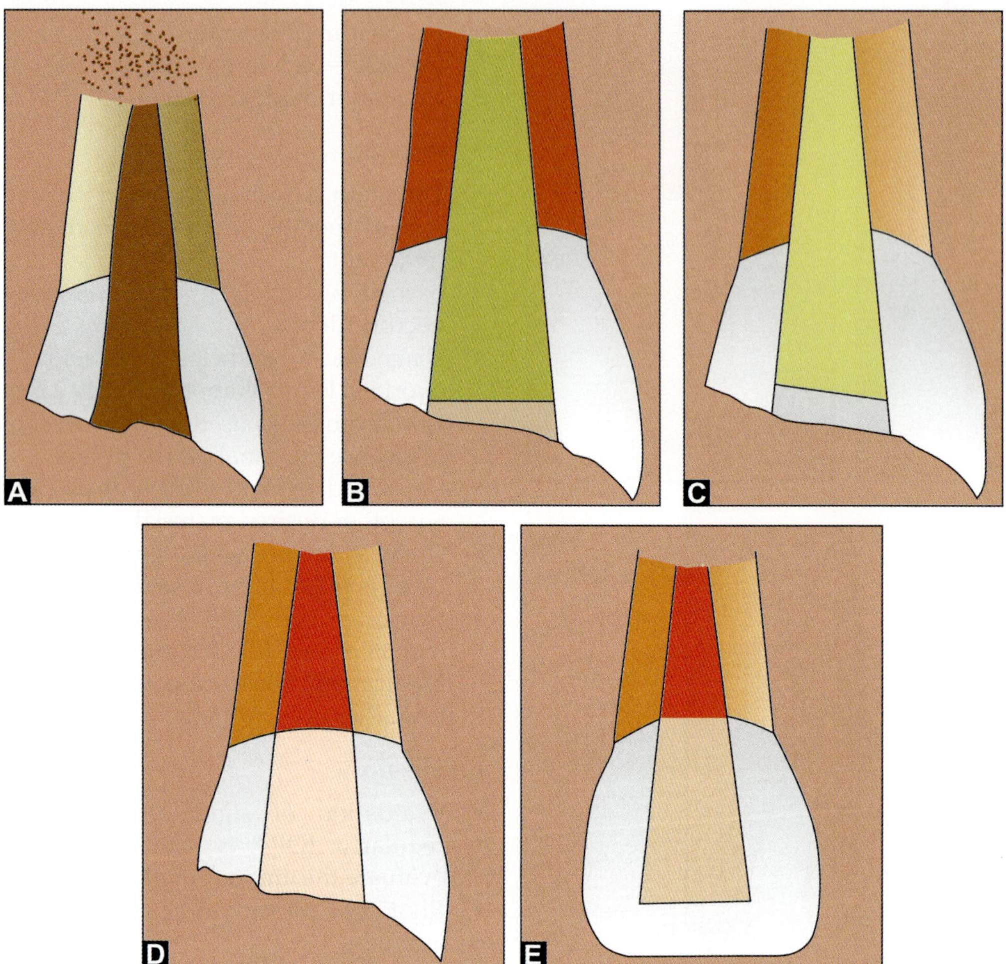

Figs 8.24A to E: Apexification procedure: (A) Nonvital tooth with open apex; (B) Root canal debrided and filled with calcium hydroxide; (C) Calcific barrier formed at the apical end; (D) The tooth is then obturated with gutta percha; (E) The tooth is then permanently restored either with plain crown restoration or post and core restoration depending on the amount of tooth material that is lost

- Mixed MTA is placed in the cavity using a large amalgam carrier. The material is pushed towards the apical foramen with a plugger or paper points
- The apical plug should be at least 3-4 mm thick and this should be checked radiographically
- If the apical plug could not be placed adequately, the entire material is rinsed from the canal with sterile water and the procedure repeated
- A moist cotton pellet is placed in the canal and the tooth is temporarily restored
- After 3 hours, the remaining canal is obturated with gutta percha and a permanent restoration is then placed.

Steps Involved in the Repair of Perforation

- Procedure is done under anesthesia and rubber dam
- After performing access opening, the canals are irrigated with NaOCl.

- Calcium hydroxide can be placed in the canal in between appointments which will help control hemorrhage
- Before placing MTA, calcium hydroxide should be completely removed
- The apical portion of the canal is obturated with sectional cone technique using gutta percha and root canal sealer
- MTA is placed into the defect and moist cotton pellet is placed over it. The access cavity is closed with a temporary restoration
- The remaining portion of the canal is restored with a permanent filling material after at least 3-4 hours.

Pulp Revascularization/Regeneration[110-114]

- This technique is recommended for a tooth with nonvital pulp especially following trauma. For this technique to be successful, the pulp although necrotic should be noninfected. The main theory behind this technique is that the tissues from the periapical area are able to regeneration into the pulp canal, where the necrotic non-infected pulp acts as a scaffold. The first step in this procedure is to disinfect the necrotic pulp. It is done by gentle debridement of the canal by flushing it with 5.25% sodium hypochlorite solution, followed by placement of a combination paste of antibiotic containing metronidazole, minocycline and ciprofloxacin. When the pulp is disinfected after about 15-20 days, the vital tissue at the periapical area is gently irritated with an endodontic instrument and bleeding is initiated. The blood is allowed to clot and a paste of MTA is placed over the clot and access cavity sealed permanently. Regular follow up evaluation is required. This technique may be extremely useful in young permanent teeth with necrotic pulp.

- The prior requisite for this treatment is the presence of open apex for tissue ingrowth and the presence of stem cells that have high regenerative potential as seen in young tooth. The canal walls should not be instrumented and calcium hydroxide should not be used as intracanal medicament while performing this procedure.
- Continued root development with improved pulp response has been observed following revascularization.
- Wider open apex increases the chance of revascularization.

REFERENCES

1. Bhasker SN. Orban's oral histology and embryology. 9th Ed St Louis CV Mosby, 1989.
2. Green D. Morphology of the pulp cavity of permanent teeth. Oral Surg 1955;8:743.
3. Avery JK. Structural elements of the young and normal human pulp. Oral Surg 1971;32:113.
4. Ingle JI, Bakland LK, Baumgartner JC. Inflammatory changes in the pulp, Endodontics 6th Ed BC Decker Inc 2008.
5. Seltzer S, Bender IB, Ziontz M. The dynamics of pulp inflammation: correlations between diagnostic data and actual histologic findings in the pulp. Oral Surg Oral Med Oral Pathol Oral Radiol Endod 1963;163:69-77.
6. Mjor IA, Tronstad L. Experimentally induced pulpitis. Oral Surg 1972;34:102.
7. Bergenholtz G. Inflammatory response of the dental pulp to bacterial irritation. J Endod 1981;7:100.
8. Warfringe J, Dahlen G, Bergenholtz G. Dental pulp response to bacterial cell wall material. J Dent Res 1985;64:1046.
9. Bender IB. Pulp biology conference, a discussion. J Endod 1978;4:37.
10. Tender KJ, Kvinnsland L. Micropuncture measurements of interstitial fluid pressure in normal and inflamed dental pulp in cats. I Endod 1983;9:105-9.
11. Moss SJ, Addelston H, Goldsmith ED. Histologic study of pulpal floor of deciduous molars. J Am Dent Assoc 1965;70:372-9.
12. Mc Donald RE. Diagnositic aids and vital pulp therapy for deciduous teeth. JADA 1956;53:14.
13. Fox AG, Heeley JD. Histologic study of human primary teeth. Arch Oral Biol 1950;25:103.
14. Massler M. Preventive endodontics: Vital pulp therapy. DCNA 1967;670.
15. Bernick S. Innervation of the teeth and periodontium DCNA 1959;503.
16. Rapp R, et al. The distribution of nerves in human primary teeth. Anat Rec 1967;159:189.
17. Zach J, Cohen G. Pulp response to externally applied heat. Oral Surg Oral Mod Oral Pathol Oral Radiol Endod 1966;19:515-30.
18. Lisanti V, Zander II. Thermal injury to normal dog teeth: *In vivo* measurements of pulp temperature and their effect on the pulp tissue. I Dent Res 1952;31:548-58.
19. Pernandcz-Seara MA, Wehrli Si, Wehrli FW. Diffusion of exchangeable water in cortical bone studied by nuclear magnetic resonance. Biophysics I 2002;82:522-9.
20. Garberoglio R, Brannstrom M, Scanning electron microscopic investigation of human dentinal tubules. Arch Oral Biol 1976;21:355.
21. Nagaoka S, Miyazaki Y, Liu HJ, et al. Bacterial invasion into dentinal tubules of human vital and nonvital teeth. J Endod 1995;21:70.
22. Siqueira JF Jr, Rocas IN. Exploiting molecular methods to explore endodontic infections: Part 2—Redefining the endodontic microbiota. J Endod 2005;31:488.
23. Vianna ME, Horz HP, Gomes BP, Conrads G. *In vivo* evaluation of microbial reduction after chemomechanical preparation of human root canals containing necrotic pulp tissue. J Int Endod 2006;39:484.
24. Sakamoto M, Rocas IN, Siqueira JF Jr, Benno Y. Molecular analysis of bacteria in asymptomatic and symptomatic endodontic infections. Oral Microbiol Immunol 2006;21:112.
25. Munson MA, Pitt-Ford T, Chong B, et al. Molecular and cultural analysis of the microflora associated with endodontic infections, J Dent Res 2002;81:761.
26. Siqueira JF Jr, Rocas IN. Uncultivated phylotypes and newly named species associated with primary persistent endodontic infections. J Clin Microbiol 2005;43:3314.
27. Grossman LI, Oliet S, Del Rio CE. Endodontic Practice 11th Ed. Varghese Publishers 1988;59-101.
28. Curzon MEJ, Roberts F, Kennedy DB. Kennedy's Paediatric Operative Dentistry. 4th Ed. Wright Publishers 1996.
29. Miwa Z, et al. Pulpal blood flow in vital and nonvital youg permanent teeth measured by transmitted light photoplethysmography: a pilot study. Pediatr Dent 2002;24(6):594-8.

30. Kilpatrick N, Seow WK, Cameron A, Widmer R. Pulp therapy for primary and young permanent teeth. Handbook of pediatric dentistry. 2nd Ed. Edinbergh: Mosby 2003.

31. Clinical guidelines reference manual V 30 / NO 7 08 / 09, The American Academy of Pediatric Dentistry (AAPD).

32. Barr ES, Flaitz CM, Hicks JM. A retrospective radiographic evaluation of primary molar pulpectomies. Pediatr Dent 1991;13(1):4-9.

33. Coll JA, Sadrian R. Predicting pulpectomy success and its relationship to exfoliation and succedaneous dentition. Pediatr Dent 1996;18(1):57-63.

34. Camp J. Pediatric Endodontics: Endodontic treatment for the primary and young permanent dentition. In: Cohen S, Burns RC (eds). Pathways of the Pulp. 8th ed. St Louis, Mosby Year Book, Inc; 2002.

35. Farooq NS, Coll JA, Kuwabara A, Shelton P. Success rates of formocresol pulpotomy and indirect pulp therapy in the treatment of deep dentinal caries in primary teeth. Pediatr Dent 2000;22(4):278-86.

36. Falster CA, Araujo FB, Straffon LH, Nor JE. Indirect pulp treatment: *In vivo* outcomes of an adhesive resin systems. Calcium hydroxide for protection of the dentin-pulp complex. Pediatr Dent 2002;24(3):241-8.

37. Fuks AB, Holan G, Davis JM, Eidelman E. Ferric sulfate versus dilute formocresol in pulpotomized primary molars: Long-term follow-up. Pediatr Dent 1997;19(5):327-30.

38. Marchi JJ, de Araujo FB, Froner AM, et al. Indirect pulp capping in the primary dentition: a 4 year follow-up study. J Clin Pediatr Dent 2006;31:68-71.

39. Fusayama T. Two layers of carious dentin: diagnosis and treatment. Oper Dent 1979;42:63.

40. Kuboki Y, et al. Mechanism of differential staining in carious dentin. J Dent Res 1983;62:713.

41. Fuks AB. Pulp therapy for the primary dentition. In: Pinkham JR, Casamassimo PS, Fields HW Jr, McTigue DJ, Nowak A (eds.). Pediatric Dentistry: Infancy Through Adolescence. 4th ed. St Louis, Mo: Elsevier Saunders Co 2005;375-93.

42. Sciaky I, Pisanti S. Localisation of calcium placed over amputated pulps in dogs' teeth. J Dent Res 1960;39:1128-32.

43. Barthel CR, Rosenkranz B, Leuenberg A, Roulet JF. Pulp capping of carious exposures treatment outcome after 5 and 10 years: a retrospective study. J Endod 2000;26:525-8.

44. Auschill TM, Arweiler NB, Hellwig E, et al. Success rate of direct pulp capping with calcium hydroxide. Schweiz Monatsschr Zahnmed 2003;113:946-52.

45. Cox CF, Sübay RK, Ostro E, Suzuki S, Suzuki SH. Tunnel defects in dentin bridges: Their formation following direct pulp capping. Oper Dent 1996;21:4-11.

46. Duque C, Negrini Tde C, Hebling J, Spolidorio DM. Inhibitory activity of glass-ionomer cements on cariogenic bacteria. Oper Dent 2005;30(5):636-40.

47. Lewis BA, Burgess JO, Gray SE. Mechanical properties of dental base materials. Am J Dent 1992;5:69-72.

48. Pereira JC, Manfio AP, Franco EB, Lopes ES. Clinical evaluation of Dycal under amalgam restorations. Am J Dent 1990;3:67-70.

49. Sönmez D, Durutürk L. Ca(OH)$_2$ pulpotomy in primary teeth. Part I: internal resorption as a complication following pulpotomy. Oral Surg Oral Med Oral Pathol Oral Radiol Endod 2008;106(2).

50. Carrotte P. Endodontics: Part 9 Calcium hydroxide, root resorption, endo-perio lesions. British Dental Journal 2004;197:735-43.

51. Cox CF, Suzuki S, Re-evaluating pulp protection: calcium hydroxide liners vs. cohehsive hybridization J Am Dent Assoc 1994;15:823-31.

52. Via W. Evaluation of deciduous molars by treated pulpotomy and calcium hydroxide. J Am Dent Assoc 1955;50:34-43.

53. Barnes IM, Kidd EA. Disappearing Dycal. Br Dent J 1979; 147:111.

54. Rao A, Rao A, Shenoy R. Mineral Trioxide Aggregate—A Review. J Clin Pediatr Dent 2009;34(1):1-8.

55. Srinivasan V, Waterhouse P, Whitworth J. Mineral trioxide aggregate in paediatric dentistry. Int J Paediatr Dent 2009;19:34-47.

56. Schmitt D, Lee J, Bogen G. Multifaceted use of proroot MTA root canal repair material. Pediatr Dent 2001;23: 326-30.

57. Myers K, Kaminski E, Miller. The effects of mineral trioxide aggregate on the dog pulp. J Endod 1996;22:198.

58. Islam I, Chang HK, Yap AUJ. X-ray diffraction analysis of mineral trioxide aggregate and Portland cement. Int Endod J 2006;39:220-5.

59. Kogan P, He J, Glickman GN, Watanabe I. The effects of various additives on setting properties of MTA. J Endod 2006;32:569-72.

60. Torabinejad M, Chivian N. Clinical applications of mineral trioxide aggregate. J Endod 1999;25:197-205.

61. Sluyk SR, Moon PC, Hartwell GR. Evaluation of setting properties and retention characteristics of Mineral Trioxide Aggregate when used as a furcation perforation repair material. J Endod 1998;24:768-71.

62. Torabinejad M, Hong CU, McDonald F, Pitt Ford TR. Physical and chemical properties of a new root-end filling materials. J Endod 1995;21:349-53.

63. Ford TR, Torabinejad M, Abedi HR, Bakland LK, Kariyawasam SP. Using mineral trioxide aggregate as a pulp-capping material. J Am Dent Assoc 1996;127:1491-4.

64. Andelin WE, Shabahang S, Wright K, Torabinejad M. Identification of hard tissue after experimental pulp capping using dentin sialo-protein (DSP) as a marker. J Endod 2003;29:646-50.

65. Holden DT, Schwartz SA, Timothy CK, Schindler WG. Clinical outcomes of artificial root-end barriers with mineral trioxide aggregate in teeth with immature apices. J Endod 2008;34:812-7.

66. Komabayashi T, Spångberg LSW. Comparative Analysis of the particle size and shape of commercially available

mineral trioxide aggregates and Portland cement: A study with a flow particle image analyzer. J Endod 2008;34:94-8.

67. Silva HD, Andrade VLM, Méndez GV, Medellín RFJ, et al. Physical-chemical analysis of mineral trioxide aggregate (MTA) by X-rays diffraction, colorimetry and electronic microscopy. Rev ADM 2000;17:125-131.

68. Torabinejad M, Smith PW, Kettering JD, Pitt Ford TR. Comparative investigation of marginal adaptation of Mineral Trioxide aggregate and other commonly used root-end filling materials. J Endod 1995;21:295-9.

69. Ding SJ, Kao CT, Shei MY, Hung CJ, Huang TH. The physical and cytological properties of white MTA mixed with Na_2HPO_4 as an accelerant. J Endod 2008;34:897-900.

70. Shah PMM, Chong BS, Sidhu SK, Pitt Fortd T. Radio-opacity of potential root end filling materials. Oral Surg Oral Med Oral Pathol Oral Radiol Endod 1996;81:476-9.

71. Roy CO, Jeansonne BG, Gerrets TF. Effect of an acid environment on leakage of root-end filling materials. J Endod 2001;27:7-8.

72. Bates C, Carnes DL, Del Rio CE. Longitudinal sealing ability of mineral trioxide aggregate as a root end filling material. J Endod 1996;22:575-8.

73. Valois CR, Costa ED Jr. Influence of the thickness of mineral trioxide aggregate on sealing ability of root-end filling *in vitro*. Oral Surg Oral Med Oral Pathol 2004;97:108-11.

74. Shipper G, Grossman ES, Botha AJ, Cleaton-Jones PE. Marginal adaptation of mineral trioxide aggregate (MTA) compared with amalgam as a root-end filling material: a low vacuum (LV) versus high vacuum (HV) SEM study. Int Endod J 2004;37:325-36.

75. Nandini S, Ballal S, Kandaswamy D. Influence of glass ionomer cement on the interface and setting reaction of mineral trioxide aggregate when used as a furcal repair material using laser Raman spectroscopic analysis. J Endod 2006;33:167-72.

76. Kettering JD, Torabinejad M. Investigation of Mutagenicity of Mineral Trioxide Aggregate and other commonly used root end filling materials. J Endod 1995;21:537-42.

77. Koh E, McDonald F, Pitt Ford T, Torabinejad M. Cellular response to mineral trioxide aggregate. J Endod 1998;24: 543-7.

78. Schwartz RS, Mauger M, Clement DJ, Walker WA. Mineral Trioxide Aggregate: A new material for endodontics. J Am Dent Assoc 1999;30:967-75.

79. Faraco IM Jr, Holland R. Response of the pulp of dogs to capping with mineral trioxide aggregate or a calcium hydroxide cement. Dent Traumatol 2001;17:163-6.

80. Fuks AB. Pulp therapy in the primary and young permanent dentition. Dent Clin North Am 2000;44:571.

81. Smith NL, Seale NS, Nunn ME. Ferric sulfate pulpotomy in primary molars: A retrospective study. Pediatr Dent 2000;22(3):192-9.

82. Burnett S, Walker J. Comparison of ferric sulfate, formocresol, and a combination of ferric sulfate/formocresol in primary tooth vital pulpotomies: A retrospective radiographic survey. ASDC J Dent Child 2002;69(1):44-8.

84. Ibricevic H, Al-Jame Q. Ferric sulphate and formocresol in pulpotomy of primary molars: Long-term follow-up study. Eur J Paediatr Dent 2003;4(1):28-32.

84. Loh A, O'Hoy P, Tran X, et al. Evidence-based assessment: Evaluation of the formocresol versus ferric sulfate primary molar pulpotomy. Pediatr Dent 2004;26(5):401-9.

85. Waterhouse PJ. Formocresol and alternative primary molar pulpotomy medicaments: A review. Endod Dent Traumatol 1995;11(4):157-62.

86. Shumayrikh NM, Adenubi JO. Clinical evaluation of glutaraldehyde with calcium hydroxide and glutaraldehyde with zinc oxide eugenol in pulpotomy of primary molars. Endod Dent Traumatol 1999;15(6):259-64.

87. Zurn D, Seale NS. Light-cured calcium hydroxide vs formocresol in human primary molar pulpotomies: A randomized controlled trial. Pediatr Dent 2008;30(1):34-41.

88. Peng L, Ye L, Tan H, Zhou X. Better outcomes in pulpotomies on primary molars with MTA. Evidence-Based Dentistry 2007;8:11-2.

89. Glossary of endodontic terms. 7th ed. American Association of Endodontists; Chicago, (IL): 2003.

90. Cvek M. A clinical report on partial pulpotomy and capping with calcium hydroxide in permanent incisors with complicated root fractures. J Endod 1978;4:232-7.

91. Sweet CA. Treatment for deciduous teeth with exposed pulps. Washington Univ. Dent J 1936;3:78.

92. Doyle W, Mc Donald R, Mitchell D. Formacresol versus calcium hydroxide in pulpotomy. J Dent Child 1962;29:86.

93. Spedding RH, Mitchell DH, Mc Donald R. Formacresol and calcium hydroxide therapy. J Dent Res 1965;44:1023.

94. Garcia-Godoy F, et al. Pulpal response to different application times of formacresol. J Pedod 1982;6:176-93.

95. Buckley J. Practical therapeutics: a rational treatment for putrescent pulps. Dent Rev 1904;18:1193-7.

96. Massler M, Mansokhani N. Effects of formacresol on the dental pulp. J dent Child 1959;26:277.

97. Milnes AR. Is formacresol obsolete? A fresh look at the evidence concerning safety issues. Pediatr Dent 2008;30(3):237-46.

98. Pruhs RJ, Olen G, Sharma P. Relationship between formacresol pulpotomies on primary teeth and enamel defects on their permanent successors. J Am Dent Assoc 1977;94:698.

99. Davis MJ, Myers R, Switkes MD. Glutaraldehyde: an alternative to formacresol for vital pulp therapy. J Dent Child 1982;49:176.

100. Spedding RH. In complete resorption of resorbable root canal filling in primary teeth: Report of two cases. J Dent Child 1985;52:214-6.

101. Mani SA, Chawla HS, Tewari A, Goyal A. Evaluation of calcium hydroxide and zinc oxide as a root canal filling material in primary teeth. ASDC J Dent Child 2000;67:142-7.

102. Nukro C, Garcia-Godoy F. Evaluation of calcium hydroxide/Iodoform paste (Vitapex) in root canal therapy for primary teeth. J Clin Pediatr Dent 1994;23:289-94.

103. Fuchino T. Clinical and histopathological studies of pulpectomy in deciduous teeth. Shikwa Gakubo 1980;80:971.

104. Nishino M, et al. Clinico-roentgenographical study of iodoform-calcium hydroxide root canal filling material vitapex in deciduous teeth. Jap J Pedod 1980;18:20.

105. Fuks AB, Eielman E, Pauker N. Root canal filling with Endo ß as in primary teeth: A retrospective study. J Clin Pediatr Dent 2002;27:41-6.

106. Aylard SR, Johnson R. Assessment of filling techniques for primary teeth. Pediatr Dent 1987;9:195.

107. Schroder U. Effect of an extra pulpal blood clot on healing following experimental pulpotomy and capping with calcium hydroxide. Odontol Rev 1973;24:257.

108. Kaiser JH. Presentation to the American Association of the Endodontists' meeting. Washington DC. 1964.

109. Frank AL. Therapy for the divergent pulp less tooth by continued apical formation. J Am Dent Assoc 1966;72:87.

110. Chueh LH, Huang GT. Immature teeth with periradicular periodontitis or abscess undergoing apexogenesis, a paradigm shift. J Endod 2006;32:1205-13.

111. Thomson A, Kahler B. Regenerative endodontics— biologically based treatment for immature permanent teeth: a case report and review of the literature. Australian Dent J 2010;55:446-52.

112. Hargreaves KM, Geisler T, Henry M, Wang Y. Regeneration potential of the young permanent tooth: what does the future hold? J Endod 2008;34:S51-S56.

113. Jung IY, Lee SJ, Hargreaves KM. Biologically based treatment of immature permanent teeth with pulpal necrosis: a case series. J Endod 2008;34:876-87.

114. Kling M, Cvek M, Mejare I. Rate and predictability of pulp revascularization in therapeutically reimplanted permanent incisors. Endod Dent Traumatol 1986;2:83-9.

FURTHER READING

1. Ballesio I, Marchetti E, Mummolo S, Marzo G. Radiographic appearance of apical closure in apexification: follow-up after 7-13 years Eur J Paediatr Dent 2006; 7(1):29-34.

2. Barrieshi-Nusair KM, Qudeimat MA. A prospective clinical study of mineral trioxide aggregate for partial pulpotomy in cariously exposed permanent teeth. J Endod 2006;32(8):731-5. Epub 2006 Jun 23.

3. Bawazir OA, Salama FS. Clinical evaluation of root canal obturation methods in primary teeth. Pediatr Dent 2006;28(1):39-47.

4. Bramante CM, Menezes R, Moraes IG, Bernardinelli N, Garcia RB, Letra A. Use of MTA and intracanal post reinforcement in a horizontally fractured tooth: a case report. Dent Traumatol 2006;22(5):275-8.

5. Canoglu H, Tekcicek MU, Cehreli ZC. Comparison of conventional, rotary, and ultrasonic preparation, different final irrigation regimens, and 2 sealers in primary molar root canal therapy. Pediatr Dent 2006;28(6):518-23.

6. Chien MM, Setzer S, Cleaton-Jones P. How does zinc oxide-eugenol compare to ferric sulphate as a pulpotomy material? SADJ 2001;56(3):130-5.

7. El-Meligy OA, Avery DR. Comparison of apexification with mineral trioxide aggregate and calcium hydroxide. Pediatr Dent 2006;28(3):248-53.

8. El-Meligy OA, Avery DR. Comparison of mineral trioxide aggregate and calcium hydroxide as pulpotomy agents in young permanent teeth (apexogenesis). Pediatr Dent 2006;28(5):399-404.

9. Gesi A, Hakeberg M, Warfvinge J, Bergenholtz G. Incidence of periapical lesions and clinical symptoms after pulpectomy—a clinical and radiographic evaluation of 1- versus 2-session treatment. Oral Surg Oral Med Oral Pathol Oral Radiol Endod 2006;101(3):379-88.

10. Guelmann M, Fair J, Bimstein E. Permanent versus temporary restorations after emergency pulpotomies in primary molars. Pediatr Dent 2005;27(6):478-81.

11. Kitasako Y, Shibata S, Tagami J. Migration and particle clearance from hard-setting $Ca(OH)_2$ and self-etching adhesive resin following direct pulp capping. Am J Dent 2006;19(6):370-5.

12. Liu JF. Effects of Nd:YAG laser pulpotomy on human primary molars. J Endod 2006;32(5):404-7.

13. Murray PE, Garcia-Godoy F. The incidence of pulp healing defects with direct capping materials. Am J Dent 2006;19(3):171-7.

14. Nagaratna PJ, Shashikiran ND, Subbareddy VV. *In vitro* comparison of NiTi rotary instruments and stainless steel hand instruments in root canal preparations of primary and permanent molar. J Indian Soc Pedod Prev Dent 2006;24(4):186-91.

15. Parirokh M, Kakoei S. Vital pulp therapy of mandibular incisors: a case report with 11-year follow up. Aust Endod J 2006;32(2):75-8.

16. Pinto AS, de Araujo FB, Franzon R, Figueiredo MC, Henz S, Garcia-Godoy F, Maltz M. Clinical and microbiological effect of calcium hydroxide protection in indirect pulp capping in primary teeth. Am J Dent 2006;19(6):382-6.

17. Prakash R, Vishnu C, Suma B, Velmurugan N, Kandaswamy D. Endodontic management of taurodontic teeth. Indian J Dent Res 2005;16(4):177-81.

18. Primosch RE, Ahmadi A, Setzer B, Guelmann M. A retrospective assessment of zinc oxide-eugenol pulpectomies in vital maxillary primary incisors successfully restored with composite resin crowns. Pediatr Dent 2005;27(6):470-7.

19. Rodd HD, Waterhouse PJ, Fuks AB, Fayle SA, Moffat MA. British Society of Paediatric Dentistry.: Pulp therapy for primary molars. Int J Paediatr Dent 2006;16 Suppl 1:15-23

20. Saltzman B, Sigal M, Clokie C, Rukavina J, Titley K, Kulkarni GV. Assessment of a novel alternative to conventional formocresol-zinc oxide eugenol pulpotomy for the treatment of pulpally involved human primary teeth: diode laser-mineral trioxide aggregate pulpotomy. Int J Paediatr Dent 2005;15(6):437-47.
21. Silva GA, Lanza LD, Lopes-Junior N, Moreira A, Alves JB. Direct pulp capping with a dentin bonding system in human teeth: a clinical and histological evaluation. Oper Dent 2006;31(3):297-307.
22. Suzuki M, Katsumi A, Watanabe R, Shirono M, Katoh Y. Effects of an experimentally developed adhesive resin system and CO_2 laser irradiation on direct pulp capping. Oper Dent 2005;30(6):702-18.
23. Tamarut T, Kovacevic M, Glavicic S. Influence of the length of instrumentation and canal obturation on the success of endodontic therapy. A 10-year clinical follow-up. Am J Dent 2006;19(4):211-6.

QUESTIONS

1. Enumerate the difference between deciduous and permanent pulp.
2. Classify pulpal and periradicular diseases.
3. What are the different diagnostic methods for evaluating pulp pathology?
4. Enumerate different treatment modalities for deciduous tooth with pulpal pathology.
5. Explain the difference between apexogenesis and apexification.
6. What are the different types of deciduous tooth pulpotomies?
7. Describe the steps involved in deciduous tooth pulpectomy.
8. What is formacresol? What is its role in treatment of diseased pulp?
9. What are the properties of MTA?
10. What is pulp revascularization?

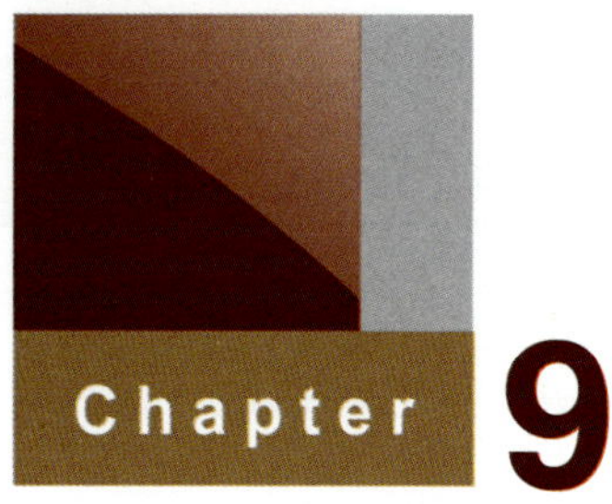

Trauma and its Management

INTRODUCTION

A child is in a dynamic state of growth, both mentally and physically. He is curious about his surroundings and is always trying to explore, and due to his lack of motor coordination is more susceptible to fall and injury.

An injury to both the primary and permanent teeth and the supporting structures is one of the most common dental problems seen in children.

The extent of injury may vary from mild chipping of the enamel to severe maxillofacial injury. Trauma is also associated with psychological impact on both the parents and the child, since these fractures may alter the child's appearance and make him the target for teasing and ridicule by other children.

Trauma to the dentition should always be considered an emergency and dealt immediately and efficiently.

EPIDEMIOLOGY

Incidence

The greatest incidence of trauma to the primary teeth occurs at 2 to 3 years of age, when motor coordination is developing.[1] The most common injuries to permanent teeth occur secondary to falls, followed by traffic accidents, violence, and sports.

On an average about 30% of all school children suffer traumatic dental injury in primary dentition, whereas 22% suffer in permanent dentition.

So slightly about >50% children will sustain a traumatic dental injury before leaving school.

Site

Majority of the injury occurred to the anterior teeth and in particular to the maxillary central incisor.

71% of trauma cases involved the maxillary central incisor and this was 3 times more frequent than maxillary lateral incisor. Out of this 56% of them involved crown fracture without pulp involvement, 13% with pulp involvement and 3% with root fracture.

Sex Distribution

Both males and females equally showed highest number of incidence between the ages of 4-5 years.

In permanent dentition similar sex distribution continues until 9 years. After this, upto 11 years boys are twice as prone to injuries of the permanent dentition as girls.

CLASSIFICATION OF TRAUMA TO ANTERIOR TEETH (FIGS 9.1 TO 9.14)

Ellis Classification (1961)[2]

- Enamel fracture
- Dentin fracture
- Crown fracture with pulp exposure
- Root fracture
- Tooth luxation
- Tooth intrusion.

Ellis and Davey Classification (1970)[3]

Class 1: Simple fracture of the crown, involving little or no dentin.

Class 2: Extensive fracture of the crown involving considerable dentin, but not the pulp.

Class 3: Extensive fracture of the crown involving considerable dentin and exposing dental pulp.

Class 4: The traumatized tooth which becomes non-vital with or without loss of crown structure.

Class 5: Loss of tooth.

Class 6: Root fracture with or without loss of crown structure.

Class 7: Displacement of a tooth without fracture of crown or root.

Class 8: Fracture of crown enmass.

Class 9: Traumatic injuries of deciduous teeth.

Hargreaves and Craig (1970)[4]

Class I: No fracture or fracture of enamel only with or without displacement of the tooth.

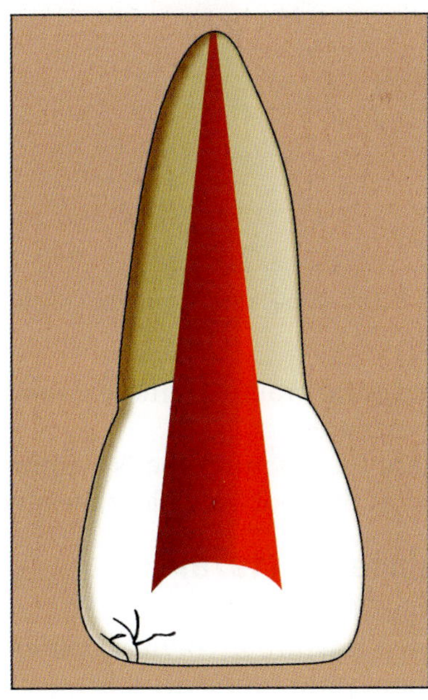

Fig. 9.1: Enamel crazing

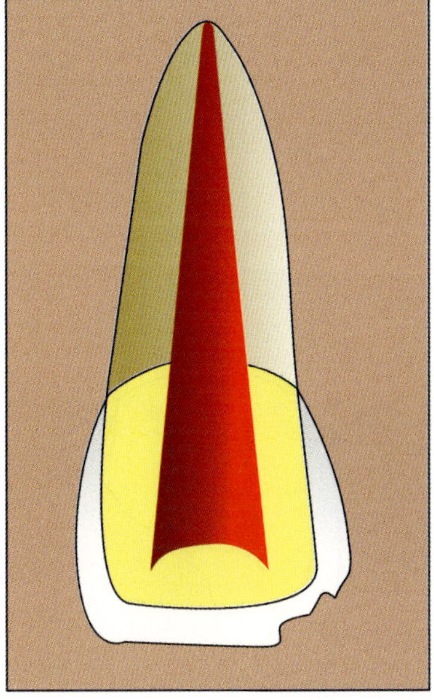

Fig. 9.2: Fracture involving only enamel

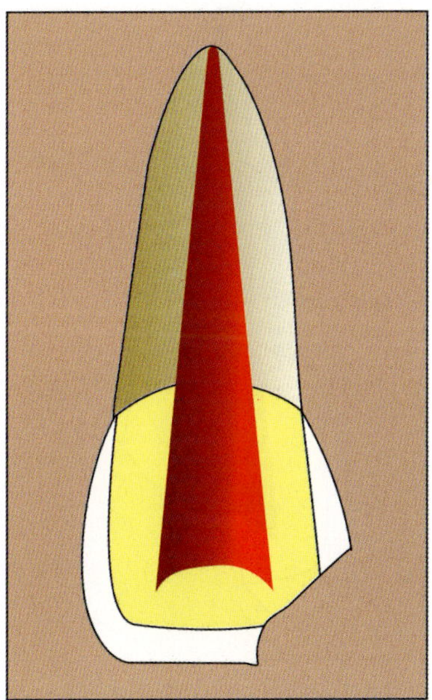

Fig. 9.3: Fracture involving enamel and dentin

Class II: Fracture of the crown involving both enamel and dentin without exposure of the pulp and without displacement of the tooth.

Class III: Fracture of the crown exposing the pulp with or without displacement of the tooth.

Class IV: Fracture of the root with or without coronal fractures, with or without displacement of the tooth.

Class V: Total displacement of the tooth.

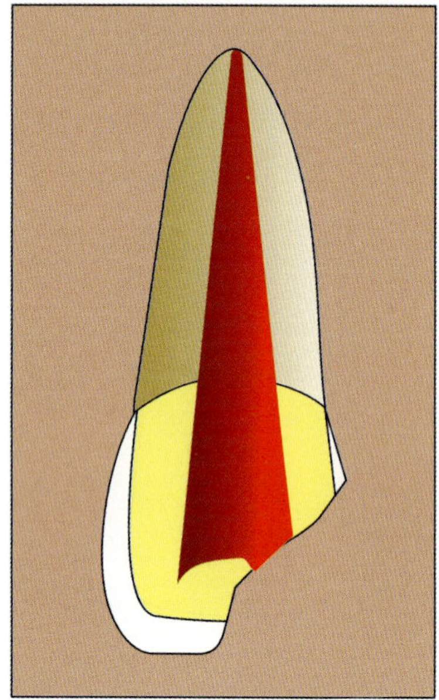

Fig. 9.4: Fracture involving enamel, dentin and pulp

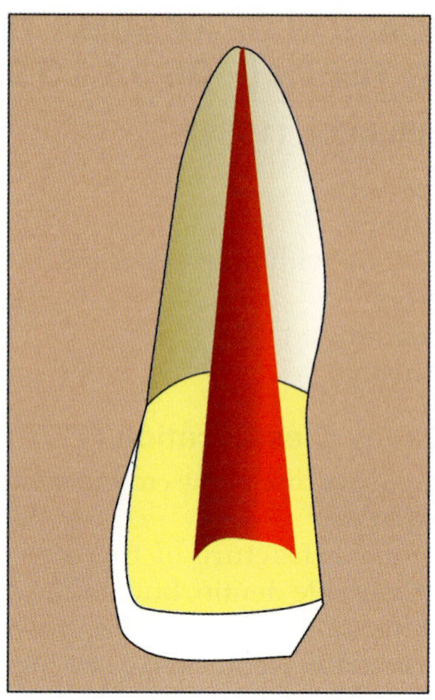

Fig. 9.6: Uncomplicated crown root fracture

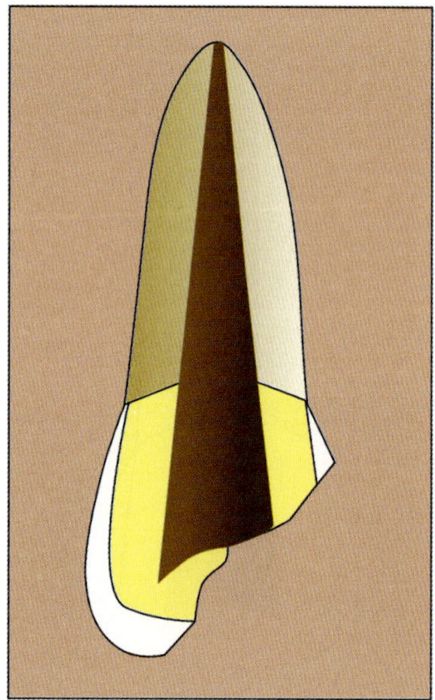

Fig. 9.5: Tooth that has become nonvital following trauma with or without fracture

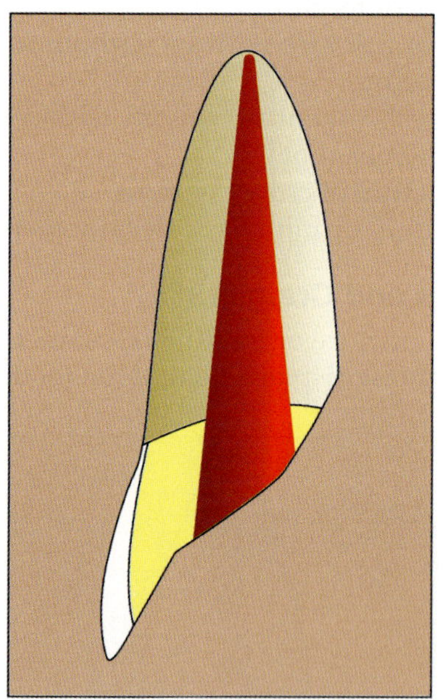

Fig. 9.7: Complicated crown root fracture

Hithersay and Morile (1982)[5]

Recommended classification of subgingival fractures based on the level of tooth fracture in relation to various horizontal planes of the periodontium.

Class 1:   Where the fracture line does not extend below the level of the attached gingiva.

Class 2:   Where the fracture line extends below the level of attached gingiva, but not below the level of the alveolar crest.

Class 3:   Where the fracture line extends below the alveolar crest.

Class 4:   Where the fracture line is within the coronal third of the root but below the alveolar crest.

WHO Classification (1978)[6]

873.60:   Enamel fracture.

873.61:   Crown fracture involving enamel and dentin without pulp exposure.

873.62:   Crown fracture with pulp exposure.

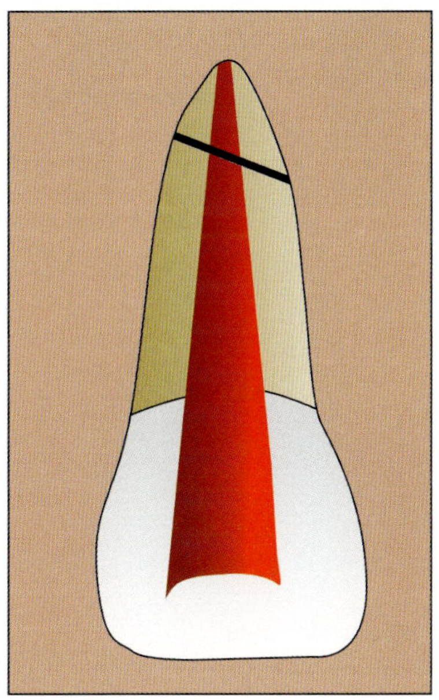

Fig. 9.8: Apical one-third root fracture

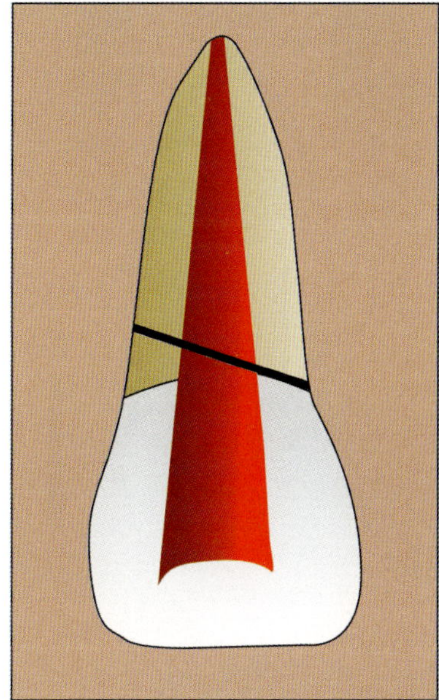

Fig. 9.10: Coronal one-third root fracture

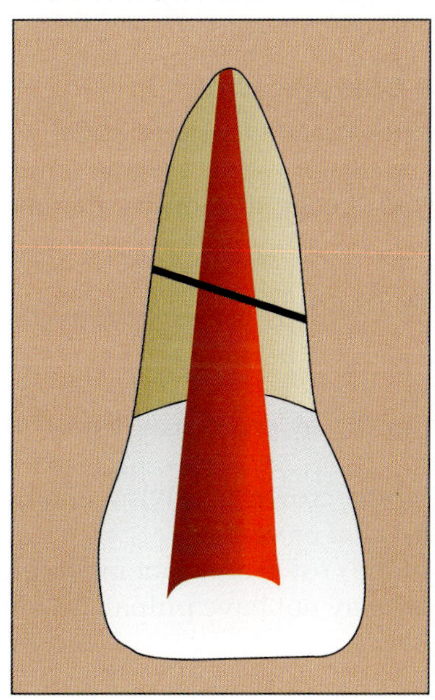

Fig. 9.9: Middle one-third root fracture

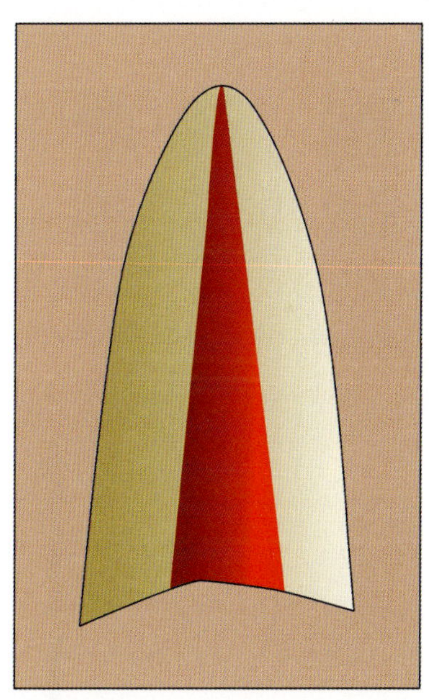

Fig. 9.11: Fracture of crown enmass

873.63:   Root fracture.
873.64:   Crown-root fracture.
873.66:   Luxation.
873.67:   Intrusion or extrusion.
873.68:   Avulsion.
873.69:   Other injuries like soft tissue injuries.

Andreasen's Modification (1981) of WHO Classification

873.64:   Uncomplicated/complicated crown-root fracture.
873.66:   Concussion/subluxation/lateral luxation.

International Classification of Diseases[7]

Injuries to Teeth

1. Enamel infarction—N 502.50.
2. Enamel fracture, uncomplicated crown fracture—N 502.50.
3. Enamel—Dentin fracture, uncomplicated crown fracture—N 502.51.
4. Complicated crown fracture—N 502.52.
5. Root fracture—N 502.53.
6. Uncomplicated crown root fracture—N 502.54.
7. Complicated crown root fracture—N 502.54.

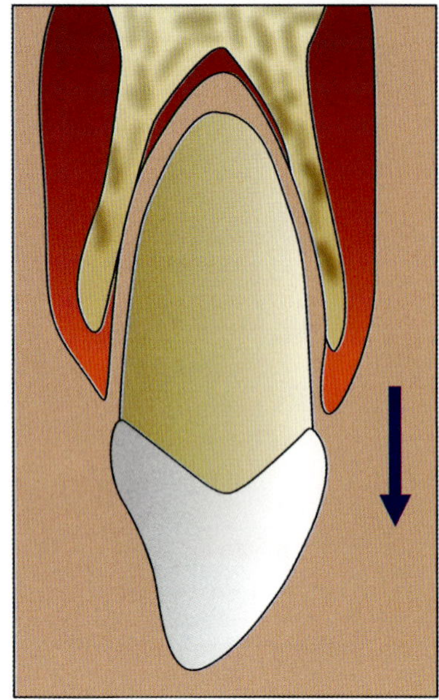

Fig. 9.12: Extrusion

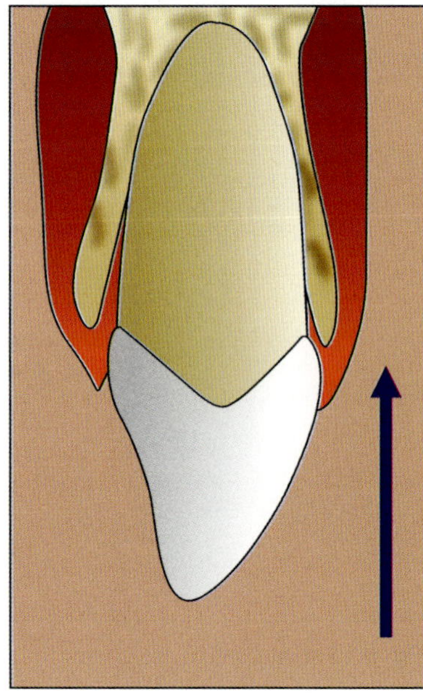

Fig. 9.13: Intrusion

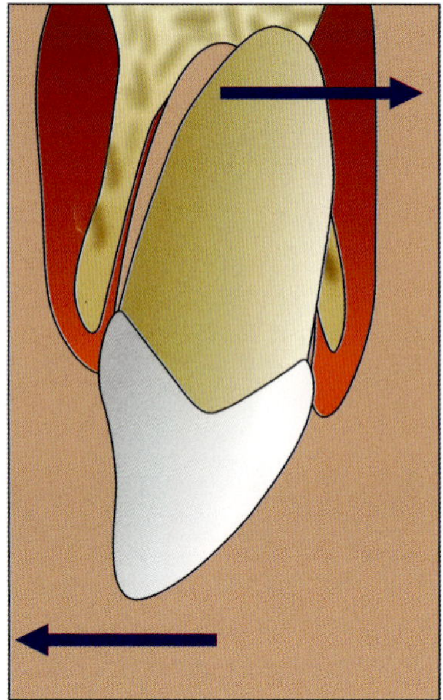

Fig. 9.14: Lingual or palatal displacement of the tooth

Injury to Periodontal Tissues

1. Concussion—N 503.20.
2. Subluxation—N 503.20.
3. Extrusive luxation—N 503.20.
4. Lateral luxation—N 503.20.
5. Intrusive luxation—N 503.21.
6. Avulsion—N 503.22.

Descriptive Classification[8]

Previous classifications were numerical which tried to give various results of dental trauma a number. In this classification, it is easy to identify the exact problem. They are:

Injuries to the Tooth

Crown

- Crack or craze of enamel without loss of tooth structure
- Fracture of the crown involving enamel, dentin or pulp (horizontal or vertical)
- Fracture of the crown and root involving cementum and may or may not have pulpal involment.

Root

- Apical 1/3rd fracture → may be horizontal or oblique
- Middle 1/3rd fracture → may be horizontal or oblique
- Coronal 1/3rd fracture → may be horizontal or oblique

Involving the whole tooth

- Concussion: Sensitivity of the tooth due to trauma without abnormal loosening or mobility. The tooth may be sensitive to percussion usually caused due to mild blow.
- Subluxation: Loosening of the tooth without displacement, due to a more severe blow resulting in injury to periodontal ligament.

- *Displacement/luxation:*
  - Intrusion: Displacement of a tooth in an apical direction. Tooth is pushed into the socket, causing fracture of the bone at the floor of the socket in most of the cases.
  - Extrusion: Displacement of a tooth in a coronal direction. The tooth is seen extruding out of the socket partially.
  - Labial/lingual/palatal: Displacement of a tooth in a labial or lingual direction.
  - Lateral: Displacement of a tooth in a mesial or distal direction.
  - Avulsion: Loss of tooth, where the entire tooth is out of the socket.

Trauma to the Supporting Bone

- Fracture of alveolar socket—due to tooth intrusion
- Socket wall fracture—labial or lingual luxation
- Fracture of alveolar process
- Fracture of maxilla
- Fracture of mandible.

Soft Tissue Injury

- Contusion
- Abrasion
- Laceration
- Deep puncture wounds
- Wide loss of tissue.

CAUSES OF TRAUMA[9,10]

Etiology of trauma may be categorized into the following:
1. Intentional injuries—child abuse and neglect
2. Unintentional accidents such as road accidents, falls or collisions, inappropriate use of teeth, handicapped children
3. Sporting activities—contact sports, bicycle or horse riding

   Trauma or injuries can also be grouped into—intentional (e.g. abuse) or unintentional (e.g. sporting activity).
   Injury to the dentition can be due to direct or indirect trauma.

Direct: When the dentition is struck directly by one of variety of objects such as a hard ball, stick, fist, etc.

Indirect: Blow to the chin may cause sudden forceful closure of mandibular teeth with their maxillary opponents, as may follow a fall, a fight or road accident.

Dental injury in young children is usually due to lack of motor coordination, i.e. during the first year of life as due to fall when the child learns to walk.

18 Months to 2 Years

The children are notoriously adventurous and inquisitive. In primary teeth, injury usually results in displacement or avulsion of teeth rather than fracture.

Fracture of the tooth is rarely observed, due to the more vertical placement of tooth, better lip protection and more pliable alveolar bone, all these yielding more readily to tooth displacement by the blow.

2-5 Years (Toddler)

At this age children are learning to walk and are very much unsteady on their feet and may result in a fall injury to anterior teeth. Common injury at this age is because of the swing, which is usually at the level of the child's teeth. The child stands in front of a moving swing and receives a blow from the moving swing.

5-10 Years

Play ground accidents, bicycle accidents are common, resulting in multiple crown fracture associated with soft tissue injuries to the upper lip and chin.

>10 Years

Injury is due to contact sports, horse riding, road traffic accidents, etc.

When a child comes with injury "Battered child syndrome" (Child abuse) must be considered. Features include:
- Children usually are under 3 years of age or are very scared and submissive.
- Presents some hours or days after accident.
- Oral trauma whose history does not coincide with clinical findings.
- Multiple bruising over the body differing in shade.
- Facial scarring, burns or bite marks.
- Other fractures.

  Details about child abuse are discussed in Chapter 10.

PREDISPOSING FACTORS[11-14]

Accident Prone Profile

a. Class II division 1 malocclusion
b. Class I type 1 malocclusion

Inadequate Lip Coverage

As observed with incompetent lip, short upper lip, mouth breathing habit, etc. Dental injuries are twice as frequent in children who have a protrusive malocclusion than those who have normal occlusion.

According to Jarvinen (1958) frequency of injury with:
A. Normal overjet   (0-3 mm)   is 14.2%

B. Increased overjet (3.1-6 mm) is 28.4%
C. Extreme overjet (>6 mm) is 38.6%

Handicapped Children

Children with cerebral palsy, mental retardation or epilepsy are more susceptible to injuries, due to the following reasons:
- They are subjected to abnormal muscle tone and function in the oral area, producing protrusion of maxillary anterior teeth.
- Because of their poor skeletal muscle coordination they are subjected to frequent fall.
- In epileptic patients, during seizures there is increased chance of trauma due to fall.

Dental Anomalies and Caries

Hypoplasia and dental caries results in weakening of the crown structure.

Mechanical Factors

According to Hallet (1953), severity of injury depends on:

Energy of Impact

Energy of impact depends upon both mass and velocity. For example, force of high velocity and low mass = gun shot injury.

High mass and low velocity = striking the tooth against the ground.

Low velocity blows cause greater damage to supporting structures and high velocity blows results in crown fractures.

Resiliency of the Impacting Object

If a tooth is struck with a resilient or cushioned object such as an elbow during play or if the lip absorbs and distributes the impact, the chance of crown fractures is reduced while the risk of luxation and alveolar fracture is increased.

Shape of the Impacting Object

A sharp impact favors clean fractures with minimum of displacement of the tooth because energy is spread rapidly over a limited area. On the other hand, a blunt impact increases the area of resistance to the force in the crown region and allows the impact to be transmitted to the apical region causing luxation and root fracture.

Angle of Direction of the Impacting Force

The impact can meet the tooth at different angles, most often hitting the tooth facially, and perpendicular to the long axis of the root. It may result in cleavage lines along with the main fracture line. It is seen that enamel is weakest parallel to enamel rod and dentin is weakest perpendicular to the dentinal tubules.

PREVENTION OF TRAUMA

1. Legislation: Compulsory use of mouth guards, seat belts, helmets, etc.
2. Education: Explaining the potential dangers.
3. Early recognition and treatment of predisposing factors.

MANAGEMENT

It includes:
1. Obtaining history
2. Clinical examination
3. Providing first aid
4. Treatment of the injury.

Obtaining History

History taking is one of the fundamental steps in routine clinical dentistry. It should be done precisely and quickly, followed by a thorough examination.
History taking includes:
1. Personal data—name, age, sex, address
2. Complaint and its history—can be related to pain, sensitivity, discomfort, etc. Pain occurring when teeth are in contact, may be due to displaced tooth. The severity of tooth mobility following trauma and chances of pulpal death is directly proportional. Pain caused by thermal change signifies pulpal inflammation.
3. Relevant medical history and history of tetanus prophylaxis should be recorded.
4. Previous dental history.
5. Neurological history—trauma may result in damage to cranial nerve. Patient is observed from the time he/she enters the dental office. Signs and symptoms suggestive of neurologic damage are:
   - Inability to sit or stand unsupported
   - Patient appears lethargic or confused
   - Presence of black eye
   - Unusual verbal response to questions
   - Nausea or vomiting
   - Headache
   - Bleeding or discharge of clear fluid from ears and nose
   - Abnormal position or movement of eye
   - Perspiration on the forehead
   - Asymmetric or decreased reaction of pupil
   - Abnormal respiratory rate
   - Level of consciousness.

Clinical Examination[15-17]

Assessment of Injury

It may be difficult in a very young child who is frightened and shocked following his accident to make him sit on a dental chair for check up. The injury can appear alarming to the mother. A little blood mixed with saliva can give the impression of copious hemorrhage and clotting of the blood on lips can suggest extensive laceration.

For an adequate clinical assessment in young children or infants—visual access to the mouth can be improved if the mother and the pedodontist sit facing each other on an ordinary chair, with the child's head on the lap of the pedodontist and legs stretched on to the mothers lap. The mother holds the child's hands with her own. Both the upper and lower arches can be readily seen and if needed, mouth prop can be used. The area to be examined is cleaned with cotton moistened with hydrogen peroxide or water.

Extraoral Examination

- Hemorrhage—subconjunctival hemorrhage may indicate fracture of zygomatic complex.
- Laceration—inspected for foreign bodies or broken tooth fragments
- Deviation in the path of mandible during mouth opening, will reveal injury to the TMJ.
- Leakage of straw colored fluid from nose, indicates fracture of the middle 1/3rd.

Intraoral Examination

Soft tissues examination

- Laceration of gingiva, labial and buccal mucosa, tongue and floor of the mouth.
- Presence of embedded tooth fragments.
- Hematoma in the floor of the mouth indicate mandibular fracture.

Hard tissues examination

- Occlusal abnormalities, which may be due to fractured dentoalveolar portion or displacement of the teeth.
- Palpation of maxilla and mandible for fracture. Mandibular fracture signs are local swelling, ecchymoses, malocclusion, and limited ability to open the mouth.
- Displacement of teeth has to be measured in millimeters.
- Mobility can be in horizontal or vertical direction. If 2 or more teeth move at a time, alveolar fracture must be suspected.

- Root fractures can be diagnosed by placing fingers against the linguopalatal and buccolabial mucosa and attempt is made to move the tooth. If independent movement of crown and root is detected, root fracture is suspected.
- Type of fracture is classified
- Color change of the crown is noted:
  - If the crown appears darkened, there are high chances that the tooth is nonvital
  - Reddish crown indicates pulpal-hyperemia, may later undergo degenerative changes terminating in pulpal necrosis.

Vitality Tests

Pulp testing by any of the conventional methods is not advisable as the response from a young child cannot be relied upon, and is of little value because a tooth that gives false responses following a trauma, may recover vitality after sometime.

Following fracture, reactions to pulp vitality test may be negative for as long as 6-8 weeks. A vital response should return within 2 weeks of the traumatic incident but sometimes may not return up to 10 months.[18,19] It is possible for trauma to injure pulpal nerves and not the blood vessels. In such a case the pulp would be healthy in having a normal blood supply, but would not respond to the stimuli. Healthy pulp responds to electrical stimulus of 150 μ Amp from a monopolar pulp tester and > 200 μ Amp may excite periodontal nerves.

Laser Doppler Flowmetry (LDF) assesses the blood supply, and hence has been found to be far better than electric pulp testing or other methods.

Recommended pulp testing—immediately, 2 weeks, 1 month, 2 months, 6 months, 12 months and then at yearly interval for next 3 years. Pulp that does not show any response by the end of 1 month, may be undergoing degeneration.

Providing First Aid

- Trauma of the orofacial region can cause profuse bleeding into oropharynx and nasopharynx, creating respiratory obstruction. It is essential to maintain the airway. If needed endotracheal intubation or tracheostomy may have to be performed.
- Deep cuts and lacerations should be sutured using chromic gut sutures (2-0) or black silk under LA.
- Fluid replacement is necessary to avoid hypovolemic shock.
- Adequate debridement of the area is important. Gentle cleaning and irrigation with normal saline solution will help to reduce the amount of dead tissue and risk of anaerobic condition. Topical antiseptics should

be used to reduce the bacterial count especially the pathogenic streptococci and staphylococci in skin or mucosa at wound site. For example, chlorhexidine, iodine, phenol, sodium hypochlorite, etc.

> **Tetanus prophylaxis:** The following regime is as follows:
> - Immunization completed previously: Booster dose within 12 months—No additional toxoid (TT) required.
> - Immunization completed within previous 10 years—administer 0.5 ml fluid tetanus toxoid booster (intramuscular).
> - Immunization completed >10 years, last booster within previous 10 years—administer 0.5 ml TT intramuscularly.
> - Immunization completed >10 years previously, no booster received within last 10 years—wound cleaned, treated promptly and adequately, 0.5 ml TT given intramuscularly.
> - Immunization completed >10 years previously, no booster within last 10 years, wound tetanus prone—administer 0.5 ml TT and 250 ml tetanus immune human globulin.
> - No history of immunization, wound not clean or treated promptly—250-500 units tetanus immune human globulin and 0.5 ml absorbed TT prophylactic use of penicillin should also be advised.

TREATMENT OF THE INJURY

Trauma to the Primary Teeth[17]

Due to the proximity of the developing succedaneous tooth, definitive treatment of the traumatized primary tooth should be instituted as soon as possible. Extent of damage to a permanent tooth depends on its developmental status at the time of injury besides the nature, extent and duration of injury to primary tooth.

Enamel Fracture

In small enamel fractures—rough enamel margins can be disked and smoothened.

In large enamel fractures—the tooth may be restored using an acid etch composite resin restoration.

Enamel and Dentin Fractures

Exposed dentin should be covered with a layer of calcium hydroxide or glass ionomer cement to prevent pulpal irritation. The tooth is then restored with acid etch composite resin restoration or by preformed polycarbonate crown or by fabricated acrylic jacket crown.

Fracture Involving the Pulp

Usually such injuries are rare in primary dentition. Treatment depends upon the vitality of the tooth. If the tooth is vital the treatment option may vary from direct pulp capping to formacresol pulpotomy. If the tooth is nonvital, pulpectomy is the choice. Final restoration is done with a celluloid crown matrix or a stainless steel crown with composite facing or window.

Root Fracture

In a primary tooth with root fracture without dislocation and excessive mobility, normal exfoliation may be anticipated. Extraction is preferred if the tooth is very mobile as it is associated with increased risk of aspiration.

Treatment depends on the level of fracture.

Apical 1/3rd fracture—is associated with good prognosis. The tooth usually maintains its vitality and normal root resorption occurs.

Middle 1/3rd and coronal 1/3rd fractures—advised extraction.

Concussion

The tooth should be made free from occlusion and is kept under observation.

Mobility

This type of trauma is very common in children. Patient is instructed to avoid eating with involved teeth and follow-up examination should occur. The bone can be remodelled around the teeth with gentle finger pressure sufficient to hold the teeth in a fairly stable position as the bone is very spongy and malleable. No splint should be placed and prognosis is good.

Intrusion

It is one of the most dangerous injuries to the developing permanent tooth bud. If the intruded deciduous tooth is contacting the permanent tooth bud, the deciduous tooth must be extracted. If it is not contacting and is placed labially, the intruded tooth is allowed to re-erupt. 90% of the teeth reerupt in 2-6 months. The tooth is kept under observation. Extraction of the intruded tooth is indicated if a fistula or a periapical radiolucency develops or does not erupt after 3-4 weeks.

Extrusion and Lateral Luxation Injuries

Most of the deciduous teeth injuries result in luxation or avulsion due to the resilient bone surrounding them.[10,20,21] In these injuries, serious damage to the PDL usually occurs. Some clinicians recommend splinting these teeth with sutures until periodontal ligament attachment occurs, which takes approximately 2 weeks. While few others prefer extraction because of the potential for aspiration of the mobile teeth or subsequent damage to developing permanent tooth bud.

*Splinting of Luxated Primary
Teeth is not Preferred*

- Cooperation is often a problem
- Bonding of the splint is difficult due to short clinical crowns and associated gingival bleeding.

Avulsion

- Primary teeth that have avulsed should not be reimplanted. The lost tooth is replaced by an artificial substitute.

Trauma to the Permanent Tooth

Treatment options of crown fractures is directly related to:

- Pulpal response to injury or restorative material
- Restorative considerations for final or definitive treatment.

> **Final restorative treatment for a traumatized permanent anterior tooth include:**
>
> - Recontouring the injured or opposite tooth
> - Composite or adhesive resin restoration
> - Reattachment of the original crown fragment
> - Laminate veneers
> - Porcelain fused to metal crowns
> - Full coverage porcelain restorations
> - Bleaching
> - Immediate needs of patient.

Crown Craze or Crack (Fig. 9.15)

These are incomplete fractures (crack) of the enamel without loss of tooth structure.

The width of the cracks are not much larger (2-5 μm) than most bacteria and they tend to become filled and sealed which is the reason why these cracks do not contribute to caries formation. But they weaken the tooth and may lead to tooth fracture.

Such cracks usually go unnoticed. Transillumination may be helpful in detection. Staining the teeth with a disclosing solution will often reveal the fracture after the residual dye is washed away. Lines of infraction exhibit a coronal pattern, depending on the direction of the force and the site of impaction.

Application of cold will elicit pain and with an electric pulp tester the tooth often responds to slightly less current than usual.

The tooth is kept under observation for vitality. Infraction lines can be sealed with unfilled resin, to prevent stains.

Fractures Involving Enamel (Fig. 9.16)

Treatment consists of smoothening the jagged edges if there is only slight chipping of the enamel. Restoration of the fractured fragment is made using acid etch composite resin restoration. The tooth should be kept under observation for 6-8 weeks for any changes in the pulp or periapical region that may occur due to deleterious effects of concussion on pulp.

*Fractures Involving Enamel and
Dentin (Figs 9.17 and 9.18)*

Although pulp is not visibly exposed, emergency treatment is necessary to protect the already traumatized pulp from further insult from excessive thermal, bacterial

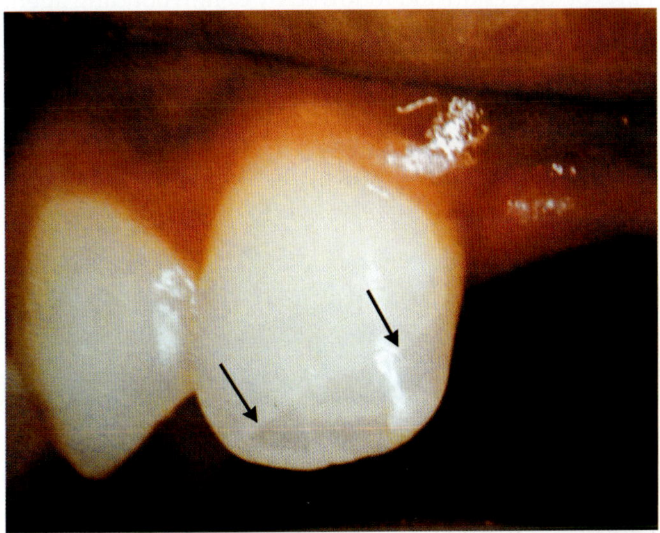

Fig. 9.15: Enamel craze line seen on the upper lateral incisor

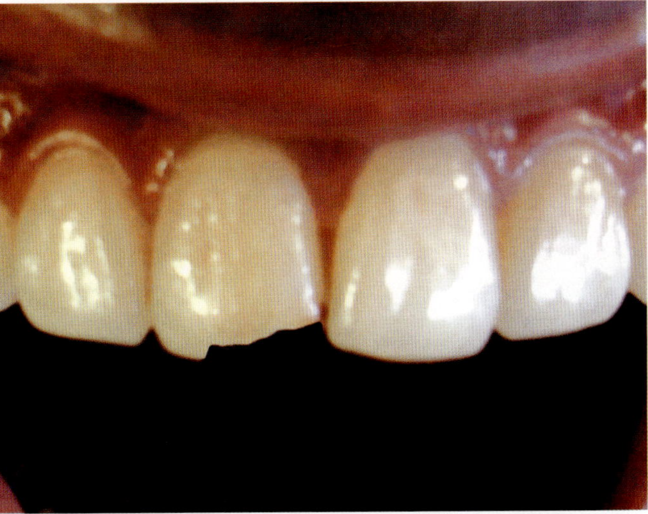

Fig. 9.16: Enamel fracture that can be restored with composite restoration

and chemical stimuli and to hasten the formation of a layer of secondary dentin in the fractured area. Dentin thickness of 2 millimeters is needed to shield the pulp. Dentinal tubules closer to the pulp are wider, therefore making it easier for the penetration of microorganisms or noxious substances. Thus deep fractures will allow more microorganisms or other substances in higher concentrations to permeate through the dentinal barrier and provoke and inflammatory response in the pulp. The traditional approach recommended includes placement of calcium hydroxide over the exposed dentin, followed by acid etch composite resin restoration. But since it is found that calcium hydroxide dissolves over a period of time, it is replaced by placement of glass ionomer to the deeper parts of the dentin and followed by dentin bonding agent to obtain a seal. Some of the advantages of using glass ionomer cements is that it does not require etching, it is hydrophilic and good biocompatibility property.[22,23]

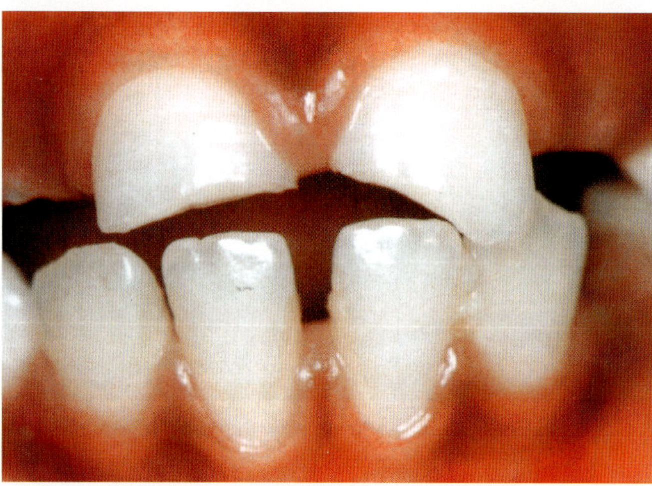

Fig. 9.17: Class II fracture of the crown

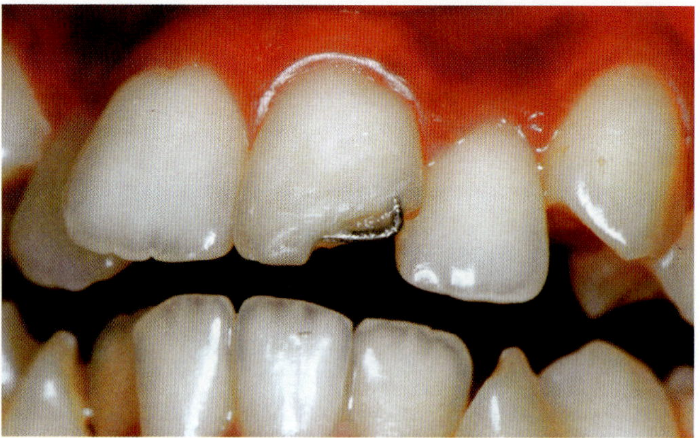

Fig. 9.18: Pin retained restoration of anterior tooth

Advantage of calcium hydroxide as a dressing material over exposed dentin

- Reduce or neutralize the acidity of cements
- Increases the local pH, provides an antimicrobial environment
- Protects the pulp by occluding open dentinal tubules
- Stimulates reparative dentin formation.

Disadvantages of calcium hydroxide

- It is soluble in water, therefore the presence of dentinal fluid may interfere with the set of the material and cause eventual dissolution.
- Soluble when exposed to 37% phosphoric acid for 60 seconds as during composite resin restoration.

Glass ionomer cement as the material to seal the exposed dentin, below the composite resin restoration

Materials used to seal dentinal tubules must be hydrophilic. Fluid flow from the tubules assist in diluting harmful chemicals or microbial products and provide a fluid movement force against which the bacteria must travel to gain access to the pulpal tissue. But this fluid affects the adherence or bonding of composite which is hydrophobic. This is not a problem with glass ionomer as it is hydrophilic. The advantage of glass ionomer cement is that it is hydrophilic, releases fluoride, chemically adheres to enamel and dentin and also has a coefficient of thermal expansion similar to dentin. Also etching glass ionomer cement does not adversely affect its properties if the minimum thickness is 0.5 mm and freshly prepared.

Methods of treatment for restoration of enamel dentin fractures

- Acid etch composite/crown restoration
- Reattachment of the fracture fragment
- Pin retained composite restoration.

Acid etch composite/crown restoration: Stainless steel crowns are not esthetically pleasing, but are extremely sturdy and durable. It is a useful restoration in cases where the fracture is close to the gingival margin and isolation is difficult and also in cases of horizontal fractures where the strength of the stainless steel crown is of great advantage. To improve esthetics a labial window can be made with a diamond bur using an air turbine. The crown must remain in place until a vital response is noted which may be for about 7-8 weeks following injury. It may then be replaced by a permanent restoration.

Reattachment of the fractured fragment: It is possible to successfully reattached the teeth fragment using resin and bonding technique. These fragments serve as esthetically perfect temporary restorations that may be retained for a long time and also no mechanical tooth preparation is needed, as the fragments are retained by enamel etch technique. If a considerable portion of dentin is exposed, modification of the fragment is done to provide space for the dressing material by removing a portion of dentin using a bur.

Pin retained composite restoration: A period of 8 weeks is allowed after injury for the pulp to recover from injury. Pin retained composite resin restorations are placed at one sitting and are esthetically satisfactory. The pins are placed in holes drilled in the dentin and serve to retain the composite restoration. Pins are usually avoided in young permanent tooth as the thickness of the dentin is very less and risk of pulp damage is high.

> In a vital dentin (dentin with dentinal tubular fluid and odontoblastic processes) during acid etching the extent of acid penetration into dentin is limited, and is not more than 10 µm. In a nonvital dentin it is about 200 µm (0.2 mm).

Fracture Involving the Pulp (Fig. 9.19)

Treatment depends upon following factors:

1. *Size of pulpal exposure:* Small pulp exposures can be managed by direct pulp caping or Cvek pulpotomy
2. *Stage of development of root apex:* The treatment procedure should be aimed at maintaining the pulp vitality.
3. *Vitality of the pulp:* Vital procedures such as direct pulp capping or pulpotomy are preferred.
4. *Time lapse:* Shorter time lapse after trauma is favorable to initiate any vital procedures. Thus prognosis of direct pulp capping is good when done immediately than done after few days.

Objectives of the treatment

1. Retain the tooth
2. Maintain its vitality, to allow apex closure in an young permanent tooth
3. Ensure root apex maturity.

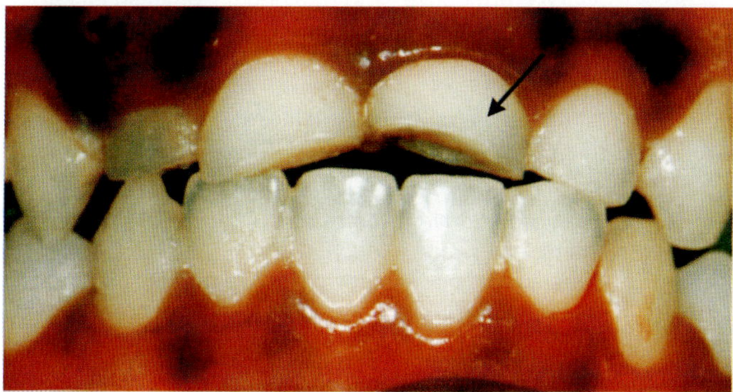

Fig. 9.19: Class III fracture of the crown

Usual treatment modalities

1. Pulp capping
2. Pulpotomy
3. Pulpectomy
4. Apexification
5. Extraction.

Pulp capping or partial pulpotomy should be done immediately in an immature tooth for better prognosis, so as to maintain its vitality.

Contamination of the pulp tissue by oral fluids directly innoculates this tissue with bacteria. Therefore the majority of complicated crown fractures require partial or complete pulpotomy.

Please refer chapter 16 for details on pulp therapy.

Pulp capping

Indicated in fractures associated with exposure of pulp and the exposure is small and not over 24 hours in duration. It is also indicated in a tooth with, incompletely formed apex.

The involved tooth is isolated with rubber dam and calcium hydroxide is placed over the exposed pulp. The tooth is then restored with a stainless steel crown or acid etch composite resin restoration. A thin layer of dentin like material should cover vital pulp tissue within 2 months.

There is some risk of failure as infection of the pulp is inevitable even with a minute exposure.

Partial pulpotomy (Shallow Pulpotomy/Cvek Pulpotomy)[24] (Figs 9.20A to E)

It is a definitive procedure that allows root closure and maintains pulpal vitality. It involves removal of 2 mm of injured coronal pulp with a sterile bur in a high speed handpiece cooled with sterile solution. Calcium hydroxide dressing is placed over the residual tissue and sealed with zinc oxide eugenol cement or glass ionomer cement. When there is radiographic evidence of development of a hard tissue barrier (3-6 months), the tooth is restored with acid etch composite resin after removing the zinc oxide eugenol cement. Cvek reported 96% success rate with this technique regardless of the stage of root development, contamination by oral fluids (up to 7 days) or size of the original exposure (up to 4 mm).

Pulpotomy

Indicated when there is moderate hemorrhage with a relatively large pulp exposure and patient is seen within 48 hours. An incisor with a wide apex and incomplete root formation is considered a good candidate for this technique because of the better recuperative powers of the young pulp.

Pulpotomy is contraindicated in a mature teeth with concurrent displacement injuries (as these procedures

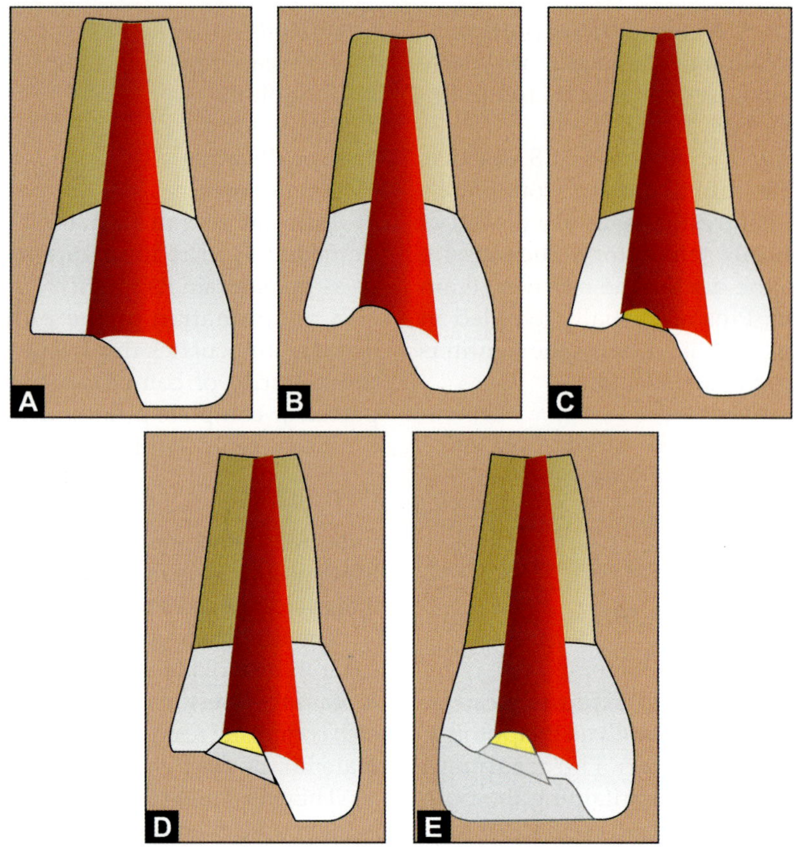

Figs 9.20A to E: Cvek pulpotomy: (A) Trauma involving enamel, dentin and pulp in an immature tooth with vital pulp; (B) Access opening is made and part of the coronal pulp is removed; (C) Calcium hydroxide is placed over the amputated pulp; (D) The tooth is then sealed with zinc oxide eugenol or glass ionomer cement; (E) The tooth is restored permanently

require the maintenance of an intact vascular supply and displacement injuries frequently involve vascular damage), teeth with other types of vascular alterations like pulpstones, degeneration or inflammatory changes and in tooth with extensive fracture requiring posts.

This procedure involves removal of the infected coronal pulp tissue leaving vital, noninfected radicular pulp tissue allowing complete apex formation.

Pulpectomy

It is indicated if the pulp is degenerated, putrescent, of questionable vitality or if the exposure period is >72 hours.

Apexification

It is the treatment of choice in the management of immature necrotic permanent teeth. It is followed by conventional root canal treatment in the management of teeth with irreversibly diseased pulp and open apices. There is formation of calcific barrier just coronal to the apex, following which routine endodontic procedure may be completed.

Treatment outline of coronal fractures in vital teeth			
Type of fracture	Emergency phase	Intermediate phase	Permanent phase
Cl I	Rounding of sharp edges	....	Cosmetic grinding, acid etch resin restoration
Cl II	$CaOH_2$ protective layer reinforced by orthodontic band, stainless steel crown, celluloid crown form	Pin retained composite, cast ¾ crown, acrylic jacket crown	Porcelain jacket crown or porcelain fused to metal crown
Cl III	Pulp capping with orthodontic band, stainless steel crown or resin and celluloid crown form	Reinforced core and acrylic jacket crown	Cast post and core, Porcelain jacket crown or porcelain fused to metal crown
	Pulpotomy or pulpectomy with same as above		
	Extraction	RPD	Fixed bridge

Fracture Involving Crown and Root

Without Pulpal Involvement

In cases when the fracture line extends only about 2 mm apical to the marginal base level, healing occurs by PDL reattachment and cementum deposition on dentin. After administering local anesthesia and the tooth is isolated with rubberdam, fractured fragment is removed using a sharp scalpel to dissect it from the attached PDL. Bleeding is easily controlled with pressure or adrenaline. The exposed dentin is covered with $CaOH_2$ and temporary crown is placed with its margin covering the fracture line. Acid etch resin restoration can also be given when isolation can be adequately maintained. Approximately 2 months is needed for periodontal fiber reattachment.

With Pulpal Involvement

Treatment options are:

In tooth with open apex

- Vital tooth = Pulpotomy, and post and crown restoration
- Nonvital tooth = Apexification followed by root canal treatment and post and crown restoration.

In tooth with closed apex

- Vital or nonvital = Root canal treatment followed by post and crown restoration.

In a tooth with open apex, pulpotomy is the treatment of choice. The fractured fragment is kept in place if the fragment is attached, to act as a temporary restoration and maintain normal esthetics. Removal of the fragment may lead to bleeding, leading to difficulty in isolation. After apex closure is complete, root canal treatment is completed and tooth restored with post and crown.

In a tooth with closed apex, RCT followed by post and crown is recommended.

Fractured area must be exposed, so that the margins of the restoration are on solid tooth structure. This can be done by extrusion or periodontal crown lengthening procedure.

If the fracture includes more than 1/3rd of the root then extraction is indicated.

Root Fracture

The fracture may be in the apical 1/3rd, middle 1/3rd, or coronal 1/3rd of the root portion.

Transverse root fractures form 6% of all dental trauma. A steep occlusal radiograph (discloses fracture in apical 1/3rd of the root) and IOPA (for identifying coronally located fracture) is recommended. The principle of management of root fractures are to reposition the coronal fragment and immobilization.

Factors important in the root fracture treatment are:
- Position of the tooth after fracture
- Mobility of the coronal segment
- Status of the pulp
- Position of the fracture line.

A tooth with root fracture and associated with a sinus tract or granulation tissue present across the fracture line is considered as nonvital. Revascularization and reinnervation of the damaged pulp are determined by the severity of the injury and by the healing capacity of the pulp, which is directly proportional to the stage of the root development.

Apical segment usually remains vital, thus treatment is rarely required and endodontic manipulation is confined to the coronal segment only. If apical segment becomes nonvital, surgical removal of the apical segment is necessary.

Healing of the root fracture: According to Andresen,[25] healing usually occurs by:
- Calcified tissue: (Bridge of dentin and cementum)—healing occurs by calcified tissue when there is minimal amount of luxation, small amount of separation, young patient, immediate splinting and tooth without restorations or marginal periodontitis.
- Interposition of connective tissue separating the 2 fragments: It is associated with increased age of the patient, presence of restoration, orthodontic band splinting of the tooth and mild mobility.
- Interposition of granulation tissue: It is associated with existing infection, fracture line communicating with oral cavity, increased luxation, decreased fracture foramen, orthodontic band splinting and antibiotic therapy at the time of the injury.
- Interposition of bone and connective tissue.

Apical 1/3rd and middle 1/3rd fractures of the root

In these fractures, there may be palatal displacement of the crown segment. The fragment is positioned under local anesthesia by digital pressure and stabilized by splinting. The tooth is observed radiographically and regular vitality test done. Endodontic treatment is instituted if the tooth becomes nonvital.

Apical 1/3rd fracture is treated by performing root canal treatment on the coronal portion and apical portion is removed surgically.

Middle 1/3rd fracture is treated by performing root canal treatment followed by intraradicular splinting with metal pin or metal endodontic implants that also serves as root canal filling.[26]

Coronal 1/3rd fractures of the root

The tooth is positioned and immobilized by splinting. If healing is uneventful, no further treatment is needed. If there is pulp necrosis or failure to heal, endodontic treatment is done. Proximity of the fracture to gingival crevice makes pulpal infection more probable. Coronal portion can be removed, endodontic treatment completed on the apical fragment and restored with post and crown.

Orthodontic extrusion of remaining apical fragment may be necessary before performing root canal treatment to improve the situation, if the fracture line is deep and difficult to access.

PERIODONTAL INJURIES

It may be associated with partial to complete severance of blood supply. This may lead to ischemic changes in the pulp and resulting in complete pulpal necrosis. If the pulp survives and becomes revascularized, there may be regressive changes seen such as calcifications, etc.

Concussion

It includes injury to the supporting structures of the tooth without loosening or displacement, with significant reactions to percussion. It usually requires no treatment. Adjustment of occlusion with regular vitality test at subsequent visits (recall at 1 or 2 weeks after trauma and at 6 month interval for a minimum of 1year) may be adequate.

Subluxation

It is associated with abnormal loosening or mobility of the tooth but no displacement. There is often hemorrhage around the gingival margin of the tooth and the tooth may be sensitive to percussion. Treatment may be confined to selective grinding and adjusting the occlusion. If mobility is extensive and involves many teeth, the teeth are splinted using the acid etch splinting technique. Periodic reviews every 3-4 weeks are essential to monitor tooth vitality and periapical changes.

Intrusion

It is associated with significant damage to the PDL, resulting in a greater incidence of external root resorption. Most of the time the treatment involves allowing the tooth to re-erupt.

Other methods of treatment

- Orthodontic extrusion and repositioning (requires about 3-4 weeks) followed by retention for about 8-12 weeks. Teeth that have been traumatized must be evaluated carefully prior to beginning or continuing orthodontic movement. Even with more simple crown/root fractures without pulpal involvement, a 3 months wait is recommended before tooth movement should begin. When there has been moderate to severe trauma/damage to the periodontium, a minimum of 6 months wait is recommended.[27,28]
- Immediate surgical repositioning followed by splinting and endodontic therapy.

The tooth with incompletely formed roots have better prognosis and usually re-erupt spontaneously.

Radiographically an intruded tooth will demonstrate an obliteration of the periodontal space. Periodic evaluation is done every 3-4 weeks for possible pulp degeneration.

Extrusion

The extruded tooth is repositioned by applying digital pressure in apical direction on the incisal edge. The tooth is then maintained in this position by splinting. Lacerated gingiva should be repositioned around the neck of the tooth and sutured. If there is no associated supporting bone fracture, period of stabilization is for 2-3 weeks, and with bone fracture, it is for 3-4 weeks to 6-8 weeks depending on the extent of bone fracture.

Lateral Luxation

It is associated with eccentric displacement of the tooth occurring in conjunction with some type of comminution or fracture of the alveolar socket. The tooth is repositioned by applying digital pressure and splinted in the new position.

Avulsed Tooth

An avulsed permanent tooth can be reimplanted and stabilized. The prognosis following reimplantation depends on the amount of time the tooth was extraorally and the medium used for its storage during that period. It is thus very important to educate the parents and the teachers about the care of an avulsed permanent tooth.

Instruction given to patients or guardians following tooth avulsion:
- The tooth should be located and should be handled by holding the crown portion.
- Rinse gently under tap water to clean the debris and not to scrub the tooth or use soap or other cleansing agents.
- To insert the tooth back after rinsing into the socket.
- The patient should gently occlude on a gauze or handkerchief for stability and should visit the dental office as soon as possible.
- If cannot be replanted, the tooth should be placed in suitable medium.

Media for storage of avulsed permanent tooth are: Saliva, milk, blood, plain water, contact lens solution, cell culture medium, Hank's balanced salt solution (commercially available as Save-A-Tooth), or the tooth can be placed in the mouth between cheek and gums or under the tongue. The vitality of the cells can be maintained by wrapping the tooth in a clean wet handkerchief and placing it in a freezer. Soaking the root portion in fluoride solution has been found to reduce the chance of root resorption.

Features that may Improve the Prognosis of Replanted Permanent Teeth

- Maintenance of the periodontal ligament
- A short time between tooth loss and replantation
- Immaturity of the tooth to be replanted
- The undertaking of root canal therapy.

The treatment of choice for an avulsed tooth is reimplantation, if done within 30 minutes of injury. If stored in a suitable medium, it should be replanted within 1 hour.

> **Storage media for avulsed permanent tooth[29,30]:**
>
> Water—least desirable due to its hypotonic environment that causes rapid cell lysis
> Saliva—incompatible osmolality and pH and presence of bacteria. But allows storage upto 2 hours.
> Milk—readily available, pH and osmolality is compatible to vital cells and relatively free of bacteria. Allows storage upto 3 hours.
> Cell culture medium—good but not readily available
> 'Save-a-tooth'—contains Hanks balanced salt solution (HBSS)-could be made readily available in schools, play grounds, ambulances, etc.
> ViaSpan—prognosis in this storage medium is found to be very effective and the healing has beengood even after 96 hours.

Emergency Management of Avulsed Tooth

The main aim of management of avulsed tooth is to establish a healthy periodontal tissue and reduce the risk of root resorption. Necrotic pulp is not of immediate concern because toxins are usually not present initially in a great enough concentration to elicit an inflammatory response. Endodontic treatment is preferably not initiated at the emergency visit if the patient reports within 30 minutes. Endodontic treatment is also considered in a tooth with closed apex. An avulsed tooth can be reimplanted and stabilized using splints before performing any endodontic treatment. Extraoral RCT has also been recommended taking care not to damage the PDL fibers on the root surface followed by reimplantation. Tooth with open apex stands a chance of revascularization if replanted early.

Treatment Modalities of Avulsed Tooth

Extraoral Dry Time Less than 30 Minutes with Closed Apex

- A chance of PDL healing is excellent
- Treatment includes cleaning the tooth off debris and rinsing followed by replantation and stabilization
- Follow-up evaluation is done at regular visits.

Extraoral Dry Time Less than 30 Minutes with Open Apex

- Revascularization of the pulp as well as continued root development is possible.

Extraoral Time of 30-60 Minutes with Either Open or Closed Apex

- Chances of revascularization is extremely poor, even in a tooth with open apex. Apexification procedure is initiated at the second visit if not done in the first.
- Root canal treatment is initiated at the second visit at 7-10 days in a tooth with closed apex.
- Treatment includes cleaning and replanting the tooth and accepting that the complications are inevitable.
- Studies reveal that soaking in storage medium can reduce ankylosis as there is increased chance of survival of cells. May be bacterial debris, necrotic debris, etc float off during soaking period (30 min).
- The tooth can be soaked in doxycycline (1mg of doxycycline mixed with 20 ml of physiologic saline) for 5 minutes before replantation for improving the revascularization significantly. Doxycycline inhibits bacteria, thus removing the major obstacle.

Extraoral Dry Time of >60 Minutes with Either Open or Closed Apex

- Soaking is ineffective as all the cells might have died.
- Here the aim is to make the root resistant to resorption.
- The tooth may be soaked in citric acid for 5 minutes, then in 2% stannous fluoride for 5 minutes and then in doxycycline for 5 minutes before replanting it.
- Endodontics can be performed extraorally taking care to preserve the remaining PDL.

Following replantation: The tooth should be stabilized by acid etch composite resin splint. Rigid splinting for longer periods should be avoided to prevent post-replantation ankylosis or resorption, one week should be sufficient.

Laceration of the gingiva is sutured around the cervical area of the tooth. Endodontic treatment should be performed 1-2 weeks after reimplantation in the case of a closed apical foramen, when total pulp necrosis is anticipated as revascularization is not possible in an avulsed tooth with closed apex. When the apical foramen is wide open and reimplantation is done within a few hours after injury, endodontic treatment can be postponed to wait for possible revascularization of the pulp. Radiographs should be taken 1-2 weeks after reimplantation, because first evidence of root resorption is seen at this time.

Healing of Reimplanted Tooth[29]

The tooth that is avulsed is associated with damage to the blood vessels and the PDL. The pulp may become necrotic.

Normal or expected healing will be complete regeneration of the periodontal ligament and may take about 4 weeks. Besides healing with a normal periodontal ligament, healing of replanted permanent teeth after accidental loss may follow 3 courses:

1. Surface resorption of cementum
2. Replacement resorption
3. Inflammatory resorption.

Surface resorption of cementum: Healing occurs by repair with normal cementum deposition. It is usually seen in areas of localized damage. If the trauma is mild it results in healing with the formation of new PDL and cemental layer. Histologically the repair of the resorption lacunae occurs with uninflamed PDL and cementum like tissue. It is symptomless and cannot be visualized on radiograph.

Replacement resorption: It is characterized by continuous replacement of root surface with bone, resulting in ankylosis. It usually follows extensive large area damage involving >20% of root surface. Initial inflammation is followed by removal of the debris and exposing the cementum. Cells start repopulating. Bone precursor cells will often move across from the socket wall and populate the damaged root rather than the slowly moving PDL cells. There is formation of bone directly in contact with root- called as dentoalveolar ankylosis. Osteoclasts that are also present resorb the dentin. Osteoblasts lay down bone in the area that was previously occupied by root. This progressive effect of ankylosis on an avulsed tooth is termed replacement resorption. Radiographically the distinction between the root and surrounding bone is lost and a moth eaten appearance results. Clinically, it presents with metallic sound on percussion and infraocclusion in the developing dentition.

Inflammatory resorption: This is characterized by development of bowl shaped areas of resorption of cementum and dentin associated with inflammatory changes consisting of granulation tissue with numerous lymphocytes, plasma cells and PMNL. Normally cementum prevents toxins from infected pulp reaching the PDL through dentinal tubules. After avulsion, the cemental covering is damaged. If the pulp becomes necrotic, toxins pass through the dentinal tubules and stimulate inflammatory response in the corresponding PDL. The result is resorption of the root and bone called as inflammatory root resorption. This continues until the irritants are removed. Radiographically it is observed as progressive radiolucent areas of the root and adjacent bone. Seen as early as 2-3 weeks after avulsion. The treatment objective is to avoid or minimize effects of two complications, the attachment damage and pulpal infection by preventing drying of the tooth, elimination of toxins from the pulp and maintaining the integrity of the periodontal fibers.

> **Prosthodontic replacement of avulsed tooth that cannot be replanted**
>
> A permanent anterior tooth, lost should be replaced with an esthetic appliance, which functions in speech and mastication and prevents tipping of adjacent teeth. In the young patient, a removable temporary appliance is constructed and worn until all permanent anterior teeth have erupted, alveolar changes have decreased and pulp chambers have receded to allow preparation for fixed replacements.

Postoperative Supportive Management

- Tetanus coverage
- Analgesics and antibiotics
- Chlorhexidine mouth wash for 7-10 days
- Management of swelling—application of ice, constricts the blood and lymph vessels.

A Traumatized Tooth is kept Under Observation

- Color change–Yellow – indicates calcific degeneration
              Gray – indicates hemorrhage into dentinal tubules
- Mobility
- Periapical pathology
- Pain
- Swelling
- Parulis

Follow-up and Evaluation

Endodontic procedure if not done earlier should be initiated, at the first sign of pathosis. Calcium hydroxide can be used as temporary obturating material, until an intact periodontal ligament space is confirmed or if radiographic evidence of resorption is present. Calcium hydroxide is changed every 3 months. Ledermix can also be used.

SPLINTING OF A TRAUMATIZED TOOTH

The purpose of splinting is to stabilize the tooth in the arch in order to prevent further damage to the pulp and periodontal tissues.

The term splint has been defined by the American Association of Endodontics (AAE)[31] as a 'rigid or flexible device or compound used to support, protect or immobilize teeth that have been loosened, replanted, fractured or subjected to certain endodontic surgical procedures.

An ideal splint for splinting a traumatized tooth should be passive and semirigid and maintain physiologic tooth mobility.[32]

The tooth is immobilized by fixing it to the two adjacent teeth. It is found that, if the distance between the splinted tooth and its neighbors is increased, it results in more elastic deviation and reduced controlled immobilization. This means that the splinting effect may not be the same between spaced arches and nonspaced arches.[33]

Properties of an Ideal Splint

1. Should be quick and easy to fabricate
2. Should be atraumatic to the teeth and gingiva
3. Should be adequately stable throughout the healing period
4. Should have access to endodontic therapy if needed
5. Should be as esthetically pleasing as possible.

Different Kinds of Splints Used

1. Wire and resin splint
2. Acid etch composite resin
3. Orthodontic brackets and wire splint
4. Interdental wiring
5. Fiber splint
6. Titanium trauma splint.

Wire and resin splint (Fig. 9.21): Round wire or rectangle wire used when 3-4 teeth are to be splinted. The wire is contoured to the arch and held in place by composite resin material. Thin flexible wire of diameter 0.3-0.4 mm is used for splint and secured by light cused compolite resin. It is a semirigid splint. This splint is easy to fabricate and provides access for root canal therapy during splinting period.

The diameter of the wire used also determines the rigidity of the splint. Lesser the diameter of the wire used, more was the flexibility of the splint.[34] It may be difficult to place this splint on a tooth with smaller crowns, artificial crowns or over a large fillings.

Acid etch composite resin splint: It consists of a thick band of composite resin that extends on the labial surface of the teeth required to be stabilized and onto at least one

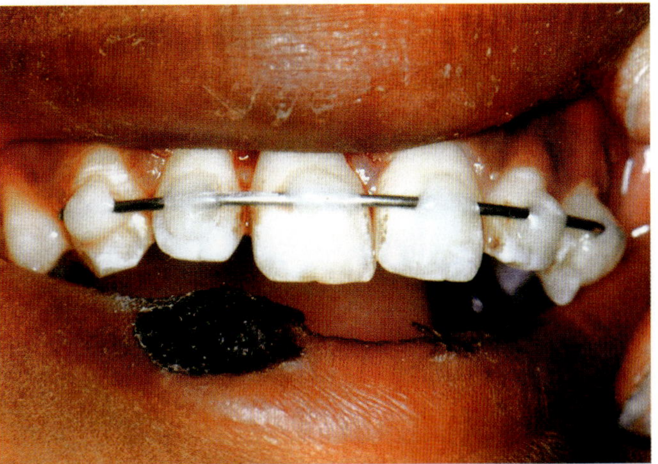

Fig. 9.21: Wire and resin splint

tooth on either side of the traumatized tooth. This splint is strong, easy to fabricate, more esthetic and provides access for root canal therapy.[35]

Orthodontic brackets and wire splint: The tooth to be splinted and the adjacent teeth on both the sides are fitted with brackets or bands. 0.3 mm soft wire is then braided from bracket to bracket to connect all the teeth.

Care should be taken to avoid orthodontic force application on the teeth.[36] But this can be advantageous if simultaneous tooth movement and tooth repositioning is needed.

Interdental wiring Essig type splint: A 15 cm length 0.020 stainless steel wire is used to ligate an injured incisor tooth to the adjacent incisor teeth and canines. The wire is placed along the labial aspect of the anterior teeth. One end rests several millimeters beyond the distal surface of the canine. The other end is passed from labial to lingual through the interproximal space between the canine and adjacent bicuspid. This end is passed around the lingual aspect of the canine, into the mesial interproximal space and emerges under the labial wire. It is then bent over the labial wire and back to the lingual aspect through the same interproximal space. This is repeated for each anterior tooth until it passes between the cuspid and the first bicuspid in the adjacent quadrant. The free ends are twisted and trimmed and turned into the interproximal embrasure.

Fiber splint (Fig. 9.22): It was introduced by Smith in 1960s and popularized by Andreasen et al in 1983.[37] The main advantage of fiber splint is that it does not require any laboratory assistance and is bonded directly onto the teeth. Fiber-reinforced composites are resin-based materials containing fibers aimed at enhancing their physical properties. The fibers commonly used are glass, ultra-high strength polyethylene fibers and Kevlar fibers.

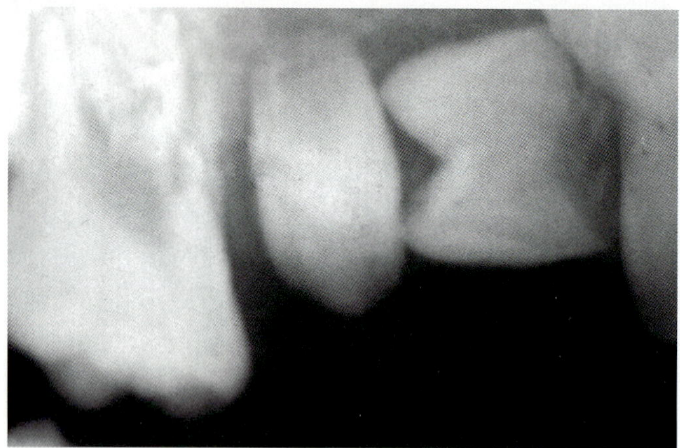

Fig. 9.22: Displacement of the developing first premolar following trauma and avulsion of the deciduous first molar

Commonly used bondable reinforced fibers in clinical practice are: Ultrahigh molecular weight polyethylene fibers-ribbond (Ribbond), Connect (Kerr), Glass Fibers-GlasSpan (GlasSpan) and fiber Splint ML(Polydentia), Fibers preimpregnated with resin Vectris (Vivadent), StickNet (StickTech) and FiberKor (Jeneric/Pentron).

Titanium trauma splint (TTS) (Fig. 9.23): It is a new device developed by von Arx et al.[38] It is made of pure titanium and is 0.2 mm thick and 2.8 mm in width (Medartis AG, Basel, Switzerland). It has a rhomboid mesh structure and can be easily adapted to the contour of the dental arch with fingers without the need of additional pliers. A thin layer of flowable composite is placed into the rhomboid opening of the splint after etching and applying the bonding agent on the tooth.

Stabilization Period

After a traumatic injury any method of stabilization is contraindicated if it involves additional force or pressure. The period of splinting is very crucial for a good prognosis. Initially, it was believed that longer the splinting period better is the healing.

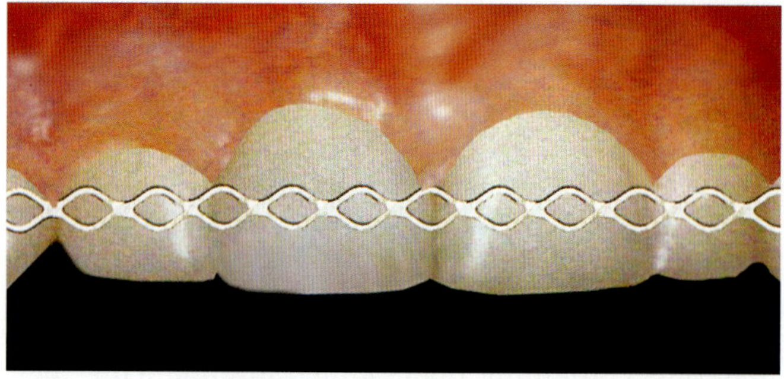

Fig. 9.23: Titanium trauma splint

Andreasen[39] has demonstrated that teeth splinted for shorter periods showed better healing than teeth that were splinted for four or six weeks. Extended splinting period may be required when there is associated injury to the marginal alveolar bone or root fractures.

The guidelines for duration of splinting for traumatic injuries is given in Figure 9.24.

REACTION OF THE PULP TO TRAUMA

Pulpal hyperemia: Even minor trauma is followed by pulpal hyperemia. Since collateral circulation is absent in the pulp hyperemic conditions may lead to infarction and pulpal necrosis. The tooth appears reddish and is often indicative of a poor prognosis.

Internal hemorrhage: Hyperemia and increased pressure may cause rupture of capillaries and the escape of RBC with subsequent breakdown and pigment formation. These may be reabsorbed before gaining access to dentinal tubules if bleeding is minute. In severe cases there is deposition of these pigments in the dentinal tubules. The change in color is evident within 2-3 weeks after injury and though is reversible, the crown may retain some amount of discoloration.

Calcific metamorphosis of dental pulp: There may be partial or complete obliteration of the pulp chamber or canal and the crown may appear yellowish opaque. Permanent tooth showing signs of calcific changes as a result of trauma should be regarded as a potential focus of infection and must be kept under observation or treated endodontically if possible.

Internal resorption: Appears as pink tooth. It is observed radiographically in the pulp chamber or canal within a few weeks or months after injury. If the progression is rapid it may cause perforation of the crown or roots within a few weeks. Such teeth should be treated endodontically as soon as diagnosed.

External root resorption: It usually results due to the damage to the periodontal structures and the pulp may not be involved—seen in severe trauma in which there has been some degree of displacement of the tooth.

Pulpal necrosis: Any type of injury especially the displacement type may cause severance of the apical vessels. This lead to loss of vascular supply to the pulp leading to autolysis and necrosis. Injured teeth with subsequent pulpal necrosis are commonly asymptomatic and the radiograph is essentially normal. The acute symptoms and clinical evidence of infection will inevitably develop at a later date. Bacteriological status of the pulp tissue of root canal of intact but traumatized teeth reveals microorganisms, including anaerobic forms

Avulsion	Root fracture	Concussion	Subluxation	Extrusion	Lateral luxation
Flexible splint for 2 weeks duration, except when the extra oral time is > 60 minutes	Stabilize the tooth with a flexible splint for 4 weeks. If the root fracture is near the cervical area of the tooth, stabilization is beneficial for a longer period of time (up to 4 months)	No treatment is needed. Monitor pulpal condition for at least 1 year	A flexible splint to stabilize the tooth for patient comfort can be used for up to 2 weeks	Reposition the tooth by gently re-inserting it into the tooth socket. Stabilize the tooth for 2 weeks using a flexible splint	Reposition the tooth with forceps to disengage it from its bony lock and gently reposition it into its original location. Stabilize the tooth for 4 weeks using a flexible splint

Fig. 9.24: The guidelines for treatment of traumatic injuries as recommended by IADT

in the pulp canal of traumatized teeth. The source of microorganisms is through gingival sulcus or blood stream or both.

Ankylosis: It is caused by injury to the periodontal membrane and subsequent inflammation which is associated with invasion by osteoclastic cells resulting in irregularly resorbed areas on the peripheral root surface. The repair may occur by fusion of alveolar bone with root surface. Radiograph shows an interruption in the periodontal membrane of the ankylosed tooth and clinically appears submerged. Ankylosed anterior primary tooth must be removed to allow eruption of the permanent tooth.

> **Risk of pulp necrosis**
>
> Concussion—2% chances of necrosis and pulp obliteration
> Subluxation—6-47% chances of pulp necrosis, 10-26% of canal obliteration, 4% of root resorption
> Extrusion—64% chances of pulp necrosis
> Lateral luxation—77% chances of pulp necrosis
> Intrusive luxation—100% chances of pulp necrosis and external root resorption.

MANAGEMENT OF DISCOLORED TEETH

Treatment options include:
1. Bleaching
2. Veneering
3. Lamination.

Only bleaching is discussed in this chapter. Other methods are discussed in Chapter 23.

Bleaching of Vital Teeth

Procedure

1. Prophylaxis with a rubber cup and unfluoridated pumice paste.
2. Lubricate the gingival tissue with petroleum jelly or topical anesthetic to prevent any tissue burning with the bleaching agent.
3. Isolate the teeth with an extra heavy rubber dam.
4. Saturate the cotton pellet with superoxol (30% hydrogen peroxide). Place the large cotton pellet on the tooth to be bleached.
5. Set the rheostat of heat source at 135°F: Apply heat to the moist pellet and ask the patient to raise the hand when the tooth begins to feel warm, then stop applying heat.
6. Repeat the procedure for each tooth. Treat each tooth on a rotating basis for 5 minutes at a time. Four or five 30 minutes appointments are usually required to complete the procedure.
7. Remove the dam and check to determine whether any of the bleaching material has leaked through. A whitish appearing gingival tissue is an indication that leakage has occurred.

Bleaching of Nonvital Teeth

The primary indication for nonvital bleaching is to lighten the teeth that have undergone discoloration after root canal therapy. Discoloration in a nonvital teeth is due to the disintegration of the by products of blood namely the hemosiderin and hematoidin from the pulp, or due to the restorative material left in the pulp chamber.

Nonvital bleachings are of two types, the in-office thermocatalytic and the walking bleach. Walking bleach is preferred due to increased risk of cervical resorption associated with in-office bleach which is due to the application of heat.

In-office Bleaching Technique

Thirty-five percent hydrogen peroxide is placed into the debrided and sealed pulp chamber and the oxidation process is accelerated by placement of a heated instrument into the pulp chamber. Recent modification is the use of pastes and gels that do not require heat application.

Walking Bleach

Following root canal obturation, the gutta percha is sealed with polycarboxylate cement. A mixture of sodium perborate and 30% hydrogen peroxide (superoxol) is placed in the pulp chamber and a temporary restoration is placed over the mixture. 7 days later the tooth is examined for color change. If required second or third procedure may be required. It is advisable to over bleach by one or two shades as there is tendency for the color to regress.

> The patient and the parent should be priorly informed that there may be little or no improvement in the color of the teeth following bleaching or that within 6 months the discoloration may begin to reappear.

EFFECTS OF TRAUMA ON DEVELOPMENT OF SUCCEDANEOUS TEETH

The roots of the deciduous incisor teeth lie just labial to the tooth germs of the permanent incisor teeth, which makes them susceptible to the pathological process as a result of trauma or the sequelae of trauma to deciduous teeth. The prevalence of disturbances to the permanent teeth as a result of trauma to the primary teeth ranges from 13-57%, and is dependent on the type and severity of the trauma, stage of permanent tooth development and the mode of treatment of the injury itself.[40-42]

- *White or yellow brown discoloration of enamel:* Usually seen on the labial surface of the tooth. There is usually no clinically detected defects in the enamel.

These are common lesions accounting for 23% of the developmental disturbances. Yellow discoloration is due to the result of breakdown products of hemoglobin from bleeding in the area at the time of injury.

- *White or yellow brown discoloration of enamel and horizontal enamel hypoplasia:* Enamel defects here is similar to the discoloration mentioned in the previous defect. In addition a narrow horizontal indentation encircles the crown cervical to the discolored area. Usually seen when the injury occurs at about 2 years of age. It accounts for about 12% of the defects and is usually associated with avulsion or intrusion of the primary tooth. The defect is probably due to localized arrest of the enamel matrix formation that occurs due to injury to ameloblasts by slight axial displacement of the tooth within its crypt.

- *Change in the position of the developing tooth bud (Fig. 9.25):* The change in tooth bud position can be in a horizontal or a vertical direction.

- *Crown dilaceration:* Occurred in 25% of the cases. The crown is usually displaced in a palatal direction for the maxillary teeth and in the opposite direction for the mandibular teeth. This injury is usually associated with intrusion and avulsion of the deciduous tooth.

- *Odontome like malformation:* It appears as conglomerate hard tissue having the morphology of a complex odontome, seen in 6% of the cases. It is usually the result of an intrusion or avulsion and occurs when one fourth or less of the crown has been formed.

- *Root duplication:* It is very rare and is due to division of the root into a mesial and distal portion, when the injury occurs at 2 years or less at the time when the crown is half or less developed.

- *Vestibular root angulation:* It consists of marked labial curvature of the root portion of the tooth. This injury occurs at 2-5 years of age and is usually the result of intrusion or avulsion.

- *Lateral root angulation or dilaceration:* It appears as a mesial or distal bending, confined to the root portion of the affected tooth. This lesion is usually the result of an avulsion.

- *Partial or complete arrest of root formation:* In spite of cessation of development, the teeth usually erupt into normal position.

- *Sequestration of the entire tooth germ:* It is an extremely rare injury.

- *Eruption disturbances:* Permanent successors can be impacted, delayed or accelerated in their eruption as a result of injuries sustained to deciduous teeth.

PREVENTION OF TRAUMA DURING CONTACT SPORTS

- Orthodontic correction of the trauma prone profile
- Use of face guards or mouth protectors.

Face and Mouth Guards[43]

Face guards are cage like protection to the entire face, attached to the helmet. It gives a total protection against facial and dental injuries.

Mouth guards or protectors are intraoral device used for protecting the teeth during contact sports to protect. They were originally made of clear, transparent material. Most of the football associations make it mandatory, that a colored mouth guards be used for easy detection to note whether players are wearing them or not and for easy retrieval if lost. Newer styles are composed of thermoplastics boiled in water and then inserted into the mouth and are custom fit.

Ideal Requirement of a Mouth Protector

1. Should be of adequate thickness to reduce impact of trauma on the tooth.
2. It should have good fit and should not fall off from the mouth during the activity nor be very tight.
3. Should not interfere with speech and breathing.
4. Material used must be nonallergic.

Classification of Mouth Protectors

1. Type 1 – Stock types
2. Type 2 – Mouth formed
3. Type 3 – Custom fabricated.

Type 1: *Stock types:* They are preformed mouth protectors and is inexpensive. They have poor retention and is held together by clenching the teeth.

Type 2: *Mouth formed:* They are of two types, thermoplastic and shell lined mouth guard. The thermoplastic type is boiled and adapted inside the mouth by biting close the teeth. In case of shell lined mouth guard, a liner is added at the borders of the appliance to improve its fit and allowed to harden inside the mouth. The liner used is ethylmethacrylate. This liner is changed before wearing to improve the fit of the device. The main disadvantage is the bitter taste of the fresh liner and extra work and time needed before each game.

Type 3: Custom fabricated: It is fabricated on the individual's cast using material like poly vinly acetate-Polyethylene. It exhibits the best fit and comfort.

Instructions to the Patient

1. Clean the mouth guard by washing it with soap and cold water before and after use.
2. Preferably dip the mouth guard in mouthwash before storing or usage.
3. Keep it securely in a box with ventilation holes so that the temperature inside the box should not increase.
4. Do not place mouth guards out side in the sun or near a oven or a fire place.
5. Do not allow others to wear your mouth guard.

REFERENCES

1. Flores MT. Traumatic injuries in the primary dentition. Dental Traumatol 2002;18(6):287-98.
2. Ellis RG. The classification and treatment of injuries to the teeth of children. 5th edn. Chicago: Year Book Medical Publishers 1970;56-199.
3. Ellis RG, Davey KW. The classification and treatment of injuries to the teeth of children 5th ed. Year Book Publishers, Chicago 1970.
4. Hargreaves JA, Craig JW. The management of traumatized anterior teeth of children, Livingstone, Edinburgh 1970.
5. Heithersay GS, Moule AJ. Anterior subgingival fractures: A review of treatment alternatives. Aus Dent J 1982;27:368-76.
6. World Health Organization. Application of the international classification of diseases to dentistry and stomatology, ICD-DA, 2nd Ed. WHO, Geneve, 1978.
7. Application of the international classification of diseases and stomatology, IDC-DA, 3ed. Geneva WHO 1992.
8. Josell SD, Abrams RG. Managing common dental problems and emergencies. Pediatr Clin North Am 1991;38:1325-42.
9. Hovland EJ, Gutmann JL, Dumsha TC. Traumatic injuries to teeth, DCNA 1995;39(1).
10. Andreasen JO, Andreasen FM, Andersson L. Textbook and color atlas of traumatic injuries to the teeth, 4th Ed. Blackwell Munksgaard 2007.
11. Forsberg CM, Tedestam G. Etiology and predisposing factors related to traumatic injuries to permanent teeth. Swed Dent J 1993;17:183-90.
12. O' Mullane DM. Some factors predisposing to injuries of permanent incisors in school children. Br Dent J 1973;134:328-32.
13. Jarvinen S. Incisal overjet and traumatic injuries to upper permanent incisors. A retrospective study. Acta Odontol Scand 1978;36:359-62.
14. Hallet GEM. Problems of common interest to the paedodontist and orthodontist with special reference to traumatized incisor cases. Eur Orthod Soc Trans 1953;29:266-77.
15. Croll TP, Brooks EB, Schut L, et al. Rapid neurologic assessment and initial management for the patient with traumatic dental injuries. J Am Dent Assoc 1980;100:530-34.

16. Andreasen FM, Andreasen JO. Diagnosis of luxation injuries: The importance of standardized clinical, radiographic and photographic techniques in clinical investigations. Endod Dent Traumatol 1985;1:160-9.

17. Wilson CFG. Management of trauma to primary and developing teeth. DCNA 1995;39:133-67.

18. Pileggi R, Dumsha T, Myslinski N. Reliability of electrical pulp testing after traumatic injuries. J Endod 1994;20:202.

19. Rauschenberger CR, Hovland EJ. Clinical management of crown fractures DCNA 1995;39(1):25-51.

20. Forsberg CM, Tedestarn G. Traumatic injuries to teeth in Swedish children living in an urban area. Swed Dent J 1990;14:115-22.

21. Galea H. An investigation of dental injuries treated in an acute care general hospital. J Am Dent Assoc 1984;109:434-8.

22. Andreasen FM, Andreasen JO. In Textbook and Color Atlas of Traumatic Injuries to the Teeth. 4th ed. Ames Iowa:Blackwell Munksgaard 2007;280-313.

23. Cox CF. Microleakage related to restorative procedures. Proc Finn Dent Soc 1992;88:83-93.

24. Cvek M. A clinical report on partial pulpotomy and capping with calcium hydroxide in permanent incisors with complicated root fractures. J Endod 1978;4:232-7.

25. Andreasen FM, Andreasen JO, Bayer T. Prognosis of root-fractured permanent incisors-prediction of healing modalities. Endod Dent Traumatol 1989;5:11-22.

26. Andreasen FM, Andreasen JO, Cvek M. Root fractures. In. Andreasen FM, Andersson L. Textbook and Color Atlas of Traumatic Injuries to the Teeth. 4th ed. Ames Iowa:Blackwell Munksgaard 2007.

27. Kindelan S, Day P, Kindelan J, Spencer J, Duggal M. Dental trauma: An overview of its influence on the management of orthodontic treatment. Part 1. J Orthod 2008;35(2):68-78.

28. Malmgren O, Malmgren B. Orthodontic management of the traumatized dentition. In: Andreasen J, Andreasen F, Andersson L. Textbook and Color Atlas of Traumatic Injuries to the Teeth. 4th ed. Ames Iowa: Blackwell Munksgaard 2007;669-716.

29. Andreasen JO, Andreasen FM, Avulsions. In Textbook and Color Atlas of Traumatic Injuries to the Teeth. 4th ed. Ames Iowa: Blackwell Munksgaard 2007;444-88.

30. Hiltz J, Trope M. Vitalilty of human lip fibroblasts in milk. Hanks balanced salt solution and Viaspan Storage media. Endod Dent Traumatol 1991;7:69-72.

31. American Association of Endodontists. An annotated glossary of terms used in endodontics 7th Edn. Chicago: American Association of Endodontists 15, 2003.

32. Rao A, Malhotra N. Splinting–When and How Dental Update 35, 2011.

33. Ebeleseder KA, Glockner K, Pertl C, Stadtler R. Splints made of wire and composite: an investigation of lateral tooth mobility *in vivo*. Endod Dent Traumatol 1995;11: 288-93.

34. Alexander PC. Replantation of teeth. Oral Surg 1956;9:110-14.

35. Oikarinen K. Tooth splinting: a review of the literature and consideration of the versatility of a wire-composite splint. Dental Traumatology 1990;6:237-50.

36. Prevost J, Louis JP, Vadot J, Granjon Y. A study of forces originating from orthodontic appliances for splinting of teeth. Endodontics and Dental Traumatology 1994;10:179-84.

37. Andersson L, Friskopp J, Blomlöf L. Fiber-glass splinting of traumatized teeth. J Dent Child 1983;38:21-4.

38. Adatia A, Kenny DJ. Titanium Trauma Splint: An Alternative Splinting Product. JCDA 2006;72:721-3.

39. Andreasen JO. Periodontal healing after replantation of traumatically avulsed human teeth. Assessment by mobility testing and radiography. Acta Odontol Scand 1975;35:325-35.

40. Andreasen JO, Flores MT. Injuries to developing teeth. In. Textbook and Color Atlas of Traumatic Injuries to the Teeth. 4th ed. Ames Iowa: Blackwell Munksgaard 2007;542-76.

41. Diab M, ElBadrawy HE. Intrusion injuries of primary incisors. Part III: Effects on the permanent successors. Quintessence Int 2000;31:377-84.

42. Odersjö ML, Koch G. Developmental disturbances in permanent successors after intrusion to maxillary primary teeth. Eur J Paediatric Dent 2001;4:165-72.

43. Sigurdsson A. Prevention of dental and oral injuries. In. Textbook and Color Atlas of Traumatic Injuries to the Teeth. 4th ed. Ames., Iowa: Blackwell Munksgaard 2007;814-41.

FURTHER READING

1. Ballesio I, Marchetti E, Mummolo S, Marzo G. Radiographic appearance of apical closure in apexification: Follow-up after 7-13 years. Eur J Paediatr Dent 2006;7(1):29-34.

2. Barrett EJ, Kenny DJ, Tenenbaum HC, Sigal MJ, Johnston DH. Replantation of permanent incisors in children using Emdogain Dent Traumatol 2005;21(5):269-75.

3. Bramante CM, Menezes R, Moraes IG, Bernardinelli N, Garcia RB, Letra A. Use of MTA and intracanal post-reinforcement in a horizontally fractured tooth: A case report. Dent Traumatol 2006;22(5):275-8.

4. Brin I, Ben-Bassat Y, Heling I, Brezniak N. Profile of an orthodontic patient at risk of dental trauma. Endod Dent Traumatol 2000;16(3):111-5.

5. Burden DJ. An investigation of the association between overjet size, lip coverage, and traumatic injury to maxillary incisors. Eur J Orthod 1995;17(6):513-7.

6. Celenk S, Ayna BE, Ayna E, Bolgul BS, Atakul F. Multiple root fracture: A case report. Gen Dent 2006;54(2):121-2.

7. Chang HH, Wang YL, Chen HJ, Huang GF, Guo MK. Root fracture of immature permanent incisors—a case report. Dent Traumatol 2006;22(4):218-20.

8. Chien MM, Setzer S, Cleaton-Jones P. How does zinc oxide-eugenol compare to ferric sulphate as a pulpotomy material? SADJ 2001;56(3):130-5.

9. Choy MM. Children, sports injuries and mouthguards. Hawaii Dent J 2006;37(5):11-3.

10. Cornwell H. Dental trauma due to sport in the pediatric patient. J Calif Dent Assoc 2005;33(6):457-61. Review.
11. El-Meligy OA, Avery DR. Comparison of apexification with mineral trioxide aggregate and calcium hydroxide. Pediatr Dent 2006;28(3):248-53.
12. El-Meligy OA, Avery DR. Comparison of mineral trioxide aggregate and calcium hydroxide as pulpotomy agents in young permanent teeth (apexogenesis). Pediatr Dent 2006;28(5):399-404.
13. Gesi A, Hakeberg M, Warfvinge J, Bergenholtz G. Incidence of periapical lesions and clinical symptoms after pulpectomy—a clinical and radiographic evaluation of 1-versus 2-session treatment. Oral Surg Oral Med Oral Pathol Oral Radiol Endod 2006;101(3):379-88.
14. Guelmann M, Fair J, Bimstein E. Permanent versus temporary restorations after emergency pulpotomies in primary molars. Pediatr Dent 2005;27(6):478-81.
15. Jackson NG, Waterhouse PJ, Maguire A. Factors affecting treatment outcomes following complicated crown fractures managed in primary and secondary care. Dent Traumatol 2006;22(4):179-85.
16. Maki K, Nishioka T, Seo R, Kimura M. Management of a root fracture in an immature permanent tooth. J Clin Pediatr Dent 2005;30(2):127-30.
17. Parirokh M, Kakoei S. Vital pulp therapy of mandibular incisors: A case report with 11 years follow-up. Aust Endod J 2006;32(2):75-8.
18. Pasini S, Bardellini E, Casula I, Flocchini P, Majorana A. Effectiveness of oral hygiene protocol in patients with post-traumatic splinting. Eur J Paediatr Dent 2006; 7(1):35-8.
19. Pinto AS, de Araujo FB, Franzon R, Figueiredo MC, Henz S, Garcia-Godoy F, Maltz M. Clinical and microbiological effect of calcium hydroxide protection in indirect pulp capping in primary teeth. Am J Dent 2006;19(6):382-6.
20. Prakash R, Vishnu C, Suma B, Velmurugan N, Kandaswamy D. Endodontic management of taurodontic teeth. Indian J Dent Res 2005;16(4):177-81.
21. Primosch RE, Ahmadi A, Setzer B, Guelmann M. A retrospective assessment of zinc oxide-eugenol pulpectomies in vital maxillary primary incisors successfully restored with composite resin crowns. Pediatr Dent 2005;27(6):470-7.
22. Raslan N, Wetzel WE. Exposed human pulp caused by trauma and/or caries in primary dentition: A histological evaluation. Dent Traumatol 2006;22(3):145-53.
23. Silva GA, Lanza LD, Lopes-Junior N, Moreira A, Alves JB. Direct pulp capping with a dentin bonding system in human teeth: A clinical and histological evaluation. Oper Dent 2006;31(3):297-307.
24. Suei Y, Mallick PC, Nagasaki T, Taguchi A, Fujita M, Tanimoto K: Radiographic evaluation of the fate of developing tooth buds on the fracture line of mandibular fractures. J Oral Maxillofac Surg 2006;64(1):94-9.
25. Tamarut T. Kovacevic M, Glavicic S. Influence of the length of instrumentation and canal obturation on the success of endodontic therapy. A 10 years clinical follow-up. Am J Dent 2006;19(4):211-6.
26. Villa P, Fernandez R. Apexification of a replanted tooth using mineral trioxide aggregate. Dent Traumatol 2005;21(5):306-8.

QUESTIONS

1. Explain classification of trauma to anterior teeth.
2. Explain Ellis and Davey classification of trauma to anterior teeth.
3. Write in detail WHO classification for traumatic injuries to anterior teeth.
4. Enumerate the causes of trauma and explain the predisposing factors.
5. Explain in detail the case history and examination procedures following trauma.
6. Write in detail the management of trauma to primary teeth.
7. What is Craze or infraction?
8. Explain the importance of sealing dentinal tubules following trauma.
9. What is reattachment?
10. What are the treatment modalities of fracture involving crown and root?
11. What is the difference between concussion, subluxation and lateral luxation?
12. Describe the immediate measures in the management of avulsed tooth.
13. Enumerate the types of healing following reimplantation of an avulsed tooth.
14. What are the different types of splints used for stabilizing a traumatized tooth?
15. Write the effects of trauma to the primary teeth on development of succedaneous teeth.
16. What are mouth guards? Explain the types.

Child Abuse and Management

INTRODUCTION

Child abuse and neglect is an international problem having victims of all ages, races, religions and socio-economic background. Formerly called battered child syndrome, child abuse and neglect have been recently described as non-accidental injury (NAI).

DEFINITION

Child abuse and neglect (CAN) is defined "as any interaction or lack of interaction between a care giver and a child resulting in nonaccidental harm to the child's physical or developmental state."

Battery is a term often associated with abuse, defined as an "unpriviledged touching of another person's body."

Henry Kempe in 1962[1] first reported the term "battered child syndrome." According to him, a child exhibiting the following features should be included under this syndrome.
1. Evidence of fracture of long bones
2. Subdural hematoma
3. Failure to thrive
4. Soft tissue swelling or skin bruising.

TYPES OF ABUSE AND NEGLECT[1-3]

1. Physical abuse
2. Sexual abuse
3. Neglect
4. Emotional abuse and neglect
5. Intentional poisoning/drugging
6. Munchausen's syndrome by proxy.

Physical Abuse

- It forms 60% of the child abuse related fatalities.
- These injuries are non-accidental and are inflicted to the body of the child, which may result in severe injury or even death.
- These type of injuries may be inflicted by the parents, relatives or baby sitters.
- Incidence of physical abuse is more in families of low socioeconomic status.
- Abusers are most of the time unhappy, angry adults under stress. They injure their children in anger for some misbehavior to relieve their frustration.
- The injuries sustained may vary from mild such as few bruises, scratches, etc. to severe ones such as burns, CNS injury, abdominal injury, multiple fractures or other life-threatening injuries.

Evidence for suspecting physical abuse

1. Injury unusual for a specific age group (e.g. fracture in an infant)

Contd...

Contd...

> 2. History of previous/recurrent injury
> 3. Unexplained injury
> 4. Bruising in unusual areas with bruising patterns (buckle marks, etc.)

Sexual Abuse

The national center on child abuse and neglect defines sexual abuse "to include contacts or interactions between a child and an adult."

Evidence for suspecting sexual abuse are:

A. Report by the patient or gaurdian
B. Early and exaggerated awareness by the patient about sex.
C. Physical trauma, if present, tearing, bruising or specific infection of the mouth, anus or genitals
D. Pregnancy.

Neglect

It consists of failure to provide the basic necessities such as adequate food, shelter, clothing and also health care needs. Some parents may not take care of their children and thus the child may be malnourished and underweighed. Common reason for such behavior is that the mother does not like or want the baby. Other reasons may include depressed mother, recent separation of the parents, parent's illness, poverty, ignorance, unusual stress on the family, etc.

Physically neglected children tend to exhibit at least several of these characteristics.

A. Dirty clothing and skin with foul smell, lice and unkempt appearance.
B. Undernourished.
C. Rampant caries, abscess, periodontal lesions, etc.
D. Uncared wounds.
E. Constant sleepiness or hunger.
F. Failure maintain appointments.

Health Care Neglect

Parents ignore or do not provide the necessary medical or dental treatment to the child even until the condition proceeds to a serious or irreversible extent. According to AAPD guidelines (2010) Dental neglect is willful failure of parent or guardian to seek and follow through with treatment necessary to ensure a level of oral heath essential for adequate function and freedom from pain and infection.[4]

Educational Neglect

Parents do not educate their children or are not bothered about the chronic absenteeism of the child from school.

They may intentionally keep the child at home and do not allow him or her to attend school.

Emotional Abuse

The child is emotionally attacked by parents, teachers or any caretakers. The child is harassed verbally and made to feel low either by direct abuse or by ridiculing the child in front of others. Severe forms may take the form of locking the child in a dark room.

Intentional Poisoning/Drugging

It is an uncommon lethal type of child abuse, involving administration of a harmful drug that is not intended to be used by the child. Parents who poison their children may have severe marital problems or may be drug abusers.

Munchausen's Syndrome by Proxy

It is also called as 'pediatric condition falsification.' Parents fabricate or induce illness and subject the child to unnecessary medical investigation, hospital admissions and treatment. Children are usually less than 6 years of age and too young to understand the deception. Parents may administer laxatives and complain to the doctors that their child is suffering from diarrhea.

INJURIES ASSOCIATED WITH ABUSE[5-7]

Orofacial Injuries (Figs 10.1 to 10.3)

- Parents hit the child on the mouth or lip to silence a crying child leading to injuries on the lip or adjoining area.

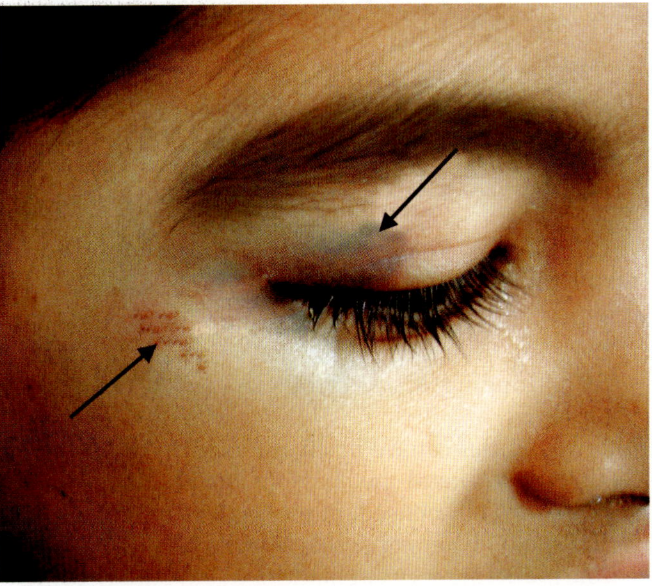

Fig. 10.1: Injury to the left eye caused due to the child being pushed onto the wall

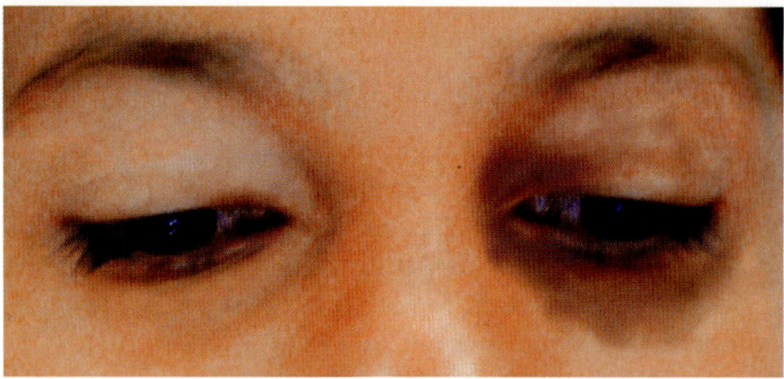

Fig. 10.2: Injury to the right eye by a blunt device

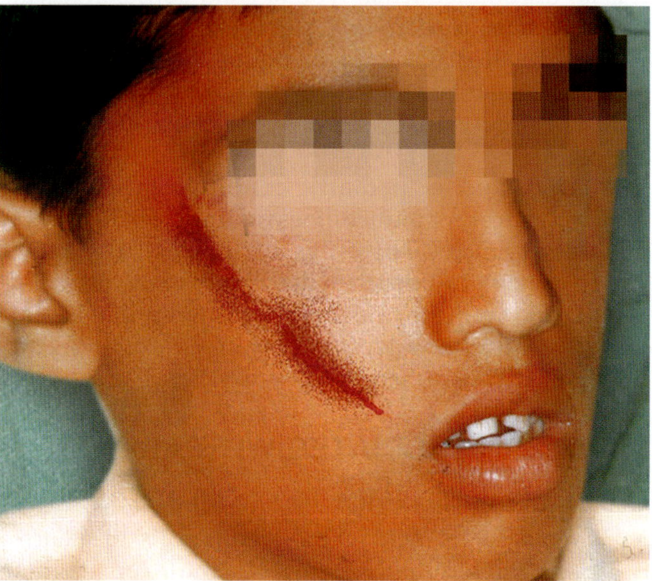

Fig. 10.3: Scratch injury on the cheek due to hitting the child's face with a pen

- Hitting hard on the face over the eyes can lead to subcutaneous hemorrhage around the eyes or any kind of injury depending on the device used to hit.
- Slapping leads to bruises on cheek, which— due to slap—where 2 or 3 parallel lines marking the finger marks may be seen.

Injury to Skin and Subcutaneous Tissues

- Marks seen on the skin are commonly due to holding the child's hand tightly or due to rope or cloth used for restraining. Marks can also be seen when hit with an object.
- Burn injuries caused by cigarette buds or hot objects are common and the shape of the injury resembles that of the object used. Burn injuries due to hot water produces blisters or scalds over the area of injury.
- Bite marks are seen as elliptic or ovoid pattern formed by the upper and lower teeth on the skin.

Head Injuries

- Such injuries are seen in cases of severe cases of abuse.
- Injuries include subdural hematoma, subarachnoid hemorrhage, etc.

Bone Injuries

- Fractures are also associated with severe cases of abuse.
- Fractures of the ribs, upper and lower limb is seen.

Abdominal Injuries

- Caused by punch and kicks that compress the organs against the spinal column and forms the second most common cause of death in cases of abuse.
- Bruises or ruptured viscera—may result in massive hemorrhage—shock and death.

CHARACTERISTICS OF AN ABUSED CHILD[8,9]

The child who has undergone abuse is emotionally hurt. Victims are at higher risk of becoming violent adult offenders. They often experience more social problems and perform less well in school. Survivors of sexual abuse tend to harbor feelings of low self-esteem and extreme depression and often experience a higher than normal incidence of substance abuse and eating disorders. The child often has characteristics that make him/her provocative, such as negativism or a difficult temperament. Some of the more offensive misbehaviors are intractable crying, wetting, soiling and spilling.

The abuser describes the abused child as difficult to control, bad or selfish. Children are most of the time passive, afraid and presents with repeated skin or other injuries.

Features of Abused Child

1. Unduly afraid or passive
2. Evidence of prolonged confinement
3. Evidence of repeated skin or other injuries
4. Inappropriate treatment of injuries by parents.
5. Under nourished child
6. Inappropriate dressing
7. May be aggressive, demanding or hyperactive or cranky, irritable or cries easily.

Abuser

Child abuse occurs in all cultural, occupational, socio-economic and ethnic groups. A proportionately higher incidence of abuse is reported in minority and low income family.

Father, mother or caretaker may be the abusers. The parents may have the following characteristics indicative of abusive behavior.

1. Poor self esteem and coping skills.
2. Violent tempers or outbursts.
3. Unrealistic expectation of child's behavior.
4. Inappropriate response to the seriousness of the child's condition.
5. Over critical behavior toward the child.
6. Avoidance of looking at or touching the child.
7. Reluctance to give the history of the accident or giving an unrealistic explanation.
8. Request for treatment long after injury has occurred.
9. Appearance of confusion or embarrassment when discussing the child's trauma.
10. Immature, depressed or demanding.

ROLE OF A DENTAL SURGEON[10]

Dental surgeons are in a unique position of seeing patients that are victims of abuse and neglect. More than 50% of the abuse occurs to the head and facial area.

Often the first medical professional to see these children routinely is a dentist. The ability to recognize the signs and symptoms when such an incident presents itself can make a difference in the child's physical, emotional and social well-being and may even save a child's life.

A dental surgeon has 3 main responsibilities towards abused children.

1. Detection
2. Reporting
3. Prevention.

Numerous dentists fail to report suspected abuse and neglect, which may be due to:

A. Lack of knowledge to identify
B. Do not know where to report such cases
C. Thinking "it is not our responsibility."

The usual controversy which exists among dental surgeons is whether they should inform the parents or caretakers that they have reported the case. The Law Enforcement Agencies stress that the parent or caretaker should not be told because of their concern for the protection of the child. If the alleged perpetrator is a member of the family, talking to the family may cause the child to suffer additional abuse or the family may move and the abuse will no doubt continue.

Once a dental surgeon is suspicious that an injury or lesion is of non-accidental origin, the findings must be collected permanently and accurately documented and presented in the court. The records must be in the form of photographs, written documents, radiographs and diagnostic study casts.

Examination

It includes obtaining a general impression as to the child's overall cleanliness, size and stature, interactions with the parent or caretaker and gait. A complete and thorough examination of the craniofacial area is essential, since these exposed areas are often involved in physical abuse.

Careful examination of the cranium and scalp can reveal battering lesions. Common finding include traumatic alopecia. Others being presence of lice, abnormalities of the ear, periorbital ecchymosis, scleral hemorrhage, ptosis, deviated gaze or unequal pupils, blood clots of the nose or presence of DNS (Deviated Nasal Septum).

Diagnosis

The evidence of physical abuse is generally easily recognized. There are types and sites of injury so common in child abuse that merely finding them is diagnostic. For example A child learning to walk may sustain injuries to shin, elbow, hands and forehead. But injuries to buttocks, lower back, genitals, inner thighs, etc. raise serious questions of non-accidental trauma. In addition, injuries to the cheeks, ears, upper lip, frenum, chest or abdomen should always be questioned.

The first step in diagnosis is taking a good history. A child's statement that some one caused an injury is usually accurate. If one parent accuses the other of inflicting the trauma on the child, even this can be taken as eyewitness account unless the child is involved in custody battle. A partial confession such as admitting to only part of or one of the multiple injuries, can be just as diagnostic as a complete confession.

It is highly suspicious when a parent is unaware or he is unable to explain an obvious injury, because most nonabusive parent know precisely how or when an injury occurred and are willing to discuss it.

REFERENCES

1. Kempe CH, et al. The battered child syndrome. JAMA 1962;181:17-24.
2. Kempe C, Helfer R. Helping the battered child and his family. Philadelphia. JB Lippincott 1972.
3. Hibbard RA, Sanders BJ. Child Abuse and Neglect. In. Mc Donald and Avery's Dentistry for the Child and Adolescent, 9th Ed Elsevier Mosby, 2011.
4. American Academy of Pediatric Dentistry. Definition of Dental Neglect. http://www.aapd.org/media/Policies_ Guidelines/D_DentalNeglect.

5. Chadwick DL, Merten DF, Reece RM. Thoracic and abdominal injuries associated with child abuse. In Child Abuse: Medical Diagnosis and Management, Lea and Febiger Philadelphia 1994.

6. Kellogg N. The Committee on Child Abuse and Neglect, Oral and Dental Aspects of Child Abuse and Neglect Pediatrics 2005;116(6):1565-8.

7. Needleman HL. Orofacial trauma in child abuse: Types, prevalence, management, and the dental profession's involvement. Pediatric Dentistry: Nol. 8 Special Issue 1, 1986.

8. Herbert CP. Family violence and family physicians. Can Fam Physician 1991;37:385-90.

9. Health Services Directorate, Health Canada. The family violence handbook for the dental community. Ottawa (ON): National Clearinghouse on Family Violence; 1994.

10. Tsang A, Sweet D, Detecting Child Abuse and Neglect—Are Dentists Doing Enough? Journal of the Canadian Dental Association 1999;65(7):387-91.

FURTHER READING

1. American Academy of Pediatric Dentistry. Clinical guideline on oral and dental aspects of child abuse and neglect. Pediatr Dent 2004;26(7):63-6.

2. American Academy of Pediatrics Committee on Child Abuse and Neglect; American Academy of Pediatric Dentistry Council on Clinical Affairs. Guideline on oral and dental aspects of child abuse and neglect. Pediatr Dent 2005-2006;27.

3. Appel JK, Kim-Appel D. Child maltreatment and domestic violence: Human services issues. J Health Hum Serv Adm 2006;29(2):228-44.

4. Becker PT. Child abuse and neglect: Attachment, development and intervention. J Adv Nur 2007;57(4): 460.

5. Chartier M, Walker J, Naimark B. Childhood Abuse, Adult Health, and Health Care Utilization: Results from a Representative Community Sample. Am J Epidemiol 2007;19.

6. Favaro A, Ferrara S, Santonastaso P. Self-injurious behavior in a community sample of young women: Relationship with childhood abuse and other types of self-damaging behaviors. J Clin Psychiatry 2007;68(1): 122-31.

7. Laraque D, DeMattia A, Low C. Forensic child abuse evaluation: A review. Mt Sinai J Med 2006;73(8):1138-47. Review.

8. McDonald KC. Child abuse: Approach and management. Am Fam Physician 2007;15;75(2):221-8. Review.

9. van der Velden A, Spiessens M, Willems G. Bite mark analysis and comparison using image perception technology. J Forensic Odontostomatol 2006;24(1):14-7.

10. Vandeven AM, Newton AW. Update on child physical abuse, sexual abuse, and prevention. Curr Opin Pediatr 2006;18(2):201-5.

QUESTIONS

1. Define child abuse and neglect.
2. What is 'battered child syndrome'?
3. Enumerate the types of abuse and neglect.
4. What are the characteristics of physical abuse?
5. Describe the injuries associated with abuse.
6. Role of dental surgeon in identification child abuse.

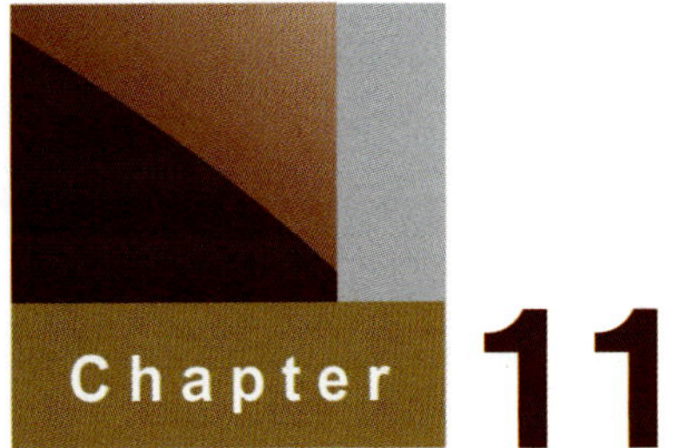

Chapter 11

Dental Management of Children with Special Health Care Needs

INTRODUCTION

Children with special health care needs are those who need extra care due to the disability they have. The disability may be in the form of physical, medical or intellectual alterations. The term 'handicapped child' was used initially which was later modified to as 'children with special health care needs.'

The American Academy of Pediatric Dentistry[1] defines individuals with special health care needs (SHCN) as those with "any physical, developmental, mental, sensory, behavioral, cognitive or emotional impairment or limiting condition that requires medical management, health care intervention and/or use of specialized services or programs."

WHO[2] defines a handicapped individual as "One who, over an appreciable time, is prevented by physical or mental condition from full participation in the normal activities of his age group, including those of a social, recreational, educational, and vocational nature."

Contd...

Contd...

American Public Health Association[3] defines handicapped child as:

"A child who cannot within limits play, learn, work or do things other children of his age can do; he is hindered in achieving his full physical, mental and social potentialities."

DEFINITIONS[4,5]

Defect: "Some imperfection or disorder of the body, intellect or personality."

Disability: The term disability has been defined as any impairment that restricts or limits daily activity in some manner. Disability is the functional limitation within the individual, caused by physical, mental, or sensory impairments and can be developmental in origin or acquired "Defect which does result in some malfunctioning but which does not necessarily affect the individual's normal life."

Handicap: Handicap is the loss or limitation of opportunities to take part in the normal life of the community on an equal level with others due to physical and social barriers. It is a disability which, for a substantial period or permanently, retards, distorts or otherwise adversely affects growth, development or adjustment to life."

> The comprehensive care required by these persons is time consuming and many patients as well as their families are uncooperative. The dentist, who extends his responsibility beyond the treatment of the 'chief complaint' however, will find great rewards in helping the disabled patient and his family adjust to and deal effectively with a long-term disability.

CLASSIFICATION

I. Nowak[6] has divided handicapping conditions into 9 categories:
   1. Physical
      a. Cerebral palsy
   2. Mental retardation
   3. Congenital defects
      a. Congenital cardiac disease
      b. Cleft lip and palate
      c. Down's syndrome
   4. Metabolic and systemic disorders
      a. Renal diseases and liver disease
      b. Diabetes mellitus
      c. Hypo/hyperpituitarism
      d. Hypo/hyperthyroidism
      e. Hypo/hyperparathyroidism
      f. Respiratory disorders
      g. Immunological disorders
   5. Convulsive disorders
   6. Childhood autism
   7. Blindness and deafness
   8. Hematological disorders
   9. Neoplasias.
II. Handicapping conditions have been divided into intrinsic and extrinsic categories:
   – Intrinsic—"one from which the person cannot be separated", e.g. all the medical and physical disability.
   – Extrinsic—"one from which the person can be removed", e.g. social deprivation.
III. Handicapping conditions can be:
   – Mental handicap
   – Physical handicap
   – Medical handicap.

Cerebral Palsy

It is characterized by paralysis, weakness, incoordination or other aberrations of motor function and have their origin either prenatally or postnatally before the CNS has reached maturity, i.e. at the age of 5 years. It may be seen in conjunction with other manifestations like seizures, mental retardation, etc. The cause may be due to congenital defects, chemical or mechanical or infections.

Definition

'Nelson'[7] described cerebral palsy as a group of non-progressive disorders resulting from malfunction of the motor centers and pathways of the brain.

Incidence

Approximately 0.6-5.9 per 1000 births.

Classification

Cerebral palsy can be 5 types, they are:
A. Spasticity
B. Athetosis
C. Ataxia
D. Rigidity
E. Tremors.

Spasticity

- Occurs in > 40% of the cases
- Caused due to lesion in the cerebral cortex
- Flexion deformities are seen which are due to tendency for the antigravity muscles to maintain a state of contraction and for the antagonists to lengthen
- Usually associated with convulsions and mental retardation
- Head movement is limited
- Hypertonicity of facial muscles and slow jaw movements
- Hypertonic orbicularis muscles
- Associated with spastic tongue thrust and drooling
- Constricted mandibular and maxillary arches
- Class II division 2 malocclusion with unilateral cross bite.

Athetosis

- Occurs in about 25% of the cases
- Caused due to a lesion in the basal ganglion
- Muscles are normal, there is no spasticity or weakness
- Involuntary movements, either tremor or rotary may be seen
- Usually associated with convulsions and mental retardation
- Excessive head movement or head drawn back with bull type neck

- Quick jaw movements with bruxism
- Hypotonic orbicularis muscles
- Grimacing and drooling
- Tongue protrudes out
- High and narrow palatal vault
- Class II division 1 malocclusion
- Presence of anterior open bite and associated with mouth breathing
- Poor swallowing, sucking, etc. due to impaired function of muscles of deglutition.

Ataxia

- Occurs in 10% of cerebral palsy patients
- Caused due to lesion of the cerebellum
- Disturbances in equilibrium is present
- No abnormal muscular involvement
- Lack of positional sensation (balance)
- Poor proprioceptive sensations
- Slow tremor like head movements
- Hypotonic oribularis muscles
- Ankyloglosia in some cases is seen
- Associated with tongue protrusion and open bite
- Grimacing and drooling.

Rigidity

- Occurs in 5% of the cases
- Caused due to lesion of the basal ganglion
- Constant rigidity of muscles seen
- Voluntary movements are slow and stiff
- Adequate mouth opening may be difficult.

Tremors

- Present in about 5% of the cases
- Caused due to lesion in the basal ganglion
- Features are—repetitive, rhythmic involuntary contraction of flexor and extensor muscles.

General disabilities associated with cerebral palsy are:
- Speech defects—50-75%
- Mental retardation—45%
- Visual defects—20-50%
- Seizures—35-60%
- Deafness—10-30%

Dental Consideration and Management

- No specific oral disease is related to cerebral palsy.
- Usual dental problems of caries and periodontal disease are often exaggerated by neglect.
- There is no significant difference in the eruption time of primary and permanent teeth.
- Routine procedures can be accomplished.

- Generally they will understand and cooperate when the dentist explains before starting a procedure, unless severely mentally retarded.
- Physical restraints can be used to control abnormal movements of head, body and the extremities.
- The dentist should at all times support or cradle the patients head to control involuntary movements.
- Premedication is very useful, but the dentist should be thorough with the patients medications and their probable interactions with each other.
- Gag, cough, bite and swallowing reflexes may be impaired or abnormal. If the Gag reflex is more exaggerated, patient should be seated in an upright position.
- Rubber dam should be used, due to increased chance of aspiration.

Communication

It forms an important aspect in the management of patients with cerebral palsy. Significant personality differences exist in each type of cerebral palsy and thus communication with the patient can be more easily attained by understanding the characteristics of each.

Behavior in Dental Clinic

Spastic patient

- Shut and introvert
- Fearful and spastic episodes may be induced by any outside stimulus, e.g. loud noises, sudden movements or even meeting strangers
- They prefer an environment devoid of excitement and stimulation.

Rigid

- Similar to spastic patient in personality
- Fear generally is not so pronounced.

Athetosis

- Without excessive fear
- Provoked to outbursts of anger
- Craves attention, affection and enjoy people's company.

Ataxic

- Resembles athetoid patient
- Has little fear
- When asked to make repeated efforts he gives up quickly.

Intellectual Disability

For a person to be diagnosed as intellectually disabled (previously called as mentally retarded), he should possess all the below mentioned three characteristics:

1. An IQ score of less than 70
2. An accompanying impairment in adaptive behavior
3. A manifestation of both before 18 years of age.

Definition

The American Association of Mental Deficiency (AAMD)[8] has defined it as follows:

"Subaverage general intellectual functioning which originates during the developmental period and is associated with impairment in adaptive behavior."

Incidence

About 0.5% of the preschool children are recognized as being retarded. The peak period of recognition is between 6-16 years, when the pressures of formal schooling seem to identify a larger number. The incidence may reach 10% or more of the school population in some areas.

Classification

The AAMD classifies retardation in 4 categories.
1. Mildly or educable mental retardation (EMR), IQ of 69-55—the educational programs are generally simplified versions of regular school programs and usually lead to literacy and attainment of skills necessary for employment. They form about 80% of the total cases.

> Etiology of intellectual disability
> *Prenatal cause:*
> - Genetic diseases
> - Maternal and fetal infections
> - Kernicterus
> - Cretinism
> - Fetal alcohol syndrome
>
> *Natal cause:*
> - Birth injuries
> - Infection
> - Cerebral trauma
> - Hemorrhage
> - Hypoxia
> - Anoxia
> - Hypoglycemia
>
> *Postnatal cause:*
> - Cerebral infections
> - Cerebral trauma
> - Poisoning
> - Cerebral vascular accidents
> - Postimmunization encephalopathy
> - Malnutrition

2. Moderately or trainable mental retardation (TMR), IQ of 54-40.
3. Severely retarded, IQ of 39-25—(nontrainable).
4. Profoundly retarded, IQ of <25—(nontrainable).

Dental Considerations

The oral cavity is generally not the primary area of concern to the patient or the family and also the patient is very uncooperative to maintain good oral hygiene. The result is poor oral health. The ideal approach is to start the patient on a good oral hygiene and preventive program and then restore the dentition.
- Premedication can be extremely helpful in allaying the anxiety.
- First visit should be limited to oral examination, oral radiographs or oral prophylaxis with fluoride application. The time taken for a procedure may vary depending on the extent of cooperation and is generally slower and requiring some modification such as the use of tongue blades, mouth props, and assistance to restrain the child.
- Radiographs are difficult to take due to gagging and uncooperation. Film holders can be used.

Modifications in Treatment Plan

A. Strong restorations such as steel crowns are preferred to large amalgam restorations.
B. Pulpotomy or preferably pulpectomy therapy should be accomplished rather than less reliable pulp capping procedure.
C. Resorbable sutures should be used after surgery.
D. It is advisable to attach floss to instruments such as files, reamers, stainless steel crown (after welding a small loop to the buccal surface), etc.

Congenital Cardiac Disease

Children with this disorder represent one of the largest groups of medically compromised patients.

> Clinical features
> 1. Clubbing of the fingers
> 2. Cyanosis of mucosa
> 3. Shortness of breath

Features and Dental Importance

- Risk of infective endocarditis is present, hence antibiotic prophylaxis should be given prior to any invasive procedure.
- Preoperative oral antiseptic mouthwash—0.2% chlorhexidine gluconate is ideal.
- Increased bleeding tendency may be present.
- Increased prevalence of enamel hypoplasia and dental caries in the primary dentition.
- Pulpotomy is contraindicated due to the possibility of subsequent bacteremia.
- There are no contraindications for the use of Lignocaine 2% and adrenaline 1: 100,000.

- Treatment under general anesthesia should be performed in hospital only.
- Sedation can be given to the patient but under careful monitoring.
- Patients with pacemakers should be identified and all dental device that may interfere with the pacemaker such as electrosurgical units, pulp testers, ultrasonic cleaning device, etc. should be disconnected.

Dental procedures requiring prophylaxis in a patient suffering from congenital cardiac disease:

Dental procedures requiring prophylaxis in a patient suffering from congenital cardiac disease	
Prophylaxis recommended	*Prophylaxis not recommended*
• Dental extractions and other surgery	• Restorative dental treatment, if bleeding is not anticipated
• Periodontal procedures including prophylaxis, subgingival procedures and probing, if bleeding is anticipated	• Intracanal endodontic obturation or postplacement
• Dental implant placement, reimplantation of avulsed teeth	• Placement of rubber dam
• Endodontic procedures	• Suture removal
• Initial placement of orthodontic bands	• Oral impressions
• Intraligamentary anesthesia	• Fluoride treatment
	• Intraoral radiographs
	• Shedding of primary teeth

Guidelines for infective endocarditis antibiotic prophylaxis[9]		
Oral route	Amoxicillin	Adults—2.0 gm Children—50 mg/kg —one hour before procedure
Unable to take oral medications	Ampicillin	Adults—2.0 gm Children—50 mg/kg, (IM or IV) —30 minutes before procedure
Allergy to penicillin	Clindamycin	Adults—600 mg Children—20 mg/kg, peroral —1 hour before procedure
	Cephalexin or Cefadroxil	Adults—2.0 gm Children—50 mg/kg, peroral —1 hour before procedure
	Azithromycin/Clarithromycin	Adults—500 mg Children—15 mg/kg —1 hour before procedure
Allergic to penicillin and unable to take oral medication	Clindamycin	Adults—600 mg Children—20 mg/kg, IV —30 minutes before procedure
	Cefazolin	Adults—1.0 gm Children—25 mg/kg, IM or IV —30 minutes before procedure

Cleft Lip and Palate

The oral cavity is bounded anteriorly by the upper and lower lip and posteriorly extends upto the oropharynx. The roof is formed by the palate and floor by the structures in the floor of the mouth. Laterally it is bounded by the cheeks.

The lower lip is formed by the fusion of mandibular process in the midline and the upper lip is formed as the maxillary processes grow medially and fuse with the lateral nasal and the medial nasal processes (Fig. 11.1). The lateral and medial nasal process fuses with each other to form the anterior nares. As growth occurs the frontonasal process becomes narrower from side to side.

The palate is formed by the fusion of the two lateral maxillary palatal shelves and the caudal portion of the frontonasal process. Initially these three processes are widely separated from each other due to vertical orientation of the lateral maxillary shelves and the developing tongue occupies this space. The primary palate includes a wedge shaped area in front of the incisive fossa and carries 4 tooth buds.

During 6th week of intrauterine life, a shelf like projection of palatine process grows medially from each maxillary process. The presence of the developing tongue prevents the palatine process from meeting each other. So they grow caudally along the side of the developing tongue.

During 7th week the mandibular arches grows more caudally and ventrally producing prominence of chin.

During the 8th week as the tongue moves downward and forward along with the developing mandible, the palatal shelves change from a vertical to horizontal position contacting each other in the midline and also with the premaxilla in the anterior region.

The fusion of 3 palatal components initially forms a 'Y' shaped suture. The site of fusion of lateral palatal shelves is traced in adults by the mid palatal suture. Ossification starts during the 8th week of IU life from the

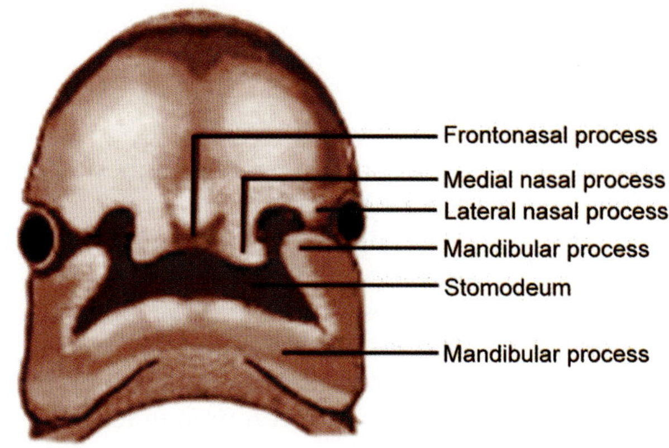

Fig. 11.1: Development of face and associated structures occur by the fusion of different processes

spread of bone into the mesenchyme of the fused palatal shelves and laterally spreading to the premaxilla. Mid palatal suture is first evident at 10½ week. Ossification does not occur in the most posterior part of the palate, which gives rise to soft palate.[10-12]

Mechanism of Cleft Formation[13,14]

A. Failure of mesoderm to unite-as the lateral growth of the face was more
B. Deficient mesoderm
C. Insufficient migration potential of mesoderm
   Failure of tongue to move downward, leads to failure of palatal shift or abnormally large tongue.

Etiology for Cleft Formation

Hereditary

If both the parents are normal, there is 4% chance and if one parent is having cleft then there is 12% chance and 45% if both of them are affected. Cleft lip and palate has a multifactorial inheritance pattern, that is, even though a susceptible gene is present it also requires exposure to adverse environmental factors conducive to cleft formation.

Environmental factors

- Riboflavin deficiency (Riboflavin is necessary for organogenesis)
- Radiation may cause chromosomal aberration
- Antimetabolites—block enzymes which interfere with DNA synthesis
- Hypoxia—may give rise to vascular deficiency
- Cortisone—inhibits palatal shelf elevation
  - reduces amniotic fluid
  - reduces RNA synthesis
  - inhibition of mitosis
- Tolbutamide—decreases uptake of glucose
- Oligohydramnios (reduced amniotic fluid) – causes hyperflexion of the head fold resulting in micrognathia. The small jaw pushes the tongue up between the palatal shelves.

Epidemiology

- *Incidence:* Cleft lip with palate—highest incidence is 45%
  Cleft palate—30%
  Cleft lip—25%
- *Race:* Negroes are affected the least and Japanese most frequently
- *Sex:* Cleft lip is higher among males but cleft palate is common in females
- *Parental age:* Increase in frequency of cleft lip with or without cleft palate with increasing parental age is seen.

- *Associated malformations:* A number of studies have shown that in individuals born with cleft lip and or palate there is increased likelihood of other congenital malformation. 10-20% have other congenital abnormalities like defects of extremities and congenital heart diseases. Syndromes associated with cleft palate are—cleidocranial dysostosis, craniofacial dysostosis, Pierre Robin syndrome, Marfan's syndrome.

Classification of Cleft Lip and Palate[15-19]

There are various classification systems available:
1. Morphologic classification:
   a. Davis and Ritchie
   b. Veau's—palate
            —lip
2. Embryologic classification—Fogh and Andersons
3. Symbolic classification—Kernahans striped 'Y'
4. Kernahan and Starte's classification.

Davis and Ritchie	
Code	*Location*
Group 1 (Pre-alveolar cleft)	Lip—unilateral, median, bilateral
Group 2 (Post-alveolar cleft)	Soft and hard palate—various degree of involvement up to the alveolar ridge
Group 3 (Alveolar cleft)	Palate, alveolus and lip—unilateral, median and bilateral
Veau's classification	
Code	*Location and type of defect*
Group 1	Palate—soft
Group 2	Palate—soft, hard up to incisive foramen
Group 3	Palate—soft, hard, alveolus, lip-unilateral
Group 4	Palate—hard, soft, alveolus, lip-bilateral
Classification of lip	
Code	*Location and type of defect*
Group 1	Lip—notching
Group 2	Lip—up to nasal septum
Group 3	Lip—involving nasal septum bilaterally
Embryologic classification—Fogh and Andersons	
Code	*Location and type of defect*
Group 1	Hare lip – single, double
Group 2	Hare lip and cleft palate- single, double
Group 3	Cleft palate

Symbolic Classification—Kernahans Striped Y

Upper arm – alveolus, hard palate upto incisive foramen
Lower arm – represents hard and soft palate
Area involved is shaded.

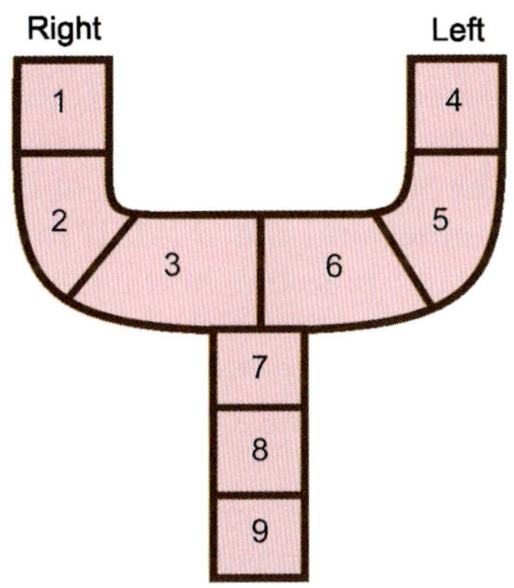

Kernahan and Starte's classification			
	Unilateral	*Median*	*Bilateral*
Cleft palate only	Complete	Complete– Premaxilla is absent	Complete
	Incomplete	Incomplete – Rudimentary premaxilla	Incomplete
Cleft of secondary palate only	Complete	Incomplete	Submucous
Cleft of primary and secondary palate	Complete	Complete	Complete
	Incomplete	Incomplete	Incomplete

Clinical Features (Figs 11.2 to 11.4)

- The least unesthetic form of cleft is the mild cleft of the lip and most unesthetic form is the bilateral cleft lip and palate.
- Unilateral cleft lip and palate—major segment of alveolus is on non-cleft side, lip is distorted and nose is flattened on cleft side.
- Bilateral cleft lip and palate—premaxilla is rotated and everted out of the oral cavity.
- In case of palatal cleft there is communication between oral and nasal cavities. So there is difficulty while feeding as the fluid tends to flow out of the nose.
- There may be abnormal frenal attachment in the form of multiple webbing seen adjacent to the cleft.
- There are chances of increased incidence of congenitally missing teeth usually the lateral incisor or increased frequency of supernumerary teeth. Natal or neonatal teeth are also found.
- If the lateral incisor is present they may erupt ectopically either palatally or within the cleft. If they erupt adjacent to the cleft, there may be deficiency of the supporting alveolar bone leading to premature loss.

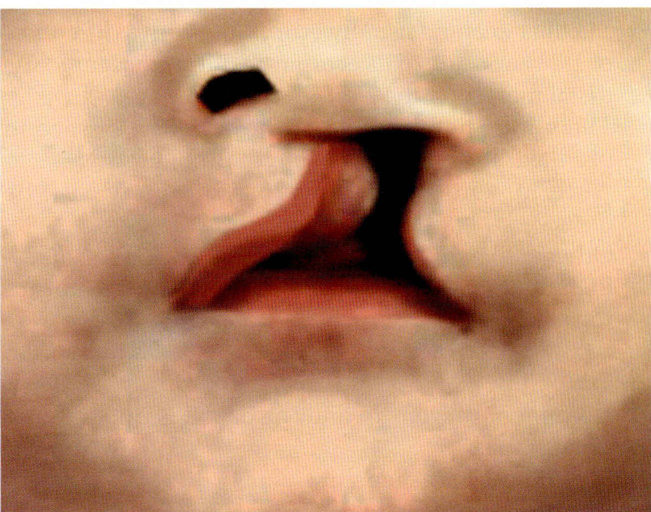

Fig. 11.2: Unilateral cleft of the lip

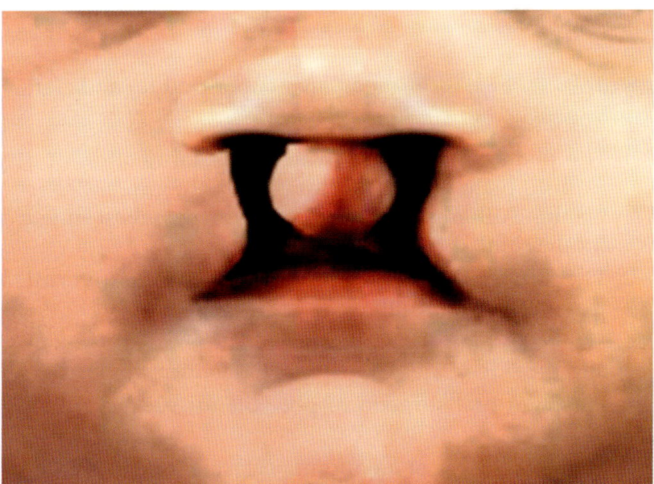

Fig. 11.3: Bilateral cleft of the lip

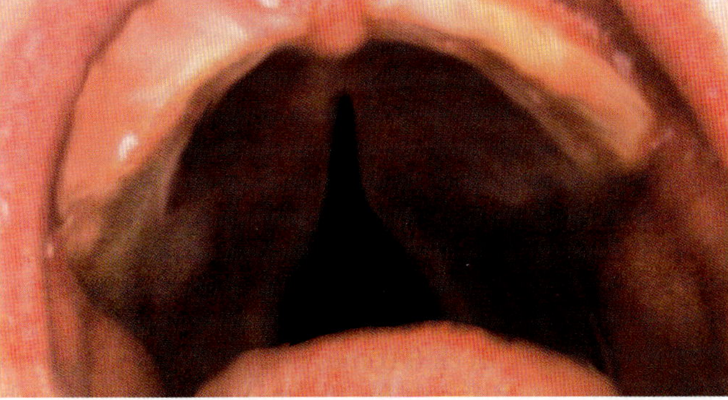

Fig. 11.4: Cleft involving only the palate

- Other changes that may be seen are hypoplastic teeth, microdontia, macrodontia, fused teeth, etc.
- The central incisor may be rotated or linguoverted.

- Maxillary canine usually erupts late with a difference of 1-2 years, due to its ectopic position adjacent to the distal margin of the cleft.
- There may be blockade of the eruption of second premolar indicating arch length problems.
- Anterior end to end or cross bite may also be observed.
- Other associated problems may be – velopharyngeal incompetence, vestibular deficiency and mid face retrusion.

Management of Cleft Lip and Palate

The treatment of cleft lip and/or palate is divided into different stages:

a. Presurgical management
b. Stage I
c. Stage II
d. Stage III
e. Stage IV.

> **Team members for the management of cleft lip and cleft palate includes:**
>
> 1. The pedodontist is involved in the fabrication of a feeding plate and obturator. He or she can assist in planning different feeding techniques that is best suited for the child.
> 2. The pediatrician responsible for patients overall maintenance of health.
> 3. The orthodontist identifies problems, predicts growth and provides comprehensive orthodontic care.
> 4. Plastic or oral surgeon responsible for surgery when needed.
> 5. Speech pathologist monitors speech and offers therapy
> 6. ENT surgeon performs test to identify any hearing difficulties, as parent will not be able to recognize hearing problems
> 7. Psychiatrist evaluates emotional, behavioral and social development. Emphasis is placed on the patients ability to cope with emotional and physical stress created by the cleft defect.

Presurgical Management

It includes counseling the parent and feeding the child.
Counseling: The parents usually are not prepared and the birth of a child with cleft comes as a shock especially to the mother. It is difficult for the mother to accept such a child with the deformed little face and it is at this time, she is in need of psychological support from her obstetrician and pediatrician initially and later from others. As Cooper has stated, the initial management is "Feed the child and treat the mother."

Feeding for infants with cleft palate: Feeding is a major problem in children with cleft palate. The mother should be encouraged to breastfeed. This is desirable from a nutritional point of view and also strengthens the bond between the mother and the child. If for some reason breastfeeding is not possible, bottle is used. Normally the infant creates a negative oral pressure while sucking the milk. But the cleft palate children cannot form a negative pressure. Mechanical feeding is thus suitable if breastfeeding is difficult.

Two main methods are employed: (a) Spoon and (b) Bottle. Both are used along with feeding plate.

Spoons can be used that are either conventional or attached to a special type of feeding bottle which acts as a reservoir. A spoon with a deep trough is recommended. It is especially useful immediately following repair of the lip because it eliminates the chances of damaging the lip. A spoon can also be fixed to a palatal attachment, such that the spoon position can be adjusted and locked in the position found to be satisfactory.

Cleft palate babies who are bottle fed, should have a teat which is soft in texture and has a large hole, to compensate for the slow draw of milk or fluid. Bottles with long nipples having opening (oblique opening) just enough to permit the milk to flow freely but not to permit milk to flow freely when inverted. Proper positioning of the child is also important. The mother should cradle the baby in her arm in a semisitting posture with the infant's body upright and tilted slightly backward. Feeding is slow and the child tends to lose major part of the feed, due to its disability. Feeding bottle to which an acrylic plate is attached can be used which closes the defect and prevents fluid from entering the nasal cavity.

Feeding Plate (Fig. 11.5)

Design: The feeding plate is made of acrylic extending over the palate covering the cleft. The plate is held in place by a 0.9 mm stainless steel wire extending from the plate out of the oral cavity on either side. The wire is then bent over the cheek without touching it. This extended wire portion prevents the accidental slippage of the feeding plate and also provides some retention.

Fabrication: The lollipop impression technique is most simple for obtaining the primary impression. As the name suggests, the tray is like a lollipop in shape. A wooden flat tongue spatula or a flattened old teaspoon also serves the purpose. Impression compound can be used to function as a tray as well as impression material. The cast is prepared and feeding plate is fabricated with self-cure or heat cure acrylic.

The feeding plate is placed in the oral cavity only during feeding.

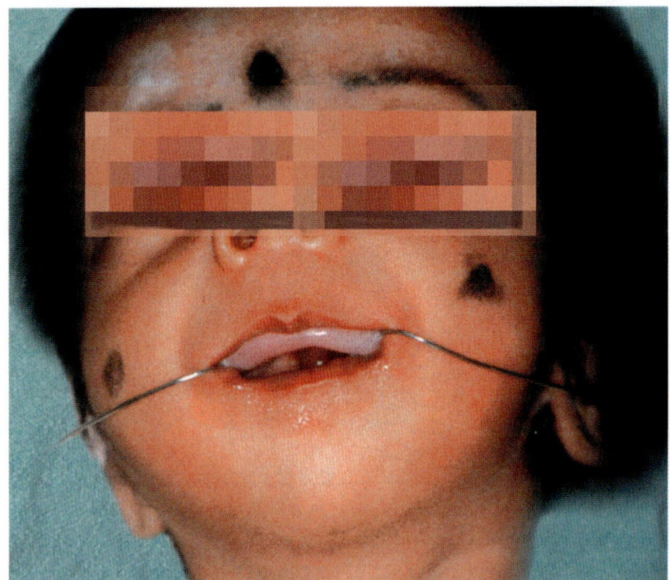

Fig. 11.5: Feeding plate in position

Stage I: Management from Birth to 18 Months

Birth to three months: Includes presurgical arch alignment, use of stimulation appliances, and cheiloplasty.

A. *Presurgical arch alignment:* In bilateral clefts the early treatment combines the expansion of the two maxillary segments and repositioning of the premaxillary segment into a position of stability between the lateral segments.

When there is a unilateral cleft, due to muscle pull, the major segment is pulled towards the non-cleft side and in the bilateral clefts the premaxillary portion moves labially and becomes everted. So if an opposing and a shearing force are applied the distortion can be minimized and the major and minor segments can be pulled together. This makes the task of the plastic surgeon easier.

This can be accomplished by the construction of a simple intraoral appliance on a series of corrected models modified progressively towards normality. Their function is to mould the deformed arch into correct anatomical alignment. This treatment begins after birth as soon as possible.

Advantage of presurgical arch alignment:
— Provides a sound basis for lip repair and affords support to the nostrils
— Restores the continuity of the lip
— Permits function of the circumoral musculature.

This appliance is fitted over the protruding and laterally displaced premaxilla and anchored to the infants head with a Bonnet appliance. By the application of the sequentially increasing forces to the premaxilla with elastic straps attached to the prosthesis, the premaxilla can be aligned in midline. The time required is about 3-4 weeks. Equal pressure is maintained for 1-2 months to retract the premaxilla in between the lateral segments.

Design and construction: Impression is made and the cast prepared. The model is examined and planned for sectioning. The model is divided with a fine saw through the cleft from the posterior border to the premaxillary region. Template can be used as an aid to the degree of correction and repositioning that is required. After sectioning, they are repositioned with wax and this model is duplicated. Baseplate is adapted over it. Blocks are made on the ridges with wax. Wings are fabricated which extend round the corners of the child's mouth and prevents the child from swallowing the appliance. The wax up appliance is tried in the child's mouth. Then final wax of the appliance is made, it is flasked, packed and acrylized. Holes are made in the ends of the wings for tapes. The appliance may be reinforced by applying extra oral strapping in the form of a bow to the premaxilla. Care is taken not to over correct by the pressure of the strapping, which will bring maxillary arch within the mandibular arch, causing malocclusion in later life.

B. *Stimulation appliances:* This technique was described by McNeil in 1955 by taking advantage of normal growth factors. Forces which are within the limit of tolerance will act to stimulate bone apposition if they are applied to a particular region and in such directions that they can be regarded as intensified normal forces.

The appliance is shaped as a spring activator which lies in contact with the palatal processes and are designed to exert a gentle pressure, which produces hyperemia of the tissues. An increase of blood supply is likely to cause proliferation of the edges of the palatal defect. The appliance is used prior to surgery of the palate. No pressure is applied to the edges of the cleft.

Construction: Impression is made and casts prepared. Teeth are selected for cribs to provide retention. The areas of pressure are marked out on the palate and covered by wax. A horse-shoe shaped wax is adapted to fit round the collor of the teeth, leaving the palate clear. 0.6 mm wire is bent and extended from horse-shoe shaped wax down into the wax pads. The waxed up pattern is sealed to the duplicated model, flasked and acrylised. After trimming and polishing the appliance is fitted.

C. *Cheiloplasty:* 3 Ten's law is a simple guide to determine if a child is ready for surgery—child should be 10 weeks old, weigh 10 lbs and should have 10 gm. Hb/100 ml. Logan's bow is given to reduce the tension in the wound following surgery. It remains in place for 5 days till sutures are removed.

Three to nine months: Management includes placement of an obturator and bone grafting procedures:

  i. Following lip closure, there is collapse of the maxillary arch, due to increased tension placed on the segments by the repaired lip. A prosthetic device termed as intraoral maxillary obturator when placed in the mouth, prevents this collapse.

  ii. When the maxillary segments are in good alignment and abutted across the cleft sides, the patient is ready for cleft bone graft, i.e. at about 6-9 months. The primary grafting is done at 6-9 months, early secondary at 2-4 years, secondary grafting at 6-15 years, late secondary grafting during adulthood.

> There may be some problems associated with early bone grafting such as:
>
> Limitation of midfacial growth, manifested as reduced anteroposterior development, increased incidence of crossbite, reduced area of upper jaw.

Obturators: They provide a false palate against which the infant can suck, reducing the incidence of feeding difficulties. It also provides maxillary cross arch stability, preventing arch collapse after lip closure. It aids in orthopedic molding of the cleft segments into approximation before primary alveolar cleft bone grafting.

- Indications for the use of obturators:
  1. To facilitate feeding prior to surgical intervention.
  2. As an interim means of treatment.
  3. Where surgery is contraindicated, because of existing disease.
  4. Where surgical procedure would result in an inferior functional result.
  5. Unwillingness of the patient to undergo surgical treatment.
  6. Where surgical correction has failed to produce a satisfactory result.
  7. Where long hospitalization is precluded by financial considerations.
- Requirements of the material used for obturators
  The material should be:
  - Nonirritating to the tissues
  - Light in weight
  - Hygienic and easily cleansable
  - Durable

- Pliable
- Poor conductor of heat
- Easy to manipulate.

- Materials used:

For palate	For velum
Acrylic	Acrylic, Latex
	Chrome cobalt, Polyvinyl chloride
Cast gold	Cast gold, rubber based material
Stainless steel	Sheet rubber

> Hinges play a very important role while fabricating the velum obturators, which enable the artificial velum to make delicate movements.

Different types of hinges available are:
1. McNeil Hinge
2. Ball and socket hinge
3. Rod and tube hinge
4. Cast hinge

Twelve months to two years: Management in this period includes palatoplasty. Closure of the palate is accomplished during this period. The main purpose being to facilitate the acquisition of normal speech.

> **Different surgical technique for palatoplasty include:**
>
> For soft palate – Three layer closure
>   – Veau-Wardill-Kilner two flap push back procedure
>   – Primary pharyngeal flap
> For complete cleft palate
>   – von Langenbeck's repair
>   – Sliding mucoperioesteal flap
>   – Bilateral Vomer flap
>   – Primary veloplasty

Stage II: Management from 18 Months to 5 Years (Primary Dentition)

Treatment during this phase is initially focused on establishing and maintaining optimal oral health. Meticulous daily oral hygiene for the child is established to reduce the possibility of developing dental caries. An increase in periodic recalled examination at 3-4 months interval enables the dentist to intercept areas of decay. Extent of malocclusion is less apparent. Treatment is difficult in the primary dentition because of the lack of good teeth for anchorage. Level of cooperation obtained by the patient is also limited and there may be relapse due to growth.

Stage III: Management from 6 Years to 11 Years (Mixed Dentition)

Treatment is concentrated at correction of traumatic occlusion and posterior segmental alignment. Maxillary expansion, to correct posterior segmental collapse is accomplished by routine palatal expansion. Secondary alveolar cleft bone grafts offer maxillary arch continuity and aids in closure of the oronasal fistula. It also supports the alar base of the nose. After 2 months healing period, tooth can be moved into the newly grafted bone and the bone will respond to the tooth movement as any normal bone would. It is observed that canines can and do erupt through the graft. If eruption is delayed surgical or orthodontic intervention is appropriate. Success rate is usually 90%.

Stage IV: Management from 12 to 18 Years (Permanent Dentition)

Treatment during this stage comprises of comprehensive orthodontic and surgical management of permanent dentition. Growth is nearing completion during this stage and magnitude of any deformity can be readily assessed. Hence it forms the appropriate time to start orthodontic or surgical procedure. Crossbite can be corrected by rapid maxillary expansion, class III malocclusion by elastic traction with fixed appliance.

Retention period required may be longer or sometimes permanent.

Speech and hearing problems associated with cleft and its management: It has been estimated that 50% of the patients suffer from some type of speech problems.

In cleft palate cases, there is defect in articulation, resonance and hearing problem. Rhythm may also be disrupted because of the nasal leakage of air that makes speaking in phrases or sentences in a single breath of air very difficult.

When there is velar insufficiency there is no distortion of the nasal sounds like—m, n, ng.

In case of severe nasal obstruction,

- Bilabial plosives [b] will be replaced by [m], e.g. Me for be.
- Linguoalveolar [d] will be substituted for n., e.g. Doe for no.
- Voiced velar g' will be substituted for linguovelar ng., e.g. rig for ring.

Hearing problems are often associated with clefts of the palate. These problems are usually caused by middle ear infection, which are inturn due to the exposure of the eustachian tube to bacteria and food in the patient with cleft palate.

Management: Speech therapist should be consulted for speech related problems. Speech therapy includes:

1. Mother is encouraged to talk to the child. This is called indirect speech therapy.
2. Direct speech therapy—patients are encouraged to produce words which stimulates tongue and lip movement.
3. Articulation therapy—proper tongue positioning and movement is shown to the child and asked to repeat.

Despite all these measures, a certain proportion of patients are left with inadequate speech. This can be related to many variables like low intelligent quotient, hearing loss, poor psychosocial family environment, presence of residual defects in the soft and hard palate and severe dento alveolar deformities.

Down's Syndrome

It is the most common chromosomal aberration seen with incidence rate of 1.5 per 1000 live births. Survival rate is very high in patients with this syndrome. The most common chromosomal abnormality seen is trisomy 21 (presence of an extra autosome 47XX in females and 47XY in males). About 4% have translocation of chromosome 21 and 1% are mosaics, i.e. there is a population of cells with both normal and trisomic chromosome numbers (a mixture of 46 and 47 chromosomes). Increased maternal age seems to be the prime cause.

Dental Management of Patient with Down's Syndrome

- Abnormalities related to Down's syndrome that can affect dental treatment are congenital heart disease and behavioral problems due to retardation.
- Patient with Down's syndrome can be treated in dental office with a tolerant and empathetic approach. The dentist should attempt to introduce dental treatment in a nonthreatening and friendly manner.
- They are very friendly and mildly affected patient are often very cooperative.
- Premedication, however, may be necessary to allay apprehension in some severely affected patients.
- Since these children have associated cardiac abnormalities, antibiotic prophylaxics is required before any invasive dental procedure.
- Detailed description is also given in chapter 18.

Renal Diseases

Renal failure leads to a drop in glomerular filtration rate, which results in progressive hypertension, fluid retention and build-up of metabolites that are not excreted normally.

Features and Dental Importance

- Children usually exhibit growth retardation.
- They are pale and anemic.
- Bleeding tendency due to capillary fragility and thrombocytopenia is positive.
- Children on dialysis are most of the time on anticoagulant therapy.
- Caries rate is lower in children with end stage renal disease, possibly caused by ammonia being released in saliva.
- Uremic stomatitis develop when serum urea is over 300 mg/ml.
- Teeth calcifying during renal failure will exhibit chronological hypoplasia or hypomineralization. They may be brown or green due to incorporation of blood products such as biliverdin.
- Additional dose of drugs should be given after hemodialysis.

Drugs to be Avoided

- Paracetamol
- Penicillin
- Tetracycline
- Chloramphenicol.

> **Prognosis of Down's syndrome**
>
> - About 25-30% die during the first year of life
> - 50% die during the first 5 years
> - The most frequent causes of death are congenital heart disease and respiratory tract infections.

Liver Disease

Features and Dental Importance

- There is reduction of production of vitamin K dependent clotting factors, which may result in increased bleeding tendency.
- Patients are usually managed with high dose steroids and are immunocompromised.
- Increased destruction of red blood cells are seen leading to anemia.
- Consultation with the pediatrician is necessary.
- Aggressive management of caries with extraction of suspected teeth should be done after replacement of clotting factors.
- Coagulopathies are usually managed with fresh frozen plasma to replace deficient clotting factors.
- Antibiotic prophylaxis required.

Drugs to be Avoided

- Acetaminophen
- Aspirin

- Lignocaine
- Mepivocaine
- Procaine
- Ampicillin
- Tetracycline
- Barbiturates
- Chloral hydrate
- Promethazine.

Diabetes Mellitus

Type I or insulin dependent diabetes mellitus is the most common form in children. This is due to damage of the pancreatic islets. The damage may be due to bacterial or viral insult. Auto immune mechanism has also been suggested in the destruction of the insulin producing β cells. The goal of treatment is to maintain blood glucose at a normal level and thereby reduce the potential complication of hyperglycemia and ketoacidosis.

> **Diagnosis of diabetes mellitus**
>
> - Fasting blood glucose level—120 mg/dl
> - Abnormal oral glucose tolerance test
> - Elevated glycosylated hemoglobin test value

Features and Dental Importance

- Periodontal disease is the most consistent oral finding in patients with poorly controlled diabetes. These patients exhibit increased alveolar bone resorption and inflammatory gingival changes. This may mimic the clinical manifestation of aggresive periodontitis.
- Xerostomia and recurrent intraoral abscesses may be present.
- Enamel hypocalcification and hypoplasia along with reduced salivary flow can predispose these patients to an increased frequency of caries.
- Altered flora with an increase in Candida albicans, Hemolytic Streptococci and Staphylococci.
- For routine dental appointments, the patient should eat a normal meal before the dental procedure and a glucose source should always be available to treat the onset of hypoglycemia.
- Fasting before a general anesthesia requires careful adjustment of hypoglycemia therapy because hypoglycemia related to anesthesia can be fatal.
- Healing can be delayed.
- All children treated under general anesthesia should be admitted to hospital and their case supervised by the pediatric endocrine team. Dextrose and insulin infusion is administered to avoid complications with fasting.
- Procedures should be done under prophylactic antibiotics.

Hypopituitarism

Features and Dental Importance

- Facial and skull measurements are smaller.
- Face appears immature with open bite.
- Skeletal development is consistently more retarded than craniofacial development, but tooth eruption and root formation can be delayed or incomplete.

Hyperpituitarism

Features and Dental Importance

- Precocious and accelerated development of the craniofacial skeleton.
- Prognathism is common.
- Accelerated dental development and eruption, enlarged tongue and facial features.
- Marked thickening of the cranium and cortical bone of the mandible.
- Overdevelopment of osseous structures with poor maturation and quality with hypercementosis.
- Management focuses on the craniofacial malformations and no contraindications exist for comprehensive dental healthcare.

Hypothyroidism

Features and Dental Importance

- Decreased vertical facial growth, decreased cranial base length and flexure, maxillary protrusion and open bite with immature facial patterns.
- Delayed eruption and increased spacing of teeth.
- Developmental retardation and hypoplasia.

Hyperthyroidism

Features and Dental Importance

- Accelerated growth and development of the craniofacial complex and skeleton.
- Precocious eruption of teeth.
- Periodontal/periapical destruction and osteoporosis
- Increased vertical facial height with open bite and mild prognathism.
- Principle risk is associated with general anesthesia as they are at risk of developing congestive cardiac failure which may be precipitated by general anesthesia.
- Untreated patient is also at risk from infection or surgical procedures since a thyroid crisis may be precipitated.
- Oral infections, directly or through toxic substances may aggravate hyperthyroidism. Oral infections should be treated aggressively.
- Antithyroid drugs may produce parotitis and agranulocytosis, which predisposes the patient to bleeding episodes, ulceronecrotic lesions and oral infection.

Hypoparathyroidism

Features and Dental Importance

- Circumoral paresthesia and spasm of the facial muscles.
- Hypoplasia of enamel, hypodontia and root anomalies.
- Delayed or arrested tooth eruption.
- Acute and chronic oral candidiasis.

Hyperparathyroidism

Features and Dental Importance

- Associated with mobility and drifting of teeth with no apparent pathologic periodontal pocketing leading to malocclusion.
- Metastatic soft tissue calcification is common.
- Radiographic features includes periapical radiolucencies and root resorption with loss of lamina dura and generalized loss of radiodensity.
- Routine treatment involves no modification unless associated with medical complication.
- May be associated with cardiac arrhythmias which increase the risk of serious problems during general anesthesia.
- Risk of pathological fractures may be a complication of oral surgical procedures and splinting of teeth may be required.

Respiratory Disease (Asthma)

Features and Dental Importance

- An acute attack during the procedure is a possibility
- If the patient is on steroid medication it may cause extrinsic staining of the teeth due to changes in oral flora and may also predispose to candidiasis and the child may also be immuno-compromised.
- Regular prophylaxis is required if extrinsic stains are present.
- Dental procedure in children who have been hospitalized for their asthma in the last 12 months and/or those managed with steroids should be done in hospital environment under pediatric care.
- There is no contraindication to the use of nitrous oxide, but should be avoided during acute illness.

Immunodeficiency

Features and Dental Importance

- Associated with candidiasis, severe gingivitis, gingivostomatitis.

- Conditions such as recurrent apthous ulceration, recurrent herpes simplex virus infection are common.
- Premature exfoliation of primary teeth.
- Recurrent bacterial infections, especially pneumonia and skin lesions.
- Prevention and regular review of oral health is important.
- Prophylactic antibiotics is required.
- Chlorhexidine 0.2% pretreatment mouth wash is recommended.

> **Classification of immunodeficiency conditions:**
>
> 1. Neutrophil disorders
> 2. Immunodeficiencies
>   — Primary—B-cell defects, T-cell defects
>   — Acquired—HIV infection, drug or chemotherapy or radiotherapy induced
>   — Combined

Acquired Immunodeficiency Syndrome

It is a condition caused by HIV type 1 or 2. T helper cells (CD4 cells) that are responsible for immunity are targeted by the virus. This results in opportunistic infections, malignancies and autoimmune disease. Patient's CD4 count and viral load is considered for estimating the disease status. Oral manifestations of HIV infection includes fungal infection (Candidiasis), Viral infection (Oral warts, HSV infections), Bacterial infections, Neoplasms (Kaposis sarcoma, non-Hodgkins lymphoma), gingivitis, periodontitis and others nonspecific lesions like salivary gland swelling, petechiae, etc.

AIDS is Diagnosed when an Individual with HIV Develops at Least one of these Conditions[20]

1. CD4+ T cell count drops below 200 cells/mm.^{3}
2. Development of one of the following opportunistic infections:
   - *Fungal:* Candidiasis of bronchi, trachea, lungs, or esophagus; *Pneumocystis carinii* pneumonia (PCP); disseminated or extrapulmonary histoplasmosis.
   - *Viral:* Cytomegalovirus (CMV) disease other than liver, spleen, or nodes; CMV retinitis (with loss of vision); herpes simplex with chronic ulcer (s) or bronchitis, pneumonitis, or esophagitis; progressive multifocal leukoencephalopathy (PML); extrapulmonary cryptococcosis
   - *Protozoal:* Disseminated or extrapulmonary coccidioidomycosis, toxoplasmosis of the brain, chronic intestinal isosporiasis; chronic intestinal cryptosporidiosis
   - *Bacterial:* Mycobacterium tuberculosis (any site); any disseminated or extrapulmonary mycobacterium, including *M. avium* complex or *M. kansasii;* recurrent pneumonia; recurrent *Salmonella septicemia*
3. Development of one of the following opportunistic cancers:
   - Invasive cervical cancer, Kaposi's sarcoma (KS), Burkitt's lymphoma, immunoblastic lymphoma, primary lymphoma of the brain, or cervical carcinoma.

Epilepsy

Epilepsy also referred to as a seizure disorder is a common neurological condition that is characterized by seizures occuring due to abnormal or excessive neuronal activity in the brain.

Classification

There are five types of epilepsy, they are:
1. Grand mal seizures
2. Petit mal seizures
3. Psychomotor seizures
4. Focal seizure (Jacksonian seizures)
5. Self-induced seizures.

Grand mal seizures

- Onset is rapid and preceded by momentary aura.
- Associated with tonic and clonic phases of muscular spasm.
- Patient losses consciousness and becomes pale. Pupils dilate, eyeballs roll upwards or to one side, the face becomes distorted and there is often rapid contraction of the jaw muscles. Micturition and defecation may occur.
- Patient may experience cyanosis during the tonic phase (continuous tension or contraction) lasting for 20-40 seconds.
- Clonic phase (alternating series of contractions and partial relaxation) may last for several minutes.
- Patient wakes up from seizure with severe headache and in a general state of confusion.
- A patient who experiences a grand mal seizure in the dental office should be handled conservatively and be put in a position in which he cannot harm himself possibly on the floor away from the dental equipment.
- If the seizure is prolonged, administration of oxygen may be necessary.
- A rubber or plastic mouth prop has to be inserted to prevent the patient from biting his tongue. A tongue blade wrapped with gauze and adhesive may be utilized.

- It is usually sufficient that the dentist wait until the seizure stops and then evaluate him.
- Recovery may be quick or patient may be irritable.

Petit mal seizures

- Appears between 3 years of age and puberty.
- More common in girls.
- Consists of transient loss of consciousness.
- May occur once or twice a month or very frequently at less intervals and lasting for less than 30 seconds.
- Other features are upward rolling of eyes, moving of the lids, drooling or rhythmic nodding of the head or slight quivering of the trunk and limb muscles.
- They may also go unnoticed.

Psychomotor seizures

- Difficult to recognize and control.
- Slight aura is manifested as a shrill of cry or an attempt to run for help.
- Child is often drowsy or sleeps for a short time after the spell.
- Seizure consists of loss of postural tone.
- 1-5 minutes of unconsciousness is followed by normal sleep or activity.
- No tonic or clonic movements present.

Focal seizure (Jacksonian seizures)

- Produced by injury to the brain.
- Seizures are clonic in nature.
- Muscles involved are the ones most specialized for voluntary movements in the hand, face and tongue.

Self-induced seizures

- It is possible for some children to induce petit mal or grand mal seizures by over breathing, watching a blinking light or by performing some other form of learned behavior.
- In such cases drug therapy alone is usually unsatisfactory
- Patient by doing so tries to draw attention to himself and is usually associated with complex family problems and psychiatric consultation is indicated.

Anti-convulsant drugs used in children and their toxic reactions		
Drug	Indications	Toxic reactions
Phenobarbital	Safest Used as adjunct and drug of choice for initial trial	Rare Drowsiness, increased excitability, dermatitis

Contd...

Contd...

Mephobarbital	Phenobarbital derivative- No advantage over phenobarbital	Same as for phenobarbital
Phenytoin (dilantin)	Good for management of grand mal and psychomotor epilepsy, may accentuate petit mal, often used with phenobarbital	Few–gingival hyperplasia, nervousness, ataxia, rash, nystagmus, nausea, vomiting
Primidone	Second choice for grand mal and complicated major seizures and psychomotor seizures	Urticaria, diarrhea, nausea, vomiting
Ethosuximide	First choice for true petit mal	Leukopenia, nausea, vomiting, headache, drowsiness, liver dysfunction

Features and Dental Importance

- Gingival enlargement.
- Precipitation of seizure during the surgery.
- Most convulsive disorders are controlled through medication and pose few problems in dental treatment. It should be made sure that the child has taken the daily dose of medicines.
- Since anxiety is a frequent precipitation factor, pre-medication with minor tranquilizers will be effective.
- These children often arrive at the dental office in a slightly sedated state due to the CNS depressed activity of anticonvulsant medications.
- Use of mouth props is mandatory during treatment because once the seizure begins, it is difficult to insert any device to prevent intraoral injury due to clenching of the jaws.
- If appliances are indicated for tooth movement or tooth replacement purposes, fixed appliance is preferred because there is less chance of dislodgement.
- Gingivectomy is the treatment of choice in case of gingival hyperplasia that usually occurs with phenytoin therapy. They usually tend to reccur. Hence the drug or the dose can be modified upon consultation with the pediatrician.
- In case an episode occurs:
  - Stop all dental procedure
  - Maintain the mouth prop in place
  - Loosen the patient's clothing
  - Turn the patient's head to the side, to prevent aspiration of oral fluids

– After the seizure, it is better to discontinue the therapy. If a cavity is already prepared, either temporize or complete the final restoration.

Childhood Autism

Kanmer in 1944—first described it as 'early infantile autism.'[21]

It was considered as a syndrome and great variations in severity and manifestations of the disturbances were observed. One symptom common to all children with the disease was an inability to relate appropriately to people and situations.

Features and Dental Importance

- Self-sufficient and introvert.
- Wants to be left alone, exhibits extreme resistance to being held. Eye contact is difficult to achieve.
- Have little or no attachment to their parents and remain detached.
- Relate poorly to persons, they frequently relate well to objects.
- They will remain occupied with moving or shiny in animate objects for hours, e.g. rotating fan, etc.
- They may typically display affection or anger with a toy.
- Language is impaired.

There are different opinions regarding the etiology of autism, such as:

- Personalities, attitudes and behavior of the child's parents, play a major role
- Autism is an early manifestation of childhood schizophrenia. But schizophrenia is a familial disease whereas infantile autism does not have familial tendency. Since most parents of autistic children are found to be highly intelligent, well educated and serious minded persons, the concept of parental causation is difficult to accept.

- Bizarre behavior makes dental management a challenge.
- Oral hygiene is often very poor because of finicky dietary habits.
- The problem with behavior modification is the time, energy and patience that are required.
- Ketamine can be used successfully as a sedative on an outpatient basis. But when there is extensive treatment required, general anesthesia is the method of choice.

Blindness

About 10% of the children below 20 years of age have visual defects.

Anyone providing treatment for these patients must first determine the degree of sight present. Overall personality defects and speech disorders are most frequently observed along with blindness.

Features and Dental Importance

- Allow the child to make full use of their tactile sense and their sense of smell when familiarizing them to the dental environment and dental procedures.
- Offer verbal and physical reassurance to the child, and remember they cannot see your smile.
- Paint a picture in the mind of your patients by describing the environment, the dental chair, equipments and the treatment and the environment throughout the procedure. A startle reflex may occur if instruments are introduced into the mouth without warning.
- Many visually impaired people are photophobic. It is important to ask parents and children about light sensitivity. Safety glasses should preferably be tinted.
- Oral hygiene education is given to the patient by introducing the surfaces of the teeth to be cleaned by having the patient first feel the teeth of a teaching model and then using his fingers in his own mouth.

Deafness

Features and Dental Importance

- Investigate how the child communicates
- A common fault is to talk loudly rather than slowly. If the patient can read the lip, face the child and speak clearly and slowly.
- It is useful to learn basic sign language.
- Deaf children may be very sensitive to vibration and so introduce high speed and low speed drills carefully.
- If a hearing aid is worn the volume may need adjustment.

Bleeding Disorder

Features and Dental Importance

- Bleeding disorders are due to failure in the initial clot formation.
- Children with thrombocytopenia will bleed immediately after trauma or surgery, unlike hemophiliacs who usually start to bleed 4 hours after the incident.
- Oral manifestations are petechiae and purpura, spontaneous bleeding and prolonged episodes of bleeding after minor trauma or tooth brushing are seen.
- Platelet level preferably should be $> 50 \times 10^9$ per liter before extraction.

- Endodontic procedures may be preferable to extractions in order to avoid the need for platelet transfusion.
- Good surgical technique and readily available local measures to control bleeding is important.
- Block injections should be avoided.
- Epsilon-aminocaproic acid 100 mg/kg loading dose and then 30 mg/kg four times a day for 7 days.

> **Bleeding disorder can be due to many reasons, they are:**
>
> 1. Platelet disorders
>   — Thrombocytopenia
>   — Thrombocytosis
>   — Platelet function disorder
> 2. Vitamin C deficiency.
> 3. Connective tissue diseases

Coagulation Disorders

Coagulation disorders can be of three types, they are:
1. Hemophilia A- factor VIII deficiency.
   (Normal level is 50-200%, Mild deficiency occurs when the level fall to 5-25%, moderate when it is 2-5% and severe when it is less than <1%).
2. von Willebrand's disease
3. Christmas disease.

Features and Dental Importance

- Consultation with physician.
- Local measures to control hemorrhage should be initiated.
- There should be minimal trauma during procedures.
- No block anesthesia without factor cover should be given, due to risk of hematoma.
- Intraperiodontal injections may be used but with great caution.
- Nitrous oxide sedation can be effective during restorative procedures.
- Extractions must never be performed without consultation.
- Endodontic procedures can be safely carried out without factor cover.
- Periodontal therapy with scaling and subgingival curettage requires factor replacement.
- Rubber dam should be used to protect soft tissues.

Hemophilia A

The coagulative disorder is characterized by deficiency of factor VIII.

Features and Dental Importance

- Dental treatment should be done following replacement therapy.
- Minor bleeding can be controlled with 30 to 50% of replacement but severe hemorrhage requires 100% replacement.
- Half-life of factor VIII is 10-12 hours.
- Emphasis should be given for prevention of oral disease.
- Increased risk of hematoma formation, hence nerve blocks are avoided.
- General anesthesia also carries the risk of bleeding similar to surgery, during endotracheal intubation
- Epsilon-aminocaproic acid should be administered prior to any procedure.
- Microfibrillar collagen hemostat (MCH) is advocated as local hemostatic agent.

> **Local hemostatic agents that can be used in dentistry:[22]**
>
> 1. Hemostatic Collagen: (Colla Tape, Helistat). They resorb within 14-56 days
> 2. Gelatin: (Gelfoam). They are resorbed in about 4-6 weeks
> 3. Bone wax: (Ethicon). It is nonresorbable
>   Cellulose: (Surgicel, ActCel). Dissolves in about 1-2 weeks

Sickle Cell Anemia

It is a hereditary type of chronic hemolytic anemia, characterized by peculiar microscopic appearance of sickle or crescent shaped erythrocytes in the blood (Figs 11.6A and B). There is substitution of valine for glutamine in the β globin chain of the hemoglobin. It is common in females and manifests before the age of 30 years. The patient is weak, short of breath, and easily fatigued. Pain in the joints, limbs, and abdomen, nausea and vomiting is common. Other features are systolic murmur and cardiomegaly.

Features and Dental Importance

- Mild to severe generalized osteoporosis and a loss of trabeculation of the jaw bones with the appearance of large, irregular marrow spaces.
- Lateral skull radiograph demonstrates 'hair on end' appearance.
- Dental treatment should be scheduled shortly after blood transfusion.
- Stress should be minimum, as significant stress might decrease the child's ability to oxygenate tissues adequately.
- Control of infection is important as most of the patients with sickle cell disease have generalized osteoporosis of the mandible and greater tendency

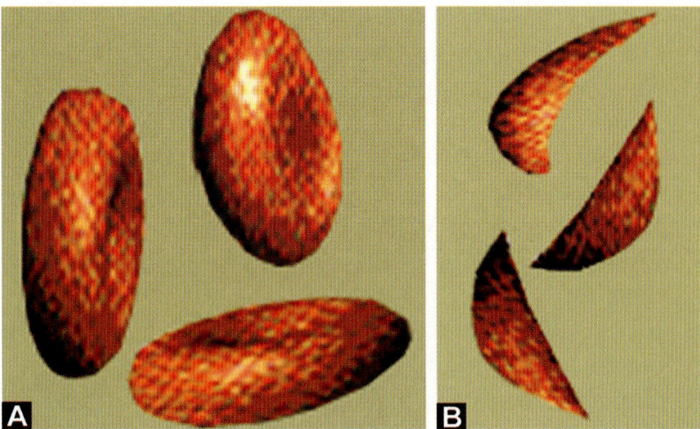

Figs 11.6A and B: Changes seen in red blood cells; (A) Normal Red blood cells; (B) Sickle shaped cells

to develop infection, which could in turn precipitate a sickle cell crisis.

- Functional asplenia may result due to chronic fibrosis of the spleen.
- For sedation, only drugs that do not depress respiration should be used.
- Local anesthesia is not contraindicated, but drugs that tend to cause methemaglobin should be avoided.

Thalassemia

- Two types of thalassemia exists—α thalassemia (minor) and β thalassemia (major).
- There is production of unstable hemoglobins that damage the erythrocytes and increase their vulnerability to destruction. It is observed within the first two years of life. The child has a yellowish pallor of the skin with fever, chills, malaise and generalized weakness. Splenomegaly and hepatomegaly may cause protrusion of the abdomen. Intercurrent infection are seen and the child may die within a few months.

Dental Implications and Management

- Mongoloid face with prominent cheek bones and protrusion of maxillary anterior teeth and depression of the nasal bridge.
- Hair on end appearance in the lateral skull radiograph.
- Osteoporotic changes are seen.
- Consultation with the hematologist. Treatment is avoided if hemoglobin is less than 100 g/L.
- Dental treatment should be scheduled shortly after blood transfusion.

Leukemia

There are basic 2 types of leukemia. They are lymphoblastic and myeloid leukemia. They can be acute or chronic. Acute lymphoblastic leukemia is common in children.

Management of leukemia includes use of anti-leukemic drugs in the first phase. The second phase includes chemotherapy and irradiation. The third phase is the use of relatively nontoxic drugs.

Clinical features of leukemia

It can be attributed to anemia, granulocytopenia and thrombocytopenia resulting from the replacement of normal bone marrow by undifferentiated blast cells.

- Fatigue and weight loss
- Anemia
- Purpura
- Infection and febrile episodes
- Hepatosplenomegaly and lymphadenopathy
- Bone pain
- Regional lymphadenopathy
- Gingival bleeding and hypertrophy
- Candidiasis
- Loose teeth

Dental Management

- Consultation with the oncologist.
- All elective dental treatment to be deferred in children whose first remission is not obtained.
- If the child is still undergoing chemotherapy but is in complete remission, routine preventive, restorative and surgical procedure can be done.
- Routine blood profile is preferred to reduce the risk of hemorrhage and infection. But if the child is under remission for not less than 2 years and is not undergoing any therapy, then the child can be treated like routine patient.
- Pulp therapy in deciduous teeth is contraindicated even in remission stage.
- Platelet count should be more than $50,000/mm^2$ prior to any routine preventive and restorative treatment that does not require injections. If the count is less than $20,000\ mm^2$, platelet transfusion is a must before any treatment, even prophylaxis.
- Absolute neutrophil count is a better indicator of the child's susceptibility to infection. If it is less than $1000/mm^2$, (Normal is >1500), elective dental treatment should be deferred and may require broad spectrum antibiotic therapy.

Dental Effects of Radiation Therapy

- Salivary gland damage and xerostomia is temporary in children, because of the lower dosage of radiation and greater regenerative capacity.
- Lower incidence of radiation caries.
- Enamel hypoplasia, altered crown morphology, shortness and tapering of roots, abnormal root

curvature, rootless teeth and tooth agenesis are common side effects.
- Micrognathia and retrognathia.

Dental Effects of Chemotherapy

- The chemotherapeutic agents do not differentiate the normal from the abnormal cells. Their target are the rapidly differentiating cells. Unfortunately even other cell such as the ameloblasts and the odontoblasts are damaged resulting in abnormalities of dental development.
- Microdontia, enlarged pulp chambers, shortening, thinning and blunting of root and delayed eruption have been found.
- Enamel opacities, hypocalcification and a high caries rate have also been noted.

Organ Transplantation

Dental Implication and Management

- Immunosuppressive agents such as corticosteroids and cyclosporine are given to prevent the organ rejection following transplant. Cyclosporin is nephrotoxic and hepatotoxic and also causes hypertension. Gingival overgrowth results from treatment with cyclosporin.
- Elimination of all possible sites of infection is very important through meticulous oral hygiene program
- Teeth with large carious lesions even if not pulpally involved should be extracted. Primary teeth soon to exfoliate should also be removed.
- Gingivectomy is done to manage gingival overgrowth
- Antibiotics for invasive treatment should be prescribed.

Bone Marrow Transplantation

Dental Management

- Dental treatment should be performed at least 2 weeks prior to induction of chemotherapy or total body irradiation to allow adequate healing.
- Chlorhexidine 0.2% mouthwashes and gels applied to the mucosa with toothettes to reduce mucositis.
- Local hemorrhage can be controlled with topical thrombin, Epsilon-aminocaproic acid.
- Epsilon Antibiotic coverage for all procedures.

Children on Anticoagulants

They are used for children with valvular heart disease and prosthetic valves.

Commonly used anticoagulant drugs are:

Warfarin—vitamin K antagonist (factor II, VII, IX and X) 3-4 days are required for full onset, and assesed by prothrombin level.
Heparin—Shorter acting, immediate onset, given IV—inhibits factors IX, X, XII.

Dental Management

- Prevention of infection is very important.
- Local measures to prevent excessive bleeding includes application of topical thrombin, packing with microfibrillar collagen hemostat or oxidized cellulose.
- Admission to hospital.

DENTAL OFFICE ACCESS

- Wider width of the doorways to allow easy movement of the wheelchair, etc.
- Equipments can be arranged on a trolley so that it is convenient to bring them near the patient.
- Dental chair should be adjustable for height to match different wheel chair designs.
- Additional time with the parent and the child is needed to establish rapport and dispel the child's anxiety.
- If patient cooperation is difficult to obtain then physical restraints or sedatives should be considered. Sedatives and physical restraints are considered in chapter 8.

Protective stabilization for special child:

Consent of the parents should be taken prior to the use of physical restraints. They are useful and effective in facilitating the delivery of dental care for patients who need help controlling their extremities and for managing extremely resistant patients who need dental care but who are not candidates for general anesthesia.

SPECIAL CONSIDERATIONS IN DENTAL MANAGEMENT

- Special attention should be given. Names and addresses of medical or dental personnel who have previously treated the patient are necessary for consultation purpose.
- Patients should be scheduled early in the day and sufficient time should be allowed to talk with the parents and the patient before initiating any dental care.

Radiographic Examination

- Modification needed to hold the child should be considered. Assistance may be required from the parents or the dental auxillary. Floss may be attached to the film through a hole made in the bite tab.
- Adequate protection with lead apron and thyroid collar should be provided to the patient and the assistant.

Preventive Methodologies

Preventing oral disease is the most desirable way of ensuring good dental health for any dental patient.

Home Care

- Parents or the guardian have the initial responsibility.
- Reinforcement of good home dental care and constant evaluation is required.
- Home dental care should begin in infancy with a soft cloth or an infant toothbrush.
- Parents should be taught the correct brushing techniques by safely restraining the child when needed.
- Wrapped tongue blades may be used to keep the child's mouth open.
- A plaque program for the disabled should be simple and yet effective. One method recommended is the horizontal scrub as it is easy and can yield good results.
- Some modifications can be made to the brush to help persons with poor fine motor skills improve their brushing techniques (Figs 11.7A to C). Electric tooth brushes can also be used effectively.

Diet and Nutrition

- It should be kept in mind the eating pattern of a child and the extent of disability while prescribing diet. For example a child with cerebral palsy may require the intake of pureed diet.
- Particular emphasis should be made on the discontinuation of the bottle feed by 12 months of age to decrease the likelihood of nursing caries.

Fluoride

- The judicious use of systemic fluoride is very important in the comprehensive management of any dental patient.
- Fluoride level of the patient's daily water supply should be estimated and the recommendation of the systemic fluoride depends upon this.
- Whether the patient lives in a fluoridated area or a non-fluoridated area, topical fluoride should be applied.
- Fluoride dentifrice and rinses should be prescribed to be used daily and depends on individual patient's ability to expectorate. Fluoride varnish are ideal for children who do not expectorate.

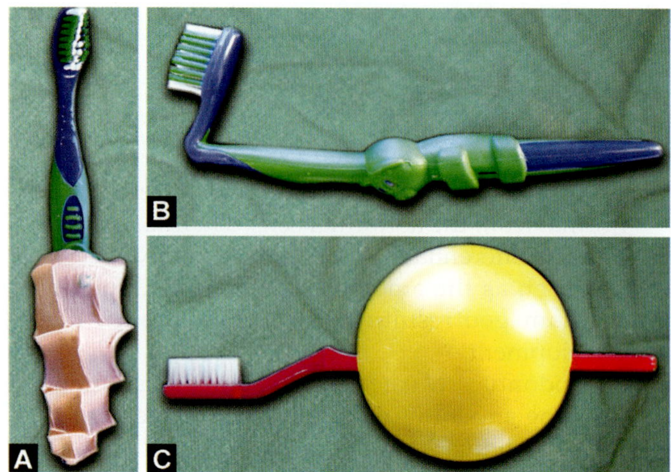

Figs 11.7A to C: Modifications made to a normal toothbrush to be used by disabled child: (A) Impression of the hand grip in acrylic molded on to the handle; (B) Additional angulation provided to the brush as per necessary; (C) Rubber ball is perforated and the handle is passed through it

Pit and Fissure Sealant

It is shown to reduce occlusal caries effectively and should be used whenever indicated.

Disabled Children can be Divided into three Groups for the Purpose of Teaching Oral Hygiene

A. Self-care group
B. Partial care group
C. Total care group.

Self-Care Group

- Those able to brush their own teeth but needing some encouragement and minimal supervision.
- Easiest to work with.
- Modification of brushes may be necessary.
- Communication must be maintained with the parents and teachers, since the parents are usually the ones who supervise the individual in the daily care.

Partial Care Group

- Those able to carry out only part of their oral hygiene needs and requiring considerable training and direct supervision to complete the job properly.
- Individuals of this group will be moderately disabled and often retarded.
- They require close supervision and direct assistance to perform the routine tasks of everyday living.
- Patients of this group will not understand the long-term benefits of brushing their teeth.

- In teaching this group, one must not expect rapid learning. Every step has to be repeated until it is mastered.

Total Care Group

- Those unable to assist in any way in their own care and must be assisted by a second party.
- Composed of mainly severely disabled who may never be able to be of much assistance in cleaning their own teeth.
- Electric tooth brush may be superior to conventional brushes and makes it easier for the parent or caretaker to master brushing the individual's teeth.

Position of the Child and the Caretaker

1. *Standing:* Caretaker stands behind the child and cradles the child's head in one arm, holding the lower jaw open in the same arm and brushing with the other. Usually used for the larger child or an adult.
2. *Sofa:* Caretaker sits on the sofa and the child lies with his head on the caretaker's lap.
3. *Lap:* Caretaker sits on the chair and the child, usually a toddler lies on the lap with head slightly hanging down to assist in opening the mouth.
   Extra assistance in each position may be advantageous.

Modification of Toothbrushes

This may be required as the children may find it difficult to hold the normal brush:
- Banded to the hand by the velcro strap.
- Handle of the brush can be lengthened by attaching a stick.
- Rubber ball perforated to hold the brush.
- Foam rubber can be rolled around the handle.
- Self-cure acrylic handle can be added and hand impression made.
- Angulation can be given to the head of the brush.
- Bicycle handle bar.

Different types of responses exhibited by a special child may be as follows:

- Overwhelming fear—fight strenuously
- Relaxed and happy—have no fear and enjoy the entire session
- Some may tolerate only superficial examination and will not voluntarily set foot outside the waiting room area
- They may come to the dental operatory quite happily, show curiosity about the equipment, enjoy a ride on the chair yet resist an examination. They may clamp their mouth shut, purse their lips, gag, grab the examiners hands and pull them away or even resist more actively by biting, kicking or scratching.

REFERENCES

1. American Academy of Pediatric Dentistry. Guideline on management of dental patients with special health care needs. Pediatr Dent (Supp Issue: Ref manual 2008-09); 30:15.
2. World Health Organization. International Classification of Impairments, Disabilities and Handicaps: a manual of classification relating to the consequences of disease. Geneva, 1980.
3. Troutman KC. The handicapped child as a dental problem. Temple Dent Rev 1970;40:4.
4. Waldman HB. Almost four million children with disabilities. J Dent Child 1995;62:205-9.
5. Tesini DA, Fenton SJ. Oral health needs of persons with physical or mental disabilities. Dent Clin North Am 1994;38:483-97.
6. Nowak AJ. Dental disease in handicapped persons. Spec Care Dent 1984;4:66-9.
7. Nelson KB, Ellenberg JH. Children who "outgrew" cerebral palsy. Pediatrics 1982;69:529-36.
8. American Psychiatric Association. Diagnostic and statistical manual of mental disorders. 4th edition, Washington DC 1994.
9. Dajani AS, Taubert KA, Wilson W, et al. Prevention of bacterial endocarditis: recommendations by the American Heart Association. J Am Dent Assoc 1997;128: 1142-51.
10. Verrusio AC. A mechanism for closure of the secondary palate. Teratology 1970;3:17.
11. Trasler PG, Fraser FC. Role of tongue in producing cleft palate in mice with spontaneous cleft lip. Dev Biol 1963;6:45.
12. Avery JK. Prenatal growth in Moyers RE. Handbook of Orthodontics 4th Ed. Year Book Medical Publishers, Inc. Chicago 1988.
13. Fraser FC, Walker BE, Trasler DG. Experimental production of congenital cleft palate, genetic and environmental factors. Pediatrics 1957;19.
14. Warkany J, Kalter H. Congenital malformations. N Engl J Med 1961;265:993.
15. Davis JS, Ritchie HP. Classification of congenital clefts of the lip and palate. J Amer. Med Ass 1922;79:1323.
16. Anderson F. Inheritance of Harelip and Cleft Palate. Arnold Busck 1942.
17. Veau V. Division Palatine. Masson. Paris. 1931.
18. Kernahan DA. The striped Y – A new classification for cleft lip and palate. Plast Reconstr Surg 1971;47:469-70.
19. Kernahan DA, Stark RB. A new classification for cleft lip and palate. Plast Reconstr Surg 1958;22:435.
20. Centers for Disease Control and Prevention (CDC): Recommendations and Reports: classification system for HIV infection and expanded surveillance case definition for AIDS among adolescents and adults. MMWR 1992;41(RR-17):1.
21. Kanner L. Early infantile autism. Journal of Pediatrics 1943;25:211-7.
22. Mc Bee WL, Koemer KR. Review of Hemostatic Agents Used in Dentistry. Dentistry Today 2005;62-5.

FURTHER READING

1. American Academy of Pediatric Dentistry Clinical Affairs Committee. Guideline on dental management of pediatric patients receiving chemotherapy, hema-topoietic cell transplantation, and/or radiation. Pediatr Dent 2005-2006;27(7 Reference Manual):170-5.

2. American Academy of Pediatric Dentistry Council on Clinical Affairs. Policy on management of patients with cleft lip/palate and other craniofacial anomalies. Pediatr Dent 2005-2006;27(7 Reference Manual):187-8.

3. American Academy of Pediatric Dentistry Council on Clinical Affairs. Guideline on the role of dental prophylaxis in pediatric dentistry. Pediatr Dent 2005-2006;27(7 Reference Manual):87-9.

4. American Academy of Pediatric Dentistry Council on Clinical Affairs. Guideline on management of persons with special health care needs. Pediatr Dent 2005-2006;27(7 Reference Manual):80-3.

5. Boyle N, Gallagher C, Sleeman D. Antibiotic prophylaxis for bacterial endocarditis—a study of knowledge and application of guidelines among dentists and cardiologists. J Ir Dent Assoc 2006 Spring; 51(5):232-7.

6. Chuang SF, Sung JM, Kuo SC, Huang JJ, Lee SY. Oral and dental manifestations in diabetic and nondiabetic uremic patients receiving hemodialysis. Oral Surg Oral Med Oral Pathol Oral Radiol Endod 2005;99(6):689-95.

7. Cogulu D, Sabah E, Kutukculer N, Ozkinay F. Evaluation of the relationship between caries indices and salivary secretory IgA, salivary pH, buffering capacity and flow rate in children with Down's syndrome. Arch Oral Biol 2006;51(1):23-8. Epub 2005 Jul 22.

8. Frachon X, Pommereuil M, Berthier AM, Lejeune S, Hourdin-Eude S, Quero J, et al. Management options for dental extraction in hemophiliacs: a study of 55 extractions (2000-2002). Oral Surg Oral Med Oral Pathol Oral Radiol Endod 2005;99(3):270-5.

9. Frezzini C, Leao JC, Cedro M, Porter S. Aspects of HIV disease relevant to dentistry in the 21st century. Dent Update 2006;33(5):276-8, 281-2, 285-6.

10. Gill DS, Gill SK, Tredwin CJ, Naini FB. Adult and paediatric basic life support: An update for the dental team. Br Dent J 2007;202(4):209-12.

11. Latham RA. Bilateral cleft lip and palate: Improved maxillary and dental development. Plast Reconstr Surg 2007;119(1):287-97.

12. Milano M, Lee JY, Donovan K, Chen JW. A cross-sectional study of medication-related factors and caries experience in asthmatic children. Pediatr Dent 2006;28(5):415-9.

13. Nomura R, Nakano K, Nemoto H, Fujita K, Inagaki S, Takahashi T, et al. Isolation and characterization of *Streptococcus mutans* in heart valve and dental plaque specimens from a patient with infective endocarditis. J Med Microbiol 2006;55(8):1135-40.

14. Piot B, Sigaud-Fiks M, Huet P, Fressinaud E, Trossaert M, Mercier J. Management of dental extractions in patients with bleeding disorders. Oral Surg Oral Med Oral Pathol Oral Radiol Endod 2002;93(3):247-50.

15. Pomarico L, Souza IP, Rangel Tura LF. Sweetened medicines and hospitalization: Caries risk factors in children with and without special needs. Eur J Paediatr Dent 2005;6(4):197-201.

16. Press N, Montessori V. Prophylaxis for infective endocarditis. Who needs it? How effective is it? Can Fam Physician 2000;46:2248-55.

17. Roberts GJ, Jaffray EC, Spratt DA, Petrie A, Greville C, Wilson M, et al. Duration, prevalence and intensity of bacteraemia after dental extractions in children. Heart. 2006;92(9):1274-7. Epub 2006 Feb 17.

18. Suzuki Y, Daitoku K, Minakawa M, Fukui K, Fukuda I. Infective endocarditis with congenital heart disease. Jpn J Thorac Cardiovasc Surg 2006;54(7):297-300.

19. Zaromb A, Chamberlain D, Schoor R, Almas K, Blei F. Periodontitis as a manifestation of chronic benign neutropenia. J Periodontol 2006;77(11):1921-6.

QUESTIONS

1. Define the American Academy of Pediatric Dentistry definition for individuals with special health care needs.
2. What is the difference between defect and disability?
3. Classify handicapping conditions.
4. Define cerebral palsy and explain its different types.
5. Classify intellectual disability and explain its types.
6. Give the antibiotic prophylaxis for congenital cardiac disease.
7. Classify cleft lip and palate.
8. What is a feeding plate?
9. What are the precautions to be taken in a child with leukemia?
10. Dental considerations in a child with HIV infection.
11. Give the preventive strategy for a child with special health care needs.

Radiology in Pedodontic Practice

INTRODUCTION

Radiographs act as an important diagnostic tool in the treatment of children. Dental pain and other related complications can be avoided if the caries is diagnosed early. Developmental problems related to eruptive abnormalities or associated with growth can be identified with the use of radiographs and early management of these problems may reduce the need for prolonged orthodontic procedures in the later life.

Selection of the appropriate radiograph for the child patient depends on the age of the child, the size of the oral cavity and the level of patient cooperation. Ideal technique should expose the patient to a minimum amount of radiation, require as few radiographs as possible, take as little time as possible and provide an adequate examination of the dentition and supporting structures.

POINTS TO BE CONSIDERED BEFORE PLANNING FOR RADIOGRAPHS

- Avoiding retakes by obtaining the previous radiographic history, following the appropriate guidelines for the correct size, number and type of film used, all area to be radiographed should be included within the film borders, avoiding cone cut, overlapping, elongation, shortening and correctly processing the film.
- Radiographs should be an adjunct for clinical examination and should not replace full mouth clinical examination.
- Determination of appropriate number and size of films required to take radiographs of the particular region and unnecessarily not the whole mouth.
- Placement of lead apron and thyroid collar on the patient and parent.

Components of X-ray machine (Fig. 12.1)

1. The X-ray tube head and the positioning device.
The tube head consists of:
A. The cathode which serves as a source of electrons. It consists of a filament and a focusing cup. The focusing cup directs the electrons generated by the filament to the focal spot (spot on the target).
B. The anode or the target at which the beam of high speed electrons is directed. It is composed of tungsten

Contd...

Contd...

target and copper stem. It helps to convert the kinetic energy of the electrons into X-ray photons.

The positioning device is used to position the tube head in correct position while taking the radiographs.

2. Power supply:

The primary function of power supply is:

A. To provide a current to heat the X-ray tube filament (achieved by a step down transformer).

B. To create a potential difference between the anode and cathode (achieved by a high voltage transformer).

3. Timer:

It is a timing device. It controls the X-ray production time by controlling the time that the high voltage is applied to the tube.

An IOPA film packet consists of (Fig. 12.2): From the side facing the X-ray tube

1. Outer wrapper made of plastic material
2. A black paper on either side of the film protects it from light
3. Film
4. A thin sheet of lead foil placed behind the film prevents residual radiation passing beyond the film and prevents back scatter radiation.

For young children, where movement during filming is a problem, the need for short exposure time is a first priority. When exposure time is shortened, compensation must be made in terms of increased mA or kVp. If mA cannot be increased then it is necessary to use high kVp.

Factors affecting radiographic quality:

Quality of the radiograph depends upon the density, contrast, sharpness, distortion and speed.

i. Density:

The density of a radiograph is a measure of its blackness. It is determined by the amount of radiation reaching the film and the sensitivity of the film to radiation. Factors that affect film density are:

a. Exposure: Increasing milliamperage (mA), Operating voltage, kVp or time of exposure will increase the density.

b. Subject thickness: The thicker the object the more attenuation of the beam is seen.

c. Object density: Greater the density of an object or an area within the object, the greater is the attenuation of the X-ray beam directed through the object or area.

d. Film speed

e. Source-to-film distance.

Contd...

ii. Contrast:

It is defined as the difference in densities between various regions on Film. A film has high contrast if the radiolucent portions are quite black and the radiopaque lesions are very white. Factors determining level of film contrast include:

a. Tube voltage: Increased kVp decreases film contrast. The X-rays produced at higher tube voltage have greater penetrating power. Selection of kilovoltage depends on the age of patient.

b. Film contrast capability (built in by manufacturer)

c. Film-processing technique.

iii. Distortion:

Variations in distortion include:

a. True (Proportional) enlargement

b. Elongation or foreshortening

c. Superimposition

d. Overlapping of structures

iv. Sharpness:

Factors important in obtaining a sharp image are:

a. Small X-ray source

b. Appropriate source object—film distances.

c. Lack of motion of cone, patient or films during exposure.

v. Speed:

Speed refers to the amount of radiation required to produce a radiographic film of standard density. The speed of a dental X-ray film is indicated by letter designating its speed group. Only films with speed D or E are indicated for intraoral radiography. A fast film relatively requires a low exposure.

General recommendations for radiologic dental examination of children

1. Exposure should be made only after taking a history and completing clinical examination and should be to supplement and not substitute for this clinical examination. If the child is a new patient but has been earlier seen by another dentist then access to, or copies of previous radiographs should be sought.

2. X-ray equipment and darkroom procedures should be well controlled to minimize unnecessary radiation and poor quality processing.

3. Fast film and rectangular collimination should be used. Correct size and number of films should be used.

4. Long cone technique with a 70-90 kVp is encouraged wherever possible. If a child does not tolerate film holders in the mouth, then the bisecting angle technique may be used.

5. Operators should be well trained to minimize the likelihood of unnecessary retakes.

6. Lead apron and thyroid collars must be used.

Contd...

Factors controlling X-ray beam:

i. Tube voltage:
Tube voltage is measured in kVp. As the kVp increases it results in an increased efficiency of conversion of electron energy into X-ray photons. High energy X-ray photons (short wavelength) are preferred as they have a greater probability of penetrating matter.

ii. Exposure time:
When the time of exposure is doubled the number of photons generated is doubled, but the range of photon energies is unchanged. Thus, the effect of increasing the exposure time helps to increase the number of photons that are generated and thus to control the "quantity" of the exposure.

iii. Tube Current:
There is a linear relationship between tube current and tube output. Thus, doubling the tube current should double the number of photons produced.

iv. Filtration:
Out of the X-ray photons of different energy levels only those with sufficient energy to penetrate anatomic structures are useful for diagnostic radiology. Photons with low penetrating powers (long wavelength) contribute only to the patient exposure and not for the quality of the film. Low power photons are removed for the safety of the patients by placing aluminium filter in the path of beam.

v. Collimation:
When X-ray beam is directed at a patient, only about 10% pass through as the information carrying beam and are available to form an image on a film whereas 90% of the X-ray photons are absorbed by the tissues and generate scattered radiation within the exposed tissues. They also tend to fog the film and degrade the image. The detrimental effect of scattered radiation on the formation of image can be minimized by reducing amount of scattered radiation formed and by preventing this radiation from reaching the film through collimation. Collimation reduces the size of X-ray beam and thus the volume of irradiated tissue. Diaphragm, tubular and rectangular collimation are used in dentistry.

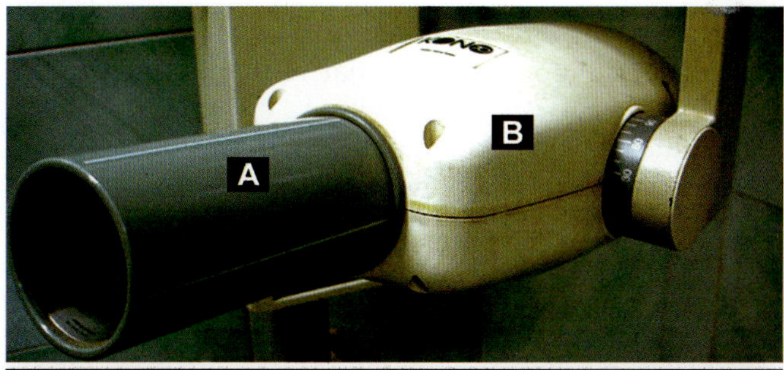

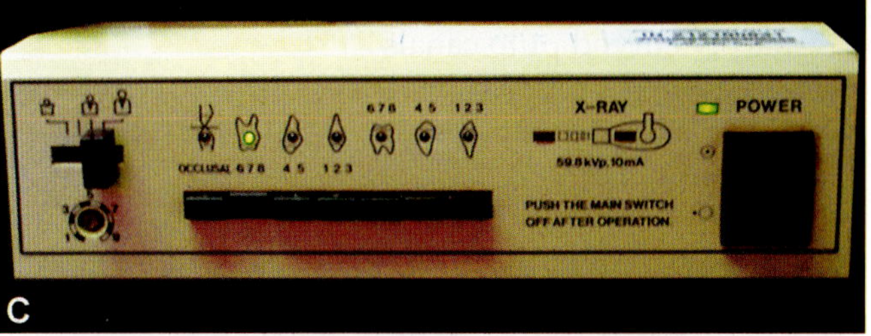

Fig. 12.1: Dental X-ray machine: (A) Positioning device; (B) Tube head; (C) Control panel or the timer

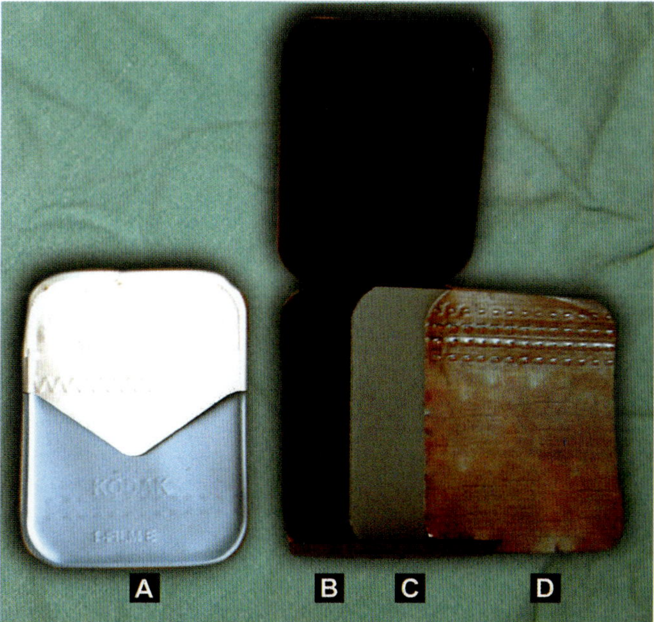

Fig. 12.2: Components of IOPA film packet: (A) Outer plastic wrapper; (B) Black paper; (C) Film; (D) Lead foil

PURPOSE FOR PRESCRIBING RADIOGRAPHS

It depends on the following criteria:

Evaluation of the Development of Dentition

This can be done by observing the radiographs for the following:

A. Stages of development, eruption and exfoliation of teeth
B. Amount of root formation
C. Physiologic root resorption
D. Amount of bone over the erupting tooth
E. Degree of pulp maturity.

Pathologic Evaluation

It includes:

A. Caries detection
B. Evaluation of traumatic injuries

C. Degree of pulp involvement such as proximity of caries to pulp horn, internal resorption or calcific degeneration
D. Evaluation of periodontal health by observing thickness of periodontal ligament, furcation involvement, bone loss, external resorption, etc.

Detection of Developmental Anomalies

Commonly observed anomalies are:
A. Widely divergent roots
B. Sharply curved pulp canals
C. Alterations in the number and length of roots
D. Ectopically positioned teeth
E. Ankylosis
F. Supernumerary teeth
G. Congenitally missing teeth
H. Malformed teeth such as microdontia, macrodontia, dens in dente, taurodontism, gemination, fusion, root dilacerations, etc.

Post-treatment Evaluation

It is done to evaluate:
A. Accuracy of treatment
B. Type and success of pulp treatment
C. Postsurgical healing
D. Treatment failure.

Routine Evaluation based on Risk Assessment

Low-risk Child

Healthy, asymptomatic patient (no evidence of caries, trauma, anomalies or malocclusion), exposed to optimum levels of fluoride, performing daily preventive technique, consuming a diet with few exposures to retentive carbohydrates between meals
- With closed proximal contact: Bite wing radiograph is taken on the first visit and when there are no caries, radiograph may be taken once a year for early intervention.
- With open proximal contact: Radiographs may be taken once in two years.

High-risk Child

- Radiographs are taken more often as twice a year. Bite wing radiographs should be taken as soon as the deciduous molars are in proximal contact.

Due to the relatively high frequency of caries among 5-year-old children, it is recommended to consider dental radiography for each child even without any visible caries or restorations. Furthermore, radiography should be considered at 8-9 years of age and then at 12-14, that is 1-2 years after eruption of premolars and second molars. Additional bitewing controls should be based on an overall assessment of the caries activity/risk. The high-risk patient should be examined radiographically annually, while a 2-3 years interval should be considered when caries activity/risk is low. Routine survey by radiographs, except for caries, has not been shown to provide sufficient information to be justified considering the balance between cost (radiation and resources) and benefit. (EAPD guidelines for use of radiographs in children [Eur J Paediatr Dent. 2003;4:40-8)]

Radiographs taken for routine evaluation		
Age (years)	*Consideration*	*Radiograph*
3-5	Nothing Abnormal - open contact - closed contact Extensive caries Deep caries	None None 4 film survey 4 film survey + IOPA of selected tooth
6-7	Nothing abnormal Extensive caries, deep caries	8 film survey 8 film survey+ IOPA of selected tooth
8-9	-do-	12 film survey
10-12	-do-	12 or 16 film survey

Film Surveys

- 4 film—2 anterior occlusal + 2 bite wing.
- 8 film—4 posterior IOPA + 2 anterior occlusal + 2 bite wing.
- 12 film—4 posterior IOPA + 4 canine IOPA + 2 incisor IOPA + 2 bite wing.
- 16 film—12 film survey + 4 permanent molar radiographs.

CHILD PREPARATION AND MANAGEMENT (FIGS 12.3A TO C)

Taking a radiograph may be the child's first dental experience. So it has to be made as pleasant as possible. Euphemisms should be used with TSD technique. (By bringing the X-ray tube near the parents face or a doll's face first, helps to dispel any fear the child may have). Modelling behavior management technique will also help reduce fear. Parents or siblings can play the role of a model. Children are also more willing or cooperative if they know that they are required to hold the film in the mouth for a limited period of time.

Tips to assist radiographic process

- Dampen the film, as it removes the taste of the packet
- Do not insert the film directly but take it horizontally and then slowly rotate it into vertical position (Fig. 12.4)

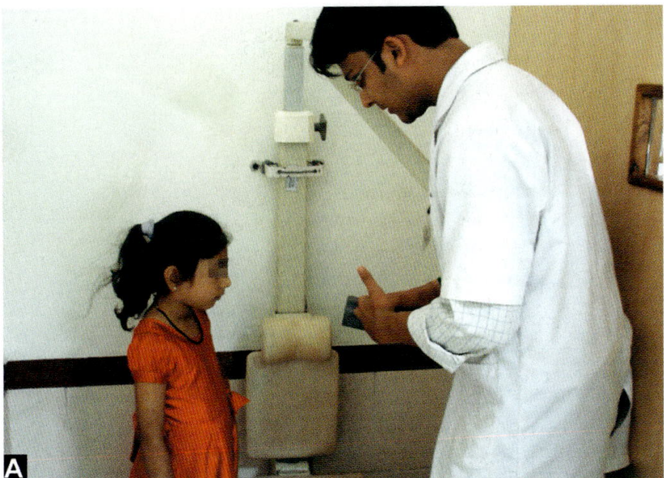

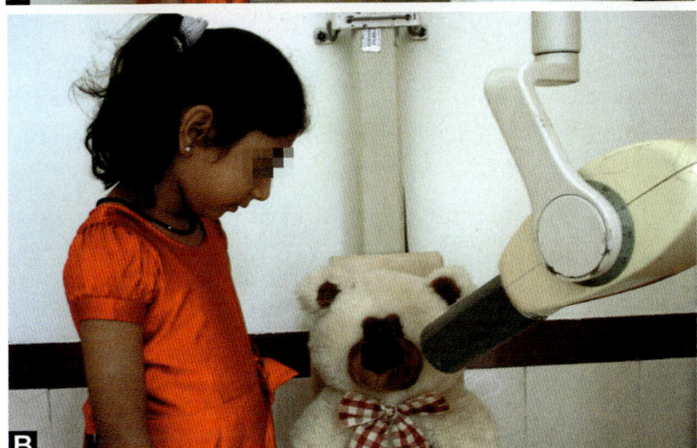

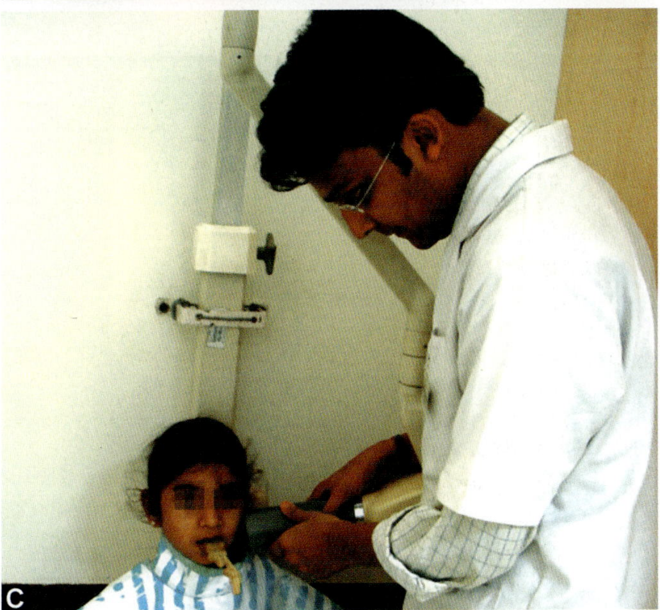

Figs 12.3A to C: Tell show do (TSD) technique for preparing the child to be radiographed: (A) The child is explained and the X-ray machine is compared to a camera; (B) The X-ray tube is placed near doll's mouth; (C) The X-ray is taken once the child is cooperative and ready

- Before inserting, curve the film slightly so that it will not impinge on the tissues.

METHODS OF REDUCING RADIATION EXPOSURE

Children are at higher risk from radiation exposure because of the following reasons:

1. Tissues are in growth and hence more sensitive for radiation
2. Longer life span of children making them more susceptible for tumors
3. Effects of radiation are cumulative
4. Because of their smaller stature, children are closer to the central beam of X-ray.
5. Due to increased caries activity, children my need more frequent radiographs
   - Wearing lead apron and thyroid collar (Fig. 12.5)
   - Use of faster speed film (F speed film)
   - Panoramic radiography uses film screen combinations that have reduced exposure time
   - Long rectangular collimator reduces the area unnecessarily exposed to radiation by almost 4 square inches compared to a round collimator
   - Use of higher kilovolt peak (KVP) technique reduces patient exposure
   - Good dark room procedures, thus avoiding retakes.

Intraoral film size (Figs 12.6A to C)

Size 0: Used for bite wing and IOPA of small children

Size 1: Used for anterior teeth in adults

Size 2: Standard film, used for anterior occlusal, IOPA and bite wing in mixed and permanent dentition

Occlusal films: 57 × 76 mm used for maxillary or mandibular occlusal radiographs.

RADIOGRAPHIC TECHNIQUES COMMONLY USED IN CHILDREN

1. Intraoral
   - IOPA
   - Bite wing
   - Occlusal
   - Panoramic
2. Extraoral
   - TMJ and lateral oblique view (film size is 1.5 × 7 inches)

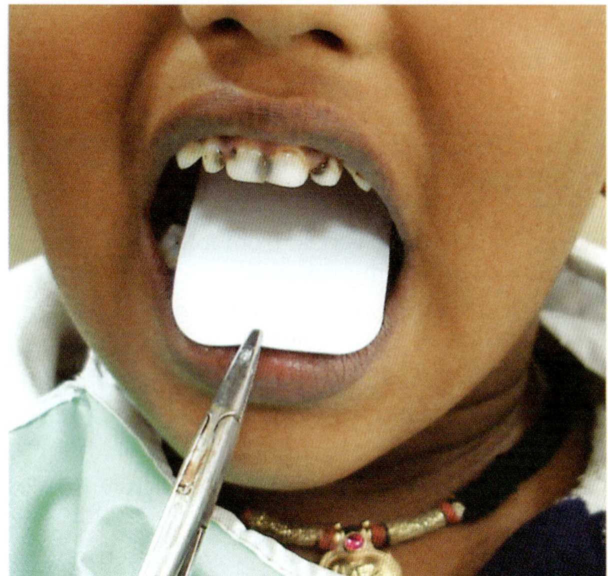

Fig. 12.4: Take the film horizontally and then rotate it to vertical direction

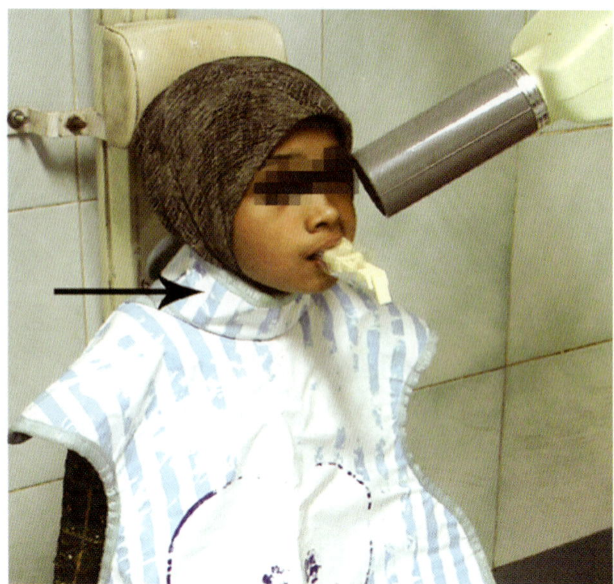

Fig. 12.5: Lead apron and thyroid collar (Arrow) in one unit

– Lateral cephalograms, PNS view (film size is 8 × 10 inches)
– Orthopantomography (film size is 6 × 12 inches)

Composition of X-ray film

1. Base: Polyester, polyethylene terepthalate
2. Adhesive layer: Attaches film emulsion to film base
3. Film emulsion: It is the image receptor system
   It consists of silver bromide crystals with some amount of silver iodide
4. A protective layer of clear gelatin to shield the emulsion from mechanical damage.

Intraoral Periapical (IOPA) Radiographs

Indications (Figs 12.7A to E)

1. To evaluate the development of the root end and to study the periapical tissue
2. To detect alterations in the integrity of the periodontal membrane
3. To evaluate the prognosis of the pulp treatment by observing the health of the periapical tissues
4. To identify the stage of development of unerupted teeth
5. To detect developmental abnormalities like supernumerary, missing or malformed teeth
6. For early detection of pathologic changes associated with teeth
7. For space analysis in the mixed dentition
8. To assess the path of eruption of permanent teeth
9. To evaluate the extent of traumatic injuries to the root and alveolus.

Loss of cancellous bone is undetectable until at least 6.6% of the mineral content of the cortical bone in the direct path of the X-ray beam has been lost. Hence a periapical lesion is usually larger than its radiographic image.

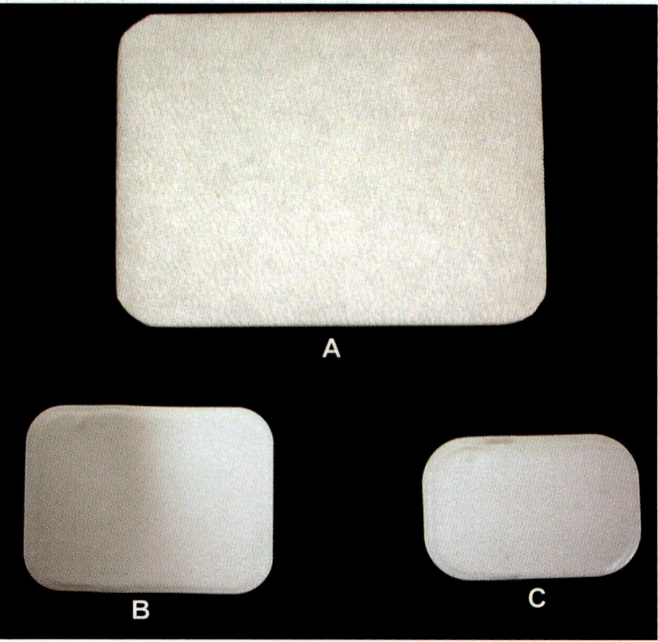

Figs 12.6A to C: Films of different sizes: (A) Occlusal film; (B) Adult or standard film; C: Pedodontic film

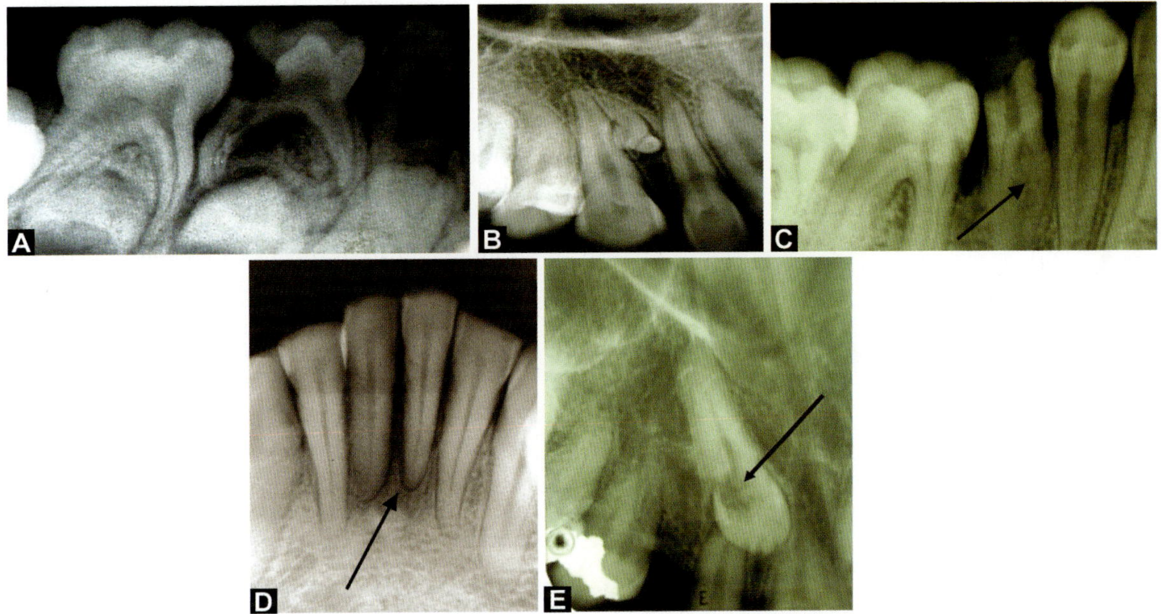

Figs 12.7A to E: Some of the indications of IOPA: (A) Evaluate the extension of caries; (B) Odontome; (C) Bifid premolar root; (D) Pathologic root resorption of lower central incisors; (E) Pre-eruptive caries

Techniques for taking IOPA

Two techniques are recommended for taking IOPA projections. They are:
1. The paralleling technique (Fig. 12.8A)
2. The bisecting angle technique (Fig. 12.8B)
    i. The paralleling technique: The film is positioned in the mouth using extension cone parallel (XCP) instruments (Figs 12.9A and B) or precision film holders such that the film is held parallel to the long axis of the tooth to be radiographed. The X-ray tube head is aimed at right angles to the tooth and the film.
    Advantage
    - Little magnification
    - Periodontal bone level are well represented
    - Radiographs are accurately reproducible by different operators
    Disadvantage
    - Difficult to position the film
    - May not be possible to place the film in shallow palates
    - Apex of the root usually appear at the edge of the film, thus periapical region is not covered adequately
    - Increased radiation exposure.
    ii. The bisecting angle technique: The film is placed close to the tooth to be radiographed using snap a ray film holder (Fig. 12.10) or hemostat (endoray film holder (Fig. 12.11) if endodontic instruments

are placed in the tooth). The X-ray tube is adjusted such that the central ray of the X-ray bisects the angle formed between the long axis of the film and the tooth.
Advantage:
- Film positioning is easy and comfortable for the patient
- If positioned based on correct angulations, the image size does not alter
Disadvantage:
- Variables are many in this technique making it difficult to reproduce accurately every time
- Incorrect vertical angulation results in elongation of the image and incorrect horizontal angulation results in overlapping of the images of the crown and root or cone cut
- Periodontal bone level are not clear
- Detection of proximal caries is difficult

Gagging in children is common while placing the film in the mouth. Some of the common remedies are:

1. Distract the child by asking to count numbers, alternately moving the right and left leg, etc
2. Patient can suck a topical anesthetic lozenge
3. Wetting the Polythene (film packet)
4. Never mention to relax tongue
5. Never slide the film along the palate or tongue
6. Advise patient to breathe rapidly through nose.

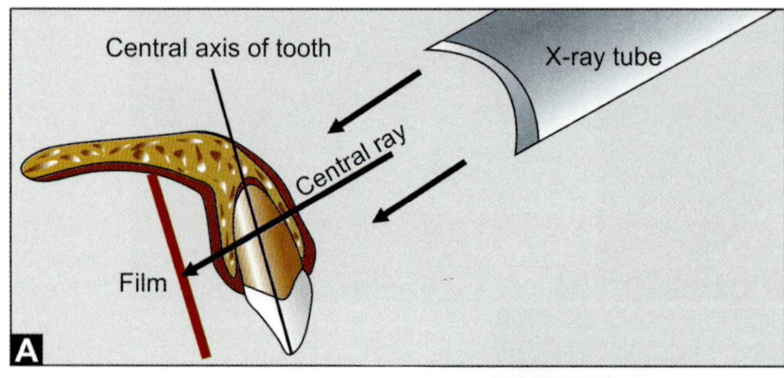

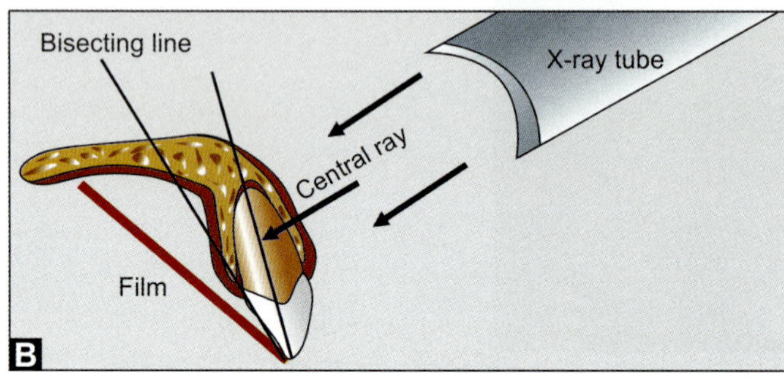

Figs 12.8A and B: Diagrammatic representation of the film and X-ray tube position: (A) Paralleling technique; (B) Bisecting angle technique

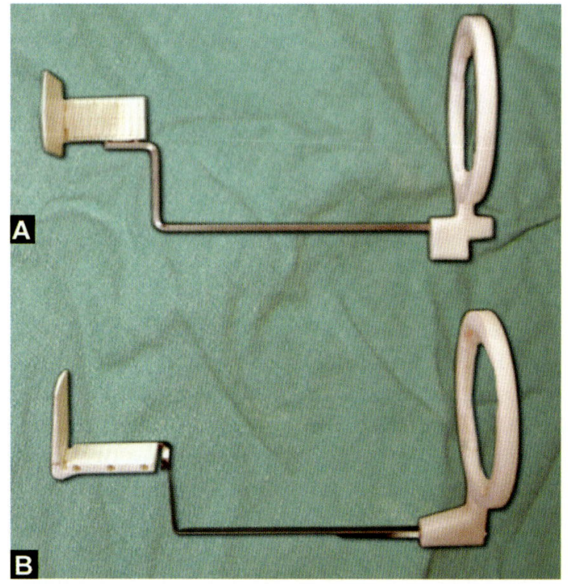

Figs 12.9A and B: XCP instrument: (A) For posterior teeth; (B) For anterior teeth

Procedure steps

- *Behavior management:* Tell Show Do technique is used to obtain the cooperation of the patient.
- *Maxillary teeth (Figs 12.12A and B):* Head of the patient is upright. The film is positioned on the palatal aspect of the teeth by using film holders. The tooth in question will occupy center of the film.

The X-ray cone is kept at the correct angulation and the central X-ray beam is directed perpendicular to the film while using long cone technique. When bisecting angle technique is used the central beam is directed perpendicular to an imaginary bisector that bisects the angle formed by the long axis of the tooth and the film.

- *Mandibular teeth (Figs 12.13A and B):* The film is kept on the floor of the mouth, on the lingual side. The tooth in question will occupy center of the film. The X-ray cone is kept at the correct angulation and the central X-ray beam is directed perpendicular to the film while using long cone technique. When bisecting angle technique is used the central beam is directed perpendicular to an imaginary bisector that bisects the angle formed by the long axis of the tooth and the film.

Angulations used for IOPA projections		
(White and Pharaoh):		
	Maxilla	*Mandible*
Anterior teeth	+ 40	− 15
Canines	+ 45	− 20
Premolars	+ 30	− 10
Molars	+ 20	− 5

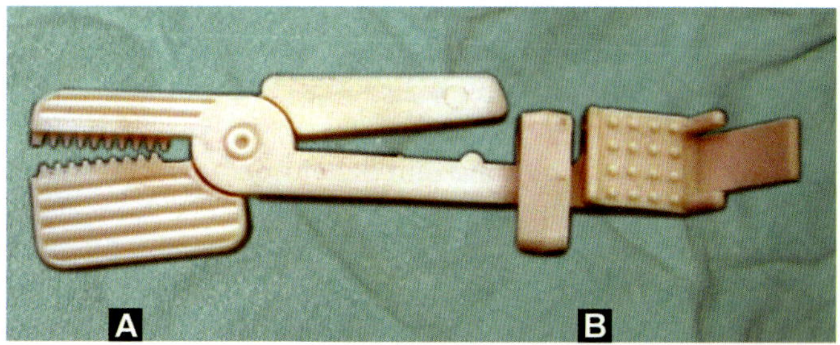

Fig. 12.10: Snap A ray film holder. It has two ends for Posterior (A) and Anterior (B) teeth

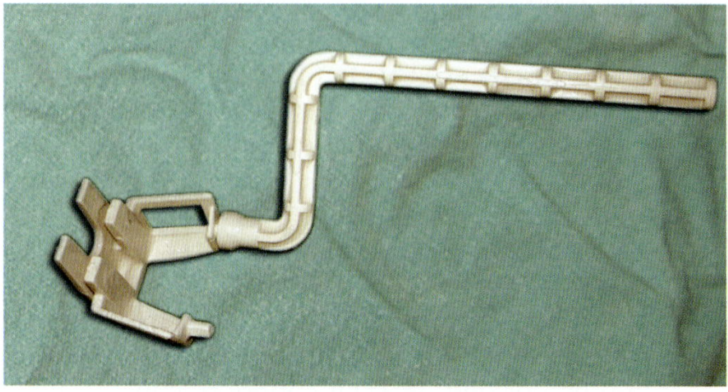

Fig. 12.11: Endoray film holder

Bite Wing Radiographs

Indications (Fig. 12.14)

- Early detection of incipient interproximal caries
- To understand the configuration of the pulp chamber
- Record the width of spaces created by premature loss of deciduous teeth
- Determine the presence or absence of premolar teeth
- To determine the relation of a tooth to the occlusal plane for possibility of tooth Ankylosis
- Detect levels of periodontal bone at the interdental area
- Detect secondary caries

Technique

The head is positioned such that the midsagittal plane is perpendicular and the ala-tragus line is parallel to the floor. The lower edge of the film is placed in the floor of the mouth between the tongue and the lingual aspect of the mandible and the bite tab is placed on the occlusal surfaces of the mandibular teeth. The film is positioned to cover all the region of concern. The central ray enters at the occlusal plane at a point below the pupil, vertical angle being +8 degrees. A tab or bite platform or unibite film holders can be used to postion the film parallel to the occlusal plane (Figs 12.15A and B).

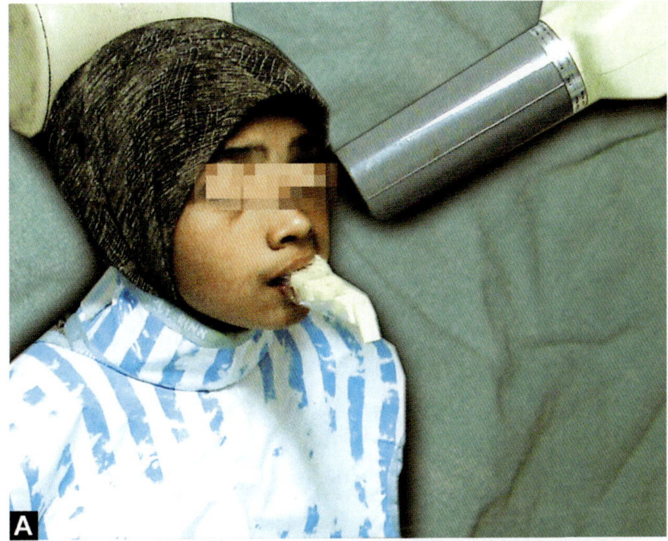
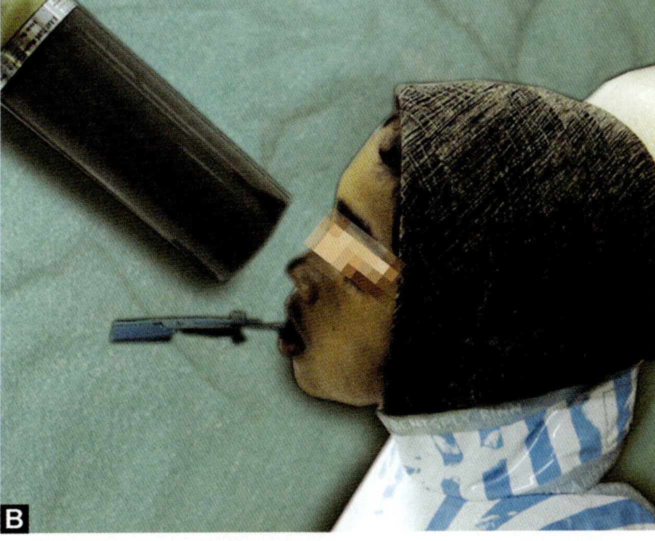

Figs 12.12A and B: Recording the X-ray for maxillary teeth: (A) Posterior teeth; (B) Anterior teeth

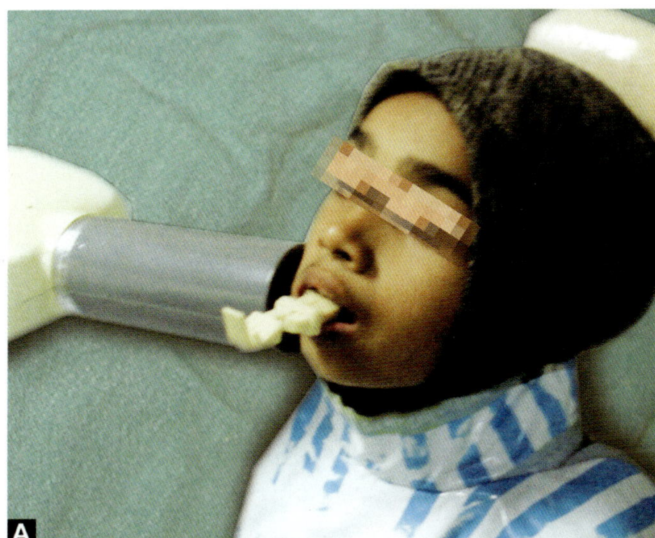
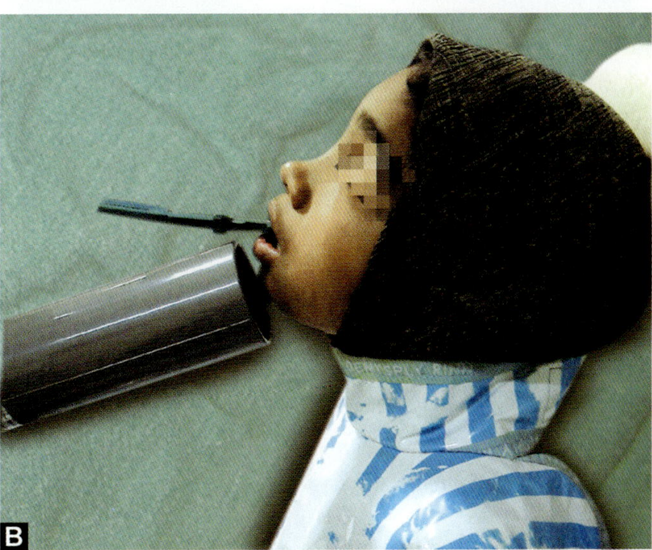

Figs 12.13A and B: Recording the X-ray for mandibular teeth: (A) Posterior teeth; (B) Anterior teeth

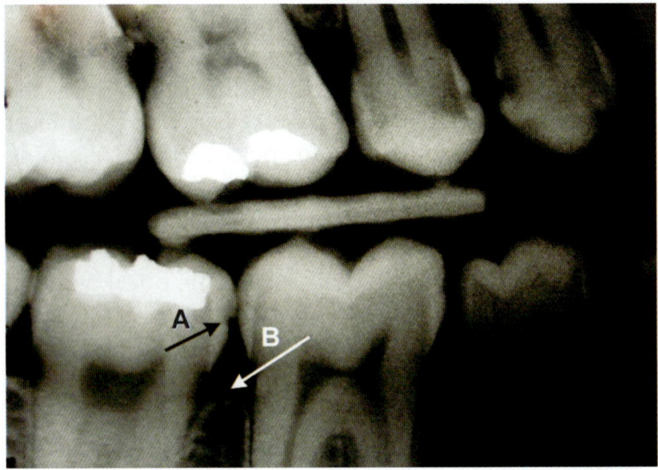

Fig. 12.14: Indications of bite wing radiograph: (A) Interproximal caries detection; (B) Evaluate the interdental bone

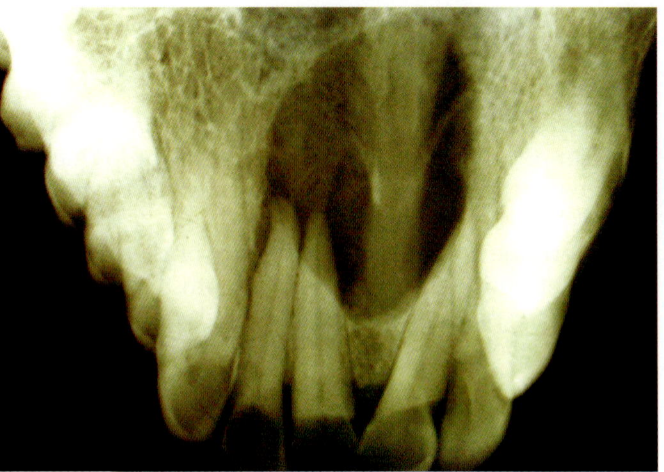

Fig. 12.16: Palatal cyst can be easily diagnosed in an occlusal radiograph

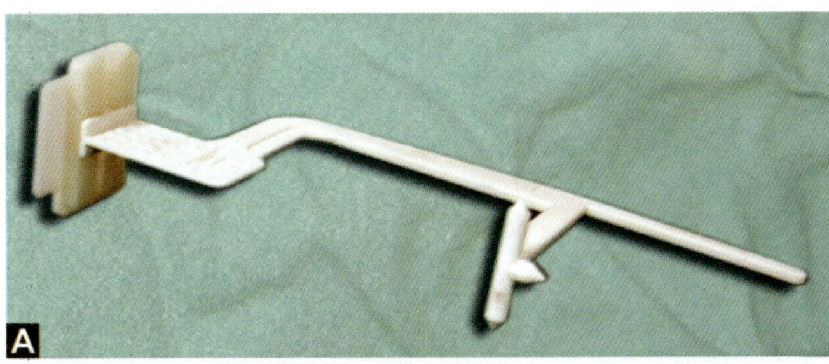

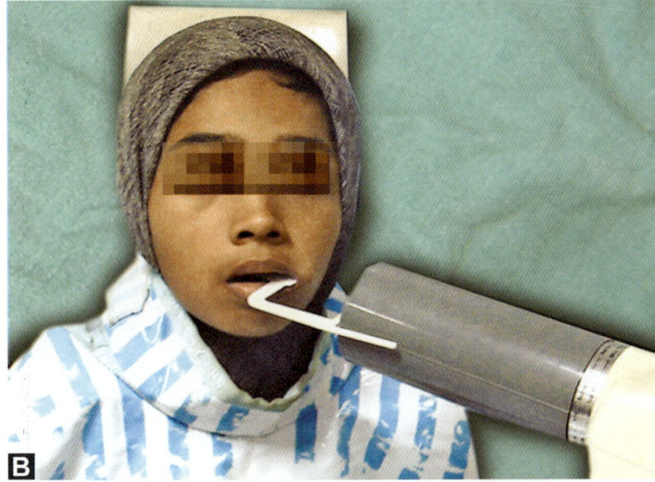

Figs 12.15A and B: Obtaining a bite wing radiograph: (A) Film holder used for recording bite wing radiograph; (B) Film and X-ray tube in position

Occlusal Radiograph

Indications (Fig. 12.16)

- Determine the presence, shape and position of midline supernumerary teeth
- Determine impaction of canines
- Determine the presence or absence of incisors
- Assess the extent of trauma to teeth and anterior segments of the arches
- In case of trismus and trauma, where the patient cannot open the mouth completely
- Determine the medial and lateral extent of cysts and tumors.

Technique (Figs 12.17A to D): Occlusal radiographs can be either maxilla or mandible.

Maxillary and mandibular occlusal radiographs can be of 3 types:

1. Anterior topographic view
2. Cross sectional view
3. Lateral topographic view

    i. *Maxillary anterior topographic radiograph:* Maxillary anterior topographic radiograph is indicated to view anterior maxilla and its dentition. While taking the radiograph the patient's head is adjusted so that the occlusal plane is horizontal to the floor. The film is placed crosswise in the mouth with exposure side towards maxilla and the posterior border touching the rami horizontally. The patient is asked to close the mouth gently. Central ray is directed through the tip of the nose toward the middle of the film with approximately +45 degrees vertical angulation and 0 degrees horizontal angulation.

   ii. *Maxillary cross-sectional view:* Maxillary cross-sectional view shows palate, zygomatic process of maxilla, nasolacrimal canals, anteroinferior aspects of antrum and nasal septum. The patients head is

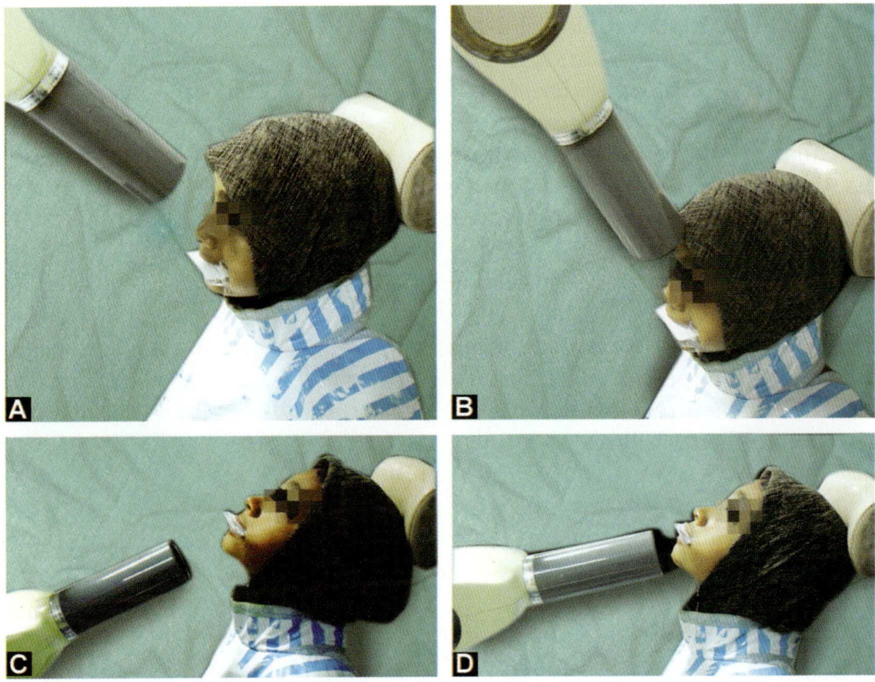

Figs 12.17A to D: Obtaining an occlusal radiograph: (A) Maxillary anterior topographic radiograph; (B) Maxillary cross-sectional radiograph; (C) Mandibular cross-sectional radiograph; (D) Mandibular anterior topographic radiograph

adjusted so that the occlusal plane is horizontal to the floor. The film is placed in the mouth crosswise with exposure side towards maxilla and the posterior border touching the rami horizontally. The patient is asked to close his mouth gently. The central ray is directed at a vertical angulation of +65 and a horizontal angulation of 0 degrees to the bridge of the nose just below the nasion, towards the middle of the film.

iii. *Maxillary lateral topographic view:* Maxillary lateral topographic view shows a quadrant of the alveolar ridge of the maxilla, tuberosity, inferolateral aspect of antrum, zygomatic process of maxilla. Here the film is placed with its long axis parallel to the sagittal plane on the side of interest till the film touches the ramus of that side. The lateral border of film is positioned parallel to the buccal surfaces of the posterior teeth, extending 1cm laterally behind the buccal cusps. The patient is asked to close and gently hold the film in position. Central ray is projected with a vertical angulation of +60 degrees to a point 2 cm below the lateral canthus of the eye, directed towards the center of the film.

iv. *Mandibular anterior topographic view:* Mandibular anterior topographic occlusal view includes the anterior portion of the mandible and inferior cortical border of the mandible. The film placement is similar to maxillary occlusal (exposure side towards mandible) and the head is placed so that the occlusal plane is at –45 degrees to the floor and central ray has –10 degree vertical angulation and is directed through the chin towards the middle of the film.

v. *Mandibular cross-sectional view:* Mandibular cross sectional view includes soft tissues of the floor of the mouth, lingual and buccal cortical plates of the mandible from second molar to second molar. The patient is seated in a semi reclining position with the head tilted back so that the ala-tragal line is almost perpendicular to the floor. The film is placed in the mouth as described for mandibular cross sectional view. The anterior border of the film should be approximately 1 cm beyond the mandibular central incisors. The central ray is directed at the midline through the floor of the mouth approximately 3 cm below the chin, at right angles to the center of the film.

vi. *Mandibular Lateral topographic view:* Mandibular lateral topographic view covers half the floor of the mouth, buccal and lingual cortical plates of half the mandible and teeth. The patient position is same as mandibular anterior topographic occlusal view. Film is placed with its long axis placed parallel to the sagittal plane and 1 cm laterally to the buccal surfaces of the teeth. The central ray is directed perpendicular to the center of the film through a point beneath the chin approximately 3 cm posterior to the point of the chin and 3 cm lateral to the midline.

Panoramic Radiographs (Figs 12.18 and 12.19)

1. It is an extraoral radiograph in which the X-ray film and the X-ray source move in opposite directions.
2. It can be used to visualize the entire dentition.
3. This reduces the total number of films and thus reduces the radiation exposures.
4. This can also be used to introduce the child to radiography as it is an extraoral radiograph.
5. It requires a total of 15 to 22 seconds to record.
6. Although it is considered as a supplement it cannot substitute intraoral radiographs in the diagnosis of caries or for viewing the periapical region.
7. This view can be useful in handicapped children and for viewing a wide area of the TMJ and associated region.

Commonly used localization techniques

1. Clark's technique
   The purpose is to locate or determine the buccolingual relationship of impacted tooth or foreign body within the alveolar process relative to erupted teeth in the maxilla.
   The rationale is that when shadows of two objects of equal size are projected in a straight line with each other and the observer, the shadow of the more distant object will be obscured from the observers view by shadow of the near object. On moving to the right, the shadow of the far object also moves to the right, i.e. in the direction the observer moves. Similarly, if the observer moves to the left, the object moves to the left. In each case the shadow of the near object will appear to move in a direction away from (opposite to) the observer movement.
   Procedure: Two radiographs of the same area are required. Radiograph 1 utilizes normal, standard radiographic procedure relative to placement and tube alignment for vertical and horizontal angulation. Radiograph 2 utilizes exactly same placement and vertical angulation as in radiograph 1. The only difference is that the horizontal angulation of the central ray is altered to a more exaggerated mesial direction.

Contd...

Contd...

The localization is accomplished through the use of buccal object rule which states that an object buccal to its adjacent structures will appear to move in a direction opposite the moving X-ray source, on the other hand an object lying lingual to its adjacent structures will appear to move in the same direction as moving X-ray source.

2. Miller' technique
   The rationale for this procedure is that in order to locate an object in space relative to another object it is necessary to take a minimum of two observations from different positions, 90° apart. This can usually be accomplished by observing directly from the side and then viewing the object from the top or bottom.
   Procedure: Two radiographs are utilized for this technique. Radiograph 1 is standard periapical radiograph utilizing the paralleling principle. This demonstrates the superior-inferior relationship of the impacted object to the adjacent teeth and alveolar crest. Radiograph 2 is a standard cross-section occlusal radiograph taken 90° to the first film. This radiograph subsequently demonstrates the buccal-lingual relationship of impacted object to the teeth and buccal and lingual cortical plates of mandible.

SPECIAL TECHNIQUE FOR THE HANDICAPPED CHILD

The physically handicapped child cannot usually hold a film in his\her mouth with fingers. In such a child radiograph can be taken by the parent holding the child or by the use of film holding devices. If the child is unable to open the mouth, extraoral radiographs such as panoramic view, lateral jaw projections, anterior occlusal screening, should be preferred.

Children are at higher risk for radiation exposures than adults. The reasons are:

- Tissues are in growth period, so more sensitive to radiation.
- Children have longer life span with greater susceptibility to tumors
- Effects of radiation are cumulative
- Because of their small stature, children are closer to the central X-ray beam
- Because of increased caries, children might require more number of radiographs.

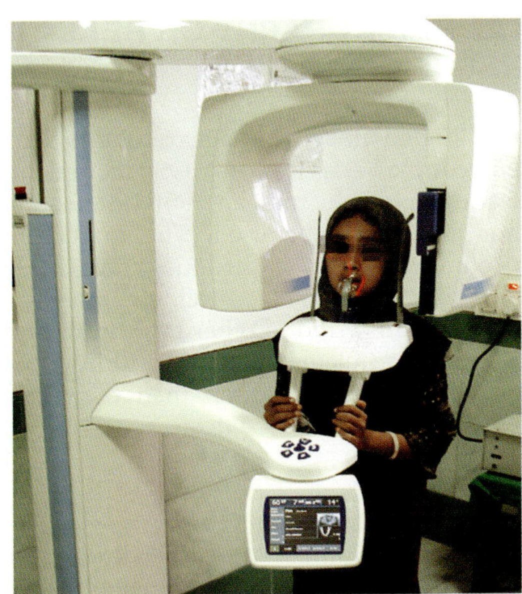

Fig. 12.18: Panoramic radiographic machine

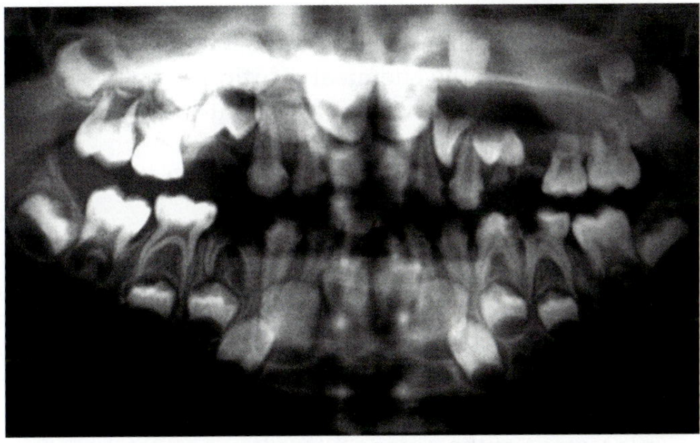

Fig. 12.19: Panoramic radiograph

HAND-WRIST RADIOGRAPHS (FIGS 12.20 AND 12.21)

- Estimates the skeletal age.
- Carpal bones, epiphysis, phalanges, metacarpals provide a clue to bone growth in the body as a whole
- Ossification occurs in these bones after birth and before maturity.
- Carpal bones ossify at different ages beginning from Capitate (3rd month), Hamate (4th month), Triquetral (3rd year), Lunate (4th year),Trapezoid and Scaphoid (5th year), Trapezium (6th year) and lastly Pisiform (12th year).
- The radiographs are inspected to assess the growth by evaluating the shape of the carpal bones, degree of ossification of the skeleton, time and order of appearance of carpals.

Indications of Hand-Wrist Radiograph

- Prior to rapid maxillary expansion- to assess the stage of growth
- When maxillomandibular changes are indicated in the treatment of Class III, skeletal Class II or skeletal open bites
- Patients with marked discrepancy between dental and chronologic age
- Orthodontic patients requiring orthognathic surgery if undertaken between the ages of 16 and 20 years.

Hand-Wrist X-ray can be Correlated

1. Dental development
2. Peak height velocity
3. Cervical vertebrae
4. Cranial base outline
5. Spheno-occipital synchondrosis

The stage of mineralization of the carpal bones are determined. Then the development of metacarpal bones and phalanges are evaluated. Standard tables and analysis of Bjork are useful which divides the maturation process of bones of the hand between the 9th to 17th year into eight developmental stages.

MRI: MAGNETIC RESONANCE IMAGING (FIG. 12.22)

It is a noninvasive technique in which high strength, static magnetic field pulsed radio waves and switched gradient magnetic fields are used to create an image. It is widely used to image the soft tissue pathologies of head and neck region.

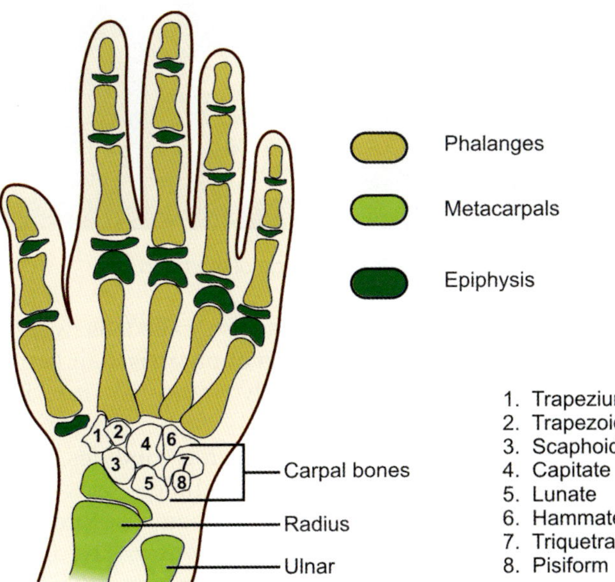

Fig. 12.20: Diagrammatic representation of hand wrist radiograph

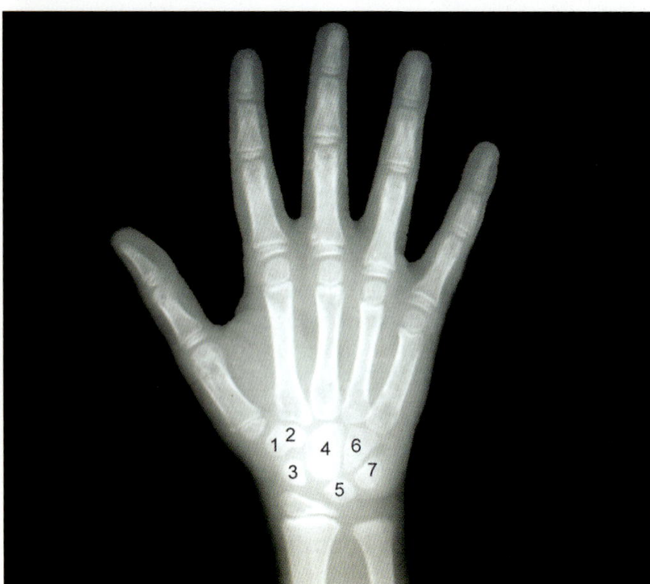

Fig. 12.21: Hand wrist radiograph of a 8-year-old-child. Note the missing pisiform bone as it begins to calcify at 12 years of age

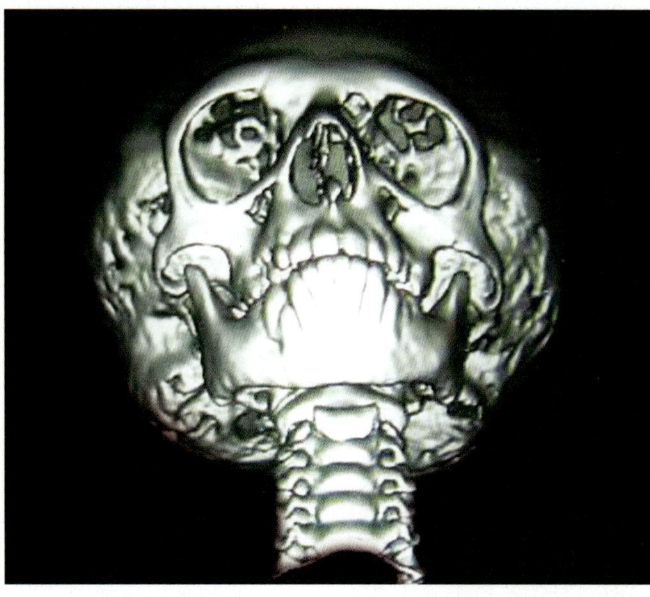

Fig. 12.22: MRI image of the head

Paranasal sinus view: It is also called as water's view, indicated for visualization of paranasal air sinus.

Reverse-Town view: Mainly indicated for TMJ visualization.

Submentovertex view: For viewing condyles, sphenoid sinus and curvature of the mandible.

RVG, RadioVisioGraphy: The image is recorded as a digital image and requires a computer. The image obtained can be modified by increasing or decreasing the brightness or contrast.

DIGITAL RADIOGRAPHY OR REAL-TIME IMAGING (FIG. 12.23)

To obtain digital images, image receptors like CCD (charged coupled device), CMOS (complementary metal oxide semiconductors) and PSP (photostimulable phosphor plates) can be used. The digital imaging system eliminates the hazardous chemical wastes like processing solutions, lead foil, etc. Images can be electronically transferred to other healthcare providers thus helping in telemedicine. In addition, digital receptors require less radiation than the films, thus lowering the patient absorbed dose.

Advantages

- Lower dose of radiation required
- Computer manipulation of the image such as alteration in contrast, resolution, image enhancement is possible
- Automated image analysis
- No need for conventional processing, thus avoiding all processing film faults and the hazards associated with handling the chemical solutions.
- Storage and archiving of patient information is easier
- Transference of images between institutions (Teleradiology) is possible.

Disadvantages

- Expensive, especially panoramic systems
- Large disk space required to store the images
- The sensor and the computer have to be connected directly, and the connecting cable can make intraoral placement of the sensor difficult.
- There can be some loss of image definition and resolution compared with film, both on the TV monitor and on the hard copy print out.
- Image manipulation can be time consuming and misleading to the inexperienced.
- It is difficult with some intraoral systems to view multiple images at once as in a full mouth survey.
- The hard copy images may fade with time - this may be a major problem in pediatric practice, since a radiograph taken of a 6-year-old child legally should be kept until the patient has reached adulthood.

DENTAL XERORADIOGRAPHY

Xeroradiography is a technique which uses the xerographic copying process to produce images generated from standard diagnostic X-rays. Xeroradiography has been successfully used in medical field. This system

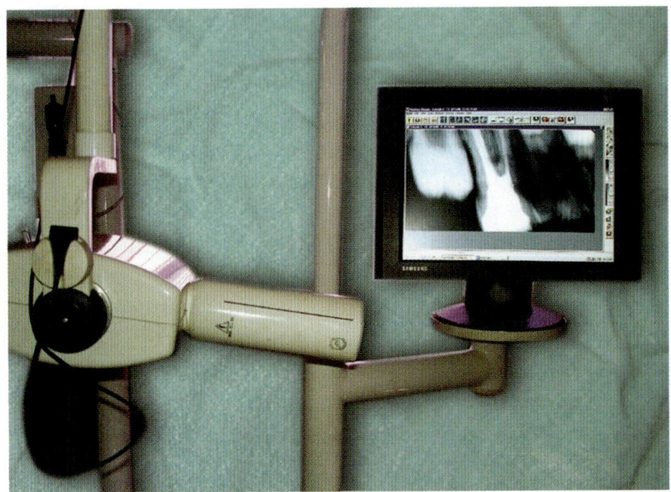

Fig. 12.23: Digital radiograph

employs a standard dental radiographic unit as the source of irradiation. Exposure settings are the same as those for conventional radiography (70 to 100 kVp and 10 to 15 mA), except that the exposure time is reduced. Xeroradiography employs a charged metal plate within a small plastic intraoral cassette. This cassette is about the size of standard No.2 radiographic packet. During exposure those portions of the plate struck by the X-ray beam are discharged in proportion to the amount of energy striking the plate and a latent image is formed.

Advantages

1. Resolution: Ability to distinctly record separate images of small objects that are placed close together.
2. Latitude: Xeroradiography has a wider latitude of exposure.
3. Edge enhancement: The advantages of resolution and latitude are a result of a special capability of xeroradiography known as edge enhancement in which the boundary is accentuated between two adjacent structures only slightly different in density.
4. The ability of xeroradiographs to display fine structural detail and a wide range of tissue densities.
5. Xeroradiographic images show both supragingival and subgingival calculus in much greater detail.
6. Amalgam and gold restorations are entirely radiopaque whereas porcelain and plastic restorations are more radiolucent. Base materials are readily distinguished from amalgam or gold.

Cone Beam CT

The recent introduction of cone-beam computed tomography (CBCT) into the medical field has allowed the nondestructive investigation of internal structures at relatively low cost and radiation exposure. The accuracy of CBCT in both two and three dimensions has been demonstrated, and CBCT has been used successfully for craniofacial anatomy. Knowing the anatomical structure of deciduous teeth is essential for clinical dentistry. Uses of CBCT in pedodontics can be:

- To evaluate the intact root form of deciduous teeth.
- To locate supernumerary root canals.
- To evaluate the changes in roots and bone during the use of orthodontic appliances.[3]
- Can be used in cases of supernumeraries because it yields accurate 3-D information relative to the orientation, sagittal position, local disorders, and neighboring anatomic structures.[4]

RADIATION PROTECTION OR RADIATION HYGIENE MEASURES

The amount of radiation produced during dental radiography is very less and conversely it may be expected that the ill-effects, also be negligible. But the risk cannot be completely ruled out. The concern is from its carcinogenic, teratogenic and mutagenic potential.

Abiding with the rules and regulation such as the Health and Safety at work act which says that every practice resulting in an exposure to ionizing radiation shall be justified by the advantages it produces. All exposures shall be kept as low as reasonably achievable (ALARA principle) and the sum of doses and committed dose received shall not exceed certain limits.

The main purpose of radiation hygiene measures are to minimize the radiation exposure to the patient and the operator. The recommendations are:

1. *Maintaining good equipment standards:* Dental radiographic equipment should be in compliance with federal and state standards and the equipment should be inspected by a person trained in radiation protection at installation, modification and at atleast five-year interval.
2. *Obtaining previous radiographs:* A thorough history of previous exposures of all children should be obtained, dentists should share existing radiographs with any other dentist when it would benefit the patient.
3. *Correct exposure time:* An accurate timer is essential to produce consistent quality diagnostic radiographs with minimal exposure to patient.
4. *Filtering of X-ray beam:* Use of aluminium filters in the X-ray tube head to absorb selectively long wavelength, poorly penetrating X-rays that are not useful in producing the radiographic image.
5. *Right type of cone to be used:* Open end, lead lined cylinders or rectangular cones are preferred.

Pointed plastic cones are not recommended because they increase scattered radiation to all areas of the patients head, neck and reproductive organ.

6. *Restricted beam of radiation:* The beam of radiation should be restricted or collimated (Fig. 12.24) no larger than 7 cm (2 3/4 inches) in diameter when measured at the patients skin or 2 1/2 inches at the end of the cone. It is useless and destructive to irradiate tissues beyond the region of radiographic interest. Collimation restricts the size of the beam so that coverage is limited to the area around the intraoral film. Rectangular field of the film is preferable to a circular filed of radiation because a smaller area of the patients face is irradiated with each exposure.

7. *Protective shielding:* The ADA recommends the use of protective shields for all patients with reproductive potential. With children, the short head-to-gonad distance and increased biological sensitivity to radiation, and use of primarily vertical cone orientation for anterior projections provide sufficient indications for use of gonadal shielding. Irradiation of thyroid may be significantly reduced by protecting the child with a lead impregnated collar.

8. *Film holding devices:* Film holding devices are recommended because they increase the stability of the film during intraoral radiographic procedures and they eliminate the need for the patient to hold the film in their mouth with fingers.

9. *Correct film processing procedures*
   These procedures include:
   a. Dark room free from light leaks
   b. Adequate darkroom safe lighting
   c. Time temperature processing.

10. *Radiation protection of operator and office personnels:* Office personnel deserve to work in an environment that is free from the potential risk of unnecessary radiation exposure. The procedures that ensure a healthful radiation environment are:
    A. Monitor office personnel: Subscribing to one of the many film badge services provides an excellent tangible way for the practitioner to express concern for reducing and monitoring radiation to office personnel.
    B. Establish radiation safety procedure: The most effective way of reducing - operator exposure to X-radiation is to enforce strict application of position and distance rule, that is, stand at least 6 feet away from the patient at an angle between 90° and 135° to Primary beam. If the operator cannot stand atleast 6 feet away from patient during exposure they should stand behind an appropriate protective barrier. Appropriate barriers includes brick wall with lead lined paneling on gypsum wall board.
    C. Films should never be held in place by operator in the patients mouth.
    D. Operator should never hold or stabilize the tube head or cone during the exposure.
    E. The operator should never stand directly in line with primary beam of radiation.

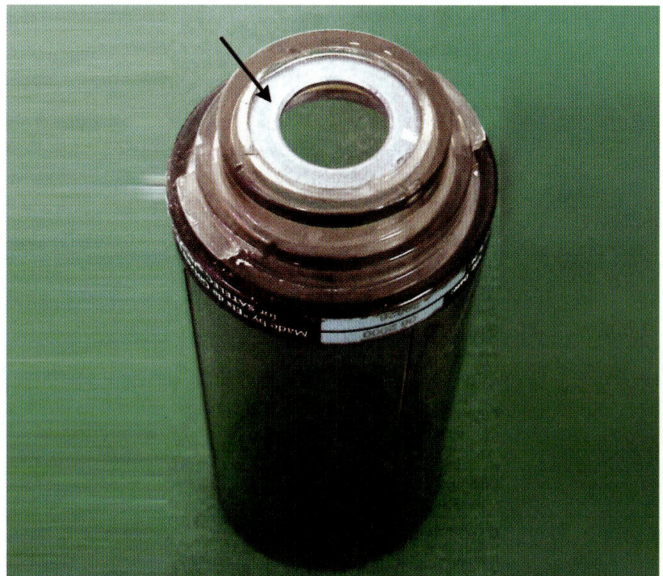

Fig. 12.24: Round collimator lined by lead (Arrow) that restricts the size of the X-ray beam

REFERENCES

1. Jung MS, Lee SP, Kim GT, Choi SC, Park JH, Kim JW. Three-dimensional analysis of deciduous maxillary anterior teeth using cone-beam computed tomography. Clin Anat. 2011 May 4. doi: 10.1002/ca.21200.
2. Manson-Hing LR, Finn SB. Roentgenography. In. Finn SB. Clinical Pedodontics. 4th Ed. WB Saunders Company, Philadelphia 1987
3. Myers DR. Dental radiology for children. Dent Clin North Am 1984;28: 37.
4. Nowak AJ. Summary on the conference on radiation exposure in pediatric dentistry. J Am Dent Assoc 1981;103:426.
5. Nurko C. Three-dimensional imaging cone bean computer tomography technology: an update and case report of an impacted incisor in a mixed dentition patient. Pediatr Dent 2010;32(4):356-60.
6. Patel S, Dawood A, Pitt Ford T, et al. The potential applications of cone beam computed tomography in the management of endodontic problems. Int Endod J 2007;40:818-30.

7. Tai K, Park JH. Dental and skeletal changes in the upper and lower jaws after treatment with Schwarz appliances using cone-beam computed tomography. J Clin Pediatr Dent 2010;35(1):111-20.

FURTHER READING

1. Akkaya N, Kansu O, Kansu H, Cagirankaya LB, Arslan U. Comparing the accuracy of panoramic and intraoral radiography in the diagnosis of proximal caries. Dentomaxillofac Radiol 2006;35(3):170-4.

2. Chrysikopoulou A, Matheson P, Milles M, Shey Z, Houpt M. Effectiveness of two nitrous oxide scavenging nasal hoods during routine pediatric dental treatment. Pediatr Dent 2006;28(3):242-7.

3. Division of Communications, American Dental Association: For the dental patient. Dental radiographs: a diagnostic tool. J Am Dent Assoc 2006;37(10):1472.

4. Ferreira RI, Haiter-Neto F, Tabchoury CP, de Paiva GA, Boscolo FN. Assessment of enamel demineralization using conventional, digital, and digitized radiography. Pesqui Odontol Bras 2006;20(2):114-9.

5. Fuhrmann AW. Current practice in conventional and digital intraoral radiography: problems and solutions. Int J Comput Dent 2006;9(1):61-8.

6. Liu DG, Zhang WL, Zhang ZY, Wu YT, Ma XC. Three-dimensional evaluations of supernumerary teeth using cone-beam computed tomography for 487 cases. Oral Surg Oral Med Oral Pathol Oral Radiol Endod 2007;103(3):403-11. Epub 2006.

7. Looe HK, Pfaffenberger A, Chofor N, Eenboom F, Sering M, Ruhmann A, Poplawski A, Willborn K, Poppe B. Radiation exposure to children in intraoral dental radiology. Radiat Prot Dosimetry 2006;121(4):461-5. Epub 2006.

8. Machiulskiene V, Nyvad B, Baelum V. Comparison of diagnostic yields of clinical and radiographic caries examinations in children of different age. Eur J Paediatr Dent 2004;5(3):157-62.

9. Makris N, Tsiklakis K, Alexiou KE, Vierrou AM, Stefaniotis T. The subjective image quality of conventional and digital panoramic radiography among 6 to 10-year-old children. J Clin Pediatr Dent 2006 Winter; 31(2):109-12.

10. Matalon S, Feuerstein O, Kaffe I. Diagnosis of approximal caries: bite-wing radiology versus the Ultrasound Caries Detector. An *in vitro* study. Oral Surg Oral Med Oral Pathol Oral Radiol Endod 2003;95(5):626-31.

11. Mejare I. Bitewing examination to detect caries in children and adolescents—when and how often? Dent Update. 2005;32(10):588-90, 593-4, 596-7.

12. Ngan DC, Kharbanda OP, Geenty JP, Darendeliler MA. Comparison of radiation levels from computed tomography and conventional dental radiographs. Aust Orthod J 2003;19(2):67-75.

13. Patel N, Rushton VE, Macfarlane TV, Horner K. The influence of viewing conditions on radiological diagnosis of periapical inflammation. Br Dent J 2000;189(1):40-2.

QUESTIONS

1. What are the factors to be considered before planning for radiographs?
2. Explain the components of a X-ray machine.
3. Enumerate the components of intraoral film packet.
4. Explain the factors affecting radiographic quality.
5. Describe different film surveys used in children.
6. Write in detail the methods of reducing radiation exposure.
7. Write the indications, disadvantage and techniques for intraoral periapical radiographs.
8. What are the indications of bite wing radiographs?
9. Explain the types, indications and techniques of occlusal radiograph.
10. What are the special techniques used in uncooperative children?
11. Explain the newer methods of radiographic techniques.
12. Radiation protection or radiation hygiene measures.

Dental Extractions in Children

INTRODUCTION

Extraction of tooth is one of the simple yet most complex procedures done on a pediatric patient. It requires extra effort for management of the child apart from the skills required for performing the procedure.

Most of the minor surgical procedures like extraction, or abscess drainage are performed under local anesthesia. In a very young child (< 3 years) or an extremely unmanageable child, procedures might have to be performed under general anesthesia, due to lack of cooperation.

Understanding the normal anatomy of the specific area, the medicament used for anesthesia and associated problems are very important before planning any procedure.

NEUROLOGIC ANATOMY

The maxillary and mandibular nerves derived from trigeminal nerve provide the main innervation for maxilla, mandible and adjoining tissues.

The terminal branches of maxillary nerve are:

1. Superior alveolar nerves
2. Greater (Anterior) palatine and Nasopalatine nerves.

The terminal branches of mandibular nerve are:

1. Inferior alveolar nerve
2. Mental and incisive nerve
3. Long buccal nerve

Superior Alveolar Branches (Fig. 13.1)

They further branch into posterior, middle and anterior branches. The posterior superior alveolar nerve branch, supplies the buccal mucosa and the mucous membrane of the cheek, posterolateral wall of the maxillary sinus and the supporting structures of the three permanent molars and their root ends with the exception of the mesiobuccal root of the permanent first molar.

The middle superior alveolar nerve innervates the epithelial surface of the sinus and the root ends and supporting structures of the primary first and second molars or permanent first and second premolars and the mesiobuccal root of the permanent first molar.

The anterior superior alveolar branch provides sensory fibers to the maxillary incisor and canine root ends and the periodontal structures.

Greater (Anterior) Palatine and Nasopalatine Branches (Fig. 13.2)

The anterior (greater) palatine nerve innervates the tissues of the soft palate and tonsillar area. The nerve also supplies sensory fibers to the tissues of the hard palate.

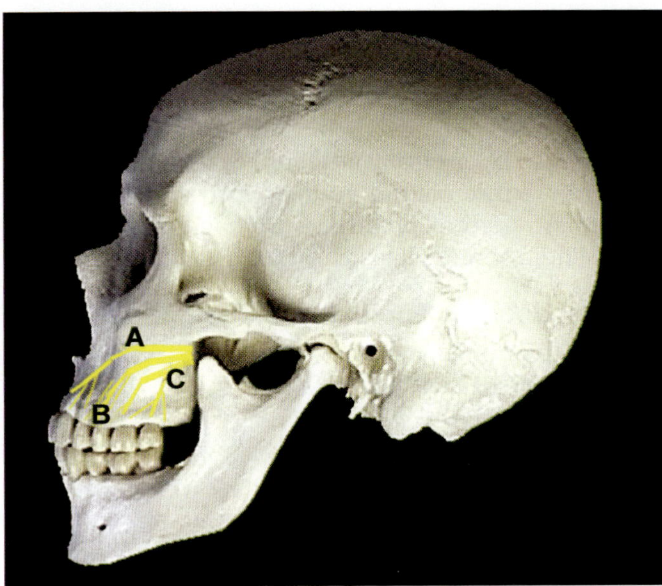

Fig. 13.1: Branches of superior alveolar branches; (A) Antero-superior alveolar nerve; (B) Middle superior alveolar nerve; (C) Posterosuperior alveolar nerve

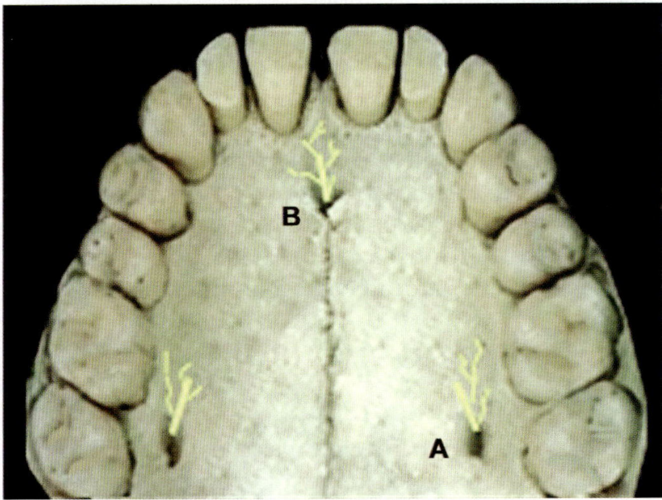

Fig. 13.2: (A) Greater palatine and (B) Nasopalatine branches emerging from greater palatine foramen incisive foramen, respectively

The nasopalatine branch of the maxillary nerve innervates the soft and hard tissues of the anterior quadrant from the midline laterally to the maxillary canine tooth. There may be accessory innervation to the incisor teeth also.

Inferior Alveolar (Mandibular) Nerve (Fig. 13.3)

The inferior alveolar nerve is the largest branch of the mandibular division of the trigeminal nerve. It arises at the level of the lateral pterygoid muscle and descends between the sphenomandibular ligament and the medial surface of the ramus of the mandible entering the mandibular canal by way of the mandibular foramen. It courses the canal anteriorly and divides into two terminal branches, the mental and incisive nerves.

Adequate pulpal anesthesia for all the mandibular teeth can be achieved by nerve block procedure. The cortical plate of bone in the mandible is thicker in the molar region and presents a barrier for an effective pulpal anesthesia during supraperiosteal infiltration technique. On the other hand, acceptable pulpal anesthesia can be achieved through supraperiosteal injections for primary and permanent incisors.

During the growth and development the shape and position of the mandible and its relation to the cranium changes. As an example, the location of the mandibular foramen in the child is inferior (lower than occlusal plane) to its site in an older individual.[1]

The mandibular ramus is narrower anteroposteriorly in the child than in an adult. This may necessitate adjustments in the nerve block procedure. The line of delivery of the syringe will be in a slightly downward direction to accommodate the more inferior location of the foramen. The needle's depth of penetration will be less in children.

Mental and Incisive Nerves (Fig. 13.4)

The mental nerve exits from the mental foramen and innervates the skin and mucosa of the lower lip and chin as well as the gingival tissues labial to the mandibular incisors. The incisive nerve furnishes sensory fibers to the first premolar, the canine, and the mandibular incisor teeth. The innervations are through a plexus of nerve branches that also decussate with like branches from the opposite side of the midline.

Long Buccal Nerve

The long buccal nerve is the first branch of the inferior alveolar nerve. Sensory fibers are distributed to the buccinator muscle, the buccal mucosa, and the buccal gingiva over the mandibular molars and second pre-molar.

Lingual Nerve

The lingual nerve is the second branch from the inferior alveolar nerve. It courses downward, lying lateral to the internal pterygoid muscle, medial to the ascending ramus and within the pterygomandibular space. The nerve courses forward in the lateral lingual sulcus, supplying the anterior two thirds of the tongue and the inferior surface of the sublingual salivary gland. There is sensory innervation to the floor of the mouth and the gingiva of the lingual surface of the body of the mandible.

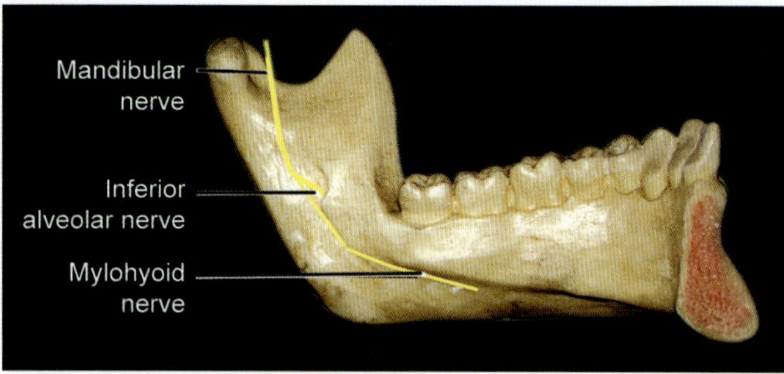

Fig. 13.3: Inferior alveolar and mylohyoid nerves

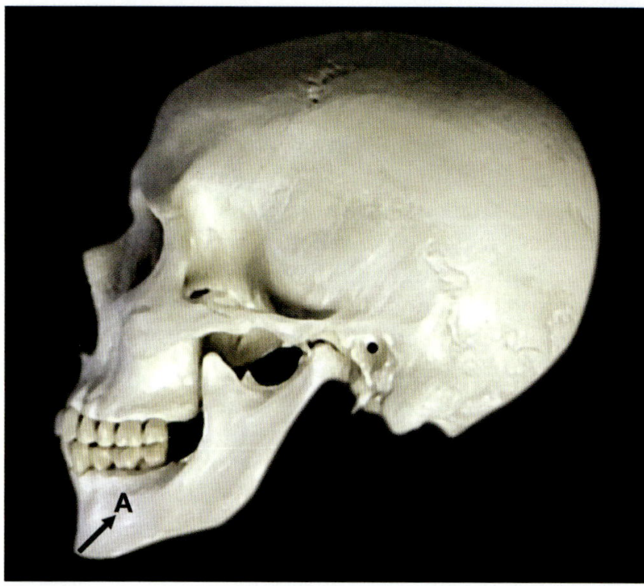

Fig. 13.4: Mental nerve emerging out of mental foramen

Mylohyoid Nerve (Fig. 13.3)

The mylohyoid nerve has both sensory and motor functions. It is a branch of the inferior alveolar nerve, arising from it and enters the mandibular foramen. Sensory fibers supply the skin about the mental protuberance, the mandibular molars and incisors.

Pain conduction	
A delta fibers	: Transmit acute pain
	: Myelinated
	: 3-5 µ diameter
	: 6-30 meters/second is the rate of conduction
C fibers	: Transmits dull, gnawing type of pain
	: Non myelinated
	: 1-3 µ diameter
	: 0.5-2 meters/second is the rate of conduction

TOPICAL ANESTHESIA

Topical anesthetic is used to minimize the discomfort caused during administration of local anesthesia. Topical anesthetic agent is effective on surface tissues (2-3 mm in depth) to reduce painful needle penetration of the oral mucosa. A variety of topical anesthetic agents are available in gel, liquid, ointment, patch, and aerosol forms.

Agents Used as Topical Anesthetics

1. Ethyl p-aminobenzoate
2. Butacaine sulfate
3. Cocaine
4. Dyclonine
5. Lidocaine
6. Tetracaine.

The topical anesthetic benzocaine is manufactured in concentrations up to 20%; lidocaine is available as a solution or ointment up to 5% and as a spray up to a 10% concentration. Ethyl p-aminobenzoate (benzocaine) is best suited in dentistry as they provide a rapid onset and longer duration of action. They are not known to produce any allergic reactions.

Method of Application of Topical Anesthetic Agent

The mucosa at the site of application is cleaned and dried. A small amount of the agent is taken on a cotton swab and applied to the tissue (Fig. 13.5). Topical anesthesia is produced in about 30 seconds.

Onset of action for benzocaine is 30 seconds, tetracaine is 60 seconds and lidocaine is 3-5 minutes.

LOCAL ANESTHESIA

Definition (Malamed,1980)[2]

"The loss of sensation in a circumscribed area of the body due to depression of excitement in nerve endings or an inhibition of conduction process."

Local Anesthetics

They are drugs that produce anesthesia in the region where it is applied or introduced. It is required that these drugs remain in the local area following their administration and gets absorbed slowly for a prolonged duration of action. Almost all of the local anesthetic agents except cocaine causes vasodilation, which means that these drugs are absorbed at a faster rate into the circulation, decreasing the duration and quality of anesthetic action and may lead to overdose. Thus a vasoconstrictor is added to the local anesthetic solution to counteract the vasodilation.

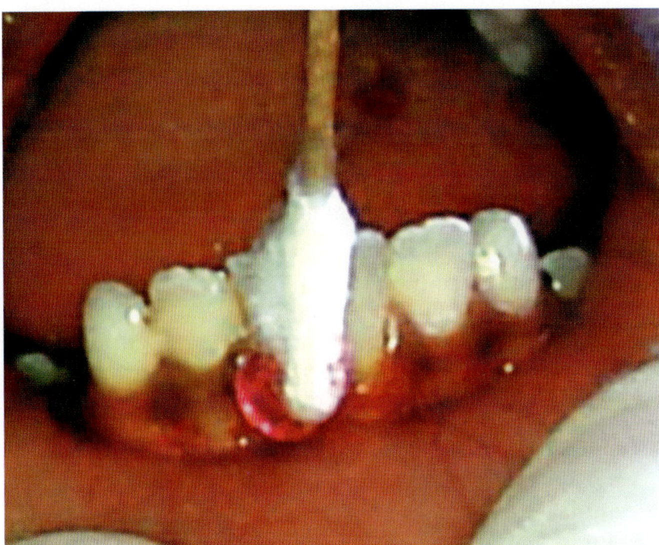

Fig. 13.5: Topical anesthesia is applied at the site of insertion of needle with a cotton swab

Vasoconstrictors slows the absorption of the local anesthetic from the site of administration into the cardiovascular system, reduces the blood flow to the area and thereby reduce bleeding at the site of surgery.

Classification of Vasoconstrictors Used with Local Anesthetics

1. Catecholamines
   - Epinephrine
   - Norepinephrine
   - Dopamine
   - Levonordefrin
2. Noncatecholamines
   - Amphetamine
   - Ephedrine
   - Methamphetamine
   - Methoxamine

The above mentioned vasoconstrictors may act directly or indirectly or both to produce the desired action. Examples of directly acting drugs are epinephrine, norepinephrine, dopamine, levonordefrin, methoxamine which act on the adrenergic receptors directly. Amphetamine and methamphetamine acts indirectly by releasing norepinephrine from adrenergic nerve terminals. Ephedrine acts in both ways that is directly on adrenergic receptors and also aid in releasing norepinephrine from adrenergic nerve terminals.

Classification of Local Anesthetic Agents

1. Ester group:
   a. Benzoic acid esters. Examples are:
      - Cocaine
      - Benzocaine
      - Butacaine
      - Piperocaine
      - Tetracaine
   b. Para-aminobenzoic acid esters. Examples are:
      - Procaine
      - Propoxycaine
      - Chloroprocaine
2. Amide group
   a. Bupivacaine
   b. Lidocaine
   c. Mepivacaine
   d. Prilocaine
   e. Etidocaine
   f. Articaine
3. Quinoline group
   a. Centbucridine: It is five to eight times as potent as lidocaine with similar onset of action and duration. It does not adversely affect the CNS and the CVS in high doses.

Composition of Local Anesthetic Solution

I. Local anesthetic agent : Lignocaine hydrochloride 2%
II. Vasoconstrictor: Adrenaline 1:50,000 to 1:2,00,000
   Uses- Delays the absorption of LA from the site
   a. Provides blood less field
   b. Prolongs the action
   c. Reduces systemic toxicity
III. Reducing agent: Sodium metabisulfite
   - Prevents oxidation of the solution
IV. Preservative: Methyl paraben, capryl hydro cuprino toxin
V. Fungicide: Thymol
VI. Vehicle: Ringer's solution

Anesthetic Agents Suitable for Children, that Rarely Evoke Allergic Reaction

1. Lidocaine hydrochloride, 2% with epinephrine 1:100,000
2. Mepivacaine hydrochloride, 2% with Levonordefrin 1:20,000. It has a more rapid onset and prolonged effect than Lidocaine HCl.
3. Prilocaine hydrochloride, 4% with epinephrine 1:200,000. It is a shorter acting agent. It should be used in sparing amounts as the metabolic product may promote the chance of developing methemoglobinemia. And therefore should be avoided in persons with anemia, cardiac failure and those who exhibit signs of respiratory failure.

Effects of overdose of anesthetic agent

- Light headedness and dizziness
- Nervous
- Twitching sensation
- Tinnitus
- Sweating
- Vomiting
- Decreased heart rate, blood pressure and respiratory rate
- Tonic clonic seizures

Articaine[3-8]

It is a local anesthetic drug most widely used in European countries and is available in many countries around the world.

This drug was first synthesized by Rusching in 1969, and brought to the market in Germany by Hoechst AG, a life-sciences German company, under the brand name Ultracain. This drug was originally referred to as "carticaine" until 1984.

It was approved by the FDA in April 2000, and became available in the United States of America two months later under the brand name Septocaine with Epinephrine 1:100,000 (Septodont).

The amide structure of articaine is similar to that of other local anesthetics, but its molecular structure differs through the presence of a thiophene ring instead of a benzene ring. Articaine is exceptional because it contains an additional ester group that is metabolized by esterases in plasma. The elimination of articaine is exponential with a half-life of 30 minutes (compared to the 90 minutes of lidocaine). Since articaine is hydrolized very quickly in the blood, the risk of systemic intoxication seems to be lower than with other anesthetics, especially if repeated injection is performed.

The toxic symptoms of the solution are:

- CNS stimulation—due to selective suppression of inhibitory neurons
- Restlessness, tremors, increased talking, increased heart rate
- Produces clonic convulsions
- Stimulation is followed by depression—fall in the BP, fall in the heart rate.
- Death is due to the respiratory failure
- In combination with sedative drugs, LA may have additive CNS depressant effect.

Ideal Requirements of the Anesthetic Agent

- Must provide adequate anesthesia
- Action must be reversible
- Non-irritating to tissues
- Low degree of systemic toxicity
- Rapid onset and sufficient duration of action
- Should not produce allergic reaction
- Readily biotransformed
- Able to be sterilized or be sterile

Potency of the anesthetic agent

- Potency is usually described in terms of the minimal anesthetic concentration that blocks impulse conduction within a specified period of time.
- Local anesthetic potency is related to a number of physicochemical properties, including intrinsic vasodilator activity, tissue diffusion characteristics but lipid solubility is the single most important determinant of local anesthetic potency.
- Highly lipid soluble anesthetics are very potent, whereas those with low lipid solubility have low potency.
- Etidocaine, has a relatively high potency, due its high lipid solubility.
- Lidocaine, is one fourth as potent as etidocaine.

Mode of Action of Local Anesthesia

- Local anesthesia is an alkaloid base that form salts when combined with acids. In solution the salt of the local anesthesia compound exists as both uncharged (as free base, which is lipid soluble) and positively charged molecule.
- The potential action of local anesthetic solution depends on the ability of the anesthetic salt to liberate free base. As pH falls, the charged molecule concentration increases more than free base concentration (The reverse happens when pH increases). That is the reason why local anesthesia is ineffective when given near an area of abscess, where the pH is acidic or low.
- Local anesthetics are suggested to interfere with the conduction of action potentials along peripheral nerve fibers by impairing the functions of sodium ion channels. Nerve impulses cannot be propagated when adequate numbers of sodium channels are not available.
- Recovery from nerve blockade is dependent on redistribution and metabolism of the local anesthetic solution.

Absorption, Metabolism and Excretion of Anesthetic Agent

Absorption

1. Increased vascular area and without adrenaline—faster is the absorption
2. Infection and low pH—slows down the absorption

Metabolism

Ester group

- Inactivated by hydrolysis in plasma by plasma cholinesterase.
- Any factor that would contribute to a decrease in plasma cholinesterase activity could allow serum concentrations of an ester linked local anesthetic to rise and thus increase the likelihood of systemic toxicity.
- The use of amino ester local anesthetics should be avoided when possible, if decreased cholinesterase activity is suspected.

Amide group

- Inactivated in the liver by microsomal enzymes.
- Prilocaine is most rapidly metabolized and this accounts for its relatively low systemic toxicity.
- Hepatic metabolism of amide linked local anesthetics can be affected by any factor that alters liver function, such as hepatic disease and drugs.
- The renal clearance of amide agents is inversely related to their protein binding capacity. Renal clearance also is inversely proportional to the pH of urine, suggesting urinary excretion by nonionic diffusion.

Excretion

- The local anesthetic agent is excreted from the kidney. Renal clearance is inversely proportional to the pH of the urine.

Duration of Action of the Anesthetic Agent

- The duration of action of local anesthetics is directly proportional to protein binding characteristics.
- Agents that are highly protein bound (for example, etidocaine and bupivacaine) have the longest duration of action.
- Those with lower protein binding capacities (for example, lidocaine and mepivacaine) have shorter durations of action.

Onset and Duration of Action of Anesthesia of 2% Lignocaine 1:100,000 Epinephrine

Onset of Action

Infiltration—2 minutes
Block—2-4 minutes

Duration of Action

Infiltration – Pulpal—1 hour
– Soft tissue—2½ hours
Block – Pulpal—1½ hours
– Soft tissue—3-5 hours

Infiltration technique is adequate for restoration of mandibular teeth, but for anesthetizing the pulp (during pulpotomy or pulpectomy) mandibular block is necessary.[9]

Contraindications for Local Anesthesia

There is no absolute contraindication, but precautions should be taken in the following conditions:

1. Very insane—mentally retarded
2. Chronic debilitating disease—septicemia, diabetes, bacteremia
3. Bleeding disorder
4. Steroid therapy—adrenal crisis. So patient should be asked to double the dose
5. Anticoagulant therapy
6. Liver or renal disorder
7. Epilepsy—initial stimulation action of lignocaine may cause seizure
8. Radiation therapy—may further reduce blood supply leading to bone necrosis
9. Hyperthyroidism—adrenaline may cause thyroid storm.

Complications Following Local Anesthetic Administration

1. *Due to the solution:* Toxicity, idiosyncrasy, allergy, anaphylactic reaction, infection, local irritation.
2. *Due to the needle:* Trismus, syncope, edema, broken needle, infection, hematoma, sloughing, and bizarre neurological symptoms.
3. *Self-inflicted injury:* The numb feeling that is produced may cause postoperative complications such as lip, tongue or cheek biting leading to severe soreness and ulcerations.

Toxicity: Ability of a drug to have deleterious effect on the living being.

Idiosyncrasy: Nonimmunological hypersensitivity to a substance

Allergy: Immunological hypersensitivity to a substance

Anaphylactic reaction: Acute type of life-threatening allergic reaction seen when a person is exposed to an allergen to which he is already sensitized.

Reversal of the effects of dental anesthesia: OraVerse (phentolamine mesylate) by Novalar Pharmaceuticals, Inc. San Diego is used to reverse the soft tissue anesthesia (lip, tongue, etc.). It is not recommended for use in children under 6 years of age or less than 15 years.[10]

TYPES OF SYRINGE

1. Jet injector syringe
2. Metal cartridge type syringe (Aspiration syringe)
3. Plastic cartridge type syringe
4. Presterilized disposable syringe (Disposable plastic syringe)
5. Computer controlled local anesthetic delivery systems (CCLD).

Jet Syringe

It is a needle less method of depositing local anesthetic agent, primarily used for topical anesthesia. The solution is forced through a very small opening, which penetrates the mucosal membrane. This method is not adequate for producing pulpal anesthesia. Other uses of jet injection are to obtain gingival anesthesia before placement of rubber dam, removal of a loose tooth or placement of the band The post-treatment soreness at the injected site and the associated cost are some of the disadvantages of this method.

Metal Cartridge Type Syringe (Aspirating Syringe)

This is a relatively safe syringe that helps prevent intravascular injections of anesthetic agent. A preloaded anesthetic carpule is used (Fig. 13.6).

Presterilized Disposable Syringe

It is the routinely used syringe made of plastic. It has a barrel to load the anesthetic solution and is calibrated. It has three parts: (1) Needle with the bevel. It is attached to the barrel through a hub, (2) Cylindrical barrel. The solution is contained inside the barrel. It has measurements marked on the outer side which aides in accurate deposition of the required drug, and (3) Plunger. It acts like a pump to push the drug out from the barrel through the needle (Fig. 13.7).

Computer Controlled Local Anesthetic Delivery Systems (CCLD)

This method of delivery system has a edge over the conventional method in providing controlled deposition of the solution. It enables the dentist in accurate placement of the needle while delivering the predeterminded amount of solution through a foot activated control. The pain perceived by the patient is also reduced compared to the traditional method.[11,12]

The Wand/CompuDent system, Comfort Control Syringe, Quick Sleeper and Anaeject are some of the CCLD systems available in the market.

Needle selection is one of the crucial steps. A good needle should allow for profound local anesthesia and adequate aspiration. Larger gauge needles cause less deflection as the needle passes through soft tissues and has more reliable aspiration. The depth of insertion varies not only by injection technique, but also by the age and size of the patient. Dental needles are available in 3 lengths: long (32 mm), short (20 mm), and ultrashort (10 mm). Gauge of the needle used—25, 27 and 30. Out of this 27 is adequate, and 25 have a larger diameter.

Rate of solution deposition—1 ml/min or at least 1 ml/30 sec.

Dilution of the vasoconstrictor

Concentration of 1:1000 indicates that there is 1 gram (1000 mg) of drug in 1000 ml of solution

To produce 1:10,000 concentration, 1 ml of 1:1000 solution is added to 9 ml of sterile water to produce 10 ml of 1:10,000 concentration of vasoconstrictor (contains 0.1mg/ml).

To produce 1: 1,00,000 concentration, 1 ml of 1:10,000 concentration is added to 9 ml of sterile water to produce 10 ml of 1: 1,00,000 concentration of vasoconstrictor (contains 0.01 mg/ml).

1:50,000 concentration contains 0.02 mg/ml of vasoconstrictor

1:2,00,000 concentration contains 0.005 mg/ml of vasoconstrictor.

Properties of Adrenaline

- Highly soluble in water
- Easily oxidized especially in the presence of heavy metal ions and heat
- Shelf life is only 18 months
- Acts directly on both α and β adrenergic receptors
- Increases the rate and force of cardiac contractions
- Causes dilatation of coronary arteries
- Increases the systolic blood pressure. Decreases the diastolic pressure in small doses and increases in large doses
- Vasoconstriction of pheripheral arteries
- Causes bronchodilatation
- In excessive dose stimulates CNS
- Stimulates glycogenolysis in liver and skeletal muscle thereby elevating blood sugar level.

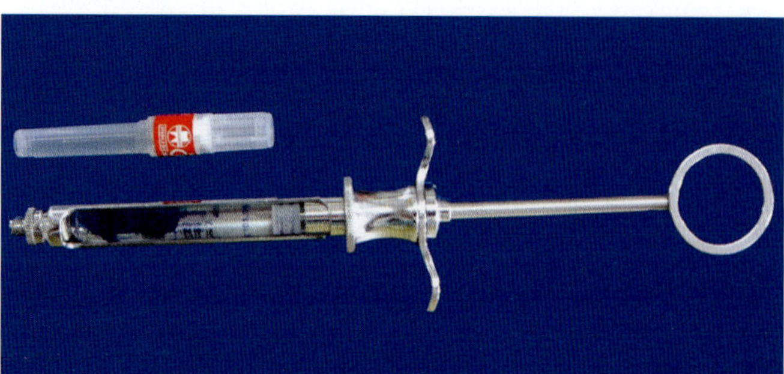

Fig. 13.6: Aspirating syringe and carpule

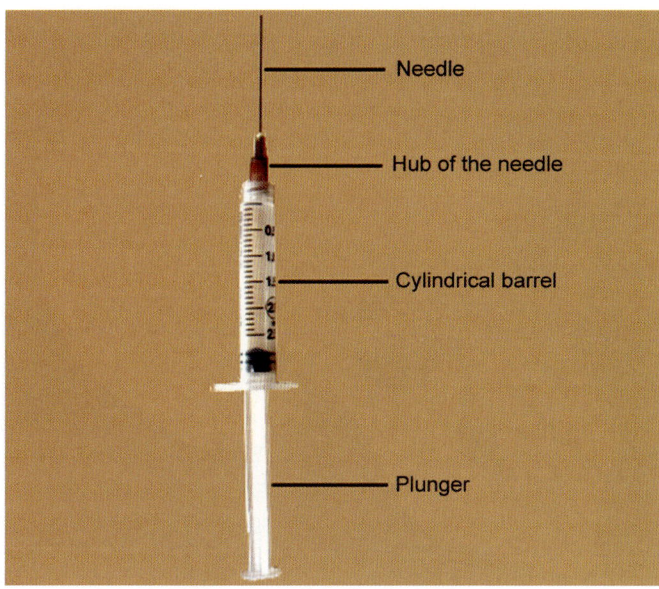

Fig. 13.7: Parts of the syringe

- Inactivated by catechol-O-methyltransferase (COMT) and monoamine oxidase (MAO) enzymes present in the liver.
- About 1% remains unchanged that is excreted in the urine.

> Maximum amount of local anesthesia that can be given is:
> 4.4 mg/kg body weight: Lidocaine, Mepivacaine
> 6.0 mg/kg body weight: Prilocaine
> 7.0 mg/kg body weight: Articaine

TYPES OF INJECTION PROCEDURES

1. *Nerve block:* The anesthetic agent is deposited near the main nerve trunk
2. *Local infiltration:* Profusion of the drug at the terminal ends of the branches
3. *Field block:* Refers to the placement of the solution around the principal terminal branches.
   For anesthetizing mandibular teeth, inferior alveolar or mental block is preferred as the bone is very thick. But with the advent of new agents like articaine, good anesthesia is achieved with infiltration itself as articaine has a high bone penetrating ability.[13]

ANESTHESIA FOR THE MAXILLARY TISSUES

A. Infiltration
B. Posterior superior alveolar nerve block
C. Middle superior alveolar nerve block
D. Maxillary anterior region block
E. Infraorbital nerve block
F. Palatal infiltration
G. Nasopalatine nerve block
H. Greater palatine nerve block

ANESTHESIA FOR THE MANDIBULAR TISSUES

A. Infiltration
B. Inferior alveolar block
C. Mental nerve block

Others

1. Periodontal ligament injection
2. Intra pulpal injection

Maxillary and Mandibular Infiltration

The needle penetration for infiltration site on the labial aspect is determined by two anatomic landmarks, the mucobuccal fold and mucogingival junction (Sweet's line). The needle penetration site is 2 to 3 mm apical to the mucogingival junction and the depth not more than 2 to 3 mm deep. About 0.5 ml of the solution is deposited. In the maxilla, palatally the needle is penetrated at the site corresponding to the root apex which is about at the junction of the horizontal and the vertical portion of the palate (Fig. 13.8).

In the mandible (Fig. 13.9) the solution is deposited in the buccal and lingual vestibule. The amount deposited is about 0.5.

Posterior Superior Alveolar Nerve Block (Fig. 13.10)

Innervates the posterior maxillary deciduous molars. They can be anesthetized as follows:
a. Needle is inserted immediately behind the buttress of the zygoma at the height of the vestibule.
b. Tip of the needle must be in close proximity to the periosteum.
c. Foramen is approximately 8 mm from the insertion point in a 3-year-old and 11 mm in a 14-year-old.

Middle Superior Alveolar Nerve Block (Fig. 13.11)

Innervates the premolars and the mesiobuccal root of the first permanent molar. The method of anestheti-zation is similar to posterior superior alveolar nerve.

Maxillary Anterosuperior Nerve Block (Fig. 13.12)

Depositing the solution in the apical region of the anterior teeth provides satisfactory anesthesia of the labial side of the maxillary anterior region in most cases.

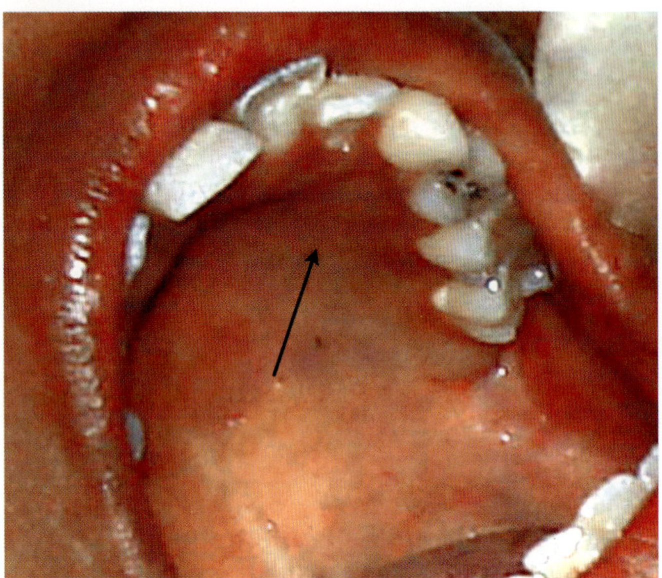

Fig. 13.8: Needle position during palatal infiltration

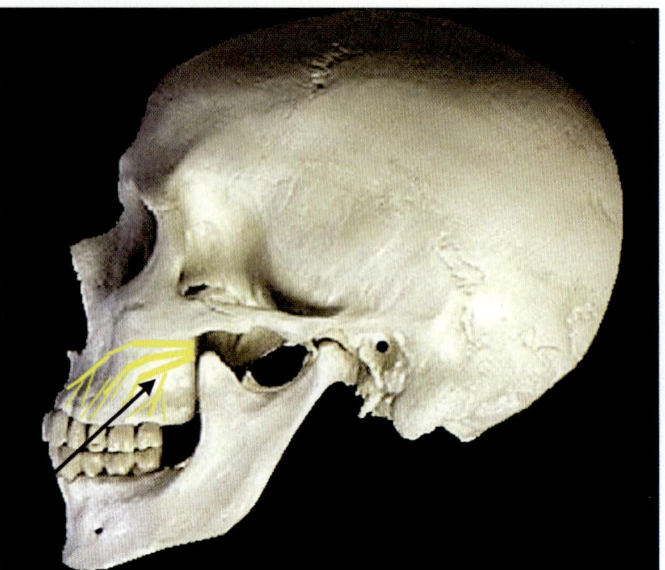

Fig. 13.10: Needle position for posterior superior alveolar nerve block

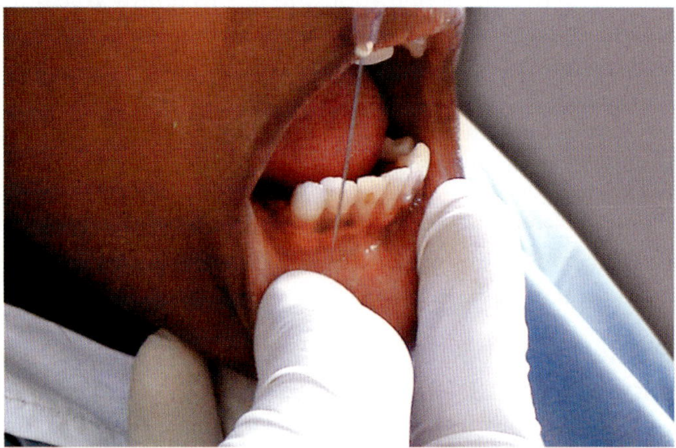

Fig. 13.9: Needle position during infiltration on the labial aspect

Infraorbital Nerve Block (Fig. 13.13)

It is given in case of swelling and when infiltration has failed. The infraorbital foramen in a 3-year-old is about 5 mm above the vestibular depth.

Palatal Infiltration

Less pain is encountered when injected into the depth of the rughae as they contain less sensory endings. The amount deposited is about 0.2 to 0.3 ml.

Nasopalatine Nerve Block (Fig. 13.14)

Nasopalatine nerve innervates the maxillary anterior teeth. It is indicated when vestibular infiltration is inadequate. About 0.2-0.3 ml of LA is administered at the entrance of the incisive foramen on the incisive papilla.

Greater Palatine Nerve Block (Fig. 13.15)

Greater palatine nerve innervates the maxillary posterior teeth in the palatal aspect. It is anesthetized at the region midway between the midline of the hard palate and the palatal surface of the posterior teeth.

MANDIBULAR ANESTHESIA

Inferior Alveolar Block (Figs 13.16 A and B)

Most common block used for anesthetizing the molars and premolars. The needle is penetrated into the pterygomandibular space and the solution is deposited close to the mandibular foramen. Factors to be considered are:

- In children the mandibular foramen is located near the posterior border of the ramus. In a 3 years old the foramen is about 5 mm from the posterior border and 20 mm from the anterior border.
- The foramen invariably aligns with the deepest concavity on the anterior border of the mandible.
- Mucosal depression on the medial aspect of the mandible formed by the medial pterygoid muscle also aligns with the inferior alveolar foramen and should be the point of insertion of the needle.

Technique of Inferior Alveolar, Lingual and Long Buccal Nerve Block

- The anterior border of the ramus is palpated, with the finger or thumb resting in its greater curvature.

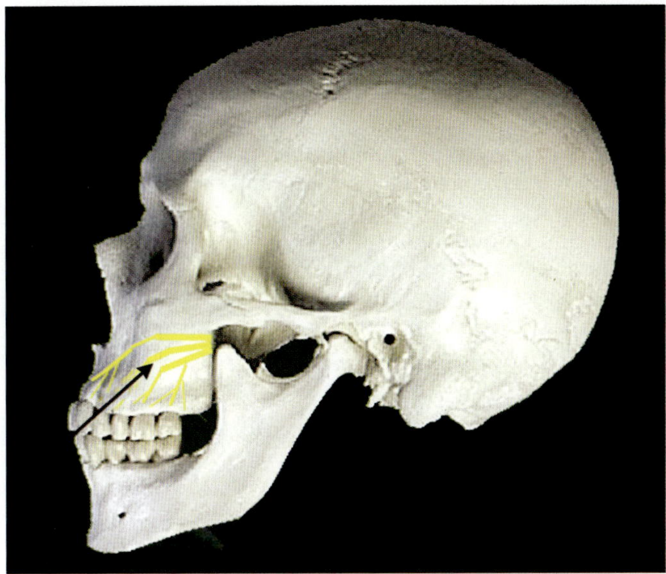

Fig. 13.11: Needle position for middle superior alveolar nerve block

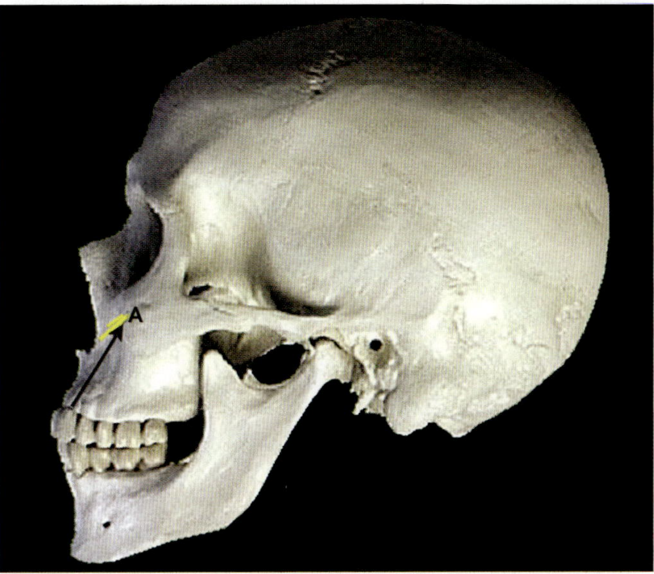

Fig. 13.13: Needle position during infraorbital nerve block: (A) Infraorbital nerves

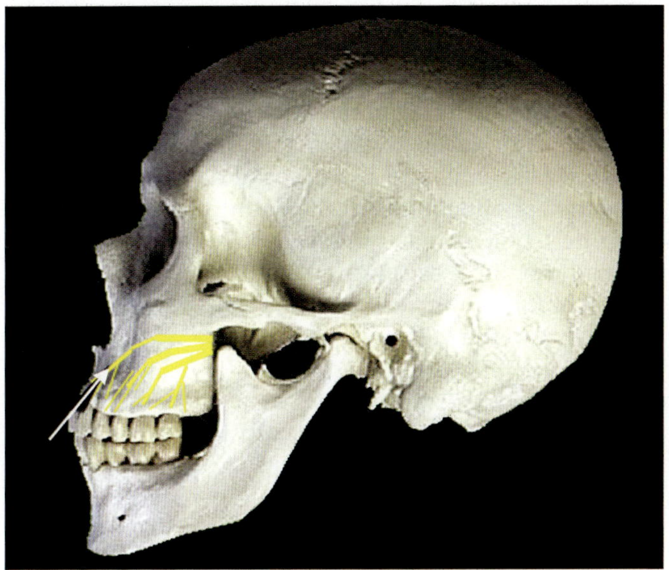

Fig. 13.12: Needle position for anterosuperior alveolar nerve block

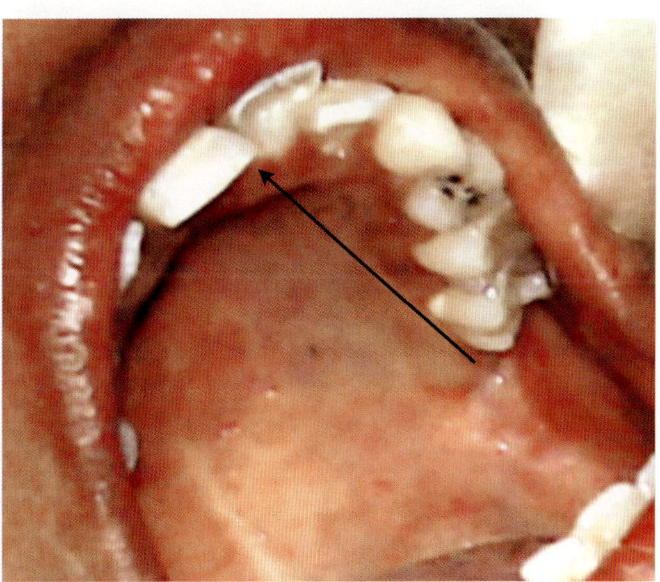

Fig. 13.14: Needle position for nasopalatine nerve block

- It should be observed that as the medial pterygoid ligament passes inferiorly and laterally to attach at the base of the mandible, a triangle is formed by the anterior border of the ramus, the medial pterygoid muscle and the lateral ptergoid muscle. The apex of the triangle is placed inferiorly. An imaginary, longitudinal line dividing the tip of the finger or thumb as it rests in the coronoid notch passes medially over a depressed area just above the apex. The penetration site of needle is the point of intersection.

- The anesthetic syringe is introduced into the oral cavity parallel with the occlusal plane of the mandibular posterior teeth.
- The needle depth is 8-10 mm from the mucosal surface. The amount deposited is 0.9 to 1.0 ml.
- Lingual nerve is anterior and medial to the inferior alveolar nerve. So the needle has to be withdrawn and solution deposited half the distance from the inferior alveolar foramen. The amount deposited is about 0.5 ml.

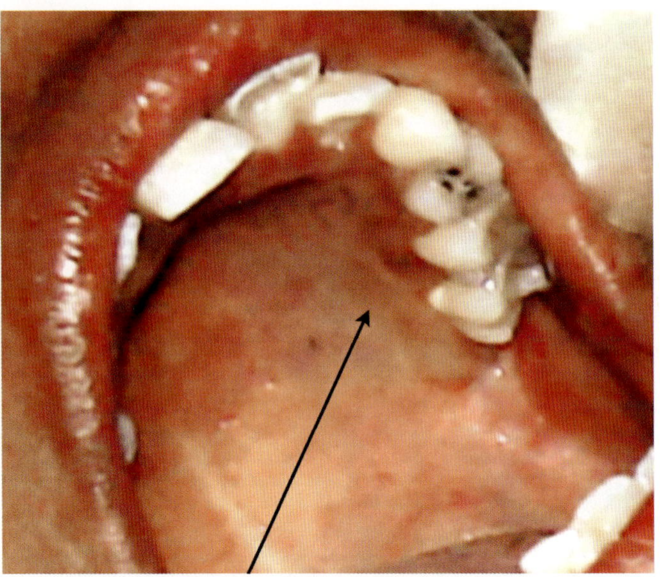

Fig. 13.15: Needle position for greater palatine nerve block

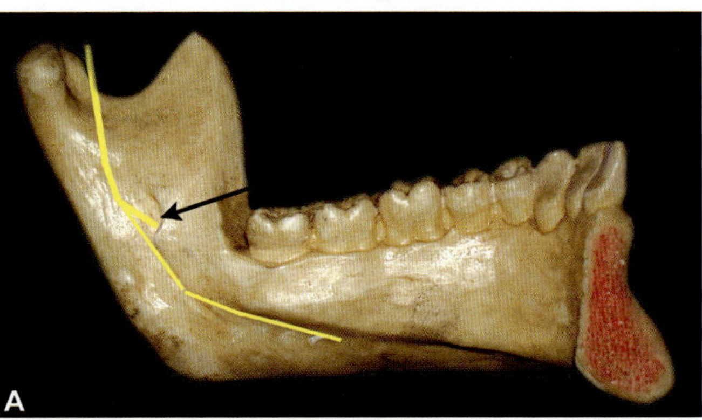

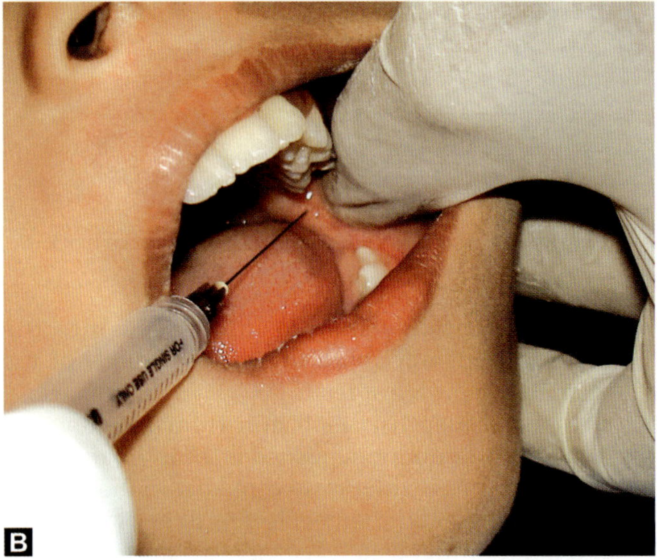

Figs 13.16A and B: (A) Needle position for inferior alveolar nerve block; (B) Needle position in the patient's mouth

- The buccal nerve can be anesthetized by infiltration in the buccal sulcus distal to the permanent teeth. The amount deposited is about 0.2 ml.

> Boundaries of pterygomandibular space
> Anterior: Pterygomandibular raphe and superior constrictor of pharyx
> Posterior: Parotid gland
> Floor and Medial: Medial pterygoid muscle
> Lateral: Ramus of the mandible
> Roof: Lateral pterygoid muscle

> Needle pathway during inferior alveolar nerve block is Mucosa, thin plate of buccinator muscle, loose connective tissue and variable amount of fat.

Mental Nerve Block (Fig. 13.17)

Is effective in producing anesthesia for the premolars and anterior teeth. The amount deposited is 0.5 to 1.0 ml.

Periodontal Ligament Injection (Intraligamentary Injection)

This is used as adjunct to the other injection techniques. The needle is placed in the gingival sulcus (preferably on the mesial side) and is advanced deeper down until resistance is obtained. About 0.2 ml of the solution is deposited. Since greater pressure is required to deposit the solution, there are syringes specifically designed for this technique. They are of two types—one of them is gun like and the other pen type.

Intrapulpal Injection

It involves anesthetizing the pulp tissues directly by depositing the solution into the pulp. It may be painful initially but the onset of action is almost immediate. It is indicated when additional pulpal anesthesia is required as during pulpectomy or root canal treatment.

Differences between a Child and Adult Patient

1. The bone in the maxilla and mandible of the adult is heavier and more compact, whereas in the child it is varyingly less dense and incompletely calcified. So diffusion of the LA agent through the layers of the bone is faster in children.
2. The anatomic structures of the child are naturally smaller than those of the adult, so the depth of penetration of the needle should be less in children.
3. Penetrating too deeply at the area of the tuberosity can produce a hematoma should the pterygoid venus plexus or posterior superior alveolar artery be injured.

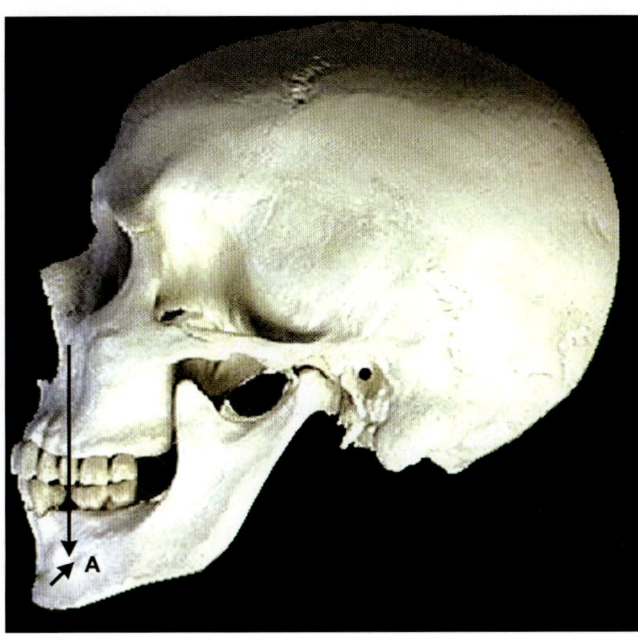

Fig. 13.17: Needle position for mental nerve block:
(A) Mental never

4. The depth of the needle penetration must be reduced because the ramus of the mandible is shorter vertically and narrower anteroposteriorly.
5. With an adult, the emotional aspect of the local anesthetic process is seldom a factor. For the child, however, the procedure is very much an emotional issue.

Factors Responsible for Successful Administration of a Local Anesthetic Agent in a Pediatric Patient

1. Able patient management
2. Concealment of the syringe
3. Appropriate use of a topical anesthetic agent
4. Effective exchange of the syringe between the assistant and the operator
5. Appropriate anesthetic agent
6. Competency of the injection process.

COMMONLY MADE MISTAKES

1. Waving the needle in front of the patient. It is important from the behavior management point of view to place the needle and other instruments behind the patient. The needle should be kept out of the direct vision of the child.
2. Not getting supportive control of the patient's head and hands. It is difficult and dangerous to administer anesthesia or perform any treatment on a child who

is hypermotive. So adequate reinforcement to restrict the movements of the head and the extremities is necessary so as to avoid complications.
3. Using long needles. Depth of penetration of a needle is very less compared to that in adults. Use of short needles will ensure that the needle does not extend into deeper tissues.
4. Using inappropriate doses. Young's rule or Clarke's rule can be used while deciding the appropriate dose for a child patient.
5. Fast injection: Care must be taken for slow administration of the solution. Time should be allowed for slow dispersion of the solution into the tissues. Ideal rate of deposition is about 1ml/min, preceded by application of topical anesthesia and aspiration to avoid intravascular injection.
6. Not advising patients or parents regarding the post anesthesia side effects. Children should be strictly told not to bite their lips or cheek until the effects subsides. Parents should be told to supervise this at home. Children usually tend to chew on the lips as it does not cause pain and feel like chewing gum and this can lead to severe laceration that can lead to ulceration (Figs 13.18A and B).

EXTRACTION OF TEETH

The principles of extraction of a permanent and a deciduous teeth are the same. But care must be taken keeping in mind the anatomic and physiologic difference between an adult and a child. The surgical instruments designed for adult procedures can be used effectively for the child patient, although forceps are available (Figs 13.19A and B) that are specifically designed for the small mouth. They are small and can be easily concealed and less fear inspiring.

Forceps such as Cowhorn and elevators that, by virtue of their design and function, threaten the underlying developing permanent teeth should be avoided. Narrow root picks and mosquito beaked forceps are the instruments of choice for root removals.

Rationale for Deciduous Tooth Removal

A number of conditions predispose the need for removal of deciduous teeth. They are as follows:

Acute Pathologic Involvement

This involvement represents an acute periapical infection of a carious deciduous tooth. The microorganisms may be virulent enough to produce an infection that is diffused and distended, such as cellulitis. The tooth is extracted if it is destroyed beyond rehabilitation (Fig. 13.20).

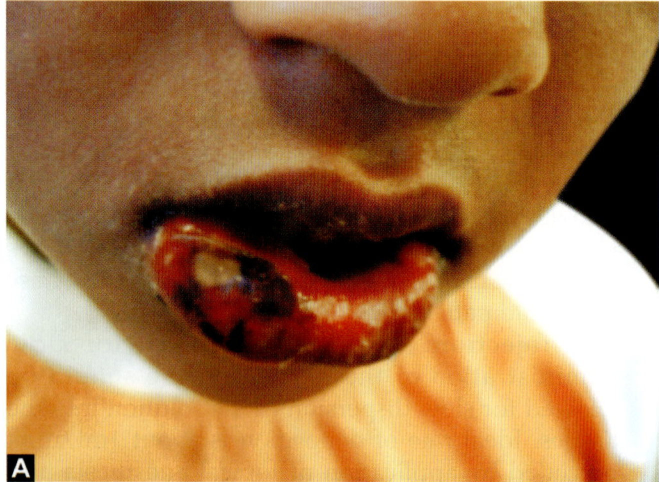

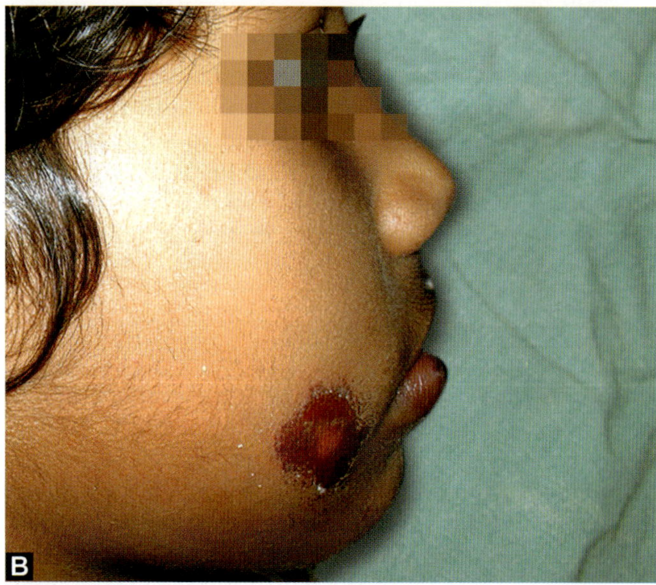

Figs 13.18A and B: (A) Ulcers on the lips due to biting following inferior alveolar nerve block; (B) Wound on the cheek that occurred due to continuous rubbing or scratching of the anesthetized area following inferior alveolar nerve block

Chronic Pathologic Involvement (Fig. 13.21)

A primary molar usually presents with furcal radiographic changes, and the deciduous anterior tooth may have changes seen in the apical portion. This presents with a parulis or a draining abscess. The risk for the normal development of the permanent tooth bud due to the infective environment warrant the extraction of the diseased deciduous tooth.

Over Retained Deciduous Tooth

The deciduous tooth may be retained for several reasons such as:
- If the erupting succedaneous tooth is malposed, the resorptive process on the deciduous tooth may be irregular.
- The resorptive process may also be affected by endocrine disturbances or vitamin deficiencies.
- Atypical resorption of a deciduous tooth root may cause it to be overretained.

Such an over retained deciduous tooth should be extracted to allow normal eruption and alignment of the permanent successor.

Ankylosed Deciduous Tooth

Such tooth shall be extracted when the cessation of vertical alveolar bone growth is observed, as evidenced by deciduous tooth submergence, followed by the placement of a space maintainer.

Cariously Involved, Nonrestorable Deciduous Tooth (Fig. 13.22)

When caries has seriously involved the clinical crown of a tooth and is non restorable, the tooth should be removed.

Natal or Neonatal Tooth

The natal tooth, which has erupted before birth, or the neonatal tooth, usually erupting within one month following birth, must be considered for extraction if:
- The tooth is mobile and there is a chance of aspiration
- The tooth is a source of mechanical irritation, causing ulceration on the ventral surface of the tongue
- There is interference with breastfeeding.
- The natal or neonatal tooth may be a supernumerary tooth.

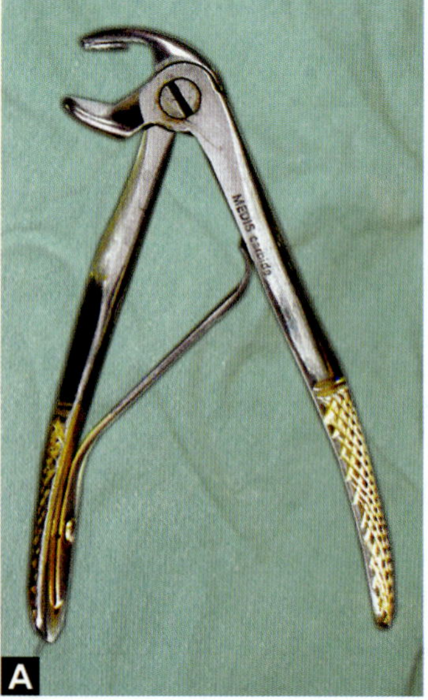
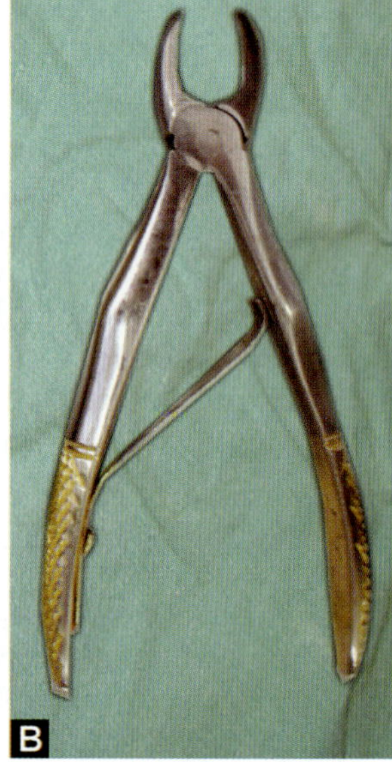

Figs 13.19A and B: (A) Forceps for extraction of lower teeth. Note the beak and the handle are perpendicular to each other; (B) Forceps for extraction of upper teeth. Note the beak and the handle are in same line

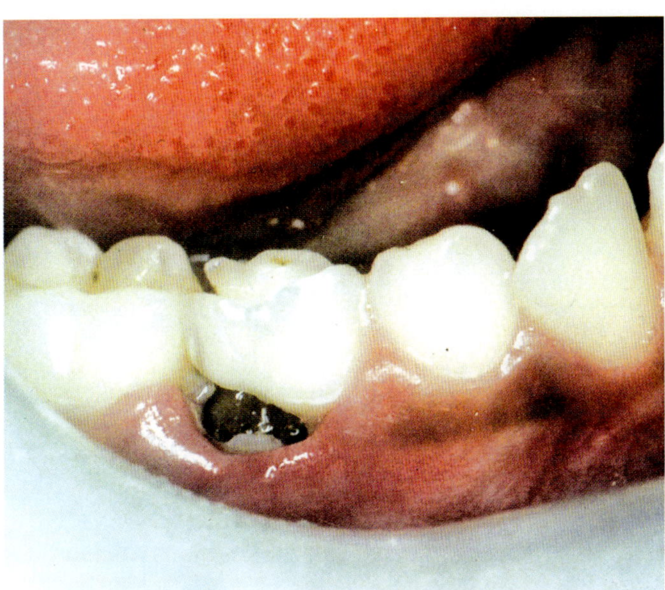

Fig. 13.20: Acute infection of first deciduous molar with furcal involvement that cannot be rehabilitated

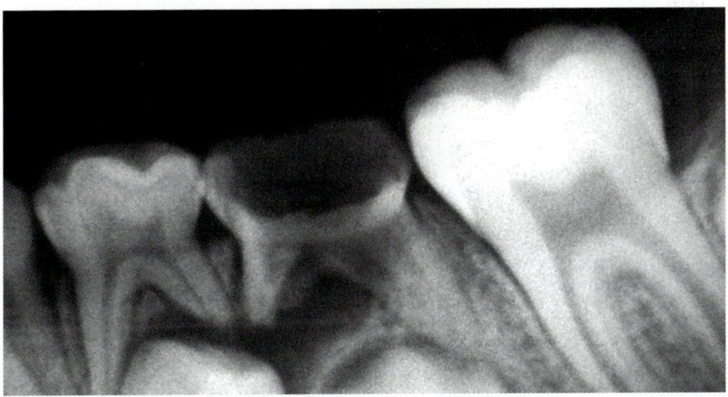

Fig. 13.21: Chronic infection of deciduous teeth as seen with relation to second deciduous molar may hinder the development of the permanent tooth

Supernumerary Tooth (Figs 13.23A to D)

The supernumerary tooth, erupted or impacted, is capable of diverting eruption of a permanent tooth from its normal path, impacting it, or delaying its eruption and should be removed.

Fractured or Traumatized Tooth

Trauma can result in various kinds of trauma to the anterior teeth. Such a deciduous tooth that imposes risk to the permanent teeth should be removed.

Impacted Tooth

The impacted tooth may be a supernumerary tooth, a malformed tooth, or an unerupted, ectopically placed tooth.

Contraindications to Tooth Removal

The removal of a tooth is contraindicated where acute symptoms of oral or systemic disease are manifested in the child patient such as:

Acute Systemic Infections

After the acute stages of systemic infections, such as glomerulonephritis, congenital heart disease, rheumatic fever, rheumatic heart disease, are reduced to chronicity, regimens of chemoprophylaxis will be required before extractions.

Blood Diseases

The hemophilic or leukemic child will require a well trained general dentist, a pediatric dentist, or an oral surgeon along with a hematologist to perform satisfactorily the measures required during tooth removal.

Uncontrolled Diabetes Mellitus

Tooth removals should be avoided. Surgical wounds heal poorly, and postoperative pain can be extreme. Recurrent hemorrhages may result.

Irradiated Bone

Tooth removal should be avoided. If an extraction is necessary, it should be accomplished before radiation therapy. Osteomyelitis usually develops following an extraction in an irradiated patient because of osseous avascularity.

Acute Oral Infection

In the presence of oral infections, such as acute necrotizing ulcerative gingivitis, acute herpetic stomatitis, acute dentoalveolar abscess, and other acute forms of oral disease, tooth removals are definitely contraindicated until the infections are eliminated.

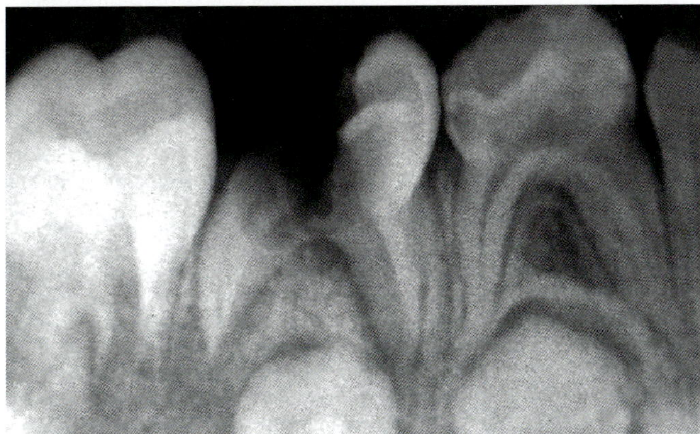

Fig. 13.22: Second deciduous molar beyond rehabilitation and is indicated for extraction

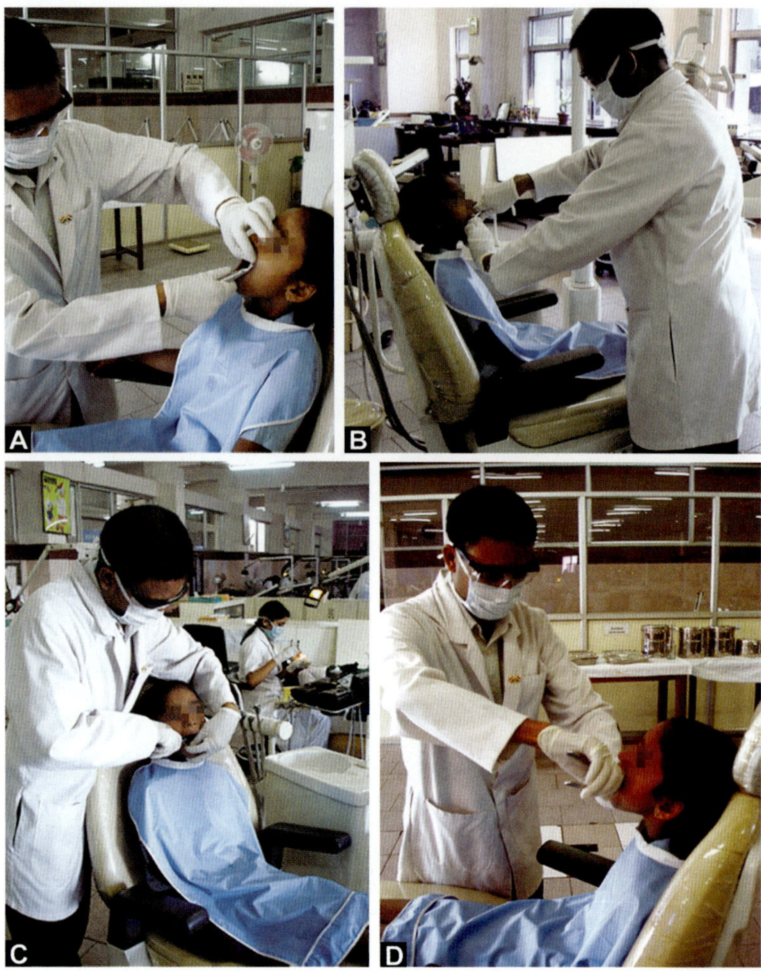

Figs 13.23A to D: Operator's and patient's position during extraction: (A) Upper teeth extraction; (B) Lower anterior extraction; (C) Lower right posterior quadrant extraction; (D) Lower left posterior quadrant extraction

Special consideration while deciding whether a primary tooth has to be extracted or retained:

- Child management: If the emergency is severe enough, the tooth has questionable prognosis and treatment may require many appointments in a child who is difficult to manage then the tooth is extracted followed by placement of a space maintainer
- Degree of root resorption: If > ½ of the root is resorbed and the tooth requires pulp treatment then it is extracted
- Space problems: If there is an existing space problem, early extraction of the tooth may allow space closure. In such cases tooth has to be retained by pulp treatment
- Degree of parental concern: If parents exhibit an obvious lack of concern over the emergency situation related to the injured tooth, the tooth is removed
- Habits: Deleterious oral habits if present will enhance the rate of space closure. In such cases tooth must be retained

Contd...

Contd...

- Speech: Early loss of the anterior teeth may have a direct effect on the speech patterns and this is another reason for maintaining the tooth in the arch
- Esthetics: For psychological purpose it is better to postpone the extraction.

Position of the Operator and the Patient (Fig. 13.24)

Patient position: The dental chair is positioned such that the back is about 45° to the floor during extraction of the upper teeth and at about 90° while extracting the lower teeth. The height of the chair is adjusted such that the operator does not need to bend nor lift his/her arm above the shoulder. Practically the operator must be able to perform the procedure without straining oneself.

The position of the operator is in front of the patient for extraction of teeth in all the quadrants except the lower right posterior quadrant. During the extraction of the teeth in the lower right posterior quadrant the operator sits or stands at about 11 O' clock position.

TECHNIQUE FOR EXTRACTION

Precautions to be Taken

The dentist should explain to the child the sensations and experiences to be encountered before administration of the local anesthetic. The child should also be informed briefly the procedure of extraction in a simple language so that the child can be prepared and be ready for the procedure. To the uninformed child the sensation of pressure from the forceps during the extraction procedure can be interpreted as pain, and extraneous noise and osseous sound conduction associated with luxation may aggravate the anxiety. Explanation and demonstration to the child that pressures and noises associated with tooth extraction need not be feared is very important as the primary step.

When a mandibular tooth is removed, it is prudent to stabilize the mandible by providing support under the mandible (Fig. 13.25).

During extraction of deciduous teeth extra care must be taken to avoid the unintentional¬ accidental removal of the permanent tooth bud.

Another measure of precaution is the use of a throat guard that acts as safety screen over the oropharynx behind the tongue to guard against swallowing or aspiration of an extracted tooth.

Primary Incisors and Canines

Procedure

1. Periosteal elevator is used to free the attached gingiva from the cervix of the tooth labially and lingually. The tooth can be luxated slightly with the same instrument, especially if the tooth is mobile.
2. Firm apical pressure is maintained with the forceps. Gently direct the initial luxative force lingually/ palatally and carefully apply the next toward the labial side. A rotative force is applied along the tooth's long axis, delivering it through its path of least resistance.
3. Mold the labial and lingual or palatal plates of the alveolar bone into normal conformity with digital pressure.
4. Fold and place a sterile gauze sponge over the wound to help establish hemostasis. Immediately before patient dismissal, place a fresh sterile gauze over

the wound with instructions to remove it after 10-20 minutes.

Primary Molars

Procedure

1. Periosteal elevator is used to free the attached gingiva from the cervix of the tooth labially and lingually. The tooth can be luxated slightly with the same instrument, especially if the tooth is mobile.
2. Firm apical pressure is applied with the forceps (Fig. 13.26). Initial luxation movement is toward the buccal side. Hold pressure momentarily, permitting buccal alveolar plate expansion. Return the luxating

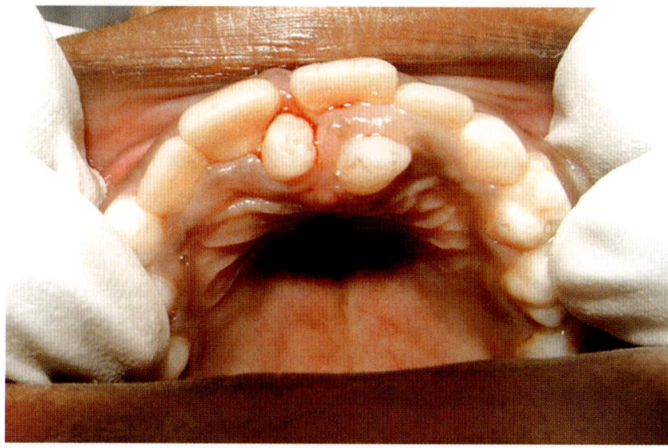

Fig. 13.24: Supernumerary teeth (mesiodens) seen erupting palatally is advised for extraction

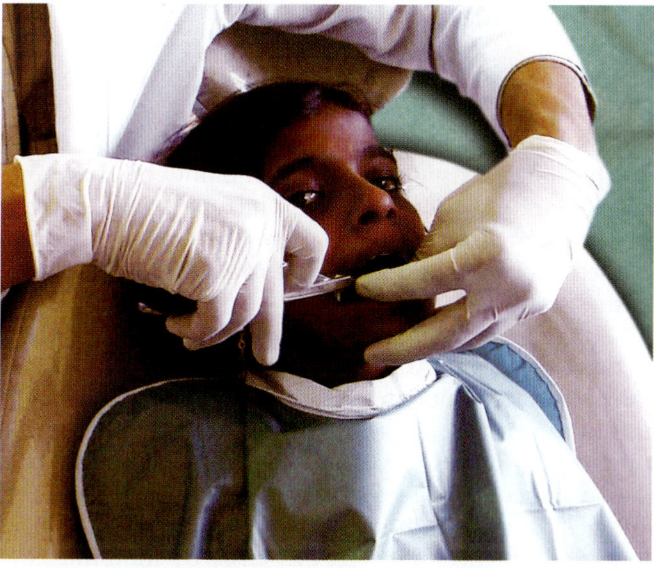

Fig. 13.25: Supporting mandible during extraction of lower teeth are very important to prevent dislocation

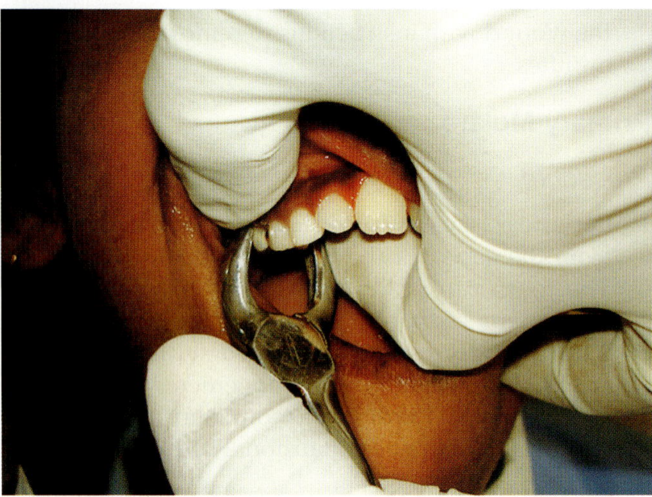

Fig. 13.26: Firm apical pressure is applied with the forceps. The crown is held at the cervical portion. Note the position of the non-operating hand used for supporting the alveolus

force lingually/palatally. Hold pressure to permit lingual alveolar plate expansion. Alternate the buccal and lingual/palatally movements to further expand the cortical plate. When there is adequate freedom of movement, deliver the tooth to the buccal side, exercising slow, firm, continuous pressure.

3. Mold the labial and palatal cortical plates into normal conformity with finger pressure. Place a folded sterile gauze over the wound during the hemostatic process.

ANALGESICS AND ANTIBIOTICS USED IN DENTISTRY

Anti-inflammatory Analgesics

Inflammation is the body's effort to inactivate or destroy microorganisms, remove irritants and aid in repair. Inflammation is triggered by the chemicals released by the injured tissue such as histamine, bradykinins, prostaglandins, interleukin, etc. The typical clinical signs that are seen during inflammation such as pain, swelling, redness and increase in temperature are due to the release of these chemical mediators.

Analgesics are drugs that are prescribed to relieve patient from pain. Analgesics are basically of two types, the opioid (Narcotic drugs) and the Nonsteroidal anti-inflammatory drugs (NSAID). The opioids are less preferred to the NSAIDs as the later do not cause any kind of drowsiness. NSAID's are effective anti-inflammatory, analgesic and antipyretic drugs and are routinely used in dental practice. They act primarily by inhibiting the cyclooxygenase enzymes that catalyze the first step in prostaglandin synthesis.

Classification of Nonsteroidal Anti-inflammatory Drugs

1. Nonselective COX inhibitors:
   – Salicylates: Aspirin
   – Propionic acid derivative: Ibuprofen
   – Anthranilic acid derivative: Mephenamic acid
   – Arylacetic acid derivative: Diclofenac
   – Oxicam derivative: Piroxicam
   – Pyrrolo-pyrrole derivative: Ketorolac
   – Indole derivative: Indomethacin
   – Pyrazolone derivative: Phenylbutazone
2. Preferential COX-2 inhibitors: Nimusulide
3. Selective COX-2 inhibitors: Rofecoxib, Valdecoxib
4. Analgesic: Antipyretics with poor anti-inflammatory action
   – Para-aminophenol derivatives: Paracetamol
   – Pyrazolone derivative: Metamizol
   – Benzoxazocine derivative: Nefopam.

> **Combination of paracetamol and ibuprofen**
>
> This combination has an addictive effect. Scientifically no extra benefit has been observed while using this combination. Though this combination is readily marketed and used, its use should be restricted to a short period.

Antimicrobial Agents Used in Dentistry

Antibiotics are drugs used to combat infections. The term antimicrobial agents are more apt as these drugs act against microbes responsible for a particular disease.

Advantage of Oral Antimicrobial Agents

1. Oral antimicrobial agents bring the infection under control faster and also prevent the progression of the disease to a more severe form.
2. Effective against most of the pathogenic microorganisms.
3. Have the ability to prevent complications of infections.
4. Reduce the need for hospitalization.
5. Most convenient and costteffective.
6. No need for frequent visits.
7. Side effects are minimum.
8. Anaphylactic reactions are rarely seen.
9. Convenient frequency of administration which can be either four, three, twice or even just once a day.
10. Easy to consume and is available in different flavors.
11. Hospitalization is avoided.

Commonly Encountered Infections in Dental Practice

1. Periapical infection
2. Cellulitis and its complication like Ludwig's angina
3. Periodontal infections
4. Gingival infections
5. Osteomyelitis

Disadvantage of injectable antimicrobial agents

- Need for frequent administration
- Fear of injection in children and even adults
- Small muscle mass in children—large doses not possible
- Complications like pain, swelling and abscess formation
- Severe complications like anaphylactic shock and syncopal attacks.

Very few antimicrobials are prescribed routinely by the dentists. But the knowledge of other oral AMAs is essential because a patient may already be taking some other oral AMAs for non-dental problems which could be good enough for dental problem as well.

Antimicrobial Agents Commonly

- Semi-synthetic penicillins: Amoxycillin.
- Cephalosporins
- Macrolides: Erythromycin, roxithromycin, azithromycin and clarithromycin
- Nitroimidazoles: Metronidazole

Advantages of amoxycillin over ampicillin

- Amoxycillin is better absorbed than ampicillin
- Serum level of amoxycillin achieved is twice more than by ampicillin
- Less diarrheal episodes with amoxycillin than ampicillin.

Amoxycillin: They are bactericidal and act by interfering with bacterial cell wall synthesis. It is well absorbed and food does not interfere with absorption. Incidence of diarrhea is less and is eliminated via urine.

Effective against gram +ve organisms such as *staphylococcus*, β hemolytic *Streptococcus*, *Streptococcus viridans*, and few gram –ve organisms such as *E. coli* and *H. influenzae.*

Dosage: 20 to 40 mg/kg body weight/day in 3 divided doses.

Cephalosporins: They are β-lactam antibiotics closely related structurally and functionally to penicillins and are effective against a wide array of bacteria, ranging from Streptococci to gram –ve bacilli including pseudo-monas.

- They are administered IV or IM due to poor oral absorption.
- Adequate distribution in the body.
- Elimination occurs through tubular secretion and or glomerular filtration.
- Adverse effects are allergic manifestations and bleeding.
- Cephalosporins have been divided into 4 generations based on the spectrum of activity
- First generation cephalosporins
  - Highly effective against gram +ve organisms that the gram –ve organisms.
  - Effective against *Streptococcus* and few *Staphylococcus* organisms.
  - Gastrointestinal side effects are rare
  - Better taste
  - Used in soft tissue infections
  - Cephalexin and Cefadroxil are the commonly used oral Cephalosporins
- Second generation cephalosporins
  - Effective against *Staphylococcus aureus*, Beta hemolyticus streptococci, *H. Influenzae, E. coli, Klebsiella and Proteus*
  - Examples are Cefaclor and *Cefuroxime axetil*
- Third generation cephalosporins
  - More useful against Gm –ve infections.
  - Convenient frequency of administration
  - Expensive
  - Examples are Cefixime, Cefpodoxime and Cefdinir
- Fourth generation cephalosporins
  - They have wider antibacterial spectrum and is active against methicillin susceptible streptococci and staphylococci, gramnegative organisms
  - Example is Cefepime

Macrolides

- Erythromycin, roxithromycin, azithromycin and clarithromycin
  - These are effective against organisms susceptible to Penicillins.
  - They act by inhibiting protein synthesis of the microorganism
  - They are available as enteric coated tablets as they are otherwise destroyed by gastric acid.
  - Metabolites are excreted in the urine.
  - Side effects include epigastric distress, cholestatic jaundice, ototoxicity.
  - Roxithromycin and azithromycin are newer macrolides.

Clarythromycin is more active against staphylococcus and streptococci than erythromycin but less effective against *H. influenzae.* Azithromycin is less effective against *Staphylococcus* and *Streptococcus* as compared to erythromycin.

Metronidazole

- Belongs to nitroimidazote group
- Highly effective in anaerobic infections
- Dosage 30 mg/kg/day in 2 to 3 divided doses.
- Metallic taste, nausea, disulfuram like action in adults
- Mechanisms of action—interferes with DNA function leading to inhibition of bacterial protein synthesis.

Selection of Antimicrobial Agents

An appropriate antimicrobial agent is selected based on the following factors:

1. *Infecting organism:* This is done based on scientific methods, by isolating organism from pus, blood or tissues. This is based on experience or knowledge of clinical presentation and probable pathogens that are unique for a particular site.
2. *Site of infection:* Adequate levels of agent must reach the site of infection. Some natural factors may act as barriers. Common barriers are blood brain barrier or the placental barrier. Other factors that determine the effectiveness of the agent at the site of infection are solubility of the drug, molecular weight of the drug and protein binding ability of the drug.
3. *Health or medical history of an individual:* For example, agents that are concentrated or eliminated by liver such as erythromycin are contraindicated in treating patients with liver disease. Patient's immune system also plays a major role in eliminating the microorganisms along with antimicrobial agents. The therapeutic effect of the antimicrobial agents may be altered in immunocompromised patients as associated with infection with HIV.
4. *Route of administration of the drug:* Oral route is selected for mild to moderate infections as it can be used on an outpatient basis and is economical. But certain drugs such as vancomycin are poorly absorbed from the gastrointestinal tract and have to be administered parenterally.
5. *Safety of the agent:* Antimicrobial agents that are specific for a particular microorganism and possess least amount of toxicity should be preferred.

Commonly used antimicrobial drugs			
Drug	Availability	Dosage	Trade names
Amoxicillin	Liquid 125 mg/5 ml, tablet 125, 250 mg, capsule 250, 500 mg injection 250, 500 mg	Children >3 months of age up to 40 kg: 20-40 mg/kg/day in divided doses every 8 hours	Amoxil, Blumox, Mox, Glamoxin, Novamox, Wymox

Contd...

Contd...

Amoxicillin clavulanate	Liquid: Amoxicillin 200 mg, clavulanic acid 28.5 mg/5 ml, tablet, Amoxicillin 500 mg, clavulanic acid 125	Based on Amoxicillin Dosage.	Acticlav, Augmentin, Blumox CA, Clamox
Erythromycin	Liquid (125 mg/5 ml), Tablet (125 or 250 or 500 mg)	30-50 mg/kg in divided dose	Althrocin, Erysoft, Eltocin
Cefalexin	Liquid 125 mg/5 ml, tablet 125,250 mg, capsule 250, 500 mg	Children: 25-100 mg/kg/day in divided doses every 8 hours	Anphexin, Neocef, cephalex, sporidex
Clindamycin	Liquid 150 mg/ml, tablet, capsule 150, 300 mg, injection 300 mg/2 ml	Oral Dose: 3-6 mg/kg every 6 hrs. Children weighing <10 kg should receive at least 37.5 mg every 8 hrs	Clinsof, Dalcinex, Pathoclin
Metronidazole	Liquid (200 mg/5 ml), tablets (200 or 400 mg)	7.5 mg/kg body weight 8 hourly	Aldezole, Flagyl, Metrogyl

Commonly used analgesics			
Drug	Availability	Dosage	Trade names
Paracetamol	Liquid (125 or 250 mg/5 ml) Tablet (500 mg)	1-5 years: 120-250 mg 4-6 hourly 6-12 years: 250-500 mg 4-6 hourly (Maximum of 4 doses in 24 hours)	Calpol, Crocin, Metacin, Febrex
Ibuprofen	Liquid (100 mg/5 ml), tablet (200 or 400 mg)	Children < 12 years: 4-10 mg/kg/dose every 6-8 hours Children > 12 years: 200 mg every 4-6 hours as needed (maximum 1200 mg/24 hours)	Brufen, Ibugesic, Ibugin

Contd...

Contd...

Diclofenac sodium	Tablets (50 mg), patch (100 mg/ 50 sq cm)	Children 6-12 years- 1-2 mg/ kg in divided doses	Diclotal, Nu-patch, Dicloact
Ibuprofen-paracetamol combination	Tablets (Ibuprofen 400 mg and paracetamol 325 mg) Syrup (Ibuprofen 100 mg and paracetamol 100 or 125 or 162.5 mg/5 ml)	Ibuprofen 100 mg and par-acetamol 125 mg/5 ml) tid	Calpol Plus, Combiflam, Ibugesic Plus, Imol

Post-treatment instructions to parents/child following extraction/surgery

1. The mouth will be numb approximately 2-4 hours. Watch to see that your child does not bite, scratch, or injure the cheek, lips, or tongue during this time.
2. Bleeding is controlled, but some occasional oozing (pink or blood-tinged saliva) may occur. Hold gauze or a clean cloth with firm pressure against the extraction site until oozing has stopped. If bleeding continues for more than 2 hours, contact us.
3. *Surgical site care:* Do not rinse vigorously, use mouthwash, or probe the area with fingers or other objects. Do not stretch the lips or cheeks. Beginning tomorrow, you may rinse with warm salt water (½ teaspoon salt with 1 cup water) after meals.
4. *Sutures:* Sutures (stitches) were placed to help control bleeding and promote healing. These sutures will dissolve and do not need to be removed OR will be removed at your follow-up visit.
5. Avoid physical exercise and exertion on the first day.
6. After all bleeding has stopped, the patient may drink cool non-carbonated liquids but should not use a straw. Cold soft foods are ideal the first day. By the second day, consistency of foods can progress as tolerated. Until healing is more established, avoid foods such as nuts and popcorn that may get lodged in the surgical areas.
7. *Oral hygiene:* Keeping the mouth clean is essential. Teeth may be brushed and flossed gently on the first day, but avoid stimulating the area of extraction.
8. *Pain:* Prescribed medicines should be given as told to avoid discomfort to your child.

REFERENCES

1. Olsen NH. Anesthesia for the child patient. J Am Dent Assoc 1956;53:548-55.
2. Malamed SF. Handbook of Anesthesia. St Louis, Mosby, 1980.
3. Oertel R, Ebert U, Rahn R, Kirch W. Clinical pharmacokinetics of articaine. Clin Pharmacokinet 1997;33(6):417-26.
4. Malamed SF. Handbook of local anaesthesia. St. Louis Mosby 2004;(5):71.
5. HornkeI, Eckert HG, Rupp W. Pharnakokinetik und Metabolismus von Articain nach intramuskularer Injektion am mannlichen Probanden. Dtsch Z Mund Kiefer Gesichts Chir 1984;8:67-71.
6. Kirch W, Kitteringham N, Lambers G, et al. Die Klinische Pharmakokinetik von Articain nach intraoraler und intramuskularer Application. Schweiz Monatsschr Zahnheilkd 1983;93:713-9.
7. Vree TB, Gielen MJ. Clinical pharmacology and the use of articaine for local regional anesthesia. Best Pract Res Clin Anesthesiol 2005;19(2):293-308.
8. Kanaa MD, et al. Articaine and lidocaine mandibular buccal infiltration anesthesia: a prospective randomized double blind cross over study. J Endodontics 2006; 32(4): 296-8.
9. Oulis CJ, Vadiakas GP, Vasilopoulou A. The effectiveness of mandibular infiltration compared to mandibular block anesthesia in treating primary molars in children. Pediatr Dent 1996;18:301-5.
10. Tavares M, et al. Reversal of soft tissue local anesthesia with phentolamine mesylate in pediatric patients. JADA 2008;139:1095-104.
11. Krochak M, Friedman N. Using a precision metered injection system to minimize dental injection anxiety. Compend Contin Educ Dent 1998;19:137-43, 146-50.
12. Allen KD, et al. Comparison of a computerized anesthesia device with a traditional syringe in preschool children. Pediatr Dent 2002;24(4):315-20.
13. Sharaf AA. Evaluation of mandibular infiltration versus block anesthesia in pediatric dentistry. J Dent Child 1997;64:276-81.

FURTHER READING

1. American Academy of Pediatric Dentistry Clinical Affairs Committee; American Academy of Pediatric Dentistry Council on Clinical Affairs: Guideline on antibiotic prophylaxis for dental patients at risk for infection. Pediatr Dent 2005-2006;27(7 Reference Manual):168-9.
2. Ashkenazi M, Blumer S, Eli I. Effectiveness of various modes of computerized delivery of local anesthesia in primary maxillary molars. Pediatr Dent 2006;28(1):29-38.
3. Burns Y, Reader A, Nusstein J, Beck M, Weaver J. Anesthetic efficacy of the palatal-anterior superior alveolar injection. J Am Dent Assoc 2004;135(9):1269-76.
4. David HT, Aminzadeh KK, Kae AH, Radomsky SC. Instrument retraction to avoid needle-stick injuries during intraoral local anesthesia. Oral Surg Oral Med Oral Pathol Oral Radiol Endod 2007;103(3):e11-3. Epub 2007.
5. Gazal G, Mackie IC. Distress related to dental extraction for children under general anaesthesia and their parents. Eur J Paediatr Dent 2007;8(1):7-12.
6. Gibson RS, Allen K, Hutfless S, Beiraghi S. The Wand vs. traditional injection: a comparison of pain related behaviors. Pediatr Dent 2000;22(6):458-62.

7. Hung PC, Chang HH, Yang PJ, Kuo YS, Lan WH, Lin CP. Comparison of the Gow-Gates mandibular block and inferior alveolar nerve block using a standardized protocol. J Formos Med Assoc 2006;105(2):139-46.

8. Lai TN, Lin CP, Kok SH, Yang PJ, Kuo YS, Lan WH, Chang HH. Evaluation of mandibular block using a standardized method. Oral Surg Oral Med Oral Pathol Oral Radiol Endod 2006;102(4):462-8. Epub 2006.

9. Malamed SF. Local anesthetics: dentistry's most important drugs, clinical update 2006. J Calif Dent Assoc 2006;34(12):971-6.

10. Maragakis GM, Musselman RJ, Ho CC. Reaction of 5 and 6 year olds to dental injection after viewing the needle: pilot study. J Clin Pediatr Dent 2006; Fall 31(1):28-31.

11. Oztas N, Ulusu T, Bodur H, Dogan C. The wand in pulp therapy: an alternative to inferior alveolar nerve block. Quintessence Int 2005;36(7-8):559-64.

12. Planells del Pozo P, Barra Soto MJ, Santa Eulalia Troisfontaines E. Antibiotic prophylaxis in pediatric odontology. An update. Med Oral Patol Oral Cir Bucal 2006;11(4):E352-7. Review.

13. Ram D, Efrat J, Michovitz N, Moskovitz M. The use of popsicles after dental treatment with local anesthesia in pediatric patients. J Clin Pediatr Dent 2006; 31(1):41-3.

14. Ram D. Postoperative pain and analgesic use in children. Br Dent J 2007;202(5):276-7.

15. Rega AJ, Aziz SR, Ziccardi VB. Microbiology and antibiotic sensitivities of head and neck space infections of odontogenic origin. J Oral Maxillofac Surg 2006; 64(9):1377-80.

16. Roberts GJ, Jaffray EC, Spratt DA, Petrie A, Greville C, Wilson M, Lucas VS. Duration, prevalence and intensity of bacteraemia after dental extractions in children. Heart 2006;92(9):1274-7. Epub 2006.

17. Schwartz-Arad D, Dolev E, Williams W. Maxillary nerve block—a new approach using a computer-controlled anesthetic delivery system for maxillary sinus elevation procedure. A prospective study. Quintessence Int 2004; 35(6):477-80.

18. Scott JK, Moxham BJ, Downie IP. Upper lip blanching and diplopia associated with local anaesthesia of the inferior alveolar nerve. Br Dent J 2007;202(1):32-3.13.

QUESTIONS

1. Write in detail the branches of maxillary and mandibular nerves.
2. What is the role of topical anesthesia?
3. Define anesthesia. Give the composition of local anesthetic solution.
4. Classification of vasoconstrictors used with local anesthetics.
5. Classification of local anesthetic agents.
6. Write in detail about articaine.
7. Explain the mode of action of local anesthesia.
8. Factors affecting absorption, metabolism and excretion of anesthetic agent.
9. Explain the complications following local anesthetic administration.
10. What are the types of syringe available for administration of local anesthesia?
11. Enumerate the types of injection procedures.
12. What are the different techniques for anesthesia of maxillary and mandibular tissues?
13. Explain in detail the inferior alveolar block.
14. What are the precautions one must take while performing extraction in child patient?
15. Give the indications for extraction of deciduous tooth.
16. Explain the position of the operator and the patient while performing extraction of the lower right quadrant.
17. Make a list of the analgesics and antibiotics used in dentistry.

Chapter 14

Gingival and Periodontal Diseases in Children

INTRODUCTION

The periodontium is a connective tissue organ covered by epithelium that attaches the teeth to the bones of the jaws and provides a continually adapting apparatus for support of teeth during function.

It comprises of (Fig. 14.1):

- Gingiva
- Periodontal ligament
- Alveolar bone
- Cementum

DIFFERENCES BETWEEN THE CHILD AND ADULT PERIODONTIUM

Features Seen in a Child[1-5]

1. Greater sulcus depth—mean depth is 2.1+/– 0.2 mm
2. Free gingiva—thicker and rounder due to cervical bulge and underlying constriction
3. Flaccid and retractable marginal gingiva due to immature connective tissue and gingival fiber system and also due to increased vascularization
4. Attached gingiva—greater width
5. Presence of interdental cleft, found in inter-radicular zone and retrocuspid papilla, 1 mm below the free gingival groove lingual to mandibular canine
6. Periodontal space is wider with few fibers
7. Alveolar bone
   - Less calcified
   - More vascular
   - Few but thicker trabeculae
   - Larger marrow space

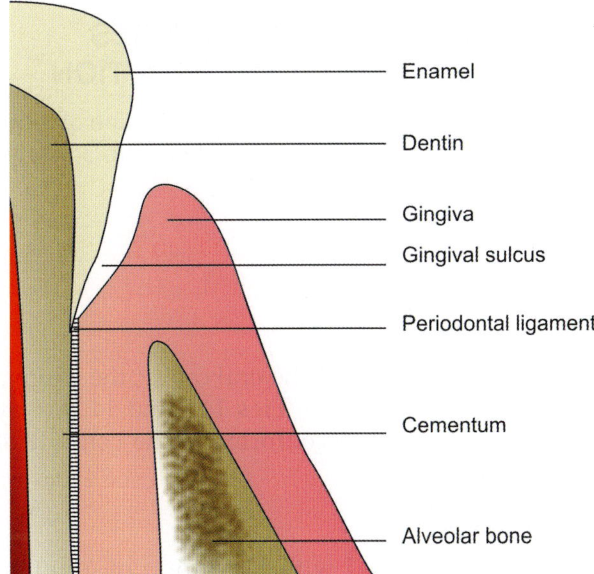

Fig. 14.1: Components of periodontium

- Prominent lamina dura
- Flattened interdental crests

8. Gingivitis is common than periodontitis and is more transient and acute, compared to progressive and chronic in adults.

It was initially thought that gingivitis rarely progressed to periodontitis in prepubertal children. The reasons given were as, more anabolic activity due to increase metabolism, absence of bacteria responsible for periodontal disease such as Spirochetes and B. melaninogenicus, altered composition of plaque and decreased leukocytic migratory rate due to low levels of immunoglobulin specific for plaque bacteria and decreased vascular inflammatory response.

But it is believed that periodontal disease seen in adults may have its origin in childhood. Therefore, American Academy of Pediatric Dentistry stress on prevention, early diagnosis and aggressive treatment of gingival and periodontal disease in children.[3]

Common periodontal diseases

1. Prepubertal periodontitis—localized and generalized
2. Early onset periodontitis—juvenile periodontitis
3. Associated with systemic diseases

Common gingival diseases

1. Acute pericoronitis
2. Eruptive gingivitis
3. ANUG
4. Gingival fibromatosis and hyperplasia

PHYSIOLOGIC GINGIVAL CHANGES ASSOCIATED WITH TOOTH ERUPTION

Gingival changes that occur during the eruption of tooth can be studied, by dividing the eruption into 3 stages, as follows:[6]

- Pre-eruptive stage
- Eruptive stage
- Posteruptive stage

Pre-eruptive Stage

Before the crown appears in the oral cavity, the gingiva presents a bulge that is firm (Figs 14.2 and 14.3), may be slightly blanched and conforms to the contour of underlying crown.

Eruptive Stage

This stage is associated with formation of gingival margin. Marginal gingiva and sulcus develop as the

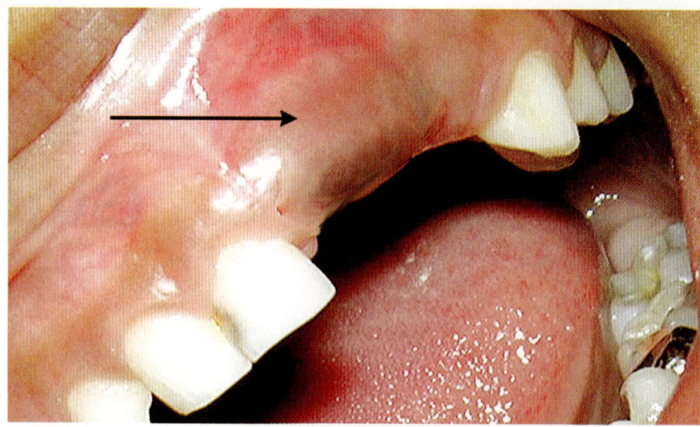

Fig. 14.2: Bulge appears on the ridge just before the tooth erupts into the oral cavity

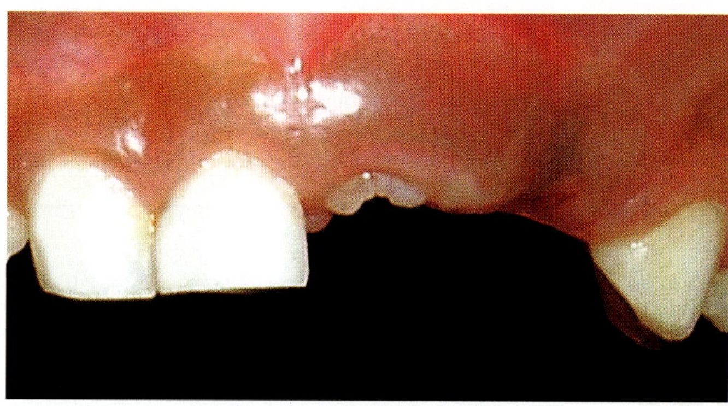

Fig. 14.3: Teeth seen just erupting through the ridge few days after the previous picture was taken

crown penetrates the oral mucosa. In the course of eruption the gingival margin is usually edematous, rounded and slightly reddened (Fig. 14.4).

During the period of mixed dentition it is normal for marginal gingiva around the permanent teeth to be quite prominent, particularly in the maxillary anterior region. At this stage in tooth eruption the gingiva is still attached to the crown and it appears prominent when superimposed on the bulk of the underlying enamel.

Posteruptive Stage

The gingiva reduces in bulk and becomes thinner and tight and firmly attached around the cervical portion of the tooth (Fig. 14.5).

Gingivitis

It is the inflammatory involvement of gingival tissue. Microscopically it is characterized by presence of inflammatory exudate and edema and destruction of collagenous gingival fibers. Ulcerations of the epithelium are also seen.

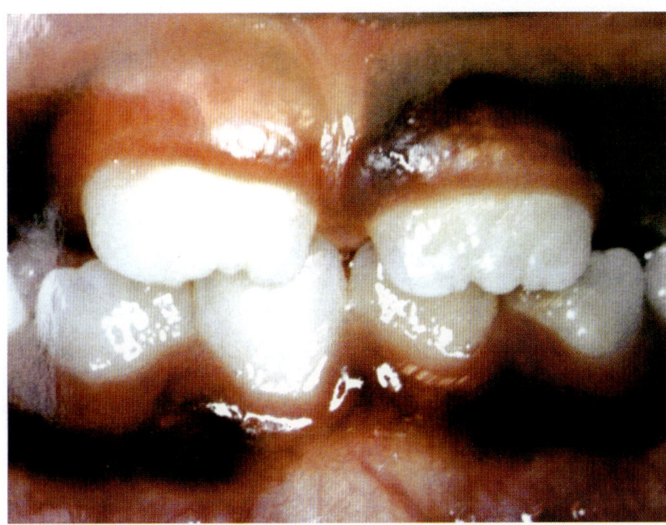

Fig. 14.4: Rounded and red gingival margin around the erupting tooth

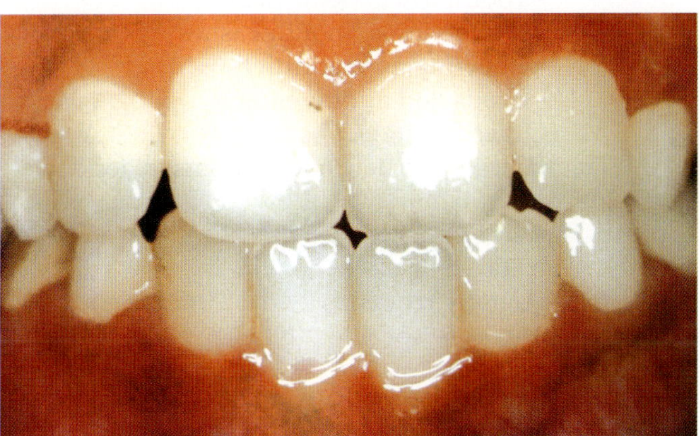

Fig. 14.5: Thin gingival margin seen around a fully erupted tooth

Stages of Gingivitis[6]

Stage I: Initial Lesion

A. Time period—2 to 4 days
B. Vascular dilatation and vasculitis is seen
C. Junctional and sulcular epithelium are seen infiltrated by polymorphonuclear cells
D. Associated with mild change in color.

Stage II: Early Lesion

A. Time period—4 to 7 days
B. Increased vascular proliferation
C. Junctional and sulcular epithelium is seen infiltrated by polymorphonuclear cells, rete pegs formation, atrophic areas
D. Lymphocytes are predominant

E. Loss of collagen
F. Clinical findings include erythema, bleeding on probing.

Stage III: Established Lesion

A. Time period—14 to 21 days
B. Increased vascular proliferation and blood stasis
C. Changes seen in the junctional and sulcular epithelium are more severe than stage II
D. Plasma cells are predominant
E. Severe loss of collagen.
F. Clinical findings include changes in color, size and texture, etc.

Stage IV: Advanced Lesion

A. The lesion extends into alveolar bone
B. Characterized by periodontal breakdown.

Clinical Features of Gingivitis

1. Gingival bleeding: Two earliest symptoms of gingival inflammation are:
   – Increased gingival fluid production rate
   – Bleeding from gingival sulcus on probing
2. Change in the color of gingiva:
   – Normal color is coral pink. Inflamed tissue is red or bluish red.
3. Changes in consistency of gingiva:
   – In chronic inflammation, both destructive (edematous) and reparative (fibrotic) changes co exist.
4. Changes in surface texture of the gingiva:
   – Loss of surface stippling is an early sign of gingivitis.
   – Chronic inflammation—the surface is either smooth and shiny or firm and nodular depending on whether changes are exudative or fibrotic.

ETIOLOGY OF GINGIVAL DISEASES

I. Local irritating factors
   A. Bacterial plaque
   B. Predisposing factors like: material alba, food debris, malalignment of teeth, dental calculus, etc.
II. Local functioning factors
   A. Malocclusion
   B. Habits: mouth breathing, tongue thrusting
   C. Eruption of teeth
III. Systemic factors
   A. Puberty
   B. Vitamin or protein deficiency
   C. Drugs and chemicals

D. Pregnancy
E. Hereditary
F. Metabolic disorders
G. Hematological disorder
H. Viral, bacterial and fungal infections.

Classification of Gingival Diseases[7]

I. As per the International Workshop for a Classification of Periodontal Diseases and Conditions

A. Dental plaque-induced gingival diseases
  1. Gingivitis associated with dental plaque only
    a. Without other local contributing factors
    b. With local contributing factors (See VIII A)
  2. Gingival diseases modified by systemic factors
    a. Associated with the endocrine system
      − Puberty-associated gingivitis
      − Menstrual cycle-associated gingivitis
      − Pregnancy-associated
        - Gingivitis
        - Pyogenic granuloma
      − Diabetes mellitus-associated gingivitis
    b. Associated with blood dyscrasias
      − Leukemia-associated gingivitis
      − Other
  3. Gingival diseases modified by medications
    a. Drug-influenced gingival diseases
      − Drug-influenced gingival enlargements
      − Drug-influenced gingivitis
        - Oral contraceptive-associated gingivitis
        - Other
  4. Gingival diseases modified by malnutrition
    a. Ascorbic acid-deficiency gingivitis
    b. Other
B. Non-plaque-induced gingival lesions
  1. Gingival diseases of specific bacterial origin
    a. *Neisseria gonorrhoeae*-associated lesions
    b. Treponema pallidum-associated lesions
    c. Streptococcal species-associated lesions
    d. Other
  2. Gingival diseases of viral origin
    a. Herpesvirus infections
      − Primary herpetic gingivostomatitis
      − Recurrent oral herpes
      − Varicella-zoster infections
    b. Other
  3. Gingival diseases of fungal origin
    a. Candida-species infections
      − Generalized gingival candidiasis
    b. Linear gingival erythema
    c. Histoplasmosis
    d. Other

4. Gingival lesions of genetic origin
    a. Hereditary gingival fibromatosis
    b. Other
5. Gingival manifestations of systemic conditions
    a. Mucocutaneous disorders
      − Lichen planus
      − Pemphigoid
      − Pemphigus vulgaris
      − Erythema multiforme
      − Lupus erythematosus
      − Drug-induced
      − Other
    b. Allergic reactions
      − Dental restorative materials
        - Mercury
        - Nickel
        - Acrylic
        - Other
      − Reactions attributable to:
        - Toothpastes/dentifrices
        - Mouthrinses/mouthwashes
        - Chewing gum additives
        - Foods and additives
      − Other
6. Traumatic lesions (factitious, iatrogenic, accidental)
    a. Chemical injury
    b. Physical injury
    c. Thermal injury
7. Foreign body reactions
8. Not otherwise specified (NOS).

Classification of Periodontal Disease[7]

Chronic Periodontitis

A. Localized
B. Generalized

Aggressive Periodontitis

A. Localized
B. Generalized

Periodontitis as a Manifestation of Systemic Diseases

A. Associated with hematological disorders
    1. Acquired neutropenia
    2. Leukemias
    3. Other
B. Associated with genetic disorders
    1. Familial and cyclic neutropenia
    2. Down syndrome
    3. Leukocyte adhesion deficiency syndromes
    4. Papillon-Lefèvre syndrome

5. Chediak-Higashi syndrome
6. Histiocytosis syndromes
7. Glycogen storage disease
8. Infantile genetic agranulocytosis
9. Cohen syndrome
10. Ehlers-Danlos syndrome (Types IV and VIII)
11. Hypophosphatasia
12. Other
C. Not otherwise specified (NOS)

Necrotizing Periodontal Diseases

A. Necrotizing ulcerative gingivitis (NUG)
B. Necrotizing ulcerative periodontitis (NUP)

Abscesses of the Periodontium

A. Gingival abscess
B. Periodontal abscess
C. Pericoronal abscess

Periodontitis Associated with Endodontic Lesions

Combined periodontic-endodontic lesions

Developmental or Acquired Deformities and Conditions

A. Localized tooth-related factors that modify or predispose to plaque-induced gingival diseases/periodontitis
   1. Tooth anatomic factors
   2. Dental restorations/appliances
   3. Root fractures
   4. Cervical root resorption and cemental tears
B. Mucogingival deformities and conditions around teeth
   1. Gingival/soft tissue recession
        a. Facial or lingual surfaces
        b. Interproximal (papillary)
   2. Lack of keratinized gingiva
   3. Decreased vestibular depth
   4. Aberrant frenum/muscle position
   5. Gingival excess
        a. Pseudopocket
        b. Inconsistent gingival margin
        c. Excessive gingival display
        d. Gingival enlargement
   6. Abnormal color
C. Mucogingival deformities and conditions on edentulous ridges
   1. Vertical and/or horizontal ridge deficiency
   2. Lack of gingiva/keratinized tissue
   3. Gingival/soft tissue enlargement
   4. Aberrant frenum/muscle position
   5. Decreased vestibular depth
   6. Abnormal color

D. Occlusal trauma
   1. Primary occlusal trauma
   2. Secondary occlusal trauma

Gingival and periodontal diseases in children may be divided as follows:[6]

Gingival Disease

1. Simple gingivitis
    a. Eruption gingivitis
    b. Gingivitis associated with poor oral hygiene
2. Acute gingival inflammation
    – Herpes simplex virus infection
    – Recurrent aphthous ulcer
    – Acute necrotizing ulcerative gingivitis
    – Acute candidiasis
    – Acute bacterial infections
3. Chronic non-specific gingivitis
4. Conditioned gingival enlargement
    a. Puberty gingivitis
    b. Fibromatosis
    c. Phenytoin induced gingival overgrowth
5. Scorbutic gingivitis

Periodontal Disease

• Pre-pubertal periodontitis
• Localized aggressive periodontitis (Localized juvenile periodontitis)
• Generalized aggressive periodontitis (Generalized juvenile periodontitis).

Eruption Gingivitis

• Seen during the eruption of teeth and subsides soon after
• Greatest incidence is 6 to 7 years when permanent teeth begin to erupt
• Reason for this is due to lack of protection to the gingiva from the coronal contour of the tooth
• It may be painful and develop into pericoronitis or pericoronal abscess
• Management includes improving oral hygiene. Some severe cases may require antibiotic therapy.

Gingivitis Associated with Poor Oral Hygiene

• Oral hygiene and gingivitis are directly related
• Adequate oral hygiene practice leading to thorough plaque removal and eating raw fiber vegetables and fruits have beneficial effect on reducing gingivitis
• It can be grouped as early, moderate and advanced gingivitis (Fig. 14.6)
• Early gingivitis is quickly reversible and treated with good tooth brushing and flossing
• Moderate and severe gingivitis requires more elaborate measures.

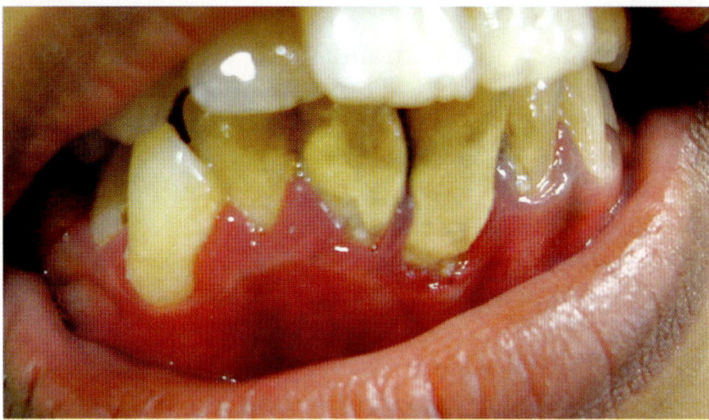

Fig. 14.6: Advanced gingivitis seen due to heavy calculus deposits

Gingivitis Associated with HSV I Infection

- Caused by the herpes simplex virus (HSV)
- Herpetic stomatitis is a common oral disease which develops in both children and young adults
- It rarely occurs before the age of six months, apparently because of the presence of circulating antibodies in the infant, derived from the mother
- The disease occurring in children is frequently the primary attack
- It is characterized by the development of fever, irritability, headache, pain upon swallowing and regional lymphadenopathy
- Within a few days the mouth becomes painful and the gingiva intensely inflamed
- The lips, tongue, buccal mucosa, palate, pharynx and tonsils may also be involved
- Shortly, yellowish, fluid filled vesicles develop. These rupture and form shallow, ragged, extremely painful ulcers covered by a gray membrane and surrounded by an erythematous halo
- They heal spontaneously within 7 to 14 days and leave no scar
- Treatment is symptomatic such as application of topical anesthetic agents on the ulcers, soft diet and adequate fluids.

Gingivitis Associated with Aphthous Stomatitis

- It can be triggered due to any stress, gastrointestinal disturbance, nutritional deficiency, hormonal imbalance, infection, allergy, etc.
- Of the three types of aphthous minor aphthae are common
- Prodromal phase of paresthesia at the site of ulceration is observed. The ulcers appear in crops of two or three and are less than 10 mm in diameter

- Ulcers are painful and are discrete or confluent
- Persists for about 12 days and heals with no scar formation
- Treatment is symptomatic. Chlorhexidine or nystatin or tetracycline can be prescribed if they are infected.

Acute Necrotizing Ulcerative Gingivitis (ANUG)

1. Caused by Borrelia vincentii and spirochetes
2. Severe ulcerating gingivitis involving the interproximal papillae, covered by a psuedomem-brane is seen
3. Associated with fetid odor
4. Recovery promptly occurs within 36 hours after penicillin therapy and application of hydrogen peroxide.

Associated with Acute Bacterial Infection

- Caused by Streptococci group of bacteria
- The gingiva is painful that bleeds easily
- Papilla is enlarged with associated gingival abscess
- Treatment includes broad spectrum antibiotics, improvement of oral hygiene and chlorhexidine mouth wash.

Associated with Chronic Nonspecific Gingivitis

- No specific etiology. May be triggered by hormonal imbalance seen in the preteenage and teenage children
- It may be localized to the anterior region or may be more generalized
- It is rarely painful, but persists for a longer period of time
- Since the cause is nonspecific the treatment is limited to maintaining the oral hygiene and regular professional prophylaxis.

Puberty Gingivitis

- Occurs in the prepubertal and pubertal period
- Gingival inflammation is confined to the anterior segment and may be limited to single arch only
- Gingiva on the lingual aspect is relatively uninvolved
- Concerned with maintenance of adequate oral hygiene, removal of local irritants, and restoration of caries.

Hereditary Fibromatosis Gingival Enlargement (Fig. 14.7)

- Characterized by slow progressive, benign enlargement of the gingiva

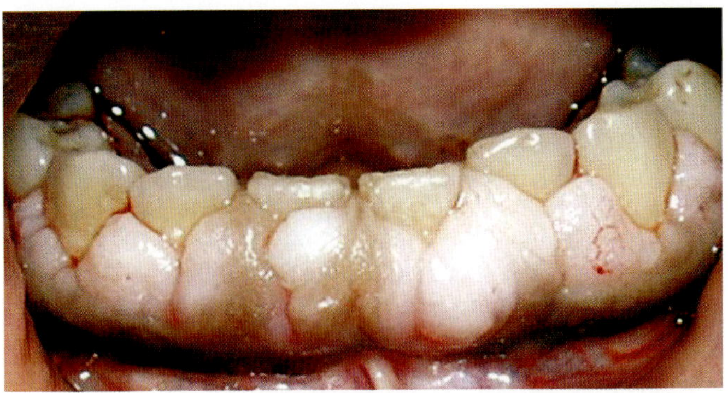

Fig. 14.7: Hereditary fibromatosis gingival enlargement

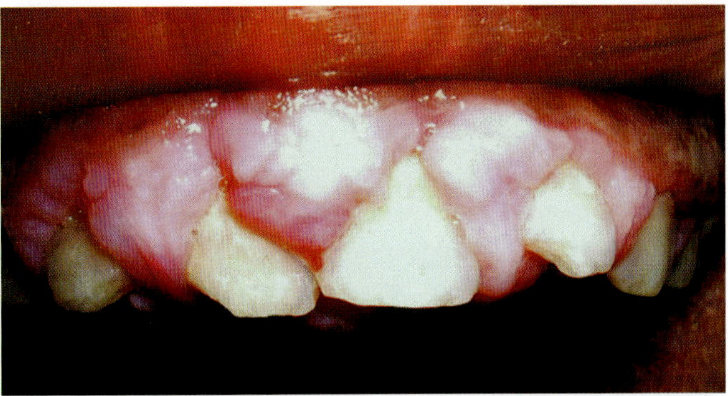

Fig. 14.8: Drug-induced hyperplasia

- The surface is normal appearing
- Appears as soon as the deciduous teeth erupt into the oral cavity and cover the teeth completely
- They are fibrous tending to displace the teeth and are nonpainful
- They regress only if the teeth are extracted
- Surgical excision is the treatment of choice but they recur to the original condition within a period of few years.

Drug-induced Hyperplasia (Fig. 14.8)

- Phenytoin, an anticonvulsant drug is the commonly seen cause of hyperplasia of the gingiva. Other drugs that induce hyperplasia are cyclosporine and Nifedipine.
- Appears as early as 2 to 3 weeks after initiation of the phenytoin therapy and peaks at 18 to 24 months.
- They cause painless enlargement of the gingiva at the interproximal aspect.
- Buccal and anterior segment are more often affected than the lingual and posterior segment.
- Gingiva appears pink and firm unless infected.
- Normally do not bleed readily
- Formation of pseudopockets
- Associated problems are during mastication, speech, etc.
- Management includes adequate oral hygiene maintenance, change of drug or dosage and surgical excision.

Scorbutic Gingivitis

- Associated with vitamin C deficiency
- Involvement is limited to marginal tissue and papillae
- Associated with severe pain, spontaneous hemorrhage
- Management includes replacement of ascorbic acid and oral hygiene maintenance.

Prepubertal Periodontitis

- Normally it is generalized, but when it occurs in deciduous dentition it is localized

- Loss of attachment and alveolar bone loss is seen in deciduous dentition in the molar and incisor region
- Plaque accumulation is minimum. Gingival inflammation may be present
- Seen soon after the eruption of the primary teeth
- Premature loss of teeth is common and all teeth may be lost by 3 years of age
- Actinobacillus actinomycetemcomitans, bacteroids, fusobacterium are found in the gingival pocket
- Management includes early diagnosis, dental curettage, prophylaxis, removal of severely mobile teeth, and broad spectrum antibiotics.

Localized Aggressive Periodontitis

- Seen in otherwise healthy children
- Characterized by rapid and severe loss of alveolar bone around more than one permanent tooth involving the first molars and incisors.
- Appears self-limiting
- No tissue inflammation is seen and little plaque or calculus is present.
- Bone loss is 3 to 4 times faster than adult periodontitis
- Caused by actinobacillus actinomycetemcomitans and bacteroids like organisms.
- Management includes early diagnosis, dental curettage, prophylaxis, removal of severely mobile teeth, and broad spectrum antibiotics.

Generalized Aggressive Periodontitis

1. Seen at around puberty
2. Affects the entire dentition (Fig. 14.9)
3. Caused by nonmotile, facultative, anaerobic, gram negative rod P. gingivalis
4. Management includes early diagnosis, dental curettage, prophylaxis, removal of severely mobile teeth, and broad spectrum antibiotics.

Papillon-Lefevre Syndrome

1. Cause is unknown, familial tendency is present
2. Primary teeth erupt at normal time

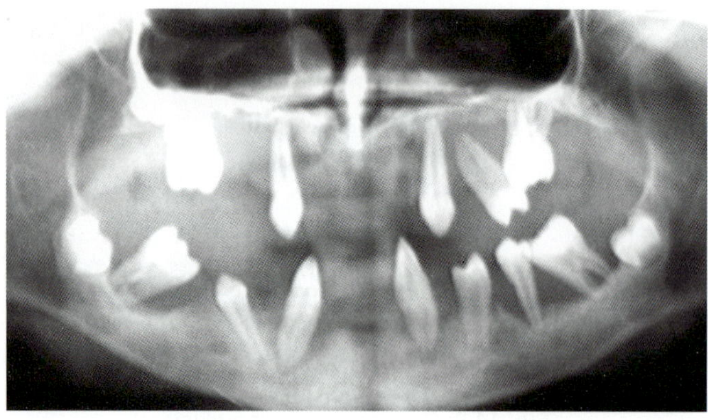

Fig. 14.9: Radiograph showing loss of many permanent teeth in generalized aggressive periodontitis

3. Increased tendency to bleed
4. Palms and soles exhibit hyperkeratosis
5. Teeth become loose with associated severe horizontal bone resorption
6. Permanent dentition may be normal
7. Management includes tetracycline therapy and extraction followed by complete denture.

REFERENCES

1. Delaney JE. Periodontal and soft tissue abnormalities. Dent Clin North Am 1995;39:837-50.
2. Delaney JE, Keels MA. Pediatric oral pathology. Soft tissue and periodontal conditions. Pediatr Clin North Am 2000;47(5):1125-47.
3. Mc Donald RE, Avery DR, Weddell JA, John V. Gingivitis and periodontal disease. In. Mc Donald and Avery's Dentistry for the Child and Adolescent, 9th Ed Elsevier Mosby. 2011.
4. Rosenblum FN. Clinical study of the depth of the gingival sulcus in the primary dentition. J Dent Child 1966;5:289.
5. Brauer JC, Highley LB, Massler M, Schour I. Dentistry for Children, 2nd Ed. Philadelphia, Blakiston 1947.
6. Carranza FA. Glickman's Clinical Periodontology. WB Saunders, Philadelphia.
7. Armitage GC. Development of a classification system for periodontal diseases and conditions. Ann Periodontol 1999;4(1):1-6.

FURTHER READING

1. Addy M, Hunter ML, Kingdon A, Dummer PM, Shaw WC. An 8-year study of changes in oral hygiene and periodontal health during adolescence. Int J Paediatr Dent 1994;4(2):75-80.
2. Bimstein E, Matsson L. Growth and development considerations in the diagnosis of gingivitis and periodontitis in children. Pediatr Dent 1999;21(3):186-91. Review.
3. Darby I, Curtis M. Microbiology of periodontal disease in children and young adults. Periodontol 2000. 2001;26:33-53. Review.
4. Kavvadia K, Pepelassi E, Alexandridis C, Arkadopoulou A, Polyzois G, Tossios K. Gingival fibromatosis and significant tooth eruption delay in an 11-year-old male: a 30-month follow-up. Int J Paediatr Dent 2005;15(4):294-302.
5. Lafzi A, Farahani RM, Shoja MA. Amlodipine-induced gingival hyperplasia. Med Oral Patol Oral Cir Bucal. 2006;11(6):E480-2. Review.
6. Matsson L, Goldberg P. Gingival inflammation at deciduous and permanent teeth. An intra-individual comparison. J Clin Periodontol 1986;13(8):740-2.
7. Matsson L, Goldberg P. Gingival inflammatory reaction in children at different ages. J Clin Periodontol 1985;12(2):98-103.
8. Meng H, Xu L, Li Q, Han J, Zhao Y. Determinants of host susceptibility in aggressive periodontitis. Periodontol 2000. 2007;43:133-59.
9. Nakagawa S, Fujii H, Machida Y, Okuda K. A longitudinal study from prepuberty to puberty of gingivitis. Correlation between the occurrence of Prevotella intermedia and sex hormones. J Clin Periodontol 1994;21(10):658-65.
10. Oh TJ, Eber R, Wang HL. Periodontal diseases in the child and adolescent. J Clin Periodontol 2002;29(5):400-10.
11. Peretz B, Machtei EM, Bimstein E. Periodontal status in childhood and early adolescence: three-year follow up. J Clin Pediatr Dent 1996 Spring;20(3):229-32.
12. Prayitno SW, Addy M, Wade WG. Does gingivitis lead to periodontitis in young adults? Lancet 1993; 342(8869):471-2.
13. Ramos-Gomez FJ, Petru A, Hilton JF, Canchola AJ, Wara D, Greenspan JS. Oral manifestations and dental status in paediatric HIV infection. Int J Paediatr Dent 2000;10(1):3-11.
14. Tsuruda K, Miyake Y, Suginaka H, Okamoto H, Iwamoto Y. Microbiological features of gingivitis in pubertal children. J Clin Periodontol 1995;22(4):316-20.
15. Ullbro C, Twetman S. Review Paper: Dental treatment for patients with Papillon-Lefevre syndrome (PLS). Eur Arch Paediatr Dent 2007;8(suppl 1):4-11.

QUESTIONS

1. Discuss the parts of the periodontium. Explain in detail the differences between the periodontium of a child and adult.
2. What are the clinical changes seen in the gingiva during tooth eruption?
3. Explain the stages of gingivitis.
4. Diagnosis of gingivitis.
5. What are the causes for gingivitis in children?
6. Acute necrotizing ulcerative gingivitis (ANUG).
7. Difference between hereditary fibromatosis gingival enlargement and drug induced hyperplasia.

Prosthodontic Considerations in Children

DEFINITION

Prosthodontics is the "art and science which deals with replacement of missing tooth and related structures in and around oral cavity with artificial substitutes."

Prosthesis is an artificial substitute.

INDICATIONS FOR PROSTHETIC REPLACEMENT/PROSTHESIS

1. Premature loss of teeth
2. Dentinogenesis imperfecta, amelogenesis imperfecta
3. Cleft lip and palate
4. Ectodermal dysplasia
5. Anodontia
6. Grossly decayed tooth.

AIMS OF PROSTHODONTIC REHABILITATION

Restoration of Esthetics

Children feel rejected or get ridiculed when they loose their anterior tooth or teeth and this may have a profound effect on the personality of a child. Such a child often exhibits a marked improvement in performance when provided with a denture.

Restoration of Masticatory Efficiency

Children become choosy about the type of food when they loose their posterior teeth as it becomes difficult to bite or chew. Masticatory efficiency is improved when dentures are provided.

Prevention and Correction of Speech Abnormality

Speech articulation is found to be poorer in children with many missing teeth especially the anterior teeth than with children with a full set of teeth. After a period of wearing complete dentures, however, the edentulous children show a significant improvement in articulation.

Prevention of Harmful Habits

When teeth are lost, the child may place the tongue into the edentulous spaces, resulting in abnormal tongue thrusting habit. Habits of sucking the lips inward can sometimes be observed in children with missing anterior teeth.

Provision of Space Maintenance

Single or multiple tooth loss in the primary dentition requires space maintenance. This may in the form of a partial denture, which in addition to preserving space for succeeding teeth, helps with mastication, speech and esthetics.

Obturation of Congenital and Acquired Defects of Orofacial Structures

Dentures or other removable prosthetic appliances may be required to provide closure of defects in the maxillofacial complex that may be developmental or acquired in origin (such as cleft palate, surgical treatment for neoplasm or trauma).

The benefits of providing such appliances depend on the site and extent of the defect and may include the facilitation of feeding and speech development and improvement in appearance.

HARMFUL EFFECTS OF PROSTHESIS AND ITS PREVENTION

Prosthesis may cause tissue damage and children may not understand or realize the early symptoms. Denture-induced tissue damage may progress very rapidly in young patients and it is therefore of great importance to institute and maintain all necessary preventive measures properly.

Caries

Increased caries risk is associated with any kind of prosthesis as it is associated with altered pattern of plaque accumulation and difficulty in maintenance of oral hygiene. The design of the prosthesis should be such that there is minimal tooth surface contact as practically possible. Good comprehensive caries prevention program should be initiated with regular monitoring.

Periodontal Disease

Gingival inflammation associated with poor oral hygiene and proximity of appliance is very common. Improved and rigorous oral hygiene measures are required to prevent damage to the periodontium that are associated with denture wear.

Effects of Growth and Development

Prosthesis in children should be changed regularly as it becomes difficult to seat the appliance in the mouth over a period of time. This is due to increase in the arch dimensions that is observed due to the normal growth and development. Care should be taken while designing prosthesis in children. It should not interfere in jaw growth and tooth eruption.

Loss of Alveolar Bone

Preservation of alveolar bone is an important consideration in young patients who requires longer periods of denture wear. Whenever possible a partial denture should be supported on fully erupted abutment teeth. Excessive movement of the prosthesis on the alveolar bone should be avoided as these will cause resorption of the alveolar bone resorption. When insufficient teeth are present to provide support, the denture base should be extended widely on the bone to distribute the loads.

Oral Mucosal Disorders

A number of mucosal disorders may be associated with denture wear. Localized pressure from an over-extended or ill-fitting denture may produce a painful area of necrosis (denture ulcer) or mucosal hyperplasia. Denture-induced stomatitis affecting the palatal mucosa is characterized by a bright red spongy appearance of mucosa in an area well demarcated by the denture margins.

These denture-induced mucosal disorders can be prevented by institution of adequate oral and denture hygiene measures in the first instance and by ensuring that features of the fitting surface that might produce mechanical irritation are relieved before denture insertion.

EXAMINATION, DIAGNOSIS AND TREATMENT PLANNING

Clinical examination of the child is carried out in the usual manner, however, radiographic examination needs particular attention. Ideally a panoramic radiograph would be desirable so that one could visualize the different stages of development at which the various succedaneous teeth, are at that particular point in time. This information helps the operator to predict the approximate time and perhaps the sequence of eruption of the succedaneous teeth and also decide whether a particular patient presents the indications for a prosthesis. The stage of treatment planning at which a prosthesis is inserted will vary in accordance with the different needs of various patients.

Mouth Preparation

It includes the procedures performed inside the mouth to create an oral environment that will provide proper support and retention for the prosthesis and that will prevent the development of forces or processes that are harmful to the remaining teeth and their supportive tissues.

A. *Surgical preparation:* Surgery may be necessary to eradicate soft tissue or osseous pathology and can range from uncomplicated extraction of teeth to complex procedures.

B. *Periodontal preparation:* Adolescents often require periodontal surgeries particularly to increase crown length and to improve tissue contours so that more ideal results in restorative and prosthetic treatment are achieved.

C. *Endodontic preparation:* Endodontic therapy may be required to preserve a tooth that is strategic to the support and retention of a proposed partial denture but grossly damaged by caries or trauma.

D. *Orthodontic preparation:* Orthodontic procedures can be used to reposition a malpositioned teeth that may serve as a abutment.

E. *Prosthetic preparation:* Placement of a crown may be required on a grossly decayed tooth acting as an abutment which will provide support and retention to the denture.

TYPES OF PROSTHESIS

A. Removable Prosthesis
   a. Partial dentures
   b. Complete dentures/over dentures
B. Fixed Prosthesis
   a. Resin bonded retainers
   b. Pin ledge and partial veneer crown retainers
   c. Inlay retainers
   d. Complete crown retainers
   e. Cantilevered prostheses
   f. Restoration for a single tooth.
C. Obturator: Discussed in Chapter 19.

Removable Partial Denture (Figs 15.1A and B)

Indications

1. As space maintainers, when there is premature loss of primary teeth. Helps to restore speech, esthetics and masticatory function.
2. When anterior deciduous teeth are missing and esthetics is a major consideration.
3. Young permanent teeth lost as a result of trauma.
4. Congenitally missing tooth/teeth, e.g. partial anodontia in ectodermal dysplasia.

5. When fixed prosthesis cannot be used, e.g. excessive span length, inability to achieve adequate retention.
6. Causes resulting in multiple extractions of primary teeth, e.g. nursing bottle caries.
7. Dentinogenesis imperfecta, amelogenesis imperfecta and cleft palate associated with multiple missing teeth either congenitally or following extraction.

Ideal Requirements

1. It should restore or improve masticatory function.
2. It should restore and improve esthetics and facial contours.
3. It should not interfere with normal growth of the dental arches.
4. Design should not interfere with speech.
5. Should allow easy placement and removal by the patient.
6. The design should permit easy adjustment and alterations if required.
7. Easily cleansable.
8. Its design should require minimal or no preparation of the abutment teeth.
9. It should prevent over eruption of opposing teeth or drift of the adjacent teeth.
10. It should prevent plaque accumulation and be nonirritating to the supporting tissues.

Design for Removable Partial Denture in Children

Two very important considerations in children are:
A. The duration for which the removable partial denture will be worn.
B. Changing nature of dental arches.

It is very important to ascertain that the force distribution on the teeth and ridge be uniform, which otherwise can cause soft tissue damage, tilting or rotation of abutment teeth. This can be ensured when maximum denture bearing area is used so that the force per unit area is minimal.

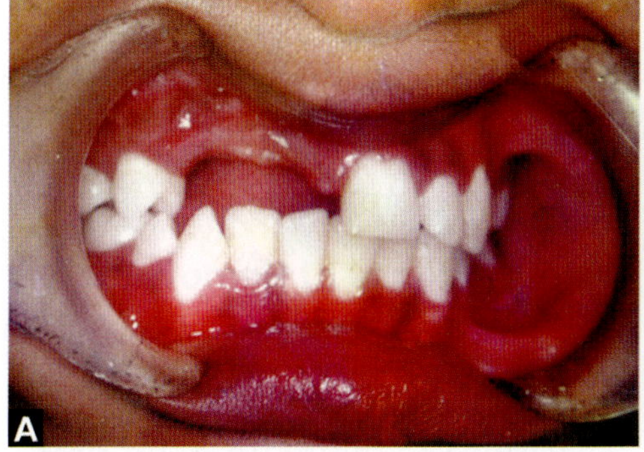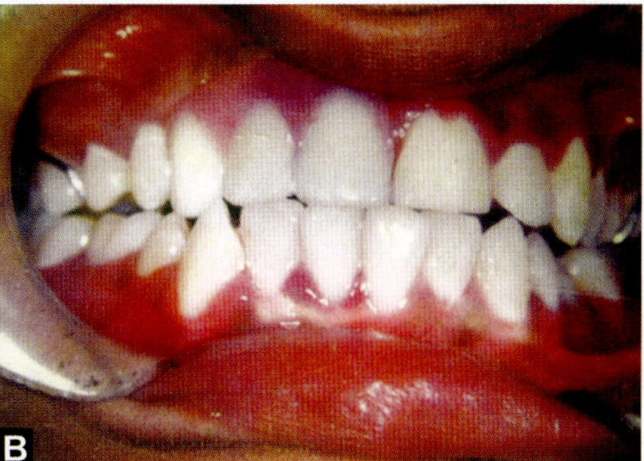

Figs 15.1A and B: Removable partial denture: (A) Pretreatment (B) Post-treatment

Parts of a Removable Partial Denture

Usually RPD for children consists of the following parts:
A. The denture base
B. Clasp
C. Artificial teeth.

The denture base: The denture base for most partial dentures are made of acrylic resin, although in some cases it may consists of metal alone or metal and acrylic resin. It provides a means for fixation of the clasps and artificial teeth. The denture base should be light and have sufficient strength to meet the functional needs.

Clasps: They are used to provide adequate fixation or retention of the denture base. They provide tooth support to the denture base. Clasps may be either cast or wrought. Commonly used clasps are 'U' clasp, ball end clasp, Adams clasp, etc. Adams clasp is very versatile and is used primarily on posterior teeth. An added aid to retention is the use of labial bow.

Artificial teeth: Commercially primary teeth are available. Teeth can be fabricated from a model by taking an impression of the teeth and duplicating them with a tooth colored resin. The teeth are cut and used as individual tooth.

Procedure for Constructing Removable Partial Denture

Making an impression: Impression trays of different sizes are available. Correct size is selected. The impression material of choice is alginate. The procedure is explained to the child by using simple terms to describe the procedure. It is common for children to gag during impression making. Gagging can be prevented by asking the patients to rinse with warm water containing some flavored surface anesthetic agent prior to impression procedure, by asking the patient to breath rapidly through nose, or any other methods to distract the child's attention.

Bite registration: A centric bite registration is necessary in order to establish an accurate relationship between maxillary and mandibular models prior to mounting them on the articulator. Bite should be registered in centric relation as some children have a tendency to approximate their incisors in an edge to edge relationship when asked to close. Children should be shown the correct method of biting before recording the bite.

Fabrication of the appliance: The working model is cast in stone and the appliance is fabricated.

Delivery or insertion of the appliance: The patient is shown the proper way to insert and remove the appliance. The patient is asked to demonstrate in front of the dental surgeon to ensure that the patient can accomplish this procedure at home.

Important considerations while designing a partial denture

A. Full palatal coverage is preferred for maxillary partial denture.
B. Buccal and lingual flanges should be relatively short and contoured.
C. Clasps when used should not interfere in tooth eruption and jaw growth.
D. Occlusal rests should be preferably placed on the permanent molars.
E. When necessary the appliance should be fabricated before extraction of teeth and used as immediate partial denture or immediate space maintainer.
F. The teeth are set with spaces and in a more vertical axis than in adult dentures.
G. The teeth may be butted to the alveolar ridge and labial flange omitted.
H. As the child grows it may be necessary to remove portions of the appliance to allow for eruption of permanent successors.
I. Teeth with shallow cusps or a zero degree teeth should be used.

Instructions to the Patient and the Parents

A. The patient is instructed to remove the partial denture during athletic activities such as swimming and contact sports and store in a small plastic box with water.
B. The partial denture should be removed at night and stored in water. It should be cleaned every day with denture cleansers or by brushing with denture cleansing paste.
C. If the denture does not fit or cause irritation the parent should be asked to call the dentist and inform him.
D. Patient is informed regarding the complications such as prolongation of treatment and extra-expenditure that will occur if the appliance is lost or broken.
E. Written copy of instruction can be provided regarding the instructions for the care of the appliance.

Advantages of Removable Denture

- Patient or the parent can always remove the denture when there is any pain or other problem.
- Good home care of both the denture and the remaining teeth is easier to accomplish.
- Material costs are minimal.
- Minimal care is required.

Disadvantages of Removable Denture

1. There is complete dependence on patient and parent cooperation. Lack of cooperation can lead to failure of the treatment.
2. Failure to maintain good oral hygiene carries increased risk of caries and gingival disease.

Complete Denture

Indications

Children with loss or missing full set of teeth as associated with certain diseases such as ectodermal dysplasia.

> **Important considerations while fabricating a complete denture**
>
> 1. The alveolar bone deposition is retarded but the face continues to grow. So the appliance has to be changed periodically to adjust for the facial growth and development.
> 2. Making a centric relation record is difficult in children and hence requires extra-effort and precaution.
> 3. Over-dentures may be fabricated using the existing teeth for retention of the denture.
> 4. Teeth with shallow cusps or a zero degree teeth should be used.

Patient Instructions

a. The child should be encouraged to wear the dentures.
b. When the dentures are first inserted, the child should be given food that is enjoyed but which requires chewing.
c. The parents should check the child's mouth for supporting tissue irritation and erupting teeth.
d. The child should be evaluated every 3 months for changes occurring due to growth.
e. The appliance should be removed at night and kept moist.
f. The appliance should be removed for sports activities.
g. The parents and patients should be instructed in home care of the appliance.

Overdentures

Occasionally congenital abnormalities or trauma result in the loss of multiple teeth and the resulting inter arch relationship does not allow conventional removable partial denture to re-establish proper occlusion with the opposing teeth. This situation may necessitate fabrication of a prosthesis that overlays all or part of the remaining teeth so that proper function and facial esthetics are established.

Fixed Partial Dentures

Types of Fixed Prosthesis

- Resin bonded retainers
- Partial veneer crown retainers
- Inlay retainers
- Complete crown retainers
- Cantilevered prostheses
- Restoration for a single tooth

> **Important considerations while fabricating a fixed prosthesis**
>
> a. When a tooth is lost, space maintenance should be provided immediately and should be continued until the fixed prosthesis is cemented.
> b. It should be kept in mind during tooth preparation the presence of large pulp chamber in a young permanent tooth.
> c. If the abutment teeth are malaligned and pulp size does not permit the amount of tooth reduction necessary to align the preparations, orthodontic repositioning of the abutment teeth will be required.
> d. For reasons of pulpal and periodontal health and to conserve tooth structure partial coverage retainers should be the first choice whenever possible.
> e. Conservative retainers are preferred over full coverage retainers.

Resin Bonded Retainers (Maryland Bridge)

Design: They are perforated metal-resin bonded appliance (Fig. 15.2).

Indications

1. Congenitally missing teeth such as lateral incisors and premolars.
2. Tooth lost to trauma.
3. Anterior teeth missing because of congenital defects such as cleft palate.
4. Carious teeth that have been extracted.

Contraindications

1. Poor oral hygiene.
2. Large carious lesions in abutment teeth.
3. Malpositioned teeth that do not allow for improved esthetics by bonding.

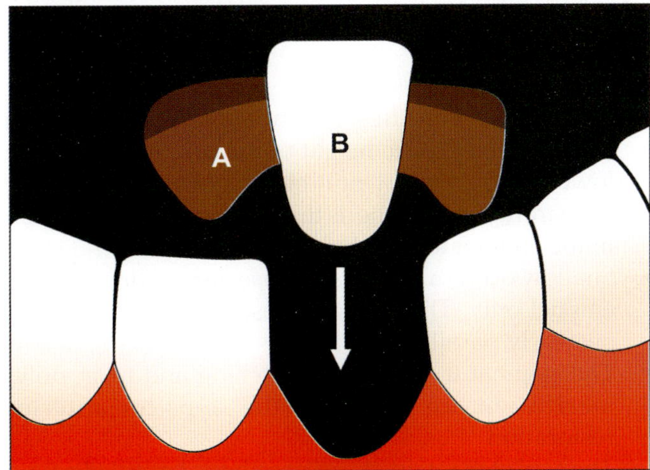

Fig. 15.2: Design of a Maryland bridge: (A) Perforated metal extension; (B) Pontic

Advantages

1. The cost is less than porcelain fused to metal restorations.
2. Conservative in enamel reduction, reducing trauma to pulp and periodontal tissue.
3. Can be done without local anesthesia.
4. Excellent esthetics.
5. Easy repair.

Disadvantages

1. Contraindicated where large restorations or carious lesions exist.
2. Technique sensitive.

Procedures—Anterior Teeth Replacement

- Lingual reduction is done using a flame shaped diamond bur. The margins are extended slightly beyond the proximal contact to provide a wrap around effect. Shallow grooves can be used. A chamfer is placed 1 mm from the gingival crest.
- An impression of the final preparation is made and model is prepared with die stone. The framework covers as much of the lingual surface as possible yet minimizing the incisal show of the material.
- Framework is tried and checked for occlusion and esthetics.
- The oral side of the casting is polished. The enamel side of the metal is etched and washed.
- Bonding must be done in a dry environment. Bonding agent is applied to etched enamel and metal surfaces. Composite resin is placed on the metal surface only.
- Seat the bridge and carefully remove all excess composite resin. Use the finishing burs for finishing,
  A patient with congenitally missing lateral incisor is an ideal candidate for these types of restorative procedure.

Posterior Teeth Replacement

- The wraparound designs should cover each tooth by 180 degrees. The height of the contour should be lowered to within 1 min of the gingival crest. The preparation should be as thick as possible yet remain in the enamel to avoid overcontouring.
- Shallow occlusal rests can be used extending into the enamel only. The walls of these occlusal rests must be nearly parallel.
- The steps of try-in, casting, etching and resin polymerization are similar to the steps for anterior restoration.
  The acid etch retained cast prosthesis has filled a void in the management of adolescents with missing teeth, whether the cause of tooth loss in trauma or congenital

defect. In the past, these tooth lost due to trauma were replaced by removable appliances that were easily broken or by extensive and expensive fixed prosthodontic appliances. The acid etch resin retained cast appliance is an excellent substitute that requires minimal tooth reduction and provides excellent esthetic results.

Partial Veneer Crown Retainers

They can be either:
1. Laminate veneers
2. Acid-etch composite veneers.

Laminate Veneers

They are of three types:
A. Preformed laminate veneers
B. Customized laboratory processed laminate veneers
C. Porcelain laminate veneers.

Indication

Patients with tetracycline stains, fluorosis, hypo-plastic or hypocalcific teeth or other unesthetic anterior teeth.

Contraindication

- Teeth with severe labial proclination
- Mouth breathers
- Exposed dentin
- Poor oral hygiene.

A. Preformed laminate veneers

These are ready made veneers adapted directly on the prepared enamel surface.

Advantages

- Surface color and finish are excellent
- Economical
- One-step procedure.

Disadvantages

- Appears slightly bulky
- Increased chair time
- Poor gingival adaptation may result in gingival inflammation
- Replacement may be difficult.

B. Customized laboratory processed veneers

Advantages

- Initially surface is very smooth
- Easy to finish
- Good shade adaptation
- Easily repairable
- Economical

Disadvantages

- It is a two appointment procedure
- Surface may roughen over time
- May fracture under-stress.
- Porcelain laminate veneers: It requires removal of sufficient tooth material. The veneer is constructed in the laboratory and attached to the tooth by mechanical and chemical methods.

Steps involved for veneer placement

- Isolation of the tooth.
- Cleaning with nonfluoride containing paste.
- Drying the tooth thoroughly and conditioning with 50% phosphoric acid.
- The tooth is then cleaned with water and dried.
- A thin layer of bonding agent is painted on the etched surface and polymerized for 20 seconds.
- Place the selected shade composite on the inner side of the veneer and place it gently on the abutment tooth.

Acid-Etch Composite Veneers

Advantages

- One appointment procedure
- The microfilled composite resins are well adapted to such procedure
- Esthetically excellent
- Economical and easily repairable.

Disadvantages

- Surface may appear rough after some months
- Stains may appear
- Method may require precise technique.

Procedure

- Isolation
- Preparing the veneer window of about 1mm in enamel. A collar of enamel is left intact around the labial aspect.
- The prepared surfaced is etched with 50% phosphoric acid, washed and dried.
- A thin layer of bonding agent is applied and dried with gentle blow of air.
- Microfilled light cured composite is adapted on the tooth surface using plastic instrument.
- The surface is then finished and polished.
- Glazing is done for the final finish.

Inlay Retainers

Second premolars and first molars sometimes may be replaced by use of inlay retainers in the abutment teeth.

Advantages

The main advantage of the inlay in the young mouth is that its subgingival extension is limited to the proximal surface, whereas adequate retention for an extracoronal retainer frequently requires total subgingival margin extension because of the short crown frequently present in adolescents.

Tooth Preparation

A. The tooth preparations are of the conventional inlay design.
B. The occlusal and proximal steps should be wider than those normally prepared for a single inlay restoration.
C. A post hole about 1.5 mm deep may be used in pulpal floor near the marginal ridge opposite to the proximal box. These modifications are made to increase retention to provide adequate bulk of metal for strength and to provide space for solder joints of proper form, location and size.

Complete Crown Retainers

When full coverage retainers are indicated but pulp size allows only minimal reduction, an all resin fixed prosthesis is the best choice. It offers good esthetics and requires only minimal axial tooth reduction (0.5 mm). Because of its inferior physical properties, it must be replaced periodically. All resin prosthesis rarely lasts more than one or two years without significant wear, color change or fracture. However, by the time replacement is needed, enough pulpal recession may have occurred that additional tooth reduction can be safely accomplished permitting use of metal ceramic retainers.

Cantilevered Prosthesis

Design

This prosthesis replaces missing tooth by taking support from only one abutment tooth.

Indications

This design can be used in selected cases of missing anterior teeth only and is not acceptable when one is replacing posterior teeth. Congenital absence of a maxillary lateral incisor is one situation where this design can be utilized with a reasonable degree of success. A two-unit fixed prosthesis can be fabricated with a lateral incisor pontic cantilevered from the canine retainer.

Requirements

The positional stability of the canine is imperative to the success of this design.

Criteria for Case Selection

1. The canine should not be mobile and the arch form should be stable.
2. The canine should not have recently undergone orthodontic repositioning that involved significant rotation.
3. There should be no centric occlusal slide and the lateral incisor pontic should be fabricated so as to be out of occlusal contact in protrusive and lateral mandibular movements.

Improved Designs

a. The positional stability of the canine can be improved by placement of a rest arm from the pontic onto the lingual surface of the central incisor.
b. Concave form can be given to the mesial aspect of the pontic so that it wraps slightly around the distolingual aspect of the central incisor.

   Both of these designs require a low caries index and meticulous oral hygiene.

Advantages

1. Less expensive than a conventional three-unit prosthesis and comparable in cast to a three unit resin bonded prosthesis.
2. Only preparation of the canine is necessary, and since this tooth is larger than an incisor and does not possess pulp horns, it can be adequately reduced with less chance of irreversible pulpal damage.
3. Avoiding the central incisors entirely renders a more esthetic result than either a conventional or a resin bonded prosthesis that includes the central incisor.

Restorations for a Single Tooth

They are:
A. Resin jacket crown
B. All ceramic crown
C. Metal ceramic crown
D. All ceramic and metal ceramic crowns supported by posts and cores.

Resin Jacket Crown (Figs 15.3 and 15.4)

Design

It is a full coverage crown made of acrylic resin and requires minimum tooth reduction.

Indications

A tooth, which requires a full coverage restoration but possess a large pulp that could be irreversibly injured during tooth reduction for an all ceramic or metal ceramic crown.

Tooth preparation

1. The minimal axial reduction depth required for an acceptable resin jacket crown is about 0.5 mm.
2. The tooth preparation for a resin jacket crown should possess a shoulder finish line, 0.5 mm in width around the entire tooth.
3. The lingual reduction for occlusal clearance is also 0.5 mm.
4. An incisal edge reduction of 1to1.5 mm is required and is biologically acceptable even in the presence of large pulps.

Advantages

1. Minimal reduction of the tooth material is required.
2. Resin jacket crowns can provide good service for a few years and thereby allow pulpal recession to occur. Then additional tooth reduction can be accomplished in a biologically safe manner allowing utilization of the longer lasting ceramic restoration.

Disadvantages

1. Poor long-term color stability.
2. Decreased resistance to wear.

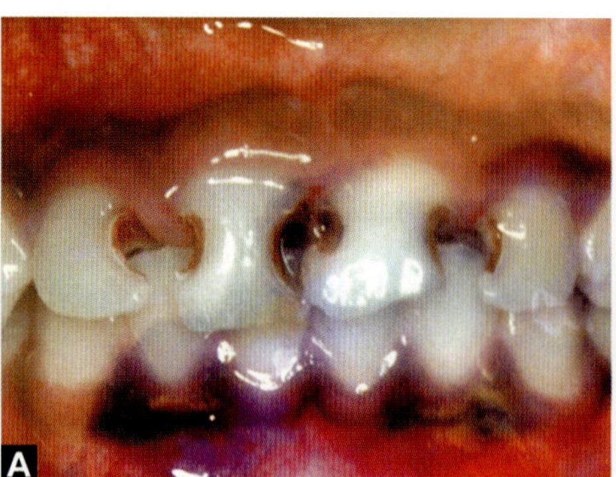
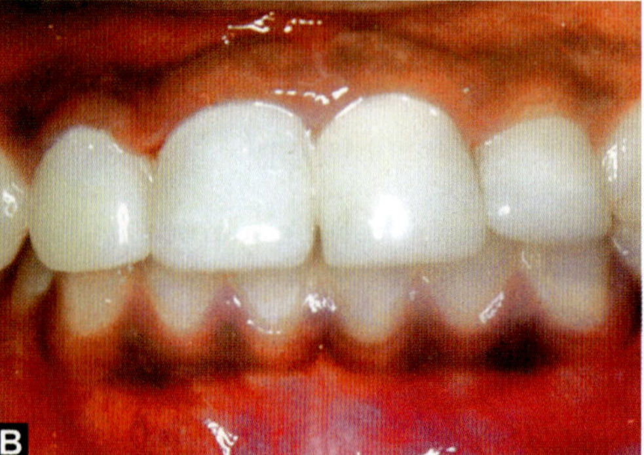

Figs 15.3A and B: Restoration of carious teeth with jacket crowns: (A) Pretreatment; (B) Post-treatment

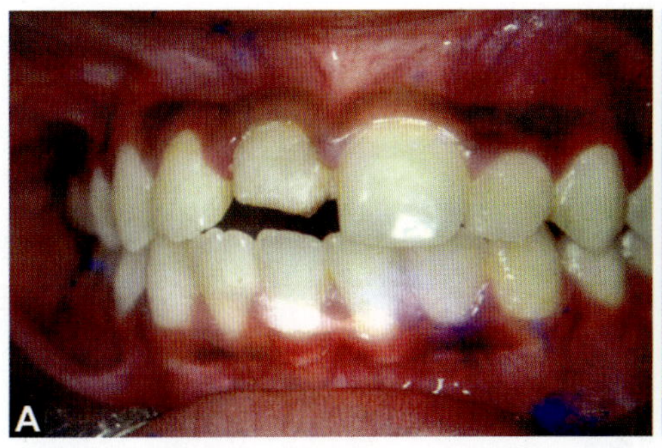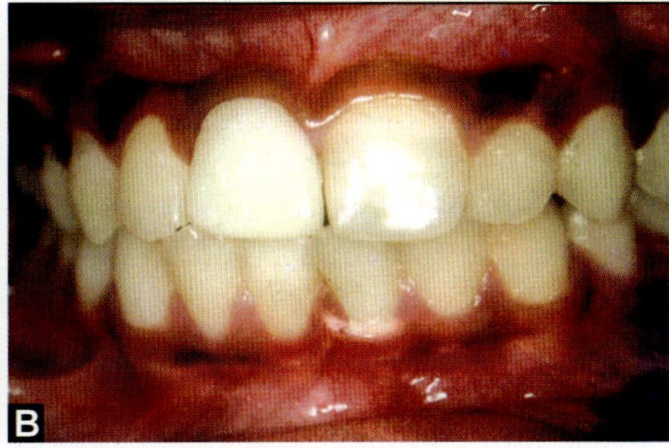

Figs 15.4A and B: Tooth restored with jacket crown: (A) Preparation of tooth;
(B) Restoration with jacket crown

3. Greater loss of surface lusture and surface form particularly in mouths where vigorous tooth-brushing occurs.

All Ceramic Crown

Indications

Used for restoration of single malformed, discolored or fractured tooth.

Requirements

1. Normal tooth preparation form is required to support the restoration.
2. There should be average or below average occlusal forces.
3. The centric occlusal contacts should occur over the concave lingual portion of the prepared tooth
4. The prepared tooth should possess average or greater incisocervical length and not be short, round or overtapered in form.

Tooth preparation

Preparation form for a porcelain jacket crown is the same as that used with the resin jacket crown except that greater reduction depths are required. Minimal axial reduction depth required is 0.8 mm.

Advantage

All ceramic crowns are the most esthetic full coverage restorations presently available in dentistry.

Disadvantages

1. Requires more tooth reduction so risk for pulpal damage is high.
2. All ceramic crowns cannot withstand greater occlusal forces and therefore cannot be used for restoration of posterior teeth.
3. Proper tooth form is required to support the restoration.

Metal Ceramic Crown

Design

The crown is backed by metal and a ceramic facing for esthetics is provided.

Indications

When inadequate preparation form or the magnitude of occlusal forces contra indicates an all ceramic crown, the stronger metal ceramic crown is indicated.

Tooth preparation

1. Minimal facial reduction of 1 mm and shoulder finish line is given on the facial surface.
2. Minimal incisal reduction of 2 mm.
3. Lingual axial reduction depths of 0.3 to 0.5 mm with a chamfer finish line.
4. Lingual reduction of 1 mm for occlusal clearance.

All Ceramic and Metal Ceramic Crowns Supported by Posts and Cores

A routine root canal treatment is done. The root canal is obturated with gutta percha occupying only apical 1/3rd of the root canal. The remaining portion of the canal is further enlarged to accommodate a post and core restoration which is cemented in the canal.

Indications

1. Fracture involving the pulp in the teeth with closed apex.
2. Pulpless permanent incisors or premolars to be restored with ceramic restorations should receive posts and cores when only a thin peripheral shell of tooth structure remains after tooth preparation.

Contraindications

a. It is contraindicated in tooth with short root, or with roots having a thin dentinal wall as in an immature tooth.

b. Tooth with internal and external root resorption.
c. Traumatic occlusion.

Post and core design

1. When post and core build up is required, the post should extend into the root canal so that its length equals or exceeds the occlusocervicallength of the proposed ceramic crown. This length provides adequate retention and optimal resistance to tooth structure.
2. Any coronal tooth structure remaining after normal preparatory procedures should be preserved and the core constructed to complete the normal coronal preparation form. Retaining coronal tooth structure helps to increase the resistance of post and core to rotational dislodging forces (Figs 15.5 and 15.6).

    Whenever possible cervical margins of crowns should not be extended into the gingival sulcus of an adolescent patient. It can lead to accelerated gingival recession in case oral hygiene is inadequate or interfere with normal cervical relocation of the gingival tissues as the patient matures. Either occurrence produces an esthetic liability.

Patient instructions

1. Every adolescent patient must be taught proper oral hygiene and home care of prosthetic restorations and be motivated until adequate performance is routinely achieved.
2. Each patient with a fixed prosthesis should be taught the use of oral hygiene aids such as the floss and the interproximal brush to enhance oral hygiene efforts.

Implant Prosthesis

The routine successful use of osseointegrated dental implants in total or partial support of prosthesis in adults has heightened interest in their use with younger patients. There are two primary concerns related to the placement of implants before growth is completed.

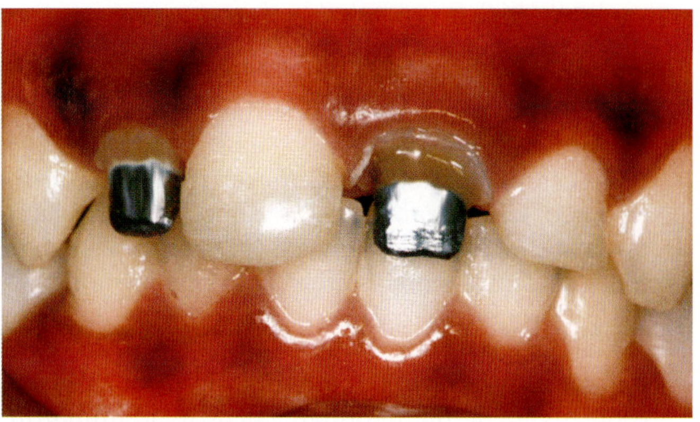

Fig. 15.5: Preformed post placed in the distal canal of a molar

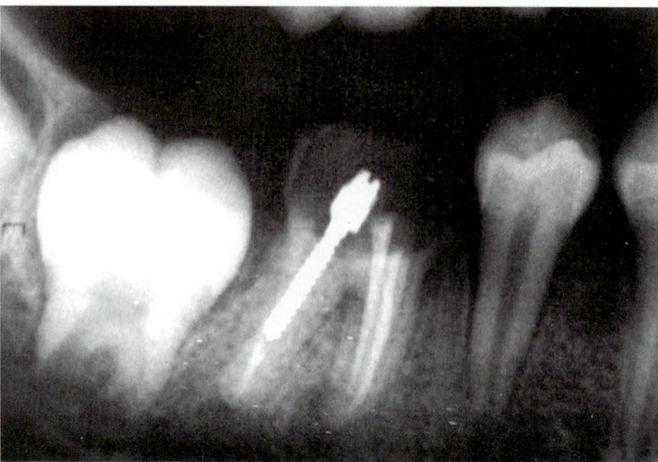

Fig. 15.6: Cast post cemented in the anterior teeth

A. The effects of growth on long-term positional stability of dental implant.
B. The effect of implant supported prosthesis on future dental and skeletal growth.

Implant Usage before Growth Completion

The clinician must understand the dynamics of positional relationship between the dental implant and its biologic environment in a growing patient.

The behavior of an osseointegrated dental implant essentially resembles an ankylosed tooth. Two facets of the relationship of the ankylosed teeth to their actively growing environment must be understood.

First, the ankylotic tooth lacking the adaptive mechanism of healthy tooth does not erupt normally and becomes buried.

Second, failing to participate in normal growth it often creates severe malocclusion secondary to tipping and associated growth changes in normal teeth adjacent to the affected ankylotic tooth.

It seems logical that an osseointegrated implant placed prematurely could elicit the same negative growth effects. An understanding of growth and development and its variability within the male and female adolescent population gives us serious concern for the premature placement of implants.

It is best to wait until maxillary and mandibular growth is completed before placing implants. Implants have been placed in anterior mandibular region in patients as young as five years of age. But the placement of dental implants should not be attempted until the accelerated phase of circumpubertal growth is close to complete.

Implants for Orthodontic Anchorage

Osseointegrated implants have been used as anchorage in cases where anchorage is required but conventional tooth anchorage is not available. Because the implants act as anklylosed teeth and are incapable of being moved by orthodontic or orthopedic forces they serve as ideal anchorage units, particularly where a large number of teeth are missing as a result of trauma or congenital anomalies. Implants are especially valuable when the prosthodontic positioning permits them to be used to support a future prosthesis.

Recall Program following Prosthodontic Replacement

A. Periodic recall appointments for inspection, maintenance, repair or replacement are a necessity if maximum longevity of service is to be expected.
B. For patients who have removable partial dentures, relining or rebasing should be performed when indicated.
C. When jacket crowns or metal ceramic restorations are used in adolescents, replacement may be needed periodically as the gingival tissue assumes its adult positions.
D. Patients with fixed partial dentures should be inspected periodically for soft tissue changes, evidence of occlusal wear and response of the supporting tissues to the added stress loads.

FURTHER READING

1. Chang TL. Prosthodontic treatment of patients with hypodontia. J Calif Dent Assoc 2006;34(9):727-33.
2. Chun NS. Esthetic primary anterior crowns. Hawaii Dent J 1998;29(2):9.
3. Croll TP, Helpin ML. Preformed resin-veneered stainless steel crowns for restoration of primary incisors. Quintessence Int 1996;27(5):309-13.
4. Heij DG, Opdebeeck H, van Steenberghe D, Kokich VG, Belser U, Quirynen M. Facial development, continuous tooth eruption, and mesial drift as compromising factors for implant placement. Int J Oral Maxillofac Implants 2006;21(6):867-78.
5. Hornbrook DS. Anterior tooth replacement using a two-component resin-bonded bridge. Compendium 1993;14(1):52-8, 59.
6. Hosoya Y, Omachi K, Staninec M. Colorimetric values of esthetic stainless steel crowns. Quintessence Int 2002;33(7):537-41.
7. Kramer FJ, Baethge C, Tschernitschek H. Implants in children with ectodermal dysplasia: a case report and literature review. Clin Oral Implants Res 2007;18(1):140-6.
8. Kupietzky A, Waggoner WF, Galea J. The clinical and radiographic success of bonded resin composite strip crowns for primary incisors. Pediatr Dent 2003;25(6):577-81.
9. Ram D, Fuks AB, Eidelman E. Long-term clinical performance of esthetic primary molar crowns. Pediatr Dent 2003;25(6):582-4.
10. Ram D, Peretz B. Composite crown-form crowns for severely decayed primary molars: a technique for restoring function and esthetics. J Clin Pediatr Dent 2000 Summer;24(4):257-60.
11. Ram D, Peretz B. Restoring coronal contours of retained infraoccluded primary second molars using bonded resin-based composite. Pediatr Dent 2003;25(1):71-3.
12. Roberts C, Lee JY, Wright JT. Clinical evaluation of and parental satisfaction with resin-faced stainless steel crowns. Pediatr Dent 2001;23(1):28-31.
13. Rocha Rde O, das Neves LT, Marotti NR, Wanderley MT, Correa MS. Intracanal reinforcement fiber in pediatric dentistry: a case report. Quintessence Int 2004;35(4):263-8.
14. Sherman G Jr, Bugg JL Jr, Carruth KR. Restoration of primary incisors with acrylic jacket crowns—one appointment procedure. J Dent Child 1966;33(3):182-5.
15. Tarjan I, Gabris K, Rozsa N. Early prosthetic treatment of patients with ectodermal dysplasia: a clinical report. J Prosthet Dent 2005;93(5):419-24.
16. Veira KA, Teixeira MS, Guirado CG, Gaviao MB. Prosthodontic treatment of hypohidrotic ectodermal dysplasia with complete anodontia: case report. Quintessence Int 2007;38(1):75-80.
17. Waggoner WF. Restoring primary anterior teeth. Pediatr Dent 2002;24(5):511-6.
18. Yilmaz Y, Kocogullari ME. Clinical evaluation of two different methods of stainless steel esthetic crowns. J Dent Child (Chic) 2004;71(3):212-4.

QUESTIONS

1. Classify the different types of prosthesis used in children.
2. Explain the design of a removable partial denture in children.
3. Write the indications and problems of complete denture in children.
4. Write in detail about Maryland bridge.
5. What are acid etch composite veneers.
6. Enumerate the different types of restorations for a missing single tooth.
7. Give the indications and tooth preparation for resin jacket crown.
8. Write in detail the metal ceramic crown used in pediatric practice.
9. Give the indications and contraindications of all ceramic and metal ceramic crowns supported by posts and cores.
10. Explain the post and core design.

Common Oral Pathologic Conditions

INTRODUCTION

Oral pathologic conditions can be discussed based on the tissue/organ involved.

DISORDERS OF THE TONGUE

Microglossia

- It is an uncommon developmental anomaly of the tongue featuring an abnormally small tongue.
- In rare cases, almost the whole tongue may be absent/missing. This is called aglossia.
- Microglossia is frequently associated with hypoplasia of the mandible and the lower incisors may be missing. It may also be associated with constricted arch and posterior cross bite.
- Treatment includes surgical correction followed by orthodontic treatment of dental defects.

Macroglossia

- Macroglossia refers to a tongue that is larger than normal.
- This condition may be either congenital or acquired in type.
- Congenital macroglossia, which is caused by an overdevelopment of the lingual musculature or vascular tissues, becomes increasingly apparent as the child develops.
- An abnormally large tongue is characteristic of hypothyroidism, in which case the tongue is fissured and may extend out of the mouth.
- Macroglossia is also commonly observed with type II glycogen storage disease, neurofibromatosis type I, and Beckwith-Wiedemann syndrome.
- It can be an isolated and sporadic (nonfamilial) trait or can be a familial (autosomal dominant) trait.
- A disproportionately large tongue may cause both an abnormal growth pattern of the jaw and malocclusion. Flaring of the lower anterior teeth and an angle class III malocclusion are occasionally the result of macroglossia.
- In infants, the large tongue is always seen protruding, causing inability to close the mouth. Drooling of saliva, noisy breathing and inability to feed are also seen.

- The treatment of macroglossia depends on its cause and severity. Surgical reduction of a portion of the tongue is occasionally necessary.

Ankyloglossia

- It is a developmental anomaly of tongue characterized by a short and thick lingual frenum, usually attached too near to the tip of the tongue (Fig. 16.1).
- Partial ankyloglossia is more common and is often called "tongue-tie."
- Complete ankyloglossia occurs as a result of fusion between tongue and floor of the mouth.
- Because of the short frenum, the movement of the tongue is restricted.
- This interferes with mastication, speech and other tongue functions.
- It may lead to anterior open-bite because it prevents the tongue from touching the roof of the mouth during swallowing. So, it pushes against the anterior teeth during swallowing.
- Stripping of the lingual gingival tissues may occur if the tongue-tie is not corrected.
- Surgical reduction of the abnormal lingual frenum is indicated if it interferes with the infant's nursing.
- In the older child a reduction of the frenum should be recommended only, if local conditions warrant the treatment.

Fissured Tongue

- A very common condition characterized by fissures, grooves or lines on the dorsal surface of the tongue.
- Etiology is uncertain, may be hereditary.
- Dorsal tongue surface exhibits multiple grooves or fissures that range from 2 to 6 mm in depth.

- Numerous fissures divide the tongue surface into multiple islands, which seem to be separated from each other by these grooves.
- Most patients exhibit a large central fissure, with smaller fissures branching outward at right angles (Fig. 16.2).
- Some patients complain of burning sensation and soreness especially on taking spicy food.
- This also occurs as part of the Melkerssen-Rosenthal syndrome.
- Treatment is not required. Tooth brushes can be used to clean the fissures, to prevent accumulation of food—debris between the fissures.

Median Rhomboid Glossitis

- It is a congenital abnormality of tongue, due to failure of tuberculum impar to withdraw before the fusion of the lateral halves of the tongue. So, a structure devoid of papilla is interposed between the 2 halves.
- Theories suggesting etiology of fungal infection by *Candida albicans* have also been put forward.
- Appears rhomboid or avoid shaped, smooth, reddish patch seen in the midline on the dorsal surface of the tongue, immediately anterior to the circumvallate papillae (Fig. 16.3).
- It stands out distinct from other areas of tongue because it has no filiform papillae (atrophied).
- Treatment includes antifungal medication if candidal infection is present. Otherwise no treatment is required.

Benign Migratory Glossitis

- A lesion of unknown etiology, characterized by migrating patches on the tongue surface.

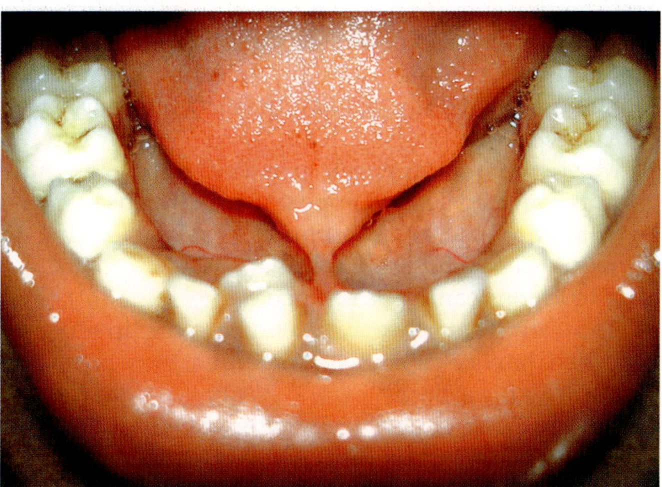

Fig. 16.1: Ankyloglossia

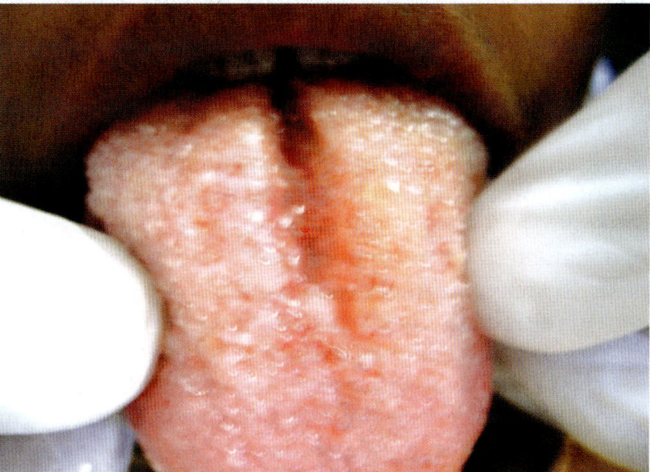

Fig. 16.2: Fissured tongue

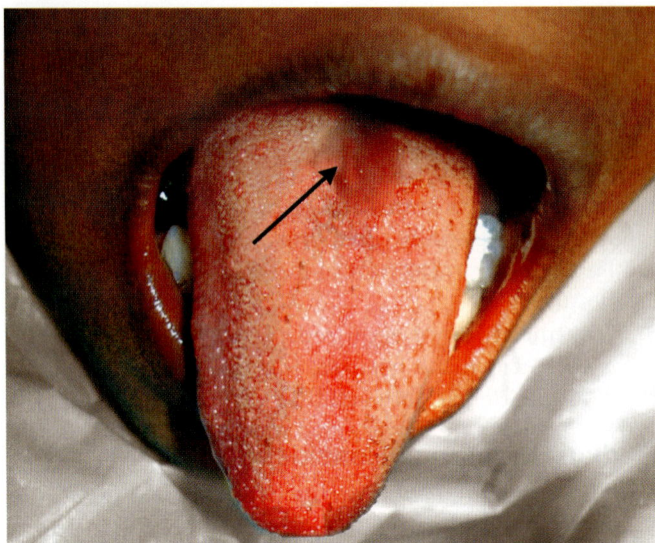

Fig. 16.3: Median rhomboid glossitis

- Shown to be stress-related. Male to female ratio = 1:2, more in 5 to 18 years of age.
- Shows multiple areas of desquamation of filiform papillae, in an irregular or circinate pattern.
- The central portion of the lesion is inflamed, while the outer part is thin and outlined by a yellowish-white band.
- The desquamated areas show fungiform papillae as red elevated dot.
- The areas of desquamation remain for a short period in one location, heal and then reappear at another location. Thus it appears to migrate, traveling the whole geography of the tongue.
- Frequently recurs, after spontaneous healing.
- Known to occur with fissured tongue
- Certain similar lesions can occur at other locations in the oral cavity like buccal mucosa, gingiva, lips, etc. They are called ectopic geographic tongue.

Hairy Tongue
- Etiology of hairy tongue is attributed to candidiasis infection and may not exactly be a developmental anomaly.
- Characterized by hypertrophy of filiform papillae, with lack of normal desquamation.
- This results in thickly matted and extensive filiform papillae on the dorsal surface.
- Their color depends on extrinsic factors like tobacco, pan, etc. and may eventually become blackish brown.
- In severe cases, these papillae will brush the palate, producing gagging.
- The entire tongue (dorsal surface) appears hairy
- Treatment is mainly concerned at keeping the tongue clean with toothbrush to avoid food accumulation and irritation.

Lingual Thyroid
- Seen in the second decade and more in females
- Characterized by a nodular enlargement with smooth or vascular surface located in the midline at the base of the tongue.
- Develop during puberty or pregnancy and normal thyroid tissue may be absent.
- If it is symptomatic, excision and thyroid hormone replacement is the choice of treatment.

DISORDERS OF THE BUCCAL MUCOSA

Fordyce's Granules
- A developmental anomaly characterized by a heterotopic/ectopic collections of sebaceous glands at various sites on the oral mucosa.
- During the development of maxillary and mandibular process, some portion of the ectoderm from the neighboring skin may get included in these sites, thereby leading to the development of sebaceous glands inside the mouth.
- Appear as multiple yellowish-white papules
- Most common on buccal mucosa (Also seen on vermilion border of upper lip, tonsils, etc.)
- May have a granular appearance of cheek mucosa because of many papules.
- Since they are asymptomatic, no treatment is indicated.

Leukoedema
- Common condition of oral mucosa, characterized by white, milky and opalescent appearance of the oral mucosa.
- Unknown etiology. Known to occur more in blacks than whites.
- Most common on cheek, producing grayish-white, milky and opalescent appearance of mucosa.
- Surface of the mucosa appears folded, leading to wrinkles or white streaks.
- The lesions cannot be scraped off.
- Typically bilateral, may extend onto the lip mucosa.
- When the cheek is stretched or tensed, the white patch tends to disappear.
- Leukoedema is not a pre-malignant condition and does not have malignant potential.
- No treatment needed.

Focal Epithelial Hyperplasia

- A condition of the oral mucosa presenting as nodular lesions, commonly on lower lip and buccal mucosa.
- May also occur on upper lip, gingiva, commissures, etc.
- Nodular, 1 to 5 mm in size with sessile base
- Soft and is of the same color as the mucosa
- Children between 3 and 18 years more affected
- May undergo regression after 6 months
- No treatment is necessary as the lesions are harmless.

DISORDERS OF THE LIPS

Commissural Lip Pits

- They are small mucosal invaginations that occur at the corners of the mouth on the vermilion borders of lips.
- Many represent a failure of normal fusion of the embryonic maxillary and mandibular processes.
- More common in adults (12–20%), while it is less in children (0.2–0.7%)
- Though they are congenital, the actual pits may develop later in life.
- Seen more in males
- May be unilateral or bilateral
- Asymptomatic
- Some of them produce fluid, when squeezed. These may represent minor salivary glands that drain into their depths.
- Not associated with any clefts of face or palate.
- No treatment required.

Double Lip

- Rare oral anomaly featured by a fold of tissue on the mucosal side of the lip
- Often congenital in origin; may be acquired also
- Upper lip is much more affected
- Both lips are rarely involved together
- Condition becomes noticeable when lips are tensed/ stretched like smiling, etc.
- No treatment required.

Cleft Lip

- Forms one of the two important components of orofacial clefts (cleft lip + cleft palate).
- Formed due to defective or failure of fusion of the median nasal process with the maxillary process.
- Frequently occurs along with cleft palate.
- They may occur singly (isolated) or, as part of syndromes (as many as 250 syndromes are identified).
- Classification:
    - Unilateral incomplete
    - Unilateral complete
    - Bilateral incomplete
    - Bilateral complete (also called "hare lip")
- The incomplete clefts extend towards the nostril and involves the palate.
- The complete clefts extends into the nostril and even more commonly involves the palate.
- Combined clefts are more frequent and severe in boys. They more frequently occur on left side.
- For detailed discussion—refer Chapter 11.

Peutz-Jegher's Syndrome

- Consists of familial intestinal polyposis, pigmented spots on the face, oral cavity, hands and feet.
- Melanin pigmentation of lips and oral mucosa is present at birth.
- Appears as small brown macules measuring 1 to 5 mm in diameter.
- Intraorally, buccal mucosa is mostly involved, followed by hard palate and gingiva.
- Tongue rarely shows pigmentation.
- Mucosal surface of lower lip is very largely involved.
- The facial pigmentation may fade later in life, but mucosal pigmentation of lip and buccal mucosa persists.
- Intestinal polyps are usually distributed through the entire intestine, but are more in small intestine.
- Thus, many patients have abdominal pain and signs of minor obstruction.
- This syndrome is not sex linked, since both sexes are equally affected and both males and females carry the factor.
- Diagnosis is often first made by dentists, through the orofacial pigmentations.

DISORDERS AFFECTING THE SHAPE OF THE TEETH

Microdontia

- This term is used to describe teeth that are smaller than normal.
- They are of three types:
    - True generalized: All teeth are smaller than normal. It is a rare condition where all the teeth are well formed but merely small.
    - Relative generalized: The teeth are of normal or slightly smaller size that are present in jaws that are somewhat larger than normal and therefore giving an illusion of microdontia. It is due to jaw and tooth size discrepancy and the role of hereditary is obvious.

– Microdontia of single tooth: A common condition affects most often maxillary lateral incisor and third molar. Most common form is the peg lateral.

Macrodontia

- Refers to teeth larger than normal.
- They are of three types:
  - True generalized: All the teeth are larger than normal. A rare condition associated with pituitary gigantism.
  - Relative generalized: It is more common: Larger than normal teeth in smaller jaws, where hereditary plays a role.
  - Macrodontia of a single tooth: Relatively uncommon, unknown etiology.

Dilaceration

- It refers to an angulation or a bend in the crown or root of a formed tooth (Figs 16.4A and B).
- Occurs due to trauma during the period in which tooth is forming with the result that the resultant tooth is calcified in the new position.
- The bend may occur anywhere along the length of the root.
- The concern is the problems that may arise during extraction or endodontic therapy.

Talon Cusp

- It is a small elevated structure resembling an Eagle's talon, projecting from the cingulum of a maxillary or a mandibular permanent incisor (Fig. 16.5).
- This cusp blends smoothly with the tooth structure except that there is a deep development groove where the cusp blends with the sloping lingual tooth surface.
- Composed of normal enamel and dentin and contains a horn of pulp tissue.
- Problems of esthetics, caries, occlusal interference
- More prevalent in persons with Rubinstein-Taybi syndrome.

Dens Evaginatus

- Appears clinically as an accessory cusp or a globule of enamel on occlusal surface between the buccal and lingual cusp of mandibular premolars.
- Unilateral or bilateral in occurrence.
- Rarely seen on molars, canines or incisors.
- There is evagination of an area of inner enamel epithelium.
- The extra-cusp may contribute to incomplete eruption, displacement of teeth and/or pulp exposure with subsequent infection following fracture or wear of surface.

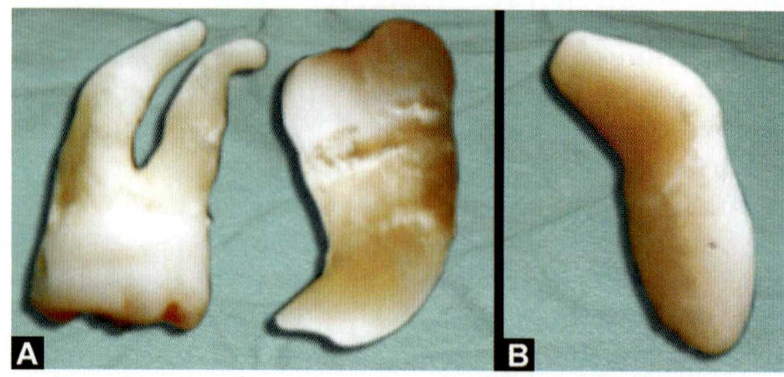

Figs 16.4A and B: Dilaceration: (A) Posterior teeth; (B) Anterior teeth

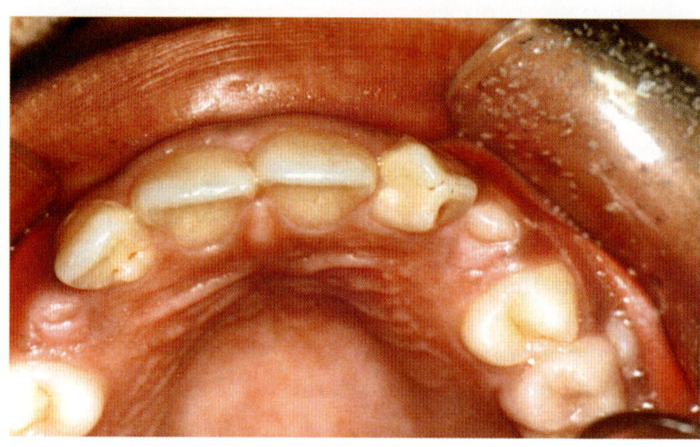

Fig. 16.5: Talon cusp seen on the maxillary left lateral incisor

Dens in Dente

- This developmental anomaly has been described as a lingual invagination of the enamel.
- This condition can occur in primary and permanent teeth.
- It is most often seen in the permanent maxillary lateral incisors.
- The condition may be inherited as an autosomal dominant trait with variable expressivity and possibly incomplete penetrance.
- Anterior teeth with dens in dente are usually of normal shape and size. In other areas of the mouth, however, the tooth can have an anomalous appearance.
- A dens in dente is characterized by an invagination lined with enamel and the presence of a foramen cecum with the probability of a communication between the cavity of the invagination and the pulp chamber.
- Application of sealant or a restoration at the opening of the invagination are the recommended treatments to prevent pulpal involvement.
- If the condition is detected before complete eruption of the tooth, the removal of gingival tissue to facilitate cavity preparation and restoration may be indicated.

Taurodontism

- Anomaly in which body of the tooth is enlarged at the expense of roots (Fig. 16.6).
- The name suggests bull like teeth due to resemblance to the teeth of cud chewing animals.
- Maybe hypo, meso or hypertaurodontism. In severe form the bifurcation or the trifurcation occurs near the apices of the roots.
- Associated with Klinefelter's syndrome.
- May affect deciduous or permanent teeth.
- Molars invariably involved.
- Clinically teeth themselves have no characteristic feature.
- The clinical significance of the condition becomes apparent, endodontic therapy is necessary.
- Radiographically-extreme large pulp chamber, pulp lacking usual constriction at cervix.

Supernumerary Roots (Fig. 16.7)

- May involve any tooth
- Clinical significance lies in exodontia where extraction may cause breakage of one root acting as a focus of infection.

Fusion (Figs 16.8 and 16.9)

- Fusion represents the union of two independently developing primary or permanent teeth.
- The condition is almost always limited to the anterior teeth and, may follow a familial tendency.
- The radiograph may show that the fusion is limited to the crowns and roots. Fused teeth will have separate pulp chambers and separate pulp canals.
- Dental caries may develop in the line of fusion of the crowns, necessitating the placement of a restoration.
- A frequent finding in fusion of primary teeth is the congenital absence of one of the corresponding permanent teeth.

Gemination

- A geminated tooth represents an attempted division of a single tooth germ by invagination occurring during the proliferation stage of the growth cycle of the tooth.
- The anomaly, which may follow a hereditary pattern, is seen in both primary and permanent teeth, though it probably occurs more frequently in primary teeth.
- The geminated tooth appears clinically as a bifid crown on a single root. The crown is usually wider than normal, with a shallow groove extending from the incisal edge to the cervical region.

Concrescence (Fig. 16.10)

- It is a form of fusion that happens after the completion of the root.

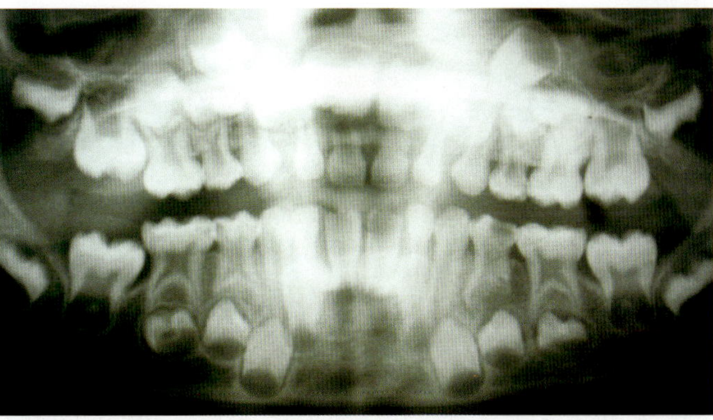

Fig. 16.6: Taurodontism of posterior teeth

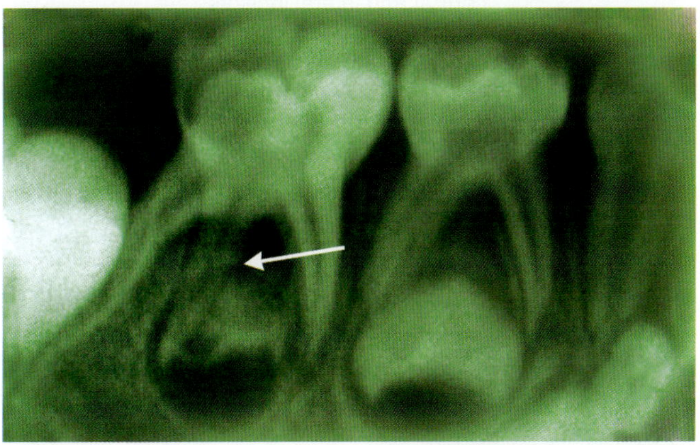

Fig. 16.7: Supernumerary root seen in the lower second deciduous molar

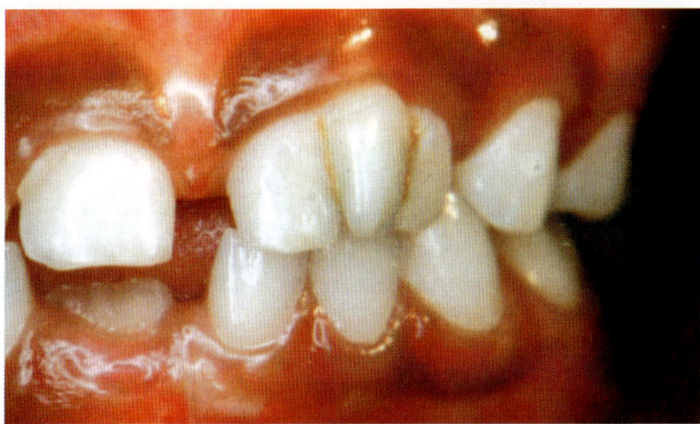

Fig. 16.8: Fusion of maxillary deciduous central and lateral incisors with a supernumerary deciduous tooth. The patient had a missing permanent lateral incisor which is a common sequelae

- The union is only at the cementum interface.
- Maybe due to traumatic injury or crowding of teeth, with resorption of interdental bone.
- It is important to diagnose this prior to extraction, otherwise both the teeth will be removed together.

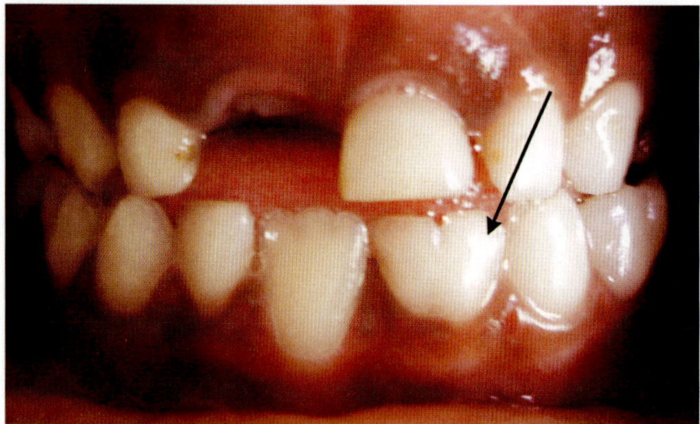

Fig. 16.9: Fusion involving deciduous mandibular central and lateral incisors

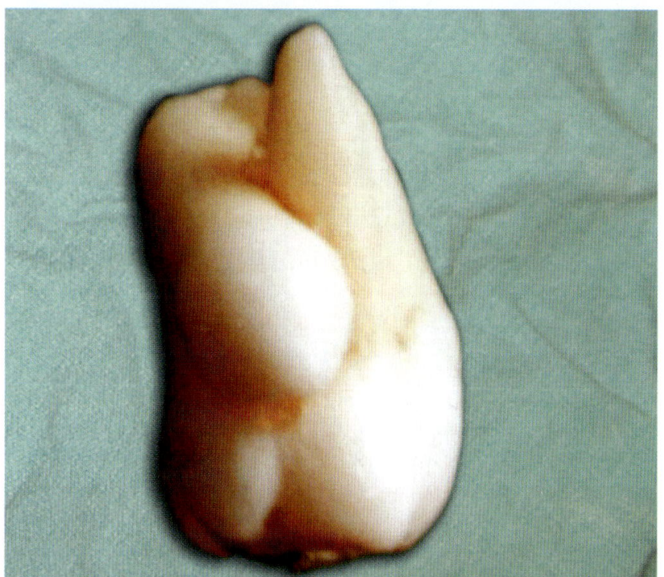

Fig. 16.10: Concrescence

Odontome

- Epithelial and mesechymal cells exhibit failure to differentiate resulting in abnormal formation of enamel and dentin.
- They are of two types: The compound composite odontoma and complex composite odontoma.
- Compound composite odontoma resembles the anatomy of the normal teeth to a certain extent.
- Complex composite odontoma appears as an irregular mass of dental tissue and bears no resemblance to normal tooth structure.
- Etiology is unknown. May be due to trauma or infection.
- It may become large and cause facial swelling and asymmetry.
- Treatment includes surgical removal.

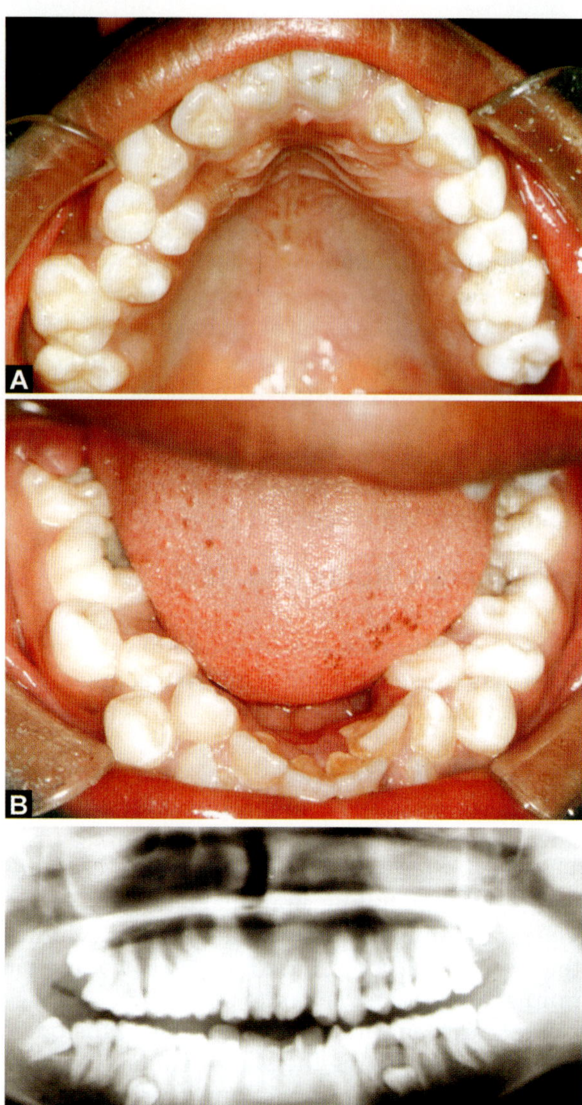

Figs 16.11A to C: Supernumerary teeth, 6 erupted and 6 unerupted: (A) Upper arch; (B) Lower arch; (C) Radiograph

DISORDERS AFFECTING THE NUMBER OF TEETH

Supernumerary Teeth (Figs 16.11A to C)

- Develops from a third tooth bud arising from the dental lamina near the permanent tooth bud, or possibly from the splitting of the permanent bud itself. In some cases a hereditary tendency has been noted.
- May be found in any location, but they have an apparent predilection for certain sites.
- Most common supernumerary tooth is the mesiodens (Figs 16.12A to C)—a tooth situated between the maxillary central incisors and occurring singly or

paired, erupted or impacted or even inverted. The mesiodens are usually small teeth with a cone shaped crown and a short root. Mesiodens is transmitted as an autosomal dominant trait.

- Maxillary 4th molar is the next most common supernumerary tooth and is situated distal to the third molar.
- Mandibular 4th molar is less common.
- Other supernumerary teeth are maxillary paramolars, mandibular premolars and maxillary lateral incisors. The paramolars are small rudimentary tooth situated buccally or lingually to one of the maxillary molars or interproximally between the first, second or third maxillary molar.
- 90% of all supernumerary teeth occur in maxilla.
- Supernumerary teeth in deciduous dentition are less common.

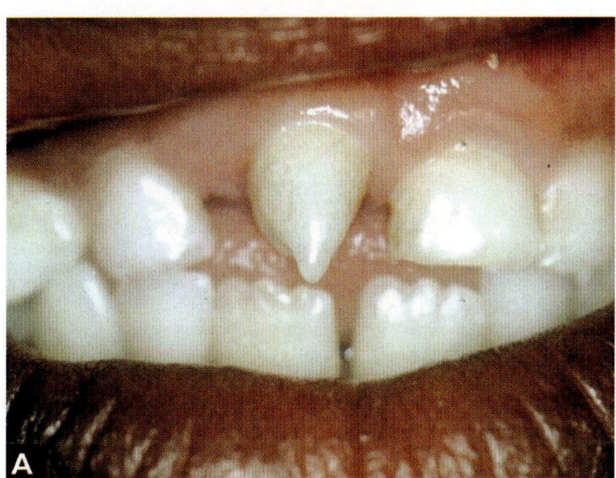
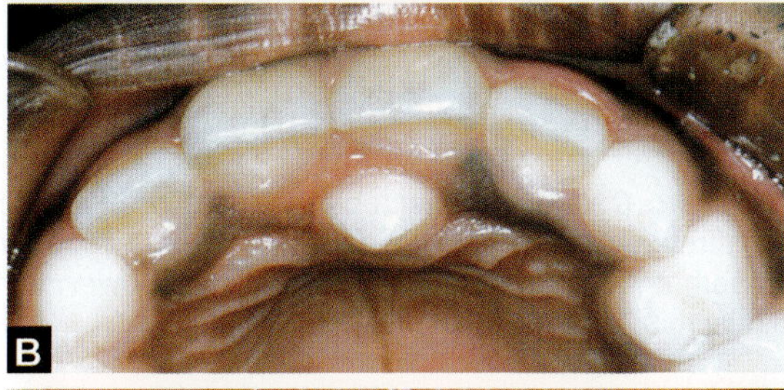
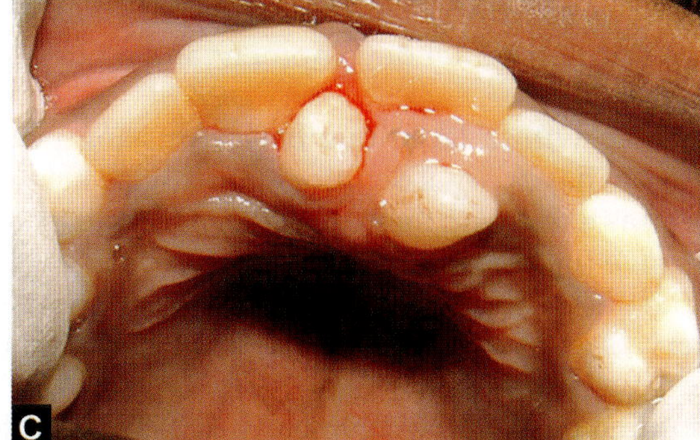

Figs 16.12A to C: Mesiodens: (A) Located in between the deciduous incisors; (B) Located behind the permanent central incisors; (C) Two mesiodens located palatally

- Cause of additional tooth bulk frequently causes malposition of adjacent teeth or prevents their eruption.

Anodontia

- Implies complete failure of the teeth to develop.
- When it occurs as an isolated trait, the primary dentition is not affected, and the inheritance is autosomal recessive.
- An overlay denture is constructed for the patient, which is the treatment of choice.

Hypodontia

- Agenesis of some teeth is referred to as hypodontia, which is same as partial anodontia. Oligodontia is used when more than six permanent teeth are missing except the third molars.
- Hypodontia may occur without a family history of hypodontia, though it is often familial.
- It may also occur as a part of a syndrome, especially in ectodermal dysplasia.
- Most frequently missing teeth are the mandibular second premolars, maxillary lateral incisors (Figs 16.13A to C), and maxillary second premolars. The absence of teeth may be unilateral or bilateral.
- Management includes replacement of the missing teeth.

Ectodermal Dysplasia

- It is characterized by varying anomalies of ectodermal derivatives including both the primary and permanent teeth, hair, nails, and skin.
- The congenital absence of primary teeth is relatively rare.
- When a number of primary teeth fail to develop, other ectodermal deficiencies are usually evident.
- Children with a number of missing primary and permanent teeth may have some or all of the signs of a type of ectodermal dysplasia and should undergo further evaluation for other systemic changes.

Anhidrotic Eectodermal Dysplasia (Figs 16.14A to C)

- It is one of the more common types of ectodermal dysplasia. Consanguinity increases the likelihood of a trait or condition that is inherited in a recessive manner to be expressed.
- Hypodontia and dental hypoplasia, as well as hypotrichosis, hypo/anhidrosis are characteristic.
- Secondary characteristics include a deficiency in salivary flow, protuberant lips and a saddle-nose appearance.
- The skin is often dry and scaly and there is fissuring at the corners of the mouth.

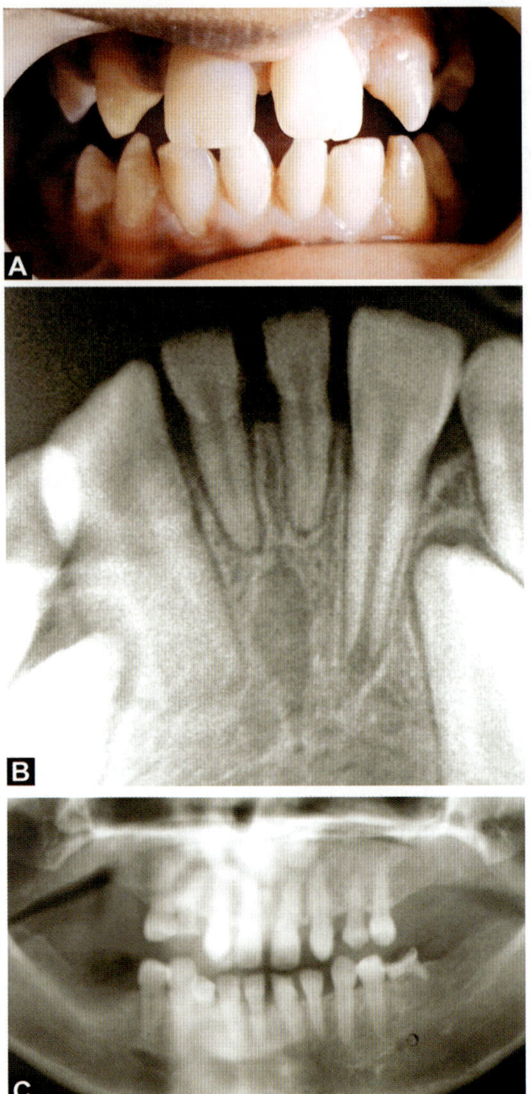

Figs 16.13A to C: Hypodontia involving: (A) Permanent maxillary lateral incisors; (B) Permanent mandibular central incisors; (C) Multiple missing teeth

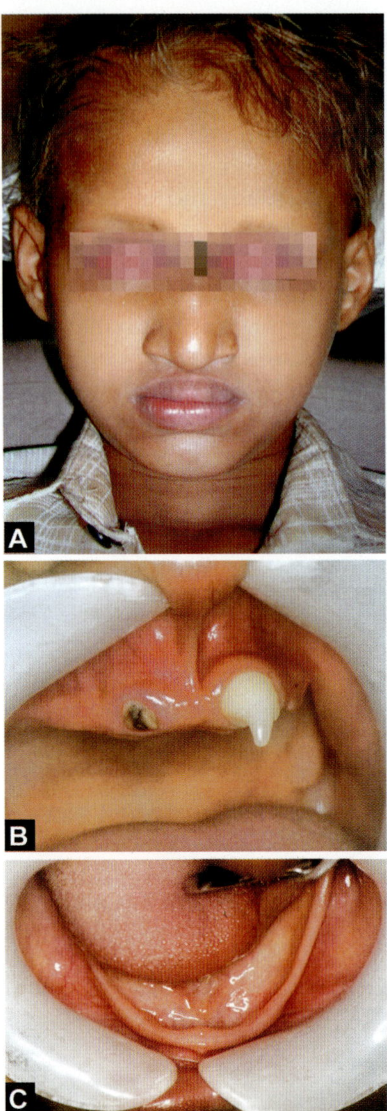

Figs 16.14A to C: Anhidrotic ectodermal dysplasia: (A) Sparse hair and stretched dry skin; (B) Upper arch with congenitally missing teeth and malformed central incisor; (C) Lower arch with congenitally missing teeth

- The absence of teeth predisposes the child to a lack in growth of the alveolar process.
- Other skeletal structures are normal.
- The size of the primary teeth that are present may be normal or reduced.
- The anterior teeth are often conical, which is characteristic of oligodontia associated with many types of ectodermal dysplasia.
- The primary molars without permanent successors have an unexplained tendency to become ankylosed.
- A deficiency in sweat glands causes a predisposition to increased body temperature, and children with hypo/anhidrosis are extremely uncomfortable during hot weather. Many of them must reside in cool climates.

- Children with an ectodermal dysplasia usually have normal mental development and a normal life expectancy.
- Children with a large number of missing primary teeth can have partial dentures constructed at an early age so as to increase their ability to masticate food and improve their nutritional status.
- A partial denture may be adjusted or remade at intervals to allow for the eruption of permanent teeth and jaw growth.
- Denture construction at an early age is desirable, to reduce the psychologic problem that may cause the child to feel "different" and to ensure masticatory efficiency.

- If the permanent teeth erupt in good position and in favorable relationship to each other, partial dentures may serve until the child is old enough for implants or fixed bridgework.

DISORDERS AFFECTING THE STRUCTURE OF THE TEETH

Enamel Hypoplasia/Enamel Hypocalcification

- Amelogenesis occurs in two stages. In the first stage, the enamel matrix forms and in the second stage, the matrix undergoes calcification. Local or systemic factors that interfere with the normal matrix formation cause enamel surface defects and irregularities called enamel hypoplasia (Figs 16.15 and 16.16). Factors that interfere with calcification and maturation of the enamel produce a condition called enamel hypocalcification.
- Postnatal hypoplasia of the primary teeth is probably as common as hypoplasia of the permanent teeth, though the former usually does not occur in as severe a form. However, hypoplasia of the primary enamel that forms before birth is rare.
- Enamel hypoplasia may be mild and may result in a pitting of the enamel surface or in the development of a horizontal line across the enamel of the crown. If ameloblastic activity has been disrupted for a long period, gross areas of irregular or imperfect enamel formation occur.
- Enamel hypoplasia is often seen as one component of many different syndromes and may occur due to many reasons such as

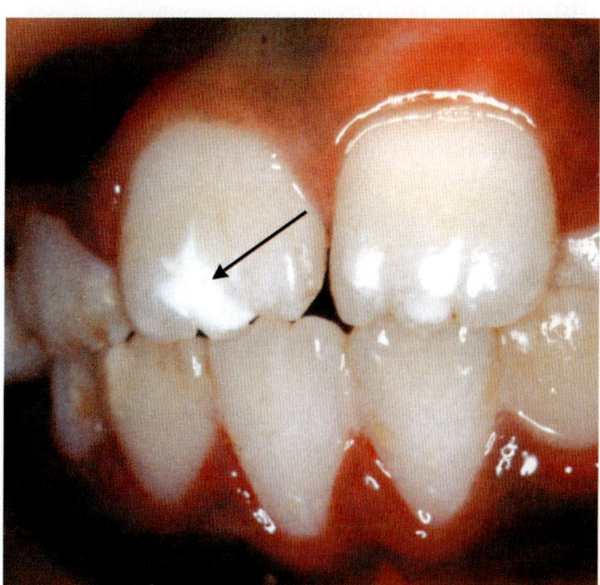

Fig. 16.15: Localized enamel hypolplasia (Arrow)

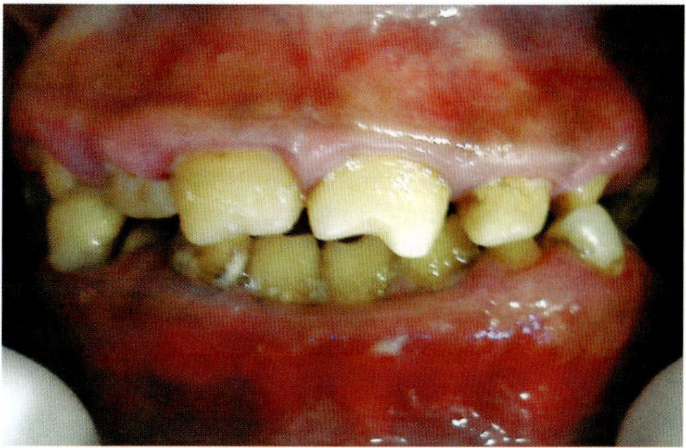

Fig. 16.16: Generalized severe enamel defect

- Hypoplasia resulting from nutritional deficiencies: such as vitamins A, C, and D, calcium, and phosphorus deficiencies.
- Hypoplasia related to brain injury and neurologic defects
- Hypoplasia associated with nephrotic syndrome
- Hypoplasia associated with allergies
- Hypoplasia associated with chronic pediatric lead poisoning
- Hypoplasia caused by local infection and trauma: such as Turner's hypoplasia
- Hypoplasia associated with cleft lip and palate
- Hypoplasia caused by X radiation
- Hypoplasia resulting from rubella embryopathy.

Dentinogenesis Imperfecta (Hereditary Opalescent Dentin)

- Dentinogenesis imperfecta is inherited as an autosomal dominant trait. Prevalence is 1 in 8000.
- The clinical picture of dentinogenesis imperfecta is one in which the primary and permanent teeth have a characteristic reddish brown to gray opalescent color.
- The enamel often breaks away from the incisal edge of the anterior teeth and the occlusal surface of the posterior teeth.
- The exposed soft dentin abrades rapidly, occasionally to the extent that the smooth, polished dentin surface is continuous with the gingival tissue.
- The roots of teeth are short.

Amelogenesis Imperfecta

- Amelogenesis imperfecta is a developmental defect of the enamel with heterogeneous etiology that affects the enamel of both the primary and permanent dentition.
- The anomaly occurs in the general population in the range of 1 in 14,000 to 1 in 16,000 and has a wide range of clinical appearances.

- At least three different clinical variations of amelogenesis imperfecta are observed—the hypocalcified type, the hypomaturation type and the hypoplastic type.
- The defective tooth structure is limited to the enamel.
- On radiographic examination the pulpal outline appears to be normal, and the root morphology is not unlike that of normal teeth.
- The difference in the appearance and quality of the enamel is thought to be attributable to the state of enamel development at the time the defect occurs.
- The defect may be due to faulty matrix formation or calcification. When the matrix is faulty the tooth appears to be imperfectly formed with normal calcification. If the fault is in calcification the enamel becomes soft.
- Treatment depends on its severity and the demands of esthetic improvement.

Dentin Dysplasia

- Dentin dysplasia is a rare disturbance of dentin formation that are of two types: radicular dentin dysplasia (type I) and coronal dentin dysplasia (type II).
- Genetic linkage has been established for dentinogenesis imperfecta.

Dentin Dysplasia (Type I)

- Both primary and secondary dentitions are affected in dentin dysplasia, type I, which is an autosomal dominant trait.
- Radiographically the roots are short and may be more pointed than normal, usually with absence of the root canals and pulp chambers.
- The color and general morphology of the crowns of the teeth are usually normal, although they may be slightly opalescent and blue or brown.
- Periapical radiolucencies may be present at the apices of affected teeth.

Dentin Dysplasia (Type II)

- It is inherited as an autosomal dominant trait in which the primary dentition appears opalescent.
- Radiographs show obliterated pulp chambers.
- The permanent dentition in dentin dysplasia, type II has normal color.
- Radiograph exhibits a thistle tube pulp configuration with pulp stones.

BENIGN TUMORS OF THE ORAL CAVITY

Hemangioma

- Seen during the first decade of life and more in females

- Commonly occurring on the lips, tongue and buccal mucosa
- They are localized to diffuse, red-blue lesion
- They are flat, nodular and soft
- Surgical excision or cryotherapy is the treatment of choice.

Lymphangioma

- Seen during the first decade with no gender predilection
- Commonly located on the tongue, lip, buccal mucosa, floor of the mouth and the neck
- Seen as localized to diffuse red-blue to translucent enlargement
- There may be multiple lesions
- Treatment of choice is excisional biopsy. Regression is rare.

Congenital Epulis

- Seen in newborn and more in females
- Located commonly in the anterior maxillary alveolar ridge area
- It appears as smooth, pedunculated swelling
- Treatment is excision.

Neurofibromatosis

- 7% of the lesions are seen in oral cavity, rest are spread throughout the body.
- Appears as nodules of neural tissue. They may be small, discrete and smooth or even pedunculated.
- No treatment is necessary.

White Sponge Nevus

- Uncommon with autosomal dominant hereditary pattern
- Buccal mucosa commonly affected
- Asymptomatic, widespread, corrugated thickening of oral mucosa
- No treatment required.

Blue Nevus

- Seen during the second decade, more in females
- Commonly occurring in the hard palate, buccal mucosa, lips and gingiva
- It is a well-delineated elevated nodule, brown black or blue in color
- It is asymptomatic
- Oral lesions are under constant irritation and at risk for malignant transformation
- Treatment includes excisional biopsy.

CYSTS OF ORAL CAVITY

Primordial Cyst

- Develops before any tooth material has been formed, thus associated with a congenitally missing tooth.
- Varies widely in size, with potential to expand the bone and displaces the adjacent teeth.
- Not painful
- X-ray shows round or ovoid, well-demarcated radiolucent lesion which may show a sclerotic border.
- It may be unilocular or multilocular.
- Treatment includes surgical removal with thorough curettage of the bone.

Dentigerous Cyst (Follicular Cyst)

- It originates after the crown of the tooth has been completely formed by accumulation of fluid between the reduced enamel epithelium and the tooth crown.
- The most common sites of this cyst are the mandibular and maxillary third molar and maxillary cuspid areas.
- The dentigerous cyst nearly always involves or is associated with the crown of a normal permanent tooth.
- Seldom is a deciduous tooth involved.
- May also be found enclosing a complex compound odontoma or involving a supernumerary tooth.
- The lesion appears as a circumscribed, fluctuant, often translucent swelling of the alveolar ridge over the site of the erupting tooth.
- X-ray shows radiolucent area associated with an unerupted tooth crown (Fig. 16.17). The dentigerous cyst is usually smooth, with unilocular or multilocular appearance.
- Smaller lesions can be surgically removed in their entirety with little difficulty. The larger cysts which

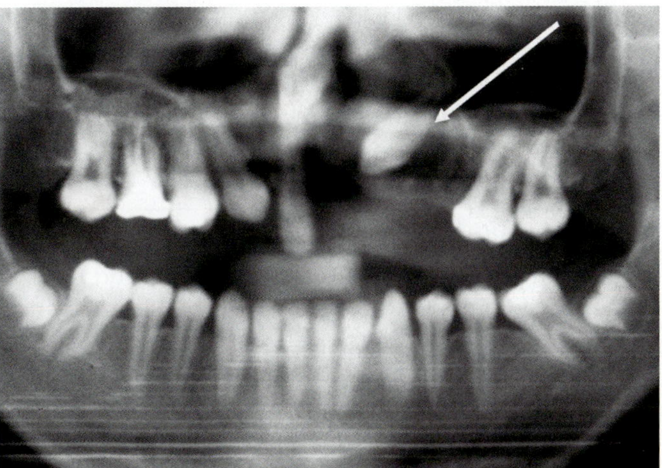

Fig. 16.17: Dentigerous cyst involving the unerupted maxillary canine (arrow)

involve serious loss of bone and thin the bone dangerously are often treated by insertion of a surgical drain or marsupialization.

Odontogenic Keratocyst

- Occurs in the second decade and seen more in males.
- Located in the posterior body and ramus of the mandible, maxillary third molar and canine region.
- It is painful.
- X-ray shows well-defined unilocular or multilocular radiolucency with thin opaque well-demarcated border.
- Can cause root resorption or displacement of adjacent roots.
- Treatment includes surgical excision with curettage.

Radicular Cyst

- Wide age distribution of occurrence. Seen more in maxilla and in association with a non vital teeth.
- X-ray shows round or ovoid radiolucency around the tooth apex.
- Treatment includes enucleation.

Nasopalatine Duct Cyst

- Originates from the cystic dilatation of the nasopalatine duct
- It is a painless soft swelling in the incisive foramen area
- X-ray shows heart shaped radiolucency in the midline of anterior maxilla
- Treatment includes enucleation.

Globulomaxillary Cyst

- It is a fissural cyst found within bone between the maxillary lateral incisor and canine.
- Treatment is enucleation.

Dental Lamina Cyst of the Newborn

(Gingival cyst of the newborn; Epstein's pearls; Bohn's nodules)
- Dental lamina cysts of the newborn are multiple, occasionally solitary, nodules on the alveolar ridge of newborn or very young infants which represent cysts originating from remnants of the dental lamina.
- Epstein's pearls are cystic, keratin filled nodules found along the midpalatine raphe.
- Bohn's nodules are keratin filled cysts scattered on the hard palate especially at the junction of the hard and soft palate.
- Appears clinically as small discrete white swellings of the alveolar ridge.
- They are painless
- No treatment is required.

DISORDERS OF THE JAW

Agnathia

- An extremely rare congenital defect characterized by absence of maxilla or mandible.
- More commonly only a portion of one jaw is missing.
- Partial absence of mandible is even more common.

Micrognathia

- It is a congenital anomaly but the condition may be acquired in later life. The mandible is most often affected.
- The cause of congenital micrognathia appears to be heterogeneous.
- Deficient nutrition of the mother and intrauterine injury resulting from pressure or trauma have been suggested as possible etiologies.
- Additionally, micrognathia may be part of the Robin sequence comprised also of cleft palate and glossoptosis.
- Infants with mandibular micrognathia have difficulty in breathing and episodes of cyanosis are seen.
- The anterior portion of the mandible is positioned so that the tongue has little if any support and can fall backward, causing obstruction.
- Because mandibular growth continues until late adolescence, it is possible to hope for an esthetically pleasing profile in adulthood.
- The nursing bottle may be used in the treatment of congenital micrognathia to help promote adequate function of the mandible.
- Acquired micrognathia may develop gradually and may not be evident until 4 to 6 years of age. Ankylosis of the jaw caused by a birth injury or trauma in later life may result in an acquired type of micrognathia. Infection in the temperomandibular joint area can also cause arrested growth at the head of the condyle and the acquired pattern of micrognathia develops. In cases of true ankylosis of the mandible, arthroplasty should be recommended.

Macrognathia

- Refers to condition of abnormally large jaws
- Associated with pituitary gigantism, Paget's disease, acromegaly
- Cases of mandibular prognathism are a common occurrence.
- Etiology is unknown although some cases may follow a hereditary pattern.
- Factors favoring mandibular prognathism are— increased height of ramus, increased mandibular body length, increased gonial angle, anterior position of glenoid fossa, decreased maxillary length, prominent chin button.

Osteomyelitis

- Seen in the first and second decade. There is no gender predilection.
- Occurs in the posterior mandibular region.
- Associated with fever, periapical abscess, a carious teeth, pain and lymphadenopathy.
- X-ray shows diffuse radiolucency with poorly defined margins.
- Treatment includes incision and drainage followed by treatment of carious teeth.

Fibrous Dysplasia

- Seen in the first and second decade, with no gender predilection.
- Maxilla is commonly affected.
- Characterized by expansion of buccal cortical plate which is unilateral and asymptomatic.
- X-ray shows radiolucent to densely opaque lesion. Ground glass appearance is the characteristic feature of fibrous dysplasia.
- Treatment is not required.

Cherubism

- Autosomal dominant mode of transmission
- Manifests early in childhood
- Painless, progressing, symmetric swelling of the jaws affecting mandible or maxilla producing a typical chubby face.
- Deciduous dentition may be spontaneously shed prematurely
- Permanent dentition may be defective
- X-ray shows bilateral destruction of bone with expansion and thinning of the cortical plate
- They regress with age. Correction other than for cosmetic reasons are not required.

DISORDERS OF THE FACE

Facial Hemihypertrophy

- Exhibit enlargement of one half of head and face.
- Etiology may be attributed to hormonal imbalance, incomplete twinning, localized alteration of intra-uterine development, chromosomal abnormalities, lymphatic, vascular and neurogenic abnormalities.
- There appears to be some relationship between hemihypertrophy and neoplasms of kidney, liver and adrenal cortex in children.

- Females are affected more.
- Permanent teeth on affected sides are enlarged, develop more rapidly and erupt before their counter parts on uninvolved side.
- Roots of teeth are short.
- Bone of maxilla and mandible are also enlarged.
- Tongue may show enlargement of lingual papillae.

Facial Hemiatrophy

- It is a progressive atrophy of some or all tissues of one side of face.
- Etiology can be attributed to malfunction of sympathetic nervous system, trauma, infection, heredity, localized scleroderma.
- Noticed in first or second decade as a white line or furrow on side of face or brow near midline.
- Lesion extends to include atrophy of skin, muscle, bone, tissue.
- Hollowing of cheek and eyes may appear depressed in orbit
- Response of atrophic facial muscles to faradic stimulation is unaltered.
- Affected skin is darkly pigmented
- Loss of facial hair is common
- Hemiatrophy of lips and tongue is reported
- Growth of teeth may be affected
- Roots of teeth may exhibit deficiency of root development
- Eruption on affected side may be retarded.

BACTERIAL INFECTIONS

Scarlet Fever (Scarlatina)

- Occurs predominantly in children during the winter months
- Caused by infection with streptococcal organisms of the beta hemolytic type that elaborate an erythrogenic toxin.
- Incubation period is of three to five days.
- The patient then exhibits severe pharyngitis and tonsillitis, headache, chills, fever and vomiting. Accompanying these symptoms are enlargement and tenderness of the regional cervical lymph nodes.
- Diffuse, bright scarlet skin rash appears on the second or third day of the illness. This rash, which is particularly prominent in the areas of the skin folds, is a result of the toxic injury to the vascular endothelium which produces dilatation of the small blood vessels and consequent hyperemia.
- The mucosa, particularly of the palate, may appear congested, and the throat is often fiery red.
- The tonsils and faucial pillars are usually swollen and sometimes covered with a grayish exudate.

- More important are the changes occurring in the tongue. Early in the course of the disease the tongue exhibits a white coating, and the fungiform papillae are edematous and hyperemic projecting above the surface as small red knobs. This phenomenon has been described clinically as a "strawberry tongue."
- The coating of the tongue is soon lost, beginning at the tip and lateral margins, and the tongue becomes deep red, glistening and smooth except for the swollen, hyperemic papillae. The tongue in this phase has been termed the "raspberry tongue"
- The skin then desquamates within a week or 10 days
- The disease is treated by antibiotic therapy.

Diphtheria

- It is an acute contagious disease caused by a gram-positive bacillus, Corynebacterium diphtheriae, or the Klebs-Loeffler bacillus.
- This infection occurs most frequently in children during the fall and winter months.
- The disease is transmitted through droplet infection or by direct contact.
- The incubation period for diphtheria is only a few days
- The disease is manifested initially by listlessness, malaise, headache, fever and occasional vomiting.
- It may be associated with sore throat, mild redness and edema of the pharynx and cervical lymph-adenopathy.
- Patchy "diphtheritic membrane" is seen on the tonsils, which later enlarges and becomes confluent over the surface. This membrane is grayish, thick, fibrinous, gelatinous-appearing exudate which contains dead cells, leukocytes and bacteria overlying necrotic, ulcerated areas of the mucosa and covering the tonsils, pharynx and larynx. It tends to be adherent and leaves a bleeding surface if stripped away.
- If the infection spreads unchecked in the respiratory tract, the larynx may become edematous and covered by the pseudomembrane and produces a mechanical respiratory obstruction.
- The disease may be prevented by prophylactic active immunization with diphtheria toxoid.
- Once the disease has developed, it is treated with antitoxin, usually in combination with antibiotics.

Tuberculosis

- Tuberculosis is an infectious granulomatous disease caused by the acid-fast bacillus Mycobacterium tuberculosis.
- Pulmonary tuberculosis is the chief form of the disease, although infection may also occur by way of the intestinal tract, tonsils and skin.

- Tuberculous infection of submaxillary and cervical lymph nodes, or scrofula, a tuberculous lymphadenitis, may progress to the formation of an actual abscess or remain as a typical granulomatous lesion. They are tender or painful, often show inflammation of the overlying skin.
- Tuberculous lesions of the oral cavity do occur secondary to a pulmonary disease.
- The organisms are carried in the sputum and enter the mucosal tissue through a small break in the surface.
- Lesions may occur at any site on the oral mucous membrane, but the tongue is most commonly affected, followed by the palate, lips, buccal mucosa, gingiva and frenula.
- The usual tuberculous lesion is an irregular, superficial or deep, painful ulcer which tends to increase slowly in size.
- The dentist may contract an infection from his contact with living tubercle.
- Bacilli in the mouths of patients who have pulmonary or oral tuberculosis is a problem of great clinical significance.
- Tuberculous gingivitis is an unusual form of tuberculosis which may appear as a diffuse, hyperemic, nodular or papillary proliferation of the gingival tissues.
- Tuberculosis may also involve the bone of the maxilla or mandible. Tuberculous osteomyelitis frequently occurs in the later stages of the disease and has an unfavorable prognosis.
- The treatment of oral tuberculosis is secondary to treatment of the primary lesions.

Actinomycosis

- Actinomycosis is a chronic granulomatous, suppurative, and fibrosing disease caused by anaerobic, gram-positive, nonacid-fast, filamentous bacteria, Actinomyces israelii, although *A. naeslundi, A. viscosus, A.odontolyticus* and *A. propionica*.
- The usual pattern of this disease is one characterized chiefly by the formation of abscesses which tend to drain by the formation of sinus tracts.
- If the pus from the abscesses is carefully examined on a clean glass slide, it shows the typical "sulfur granules," or colonies of organisms which appear in the suppurative material as tiny yellow grains.
- Actinomycosis is classified anatomically according to the location of the lesions, and thus we recognize (i) cervicofacial, (ii) abdominal, and (iii) pulmonary forms.
- Cervicofacial actinomycosis is the most common form of this disease and is of greatest interest to the dental professionals.

- It involves the salivary glands, bone or even the skin of the face and neck, producing swelling and induration of the tissue. These soft tissue swellings eventually develop into one or more abscesses which tend to discharge upon a skin surface, rarely a mucosal surface, liberating pus containing the typical "sulfur granules."
- The skin overlying the abscess is purplish red and indurated or often fluctuant.
- The infection of the soft tissues may extend to involve the mandible or, less commonly, the maxilla. If the bone of the maxilla is invaded, the ensuing specific osteomyelitis may eventually involve the cranium, meninges or the brain itself.
- The treatment of this disease is difficult and has not been uniformly successful. Penicillin and tetracyclines have been used most frequently, but the course of the disease is still often prolonged.

Tetanus (Lock-jaw)

- Tetanus is a disease of the nervous system characterized by intense activity of motor neurons and resulting in severe muscle spasms.
- It is caused by the exotoxin of the anaerobic gram positive bacillus *Clostridium tetani.*
- Clinical manifestations consist of pain and stiffness in the jaws and neck muscles, with muscle rigidity producing trismus and dysphagia.
- Rigidity of facial muscles may also occur, producing the typical "risus sardonicus."
- "Cephalic tetanus" is tetanus which is either localized or generalized, occurring in association with cranial nerve palsy, most commonly the seventh cranial nerve.
- All patients with the disease should receive antimicrobial drugs, active and passive immunization, surgical wound care.

Syphilis

- Syphilis is caused by infection with a spirochete, *Treponema pallidum.*
- Syphilis may be classified as either acquired or congenital.
- Congenital syphilis is transmitted to the offspring only by an infected mother and is not inherited.
- Manifestation of congenital syphilis are:
  - Frontal bossae
  - Short maxilla
  - High palatal arch
  - Saddle nose
  - Mulberry molars
  - Irregular thickening of the sternoclavicular portion of the clavicle

- Relative protuberance of mandible
- Rhagades
- Saber shin
- Hutchinson's triad consisting of hypoplasia of the incisor and molar teeth, eighth nerve deafness and interstitial keratitis.
- Adequate treatment of the mother before 16th week of gestation.

Noma (Cancrum Oris)

- Noma is a rapidly spreading gangrene of the oral and facial tissues that occur usually in debilitated or nutritionally deficient persons.
- Thus noma may be considered a secondary complication of systemic disease rather than a primary disease.
- It is seen chiefly in children.
- Noma appears to originate as a specific infection by Vincent's organisms, an acute necrotizing gingivostomatitis, which is soon complicated by secondary invasion of many other microbial forms, including streptococci, staphylococci and Diphtheria bacilli.
- Noma usually begins as a small ulcer of the gingival mucosa which rapidly spreads and involves the surrounding tissues of the jaws, lips and cheeks by gangrenous necrosis.
- The odor arising from the gangrenous tissues is extremely foul. The palate and occasionally the tongue may become involved by this process, but this is not common. Patients have a high temperature during the course of the disease, suffer secondary infection and may die from toxemia or pneumonia.
- The mortality rate of noma approximated 75 percent before the availability of antibiotics.
- The prognosis is considerably better if antibiotics are administered before the patient reaches the final stages. Immediate treatment of any existing malnutrition further improves the probability of saving the patient.

Pyogenic Granuloma (Granuloma Pyogenicum)

- The pyogenic granuloma is a distinctive clinical entity originating as a response of the tissues to a nonspecific infection either staphylococci or streptococci, usually triggered by local irritation.
- Occurs most frequently on the gingiva, but may also be found on the lips, tongue and buccal mucosa and occasionally on other areas.
- The lesion is usually an elevated, pedunculated or sessile mass with a smooth, lobulated or even a warty surface which commonly is ulcerated and shows a tendency for hemorrhage either spontaneously or upon slight trauma.
- Treatment includes removal of the irritant and oral hygiene measures.

VIRAL INFECTIONS

Herpes Simplex Virus Type I Infection

- Caused by the herpes simplex virus (HSV)
- Herpetic stomatitis is a common oral disease which develops in both children and young adults
- It rarely occurs before the age of six months, apparently because of the presence of circulating antibodies in the infant derived from the mother.
- The disease occurring in children is frequently the primary attack.
- It is characterized by the development of fever, irritability, headache, pain upon swallowing and regional lymphadenopathy.
- Within a few days the mouth becomes painful and the gingiva intensely inflamed.
- The lips, tongue, buccal mucosa, palate, pharynx and tonsils may also be involved.
- Shortly, yellowish, fluid-filled vesicles develop. These rupture and form shallow, ragged, extremely painful ulcers covered by a gray membrane and surrounded by an erythematous halo.
- They heal spontaneously within 7 to 14 days and leave no scar.
- Treatment is symptomatic such as application of topical anesthetic agents on the ulcers, soft diet and adequate fluids.

Herpangina

- Herpangina is a specific viral infection.
- Coxsackie group A viruses are the cause of the disease
- It is most commonly seen in young children; older children and adults are only occasionally affected.
- Herpangina is chiefly a summer disease, and many children may actually harbor the virus at this time without exhibiting clinical manifestations of the disease.
- This disease appears to be transmitted from one person to another through contact and multiple cases in a single household are common.
- The incubation period is about 2 to 10 days.
- The clinical manifestations of herpangina are comparatively mild and of short duration.
- It begins with sore throat, low-grade fever, headache, sometimes vomiting, prostration and abdominal pain.
- The patients soon exhibit small vesicles which are present for a short duration of time that later ulcerates,

each showing a gray base and an inflamed periphery on the anterior faucial pillars and sometimes on the hard and soft palates, posterior pharyngeal wall, buccal mucosa and tongue.

- The ulcers do not tend to be extremely painful, although dysphagia may occur. They generally heal within a few days to a week.
- A permanent immunity to the infecting strain usually develops rapidly.
- No treatment is necessary, since the disease appears to be self-limiting and presents few complications.

Measles (Rubeola)

- Measles is an acute, contagious, dermatropic viral infection, primarily affecting children and occurring many times in epidemic form.
- Spread of the disease occurs by direct contact with an affected person or by droplet infection, the portal of entry being the respiratory tract.
- The disease has an incubation period of 8 to 10 days.
- Characterized by the onset of fever, malaise, cough, conjunctivitis, photophobia and lacrimation. Eruptive lesions are seen on the skin and oral mucosa that appear as tiny red macules or papules which enlarge and coalesce to form blotchy, discolored, irregular lesions which blanch upon pressure. They gradually fade away in four to five days with a fine desquamation.
- The oral lesions frequently occur two to three days before the cutaneous rash, and are pathognomonic of this disease.
- The intraoral lesions are called as Koplik's spots which is a characteristic feature of measles, usually occurring on the buccal mucosa. They are small, irregularly shaped flecks which appear as bluish, white specks surrounded by a bright red margin.

Chickenpox (Varicella)

- Chickenpox is an acute viral disease, usually occurring in children and most common in the winter and spring months.
- It is caused by herpes-varicella-zoster virus.
- The incubation period is approximately two weeks.
- The mode of transmission is by airborne droplets or direct contact with infected lesions, with the probable portal of entry being the respiratory tract.
- The disease is characterized by the prodromal occurrence of headache, nasopharyngitis and anorexia, followed by maculopapular or vesicular eruptions of the skin and low-grade fever. These eruptions usually begin on the trunk and spread to involve the face and extremities.

- Small blister-like lesions occasionally involve the oral mucosa, chiefly the buccal mucosa, tongue, gingiva and palate, as well as the mucosa of the pharynx.
- The lesion is a slightly raised vesicle with a surrounding erythema, that ruptures soon after formation to form small eroded ulcers with a red margin.
- Management is symptomatic by application of topical anesthetic gel and mouth rinses.

Herpes Zoster (Shingles)

- Herpes zoster is an acute viral infectious disease caused by herpes-varicella-zoster virus.
- It is an extremely painful disease characterized by inflammation of dorsal root ganglia or extra-medullary cranial nerve ganglia, associated with vesicular eruptions of the skin or mucous membranes in areas supplied by the affected sensory nerves.
- It is now believed that a primary infection by the V-Z virus, results clinically in chickenpox, while a recurrent infection results clinically in herpes zoster.
- Initially, the adult patient exhibits fever, a general malaise and pain and tenderness along the course of the involved sensory nerves and is usually unilaterally. Within a few days the patient has a linear papular or vesicular eruption of the skin or mucosa supplied by the affected nerve.
- The triggering factors initiating the onset of an attack of herpes zoster are varied and may include trauma, development of malignancy or tumor involvement of dorsal root ganglia, local X-ray radiation or immuno-suppressive therapy.
- Herpes zoster may involve the face by infection of the trigeminal nerve.
- The newer anti-viral drugs are now under intensive clinical testing for potential effectiveness in the treatment of herpes zoster.

Mumps (Epidemic Parotitis)

- Mumps is an acute, contagious, viral infectious disease characterized chiefly by unilateral or bilateral swelling of the salivary glands, usually the parotid.
- Mumps has an incubation period of two to three weeks.
- The disease is usually preceded by the onset of headache, chills, moderate fever, vomiting and pain below the ears.
- These symptoms are followed by a firm, rubbery or elastic swelling of the salivary glands, frequently elevating the ear, which lasts for about one week.
- Management includes adequate rest and fluid intake.

AIDS—Acquired Immunodeficiency Syndrome

- Caused by human immunodeficiency virus (HIV)
- About 1/3rd to half the number of HIV positive babies are born to mothers who are infected with HIV.
- Virus transmission may occur to the fetus in pregnancy as early as the first trimester but infection is more common perinatally.
- Many of the infected children may not survive for a year.
- Children may also get the infection from blood transfusion or blood products.
- Children develop humoral immunodeficiency early, leading to recurrent bacterial infection.
- In children abnormal B cell function is seen prior to T cell abnormality. T4 helper cells that play a vital role in the induction and evolution of a normal immune response is destroyed by direct or indirect cytopathic mechanisms of HIV. They also interfere in the production of interferons. All these lead to greater susceptibility to opportunistic infections, increased propensity towards malignancy, thrombocytopenia, etc.
- Direct effect of the virus on CNS may lead to progressive encephalopathy with cognitive, behavioral and motor deficits.
- Failure to thrive, chronic diarrhea, lymphadenopathy, tuberculosis and opportunistic bacterial infections are common manifestations.
- Lymphocytic interstitial pneumonia is most commonly seen in children, while kaposis sarcoma, toxoplasmosis and cryptocococci are less common.
- The typical findings in children include pulmonary lymphoid hyperplasia, salivary gland enlargement, pyogenic bacterial infection, developmental delay, dysmorphic craniofacial features.
- Oral features include oral candidiasis, herpes simplex virus infection, recurrent apthous ulcerations, rapidly progressive periodontal disease, parotitis, oral hairy leukoplakia, petechiae, linear gingival erythema, cervical lymphadenopathy.
- Specific tests for HIV infection are antigen detection, virus isolation, polymerase chain reaction, antibody detection tests like ELISA and western blot.
- Symptomatic antiviral drugs—interferons, acyclovir, etc.

FUNGAL INFECTIONS

Acute Pseudomembranous Candidiasis (Thrush)

- Prone to occur in the debilitated or the chronically ill or in infants

- The oral lesions are characterized by the appearance of soft, white, slightly elevated plaques most frequently occurring on the buccal mucosa and tongue, but also seen on the palate, gingiva and floor of the mouth.
- The white plaque can usually be wiped away with gauze, leaving either a relatively normal appearing mucosa or an erythematous area.
- Treatment includes application of antifungal medicines such as nystatin, amphotericin B, etc.

OTHERS

Pre-eruptive "Caries"

(Pre-eruptive coronal resorption or pre-eruptive intracoronal radiolucency)

- Etiology is unknown
- These are defects on the crowns of developing permanent teeth that are evident radiographically, without infection of the primary tooth or the surrounding area.
- Such a lesion does resemble caries when it is observed clinically, and the destructive nature of the lesion progresses if it is not restored.
- As soon as the lesion is reasonably accessible, the tooth should be uncovered by removal of the overlying primary tooth or by surgical exposure. The caries like dentin is then excavated, and the tooth is restored with amalgam or a durable temporary restorative material. In some cases the lesion may be so extensive that indirect pulp therapy is justified.

Intrinsic Stains

- The primary teeth occasionally have unusual pigmentation. Factors causing these include blood borne pigment, blood decomposition within the pulp and drugs. Other causes of intrinsic staining are:
  1. Erythroblastosis fetalis
  2. Porphyria
  3. Cystic fibrosis
  4. Tetracycline therapy.

Discoloration in Erythroblastosis Fetalis

- Erythroblastosis fetalis results from the transplacental passage of maternal antibody active against red blood cell antigens of the infant, leading to an increased rate of red blood cell destruction.
- It is a significant cause of anemia and jaundice in newborn infants despite the development of a method of prevention by Rh antigens.
- An infant from an Rh-negative mother's first pregnancy rarely contracts this hemolytic disease.

- If an infant has had severe, persistent jaundice during the neonatal period, the primary teeth may have a characteristic blue-green color, though in a few instances brown teeth have been observed. The color of the pigmented tooth is gradually reduced. The fading in color is particularly noticeable in the anterior teeth.

Discoloration in Porphyria

- It is a rare genetic disturbance of porphyria metabolism occurring in humans and animals.
- Characterized by the excessive production of pigments in the body.
- The condition is often observed at birth, or it may develop during infancy.
- Children with congenital porphyria have red colored urine, are hypersensitive to light and develop blisters on their hands and face.
- Their teeth are purplish brown as a result of the deposition of porphyrin in the developing structures.
- In congenital porphyria the permanent teeth also show evidence of intrinsic staining.

Discoloration in Cystic Fibrosis

- A high percentage of children with cystic fibrosis have teeth that are dark in color, ranging from yellowish gray to dark brown.
- Patients afflicted with cystic fibrosis are usually subjected to large amounts of tetracyclines during childhood which may also contribute for the color change seen.

Discoloration in Tetracycline Therapy

- Children who have received tetracycline therapy during the period of calcification of the primary or permanent teeth show a degree of pigmentation of the crowns of the teeth.
- Tetracyclines chelate calcium salts and the drug is incorporated into bones and teeth during calcification and will be deposited in the dentin and to a lesser extent in the enamel of teeth that are calcifying during the time the drug is administered.
- The crowns of affected teeth are discolored, ranging from yellow to brown and from gray to black.
- The tooth fluoresce under ultraviolet light
- The exposure of the teeth to light results in slow oxidation, with a change in color of the pigment from yellow to brown.
- Because tetracyclines can be transferred through the placenta, the crowns of the primary teeth may also show noticeable discoloration if tetracyclines are administered during pregnancy.

- The critical period for tetracycline-related discoloration in the primary dentition is 4 months *in utero* to 3 months post partum for maxillary and mandibular incisors and 5 months *in utero* to 9 months postpartum for maxillary and mandibular canines.
- The sensitive period for tetracycline-induced discoloration in the permanent maxillary and mandibular incisors and canines is 3 to 5 months post partum to about the seventh year of the child's life. The maxillary lateral incisors are an exception because they begin to calcify at 10 to 12 months postpartum.
- Teeth with tetracycline pigmentation occasionally show evidence of enamel hypoplasia. This is true for both the primary and the permanent teeth.

Mucocele

- Caused due to traumatic severance or obstruction of salivary duct causing the pooling of mucus in the tissue.
- Seen more commonly on the lips
- Appears as raised circumscribed vesicle, several millimeters to a centimeter or more in diameter (Fig. 16.18).
- They are cyst like lesion. When present in the floor of the mouth it is termed as ranula.
- Treatment includes excision along with the involved minor salivary gland.

Ranula

- It is a form of mucocele occurring specifically in the floor of the mouth in association with the ducts of the submandibular or sublingual salivary glands.
- It is painless and slowly enlarging.

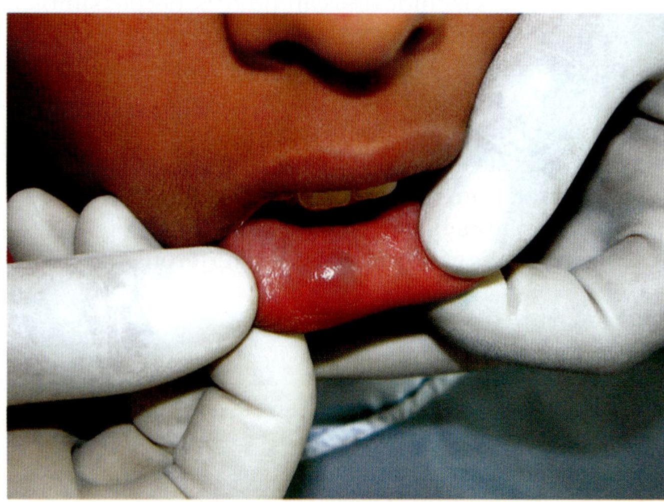

Fig. 16.18: Mucocele on the lower lip

- Incision is the treatment of choice as the lesion is deep seated.

Recurrent Aphthous Stomatitis

- It can be triggered due to any stress, gastrointestinal disturbance, nutritional deficiency, hormonal imbalance, infection, allergy, etc.
- Of the 3 types of apthous, minor apthae are common, others being aphthous major and herpetiform.
- Prodromal phase of paraesthesia at the site of ulceration is observed. The ulcers appear in crops of two or three and are less than 10 mm in diameter.
- Ulcers are painful and are discrete or confluent.
- Persists for about 12 days and heals with no scar formation.
- Treatment is symptomatic. Chlorhexidine or nystatin or tetracycline can be prescribed if they are infected.

FURTHER READING

1. Ahuja V, Shin RH, Mudgil A, Nanda V, Schoor R. Papillon-Lefevre syndrome: a successful outcome. J Periodontol 2005;76(11):1996-2001.
2. Bolan M, Gerent Petry Nunes AC, de Carvalho Rocha MJ, De Luca Canto G.: Talon cusp: report of a case. Quintessence Int 2006;37(7):509-14.
3. Crawford NL, North S, Davidson LE. Double permanent incisor teeth: management of three cases. Dent Update 2006;33(10):608-10.
4. Danesh G, Schrijnemakers T, Lippold C, Schafer E. A fused maxillary central incisor with dens evaginatus as a talon cusp. Angle Orthod 2007;77(1):176-80.
5. Glavina D, Skrinjaric T. Labial talon cusp on maxillary central incisors: a rare developmental dental anomaly. Coll Antropol 2005;29(1):227-31.
6. Hong HH, Tsai AI, Liang CH, Kuo SB, Chen CC, Tsai TP, Lu CF. Preserving pulpal health of a geminated maxillary lateral incisor through multidisciplinary care. Int Endod J 2006;39(9):730-7.
7. Kokich VG, Kokich VO. Congenitally missing mandibular second premolars: clinical options. Am J Orthod Dentofacial Orthop 2006;130(4):437-44.
8. Lo Muzio L, Bucci P, Carile F, Riccitiello F, Scotti C, Coccia E, Rappelli G. Prosthetic rehabilitation of a child affected from anhydrotic ectodermal dysplasia: a case report. J Contemp Dent Pract 2005;6(3):120-6.
9. Maroto M, Barberia E, Arenas M, Lucavechi T. Displacement and pulpal involvement of a maxillary incisor associated with a talon cusp: report of a case. Dent Traumatol 2006;22(3):160-4.
10. Prager TM, Finke C, Miethke RR.: Dental findings in patients with ectodermal dysplasia. J Orofac Orthop 2006;67(5):347-55.
11. Prakash R, Vishnu C, Suma B, Velmurugan N, Kandaswamy D. Endodontic management of taurodontic teeth. Indian J Dent Res 2005;16(4):177-81.
12. Rao A, Arathi R. Taurodontism of deciduous and permanent molars: report of two cases. J Indian Soc Pedod Prev Dent 2006;24(1):42-4.
13. Rodekirchen H, Jung M, Ansari F. Dens invaginatus type II: case report with 2-year radiographic follow-up. Oral Surg Oral Med Oral Pathol Oral Radiol Endod 2006;102(4):e121-5. Epub 2006 Jul 27.
14. Sakai VT, Oliveira TM, Pessan JP, Santos CF, Machado MA. Alternative oral rehabilitation of children with hypodontia and conical tooth shape: a clinical report. Quintessence Int 2006;37(9):725-30.
15. Schulman GS, Redford-Badwal D, Poole A, Mathieu G, Burleson J, Dauser D. Taurodontism and learning disabilities in patients with Klinefelter syndrome. Pediatr Dent 2005;27(5):389-94.
16. Shenoy SS, Dinkar AD. Pyogenic granuloma associated with bone loss in an eight year old child: A case report. J Indian Soc Pedod Prev Dent 2006;24(4):201-3.

QUESTIONS

1. What are the disorders of the tongue?
2. Write short notes on Fordyce's granules.
3. Disorders affecting the shape of the teeth.
4. Write the problems associated with microdontia, macrodontia and dilaceration.
5. Write short notes on ectodermal dysplasia.
6. Enumerate the disorders affecting the structure of the teeth and write in detail about enamel hypoplasia.
7. Explain the difference between a primordial and dentigerous cyst.
8. Dental lamina cyst of the newborn
9. What are the gingival cyst of the newborn? Explain each of them.
10. Enumerate the common bacterial infections seen in children and explain any two of them.
11. Give the clinical features and management of herpes simplex virus type I infection.
12. Acquired immunodeficiency syndrome in children.
13. Explain the etiology, clinical features and management of acute pseudomembranous candidiasis.
14. What is preeruptive "caries"?
15. Write in detail about intrinsic stains.

Infection Control

INTRODUCTION

The dental environment is associated with a significant risk of exposure to various microorganisms. These infectious agents may be present in blood or saliva and form the source of spread of infection.

ROUTES OF TRANSMISSION OF INFECTION[1-2]

Infections may be transmitted in the dental operatory through several routes such as:

1. Direct contact with blood, oral fluids, or other secretions.
2. Indirect contact with contaminated instruments, operatory equipment, or environmental surfaces.
3. Contact with airborne contaminants present in either droplet spatter or aerosols of oral and respiratory fluids.

GENERAL GUIDELINES FOR ALL DENTAL OFFICE STAFF[3-7]

1. Provide Hepatitis B immunization to employees without charge within 10 days of employment.
2. Require that universal precautions be observed to prevent contact with blood and other potentially infectious material. Saliva is considered to be a blood-contaminated body fluid in relation to dental treatments.
3. Implement engineering controls to reduce production of contaminated spatter, mists and aerosols.
4. Implement work practice control precautions to minimize splashing, spatter or contact of bare hands with contaminated surfaces.
5. Provide facilities and instructions for washing hands after removing gloves and for washing skin immediately or as soon as feasible, after contact with blood or potentially infectious materials.
6. Prescribe safe handling of needles and other sharp items.
7. Prescribe disposable or single-use needles. Wires, carpules and sharp items should be disposed as close to the place of use as possible, as soon as feasible, in hard walled, leak proof containers that are closable. Containers must be red or bear a biohazard label. Extracted teeth must be discarded in the same containers.

8. Contaminated reusable sharp instruments must not be stored or processed in a manner that requires employees to reach hands into containers to retrieve them.

9. Prohibit eating, drinking, handling contact lenses, etc. in contaminated environments. Ban storage of food and drinks in refrigerators or other spaces where blood or infectious materials are stored.

10. Place blood and contaminated specimen to be shipped, transported or stored in suitable closed containers that prevent leakage.

11. At no cost to employees, provide them with necessary personal protective equipment (PPE) and clear directions for use of appropriate universal barrier protection in treating all patients (PPE includes gloves, gowns, etc.).

12. Ensure that employees correctly use and discard PPE or properly prepare it for reuse.

13. As soon as feasible after treatments, attend to housekeeping requirements including floors, sinks, etc. that are subject to contamination.

14. Provide a written schedule for cleaning.

15. Contaminated equipment that requires service must first be decontaminated or a biohazard label must be used to indicate contaminated parts.

16. Place reusable contaminated sharp instruments into a basket in a hard-walled container for transportation to the clean-up area. Personnel must not reach hands into containers of contaminated sharps.

17. Provide laundering of protective garments used for universal precautions at no cost to employees.

BARRIER PRECAUTIONS[8-10]

- During dental procedures, dental health-care workers must wear correct sized gloves when they put their hands into any patient's mouth, and change these gloves between patients (Figs 17.1A and B). They should also wear gloves when they touch instruments, equipment, or surfaces that may be contaminated with blood or saliva.

- Hands must be washed and regloved before performing procedures on another patient. Repeated use of a single pair of gloves or washing of gloves between patients is not recommended, since such practice is likely to produce defects in the glove material, which will diminish its value as an effective barrier.

- Surgical masks and protective eyewear or chin-length plastic face shields must be worn when splashing or spattering of blood, saliva, or oral secretions is likely, as is common during dental procedures.

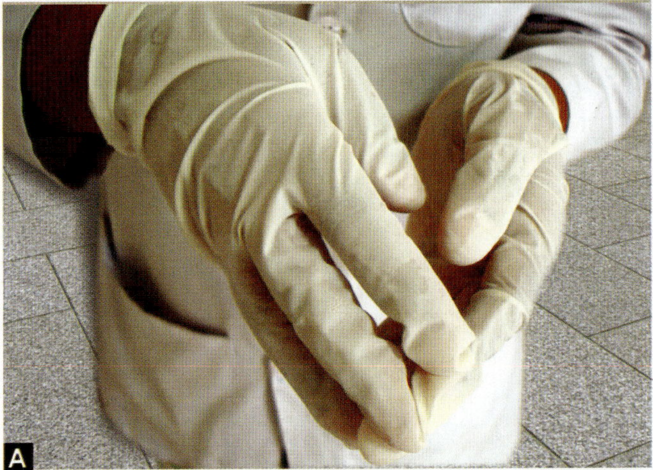
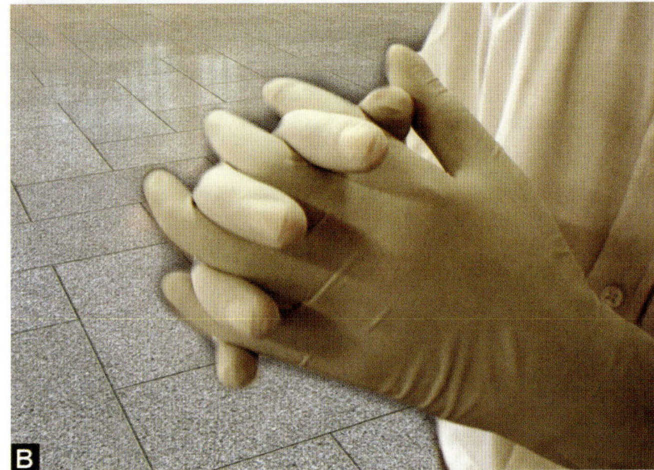

Figs 17.1A and B: (A) Loose fit gloves should not be used; (B) Gloves should be comfortable when worn with good fit

- Reusable or disposable gowns, laboratory coats, or uniforms must be worn when clothing is likely to be soiled with blood, saliva, or oral secretions. If reusable gowns are worn, they should be washed, using a normal laundry cycle. Gowns should be changed at least daily or when visibly soiled with blood.

- Disposable waterproof coverings such as impervious-backed paper, aluminum foil, or clear plastic wrap may be used to wrap hard-to-clean surfaces such as light handles or X-ray unit heads, etc. (Figs 17.2A and B). These surfaces may be contaminated by blood or saliva and are difficult or impossible to clean and disinfect. To replace the covering between patients, the coverings should be removed with gloved hands and discarded. Then, after removing the soiled gloves, the coverings can be replaced with clean material.

- Patient's case sheets, pen, desk top, etc. should not be touched with gloved hands (Fig. 17.3). Gloves should

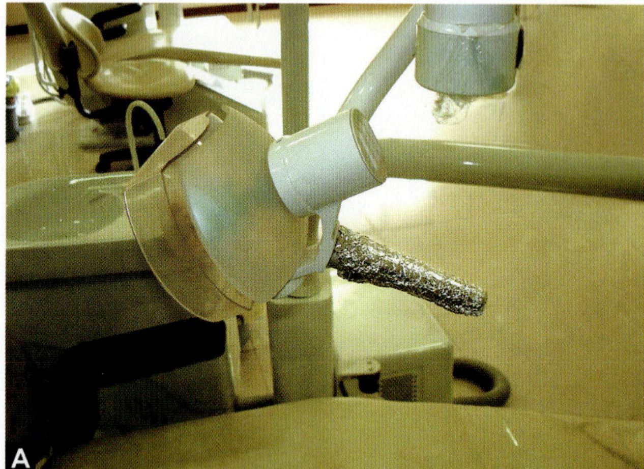

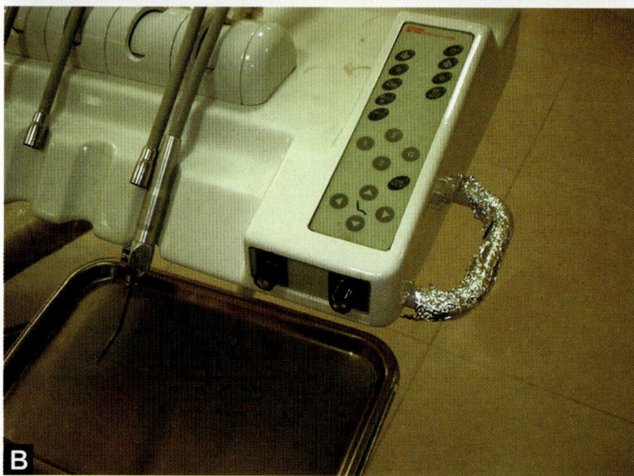

Figs 17.2A and B: Areas likely to be touched regularly during treatment such as: (A) Light handle, or; (B) Tray handle should be wrapped with aluminum foil

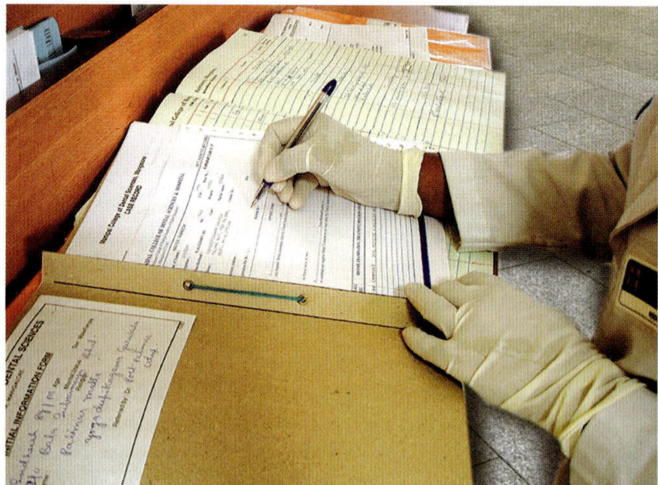

Fig. 17.3: Care should be taken NOT to touch the case sheet, pen, desk or any other areas wearing gloves

be removed before handling unsterile material. Hands should be rewashed before regloving the hands.

HANDWASHING AND CARE OF HANDS[11-13]

The hands must be washed before and after treating each patient (i.e., before glove placement and after glove removal) and after barehanded touching of inanimate objects likely to be contaminated by blood, saliva, or respiratory secretions. All the jewellery in the hand including watches should be removed (Figs 17.4A and B). The hands should be scrubbed using liquid soap and washed under tap water. The hands are then dried completely. Hands should be washed after removal of gloves because gloves may become perforated during use and may become contaminated through contact with patient material. Soap and water will remove transient microorganisms acquired directly or indirectly from patient contact. Therefore, for many routine dental procedures, such as examinations and nonsurgical techniques, handwashing with plain soap is adequate. For surgical procedures, an antimicrobial surgical handscrub should be used.

When gloves are torn, cut, or punctured, they should be removed as soon as patient safety permits. Then the hands should be thoroughly washed and regloved to complete the dental procedure. Operators who have exudative lesions or weeping dermatitis, particularly on the hands, should refrain from all direct patient care and from handling dental patient-care equipment until the condition resolves.

USE AND CARE OF SHARP INSTRUMENTS AND NEEDLES[13]

- Sharp items (e.g. needles, scalpel blades, wires) contaminated with patient blood and saliva should be considered as potentially infective and handled with care to prevent injuries.
- Used needles should not be manipulated utilizing both hands, or any other technique that involves directing the point of a needle toward any part of the body. Either a one-handed "scoop" technique (Figs 17.5A and B) or a mechanical device designed for holding the needle sheath should be employed.
- Used disposable syringes and needles, scalpel blades, and other sharp items should be placed in appropriate puncture-resistant containers located as close as is practical to the area in which the items were used.
- Bending or breaking of needles before disposal requires unnecessary manipulation and thus is not recommended.

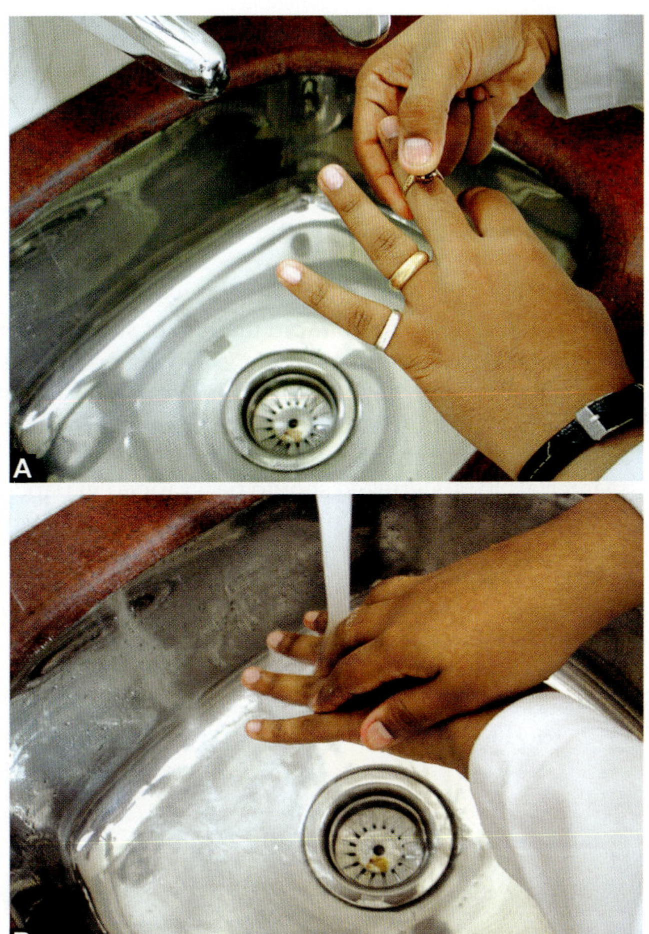

Figs 17.4A and B: Handwash: (A) All jewellery including watch should be removed first; (B) Hands should be washed with soap and water and then dried before wearing the gloves

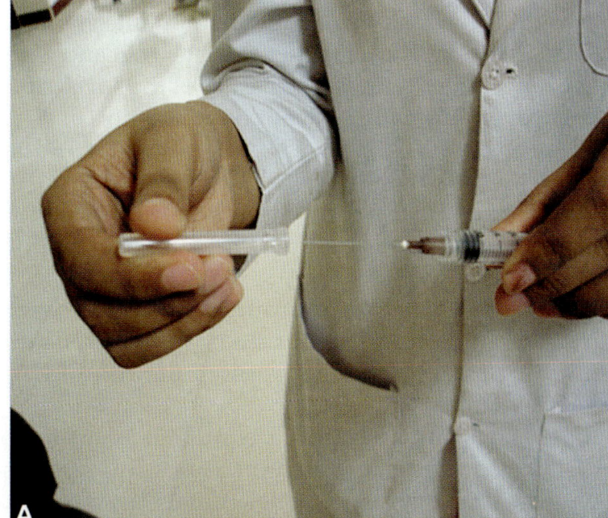

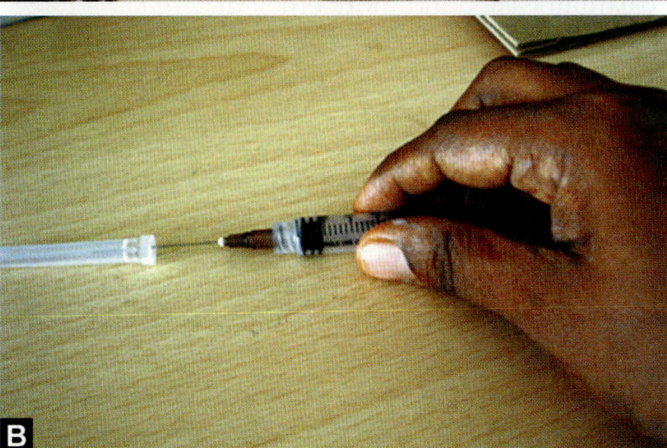

Figs 17.5A and B: Safety measures to be taken while handling the needle: (A) Wrong and unsafe method to recap the needle as there is high chance of getting pricked; (B) The correct method of placing the syringe back into the cap using 'One Hand Scoop technique'

- Before attempting to remove needles from nondisposable aspirating syringes, one should recap them to prevent injuries. For procedures involving multiple injections with a single needle, the unsheathed needle should be placed in a location where it will not become contaminated or contribute to unintentional needlesticks between injections.

STERILIZATION OR DISINFECTION OF INSTRUMENTS[14]

As with other medical and surgical instruments, dental instruments are classified into three categories, such as critical, semicritical, or noncritical, depending on their risk of transmitting infection and the need to sterilize them between uses.

Each dental practice should classify all instruments as follows:

- Critical: Surgical and other instruments used to penetrate soft tissue or bone is classified as critical and should be sterilized after each use. These devices include forceps, scalpels, bone chisels, scalers and burs.
- Semi-critical: Instruments such as mirrors and amalgam condensers that do not penetrate soft tissues or bone but contact oral tissues are classified as semi-critical. These devices should be sterilized after each use. If, however, sterilization is not feasible because the instrument will be damaged by heat, the instrument should receive, at a minimum, high-level disinfection.
- Non critical: Instruments or medical devices such as external components of X-ray heads that come into contact only with intact skin are classified as noncritical. Because these noncritical surfaces have a relatively low risk of transmitting infection, they may

be reprocessed between patients with intermediate-level or low-level disinfection or detergent and water washing, depending on the nature of the surface and the degree and nature of the contamination.

Pre-sterilization Cleaning

1. Before sterilization or high-level disinfection, instruments should be cleaned thoroughly to remove debris.
2. Persons involved in cleaning and reprocessing instruments should wear heavy-duty (reusable utility) gloves (Fig. 17.6) to lessen the risk of hand injuries.
3. Placing instruments into a container of water or disinfectant/detergent as soon as possible after use will prevent drying of patient material and make cleaning easier and more efficient.
4. Cleaning may be accomplished by thorough scrubbing with soap and water or a detergent solution, or with a mechanical device (e.g. an ultrasonic cleaner). The use of covered ultrasonic cleaners, when possible, is recommended to increase efficiency of cleaning and to reduce handling of sharp instruments.

Sterilization Methods

All critical and semi-critical dental instruments that are heat stable should be autoclaved. Dry heat, or chemical vapor can also be used following the instructions of the manufacturers of the instruments and the sterilizers. Critical and semi-critical instruments that will not be used immediately should be packaged before sterilization.

The three most commonly used methods of sterilization in dentistry are:

- The steam autoclave
- The unsaturated chemical vapor sterilizer (chemiclave)
- Dry heat ovens
  Other methods are:
a. Exposure to ethylene oxide gas
b. Boiling water
c. Ionizing radiation

Autoclave (Steam under Pressure)

It is an efficient, reliable and rapid method of sterilization except for oils, greases and powders. All living organisms are rapidly destroyed at 121°C temperature and 15 lbs pressure for 15 minutes. The major problems are excess moisture, air entrapment and severe wetting.

Materials to be sterilized should be wrapped in paper, muslin or steam permeable plastic. To check the efficiency of sterilization, colored stripped (Figs 17.7A and B) or spore containing carpules (Figs 17.8A and B) with known numbers of bacillus stearothermophilus are available that should be placed in the deepest layer of the sterilizer load.

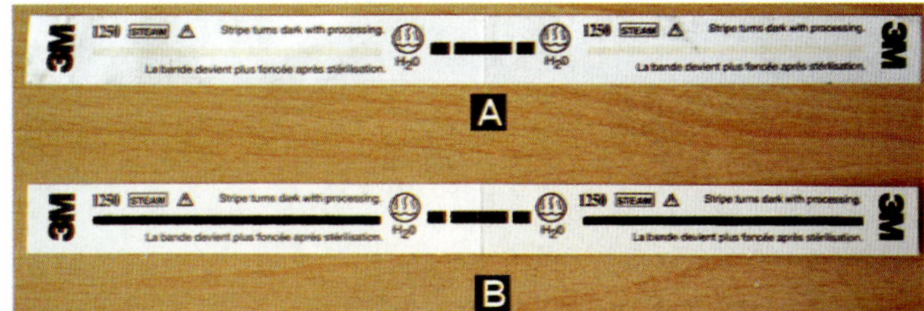

Figs 17.7A and B: Colored strips used for detecting the efficiency of sterilization: (A) Before the sterilization; (B) After the sterilization, note the change in the color to black

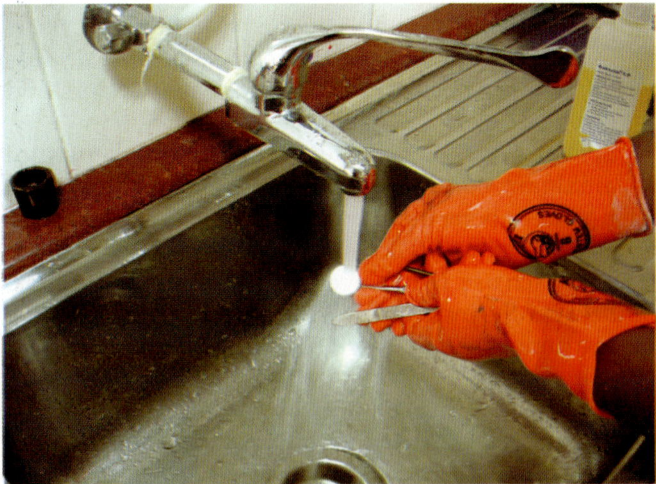

Fig. 17.6: Utility gloves should be worn while cleaning and washing the instruments

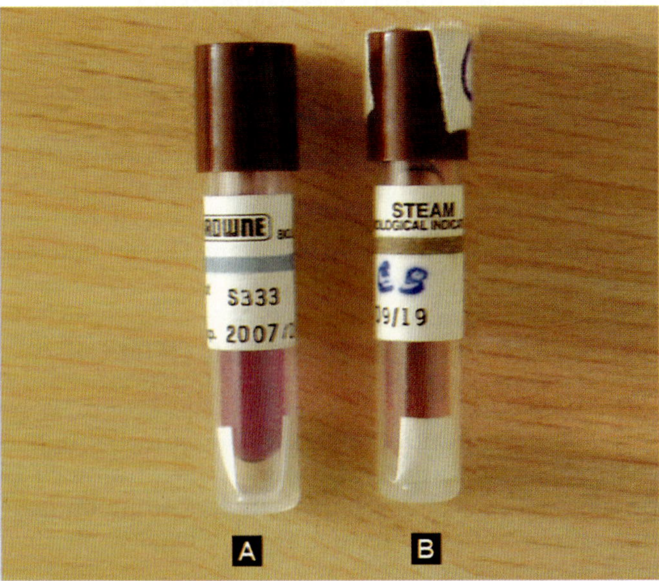

Figs 17.8A and B: Spore containing carpules: (A) Fresh carpules; (B) Used carpules which will be tested for biologic growth

After sterilization, the strips are observed for any color change. Change in the color to dark brown or black (as per the manufacturer) indicates adequate sterilization. The spore containing carpules are incubated and the presence of growth is checked. Absence of growth proves sterilization. The strips can be placed with every load of instruments and spore carpules can be placed once in a week or once in a month.

Unsaturated Chemical Vapor Sterilizer

This sterilizer uses a special chemical solution containing formaldehyde and alcohol. The major advantage is the greatly reduced corrosion of metal items. Closed containers cannot be used, as the chemical vapors must reach the surface of the items being processed. Specified wrapping material should be used.

Dry Heat Sterilizer

These sterilizers use hot air to kill microorganisms and do not cause corrosion. The standard dry heat-sterilizing oven operates at an air temperature of about 320°F for exposure times of 60 to 120 minutes. Closed containers can be used.

A second type of dry heat sterilizer (rapid heat transfer) utilizes a controlled internal air flow system. The instruments warm faster as the 375°F air is rapidly circulated within the chamber. Sterilization time is 6 minutes for unwrapped instruments and 12 minutes for wrapped instruments.

Chemical Sterilization of Instruments

"Sterilant/disinfectant" chemicals are used to attain high-level disinfection of heat-sensitive semi-critical medical and dental instruments. The product manufacturers' directions regarding appropriate concentration and exposure time should be followed closely. Liquid chemical agents that are less potent than the "sterilant/disinfectant" category are not appropriate for reprocessing critical or semi-critical dental instruments.

Post-sterilization Procedures

Post-sterilization procedures involve drying, cooling, storage and distribution. Careful handling, storage and distribution of the sterilized instrument packs or trays reduce the chances for recontamination until the instruments are reused.

If instruments are to be stored after sterilization, they should be wrapped or bagged before sterilizing, using a suitable wrap material such as muslin, clear pouches or paper as recommended by the manufacturer of the sterilizer. The wrap or bag should be sealed with appropriate tape. Pins, staples or paper clips should not be used, as these make holes in the wrap that permit entry of microorganisms. Instruments that are to be used should be kept in a sterilized tray with a lid (Fig. 17.9).

CLEANING AND DISINFECTION OF DENTAL UNIT AND ENVIRONMENTAL SURFACES

After treatment of each patient and at the completion of daily work activities, countertops and dental unit surfaces that may have become contaminated with patient material should be cleaned with disposable toweling, using an appropriate cleaning agent and water as necessary. Surfaces then should be disinfected with a suitable chemical germicide.

These disinfectants include phenolics, iodophors, and chlorine-containing compounds, quaternary ammonium compounds and fresh solution of sodium hypochlorite (household bleach) prepared daily is an inexpensive and effective intermediate-level germicide.

DISINFECTION AND THE DENTAL LABORATORY

Laboratory materials and other items that have been used in the mouth (e.g. impressions, bite registrations, fixed and removable prostheses, orthodontic appliances) should be cleaned and disinfected before being manipulated in the laboratory. These items also should be cleaned and disinfected after being manipulated in the dental laboratory and before placement in the patient's mouth.

CARE OF HANDPIECES

Routine between patient use of a heating process capable of sterilization (i.e. autoclaving, dry heat, or heat/chemical vapor) is recommended for all high-speed dental hand pieces, low-speed hand piece components

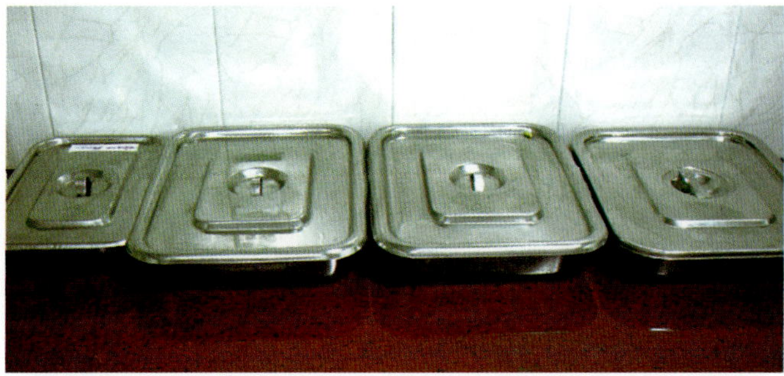

Fig. 17.9: Instruments should be kept closed ready to be used

used intraorally. Manufacturers' instructions for cleaning, lubrication, and sterilization procedures should be followed closely to ensure both the effectiveness of the sterilization process and the longevity of these instruments.

SINGLE-USE DISPOSABLE INSTRUMENTS

Single-use disposable instruments (e.g. prophylaxis cups and brushes; tips for high-speed air evacuators, saliva ejectors, and air/water syringes) should be used for one patient only and discarded appropriately. These items are neither designed nor intended to be cleaned, disinfected, or sterilized for reuse.

DISPOSAL AND TREATMENT OF HEALTH CARE WASTE MATERIALS[8,15-21]

The wastes are collected separately in color coded bags [containing the symbol of biohazard (Fig. 17.10)] depending on the method of treatment to be used for disposal. Segregation is done as follows:

Red bags: Wastes that are contaminated and cannot be incinerated. It includes gloves, suction tips and similar items.
Yellow bags: Wastes that are contaminated but can be incinerated. It includes material like cotton and gauze.
Blue plastic container: Wastes such as blade or needles.
Black bags: Wastes that are uncontaminated such as empty bottles, paper covers, etc.

Treatment and disposal technologies for health-care waste are:

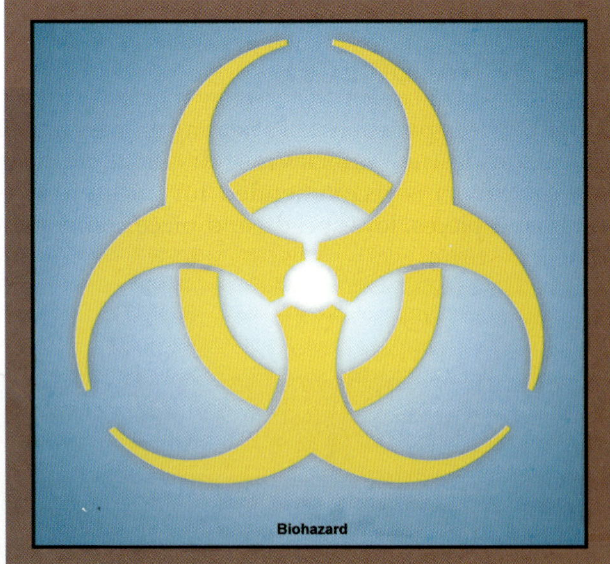

Fig. 17.10: Symbol that denotes 'Biohazard'

1. Incineration
   - Pyrolytic
   - Single chamber
   - Rotary kiln
2. Chemical disinfection
3. Wet thermal treatment
4. Microwave irradiation
5. Encapsulation
6. Safe burying
7. Inertization.

Incinerators

Incineration is a high temperature dry oxidation process that reduces organic and combustible waste to inorganic, incombustible matter and results in a very significant reduction of waste volume and weight.

This process is usually used to treat wastes that cannot be recycled, reused or disposed off in a landfill site.

Types of Incinerators

- Double-chamber pyrolytic incinerators
- Single-chamber furnaces with static grate
- Rotary kilns.

Pyrolytic Incinerators

This is the most reliable and commonly used process for health-care waste. They are also called controlled air incineration or double-chamber incineration.

The pyrolytic incinerators comprise:
- A pyrolytic chamber
- A post-combustion chamber.

In the pyrolytic chamber, the waste is thermally decomposed through an oxygen deficient medium temperature combustion process [800 to 900°C] producing solid ashes and gases. The pyrolytic chamber includes a fuel burner, used to start the process. The waste is loaded in suitable waste bags or containers. The gases produced in this way are burned at high temperature [90 to 1200°C] by a fuel burner in the post-combustion chamber, using an excess of air to minimize smoke and odors.

Drawbacks

- Relatively expensive equipment
- Expensive to operate and maintain
- Well-trained personnel are required.

Incinerators must be located at a minimum distance of 500 meters from any human settlement.

Single-chamber Incinerator

This can be used for health-care waste if a pyrolytic incinerator cannot be afforded. This type of incinerator treats waste in batches. Loading and de-ashing operations are performed manually. The combustion is initiated by addition of fuel and should then continue unaided.

Drawbacks

- Chemical and pharmaceutical residues will persist if temperatures do not exceed 200°C.
- The process will cause emission of black smoke, fly ash and potentially toxic gases.
- Exhaust gas cleaning is not practicable—can cause air pollution.

Rotary Kiln

A rotary kiln comprises a rotating oven and a post-combustion chamber. The kiln rotates 2 to 5 times per minute and is charged with waste at the top. Ashes are evacuated at the bottom end of the kiln. The gases produced in the kiln are heated to high temperatures to burn off gaseous organic compounds in the post-combustion chamber and typically have a residence time of 2 seconds.

Rotary kilns can be used for

- Infectious waste (including sharps) and pathological waste
- All chemical and pharmaceutical wastes including cytotoxic waste.

Disadvantages of rotary kilns

- Well-trained personnel are required.
- Equipment and operation costs are high.
- Energy consumption is high.
- Highly corrosive waste and by-products damage the refractory lining of the kiln.

Chemical Disinfection

In this method, chemicals are added to waste to kill or inactivate the pathogens. This method is most suitable for treating liquid waste such as blood, urine, stools or hospital sewage.

The effectiveness of disinfection is estimated from the survival rates of indicator organisms in standard microbiological tests.

Types of Chemical Disinfectants

1. Formaldehyde: It has an inactivating effect against all microorganisms including bacteria, viruses and bacterial spores [contact time: 45 minutes]
2. Ethylene oxide: It inactivates all microorganisms including bacteria, viruses and spores. It can also disinfect solid wastes at temperatures of 37 to 55°C at 60 to 80% humidity for 4 to 12 hours.
   The use of ethylene oxide is not recommended because of significant health hazards.
3. Glutaraldehyde: It is active against both bacteria and parasite eggs. It should be used as 2% aqueous solution with acetate buffer.
   Contact time: 5 minutes for disinfection of medical equipment and 10 hours to kill spores.
   Glutaraldehyde waste should never be discharged in sewers. It may be neutralized through careful addition of ammonia or sodium bisulfite. It may also be incinerated, after mixing with a flammable solvent.
4. Sodium hypochlorite: It is active against most bacteria, viruses and spores. Not effective for disinfection of liquids with high organic content such as blood or stools.
5. Chlorine dioxide: It is active against most bacteria, viruses and spores.

Wet Thermal Treatment

Wet thermal treatment or steam disinfection is based on exposure of shredded infectious waste to high-temperature, high-pressure steam. It inactivates most types of microorganisms.

This process requires that waste be shredded before treatment to increase disinfection efficiency. The process is inappropriate for the treatment of anatomical waste and animal carcasses.

Disadvantages

a. The shredder is liable to mechanical failure and breakdown.
b. The efficiency of disinfection is very sensitive to the operational conditions.

Advantages

a. Relatively low investment and operating costs.
b. The low environmental impact.

Microwave Irradiation

Most microorganisms are destroyed by the action of microwaves of a frequency of about 2450 MHz. Although this process is becoming increasingly popular, relatively high costs coupled with potential operation and maintenance problems mean that it is not yet recommended for use in developing countries.

Encapsulation

This procedure involves filling containers, made of high density polyethylene or metal drums, with waste. These containers are then filled up with a medium of immobilizing material such as plastic foam, cement mortar or clay. After the medium has dried, the containers are sealed and disposed of in landfill sites. It is a simple, low-cost and safe method but not recommended for non-sharp infectious waste.

Safe Burying

Safe burial of waste may be used when this is the only viable option available especially in establishments which use minimal programs for health care waste management.

Certain basic rules that should be followed are:

a. Access to the disposal site should be restricted to authorized personnel only.
b. The burial site should be lined with a material of low permeability like clay.
c. Only hazardous health-care waste should be buried, so as to conserve space.
d. Large quantities of chemical waste should not be buried at one time to avoid environmental pollution.
e. The burial site should be covered with a layer of earth to prevent health hazards.

Inertization

This process involves mixing waste with cement and other substances before disposal in order to minimize the risk of toxic substances contained in the waste migrating into surface water or ground water. It is especially suitable for pharmaceuticals and for incineration ashes with a high metal content. This is a relatively inexpensive method of waste disposal but it is not applicable to infectious waste.

REFERENCES

1. Centers for Disease Control and Prevention: Guidelines for infection control in dental health care settings. Morb Mortal Wkly Rep. 2003;52: 1-68.
2. Micik RE, et al. Studies on aerobiology, I Bacterial aerosols generated during dental procedures. J Dental Res. 1969;48: 49-56.
3. Updated US Public Health Service Guidelines for the Management of Occupational Exposures to HBV, HCV, and HIV and Recommendations for Postexposure Prophylaxis, CDC, Morbidity and Mortality Weekly Report June 29. 2001 / 50(RR11);1-42.
4. Immunization of Health-Care Workers: Recommendations of the Advisory Committee on Immunization Practices (ACIP) and the Hospital Infection, CDC, Morbidity and Mortality Weekly Report December 26, 1997 / 46(RR-18);1-42.
5. http://www.ada.org/1857.aspx
6. http://www.cdc.gov/oralhealth/infectioncontrol/guidelines/index.htm
7. CDC, Morbidity and Mortality Weekly Report December 19, 2003 / Vol. 52 / No. RR-17, Guidelines for Infection Control in Dental Health-Care Settings — 2003.
8. Bentlley CD, et al. Evaluating spatter and aerosol contamination during dental procedures. J Am Dent Assoc. 1994;125: 579-84.
9. Occupational safety and Health Administration: Blood borne pathogens, Fed Reg 1991;56: 64175-81.
10. Crawford JJ, Leonard RH. Infection Control. In. Roberson TM, Heymann HO, Swift EJ. Sturdevant's Art and Sciences of Operative Dentistry, 5th Ed. Mosby 2006;368-404.
11. Garner JS, Favero MS. Guidelines for handwahing and hospital environmental control, Atlanta Public Health Service, Centers for disease control, 1985.
12. Ehrenkranz NJ, Alfanso BC. Failure of bland soap handwash to prevent hand transfer of patient bacteria to urethral catheters. Infect Control Hosp. Epidemiol 1991;12: 654-62.
13. Goswami M, Patel P, Nayal S, et al. Needle stick and sharp instruments injuries among health care providers at cardiology institute, Ahmedabad, National Journal of Community Medicine. Issue 2. 2010;(1): 114-7.
14. http://www.ada.org/sections/professional resources/pdfs/cdc_sterilization.pdf - Updated July 2009, Copyright 2004 American Dental Association.
15. Rutala AW, Mayhall G. Medical Waste, Infection Control Hospital Epidemiology. 1992;38-48.
16. Arian DS, AM Asce J, HB Arian L, Mcmurray TD. Hospital Solid Waste Management- A Case Study. J Environ Eng Div. August 1980; 741-53.
17. Lee CC, Huffman GL, Nalesnik PR. Medical Waste Management. Environ. Sci. Technol.1993; 25(3):360.
18. Li C, Fu-Tien J. Physical and Chemical Composition of Hospital Waste, Infection Control and Hospital Epidemiology. 1993; 14(3):145.
19. Guerquin F. Treatment of Medical Wastes, Waste Manag Disp J. 1995;115-7.
20. EPA. Guide for Infectious Waste Management,1986; EPA/530-SW-86-014.
21. EPA, Medical Waste Management in USA, Second Interim Report to Congress,1990, EPA/ 530-SW-90-087A.

FURTHER READING

1. Centers for Disease Control and Prevention: http://www.cdc.gov
2. Cleveland JL, Barker LK, Cuny EJ, Panlilio AL. National Surveillance System for Health Care Workers Group. Preventing percutaneous injuries among dental health care personnel. J Am Dent Assoc. 2007; 138(2):169-78.
3. Gigola P, Angelillo V, Garusi G.: Effectiveness of a glutaraldehyde formulation in decontamination of dental unit water systems. Minerva Stomatol. 2006;55(7-8):437-48.
4. Gordon BL, Burke FJ, Bagg J, Marlborough HS, McHugh ES.: Systematic review of adherence to infection control guidelines in dentistry. J Dent 2001; 29(8):509-16.
5. Harte JA, Charlton DG.: Characteristics of infection control programs in US. Air Force dental clinics: a survey. J Am Dent Assoc, 2005;136(7):885-92.
6. Harte JA.: Looking inside the 2003 CDC dental infection control guidelines. J Calif Dent Assoc 2004;32(11):919-30.
7. Kohn WG, Harte JA, Malvitz DM, Collins AS, Cleveland JL, Eklund KJ; Centers for Disease Control and Prevention.: Guidelines for infection control in dental health care settings--2003. J Am Dent Assoc 2004; 135(1):33-47.
8. Mills SE.: Dental water quality--the scientific evidence for current CDC guidelines. Tex Dent J 2005; 122(10):1054-63.

9. Myers R.: Hand care and waterlines: update for the dental profession. Dent Today. 2004;23(10):132-6.

10. O'Donnell MJ, Shore AC, Coleman DC. A novel automated waterline cleaning system that facilitates effective and consistent control of microbial biofilm contamination of dental chair unit waterlines: a one-year study. J Dent. 2006;34(9):648-61. Epub 2006 Jan 24.

11. Rubin L, Hefer E, Dubnov Y, Warman S, Rishpon S. An evaluation of the efficacy of the national immunization programme for hepatitis B. Public Health. 2007 Feb 21;

12. Shulman ER, Brehm WT. Dental clinical attire and infection-control procedures. Patients' attitudes. J Am Dent Assoc 2001;132(4):508-16.

13. Vos D, Gotz HM, Richardus JH. Needlestick injury and accidental exposure to blood: the need for improving the hepatitis B vaccination grade among health care workers outside the hospital. Am J Infect Control 2006; 34(9):610-2.

14. Xavier RL, Vasconcelos BC, da Silva LC, Porto GG. Glove perforation during oral surgical procedures. Med Oral Patol Oral Cir Bucal. 2006;11(5):E433-6.

15. Zimmerman RK, Middleton DB. Vaccines for persons at high risk, 2007. J Fam Pract. 2007;56(2):S38-46.

QUESTIONS

1. Explain the routes of transmission of infection in dental setup.
2. Express in detail the general guidelines for infection control that should be followed in dental clinics.
3. What is barrier precautions in infection control?
4. Importance and method of handwashing and care of hands.
5. What care should be taken while handling sharp instruments and needles?
6. Explain the classification of dental instruments depending on their infection risk.
7. Enumerate the sterilization methods and explain autoclaving in detail.
8. What do you understand by waste disposal? What are the criteria that should be followed in dental clinic?

Genetics in Pedodontic Practice

INTRODUCTION

Genetic abnormalities comprise disorders due to defect in the genetic system comprising of the genes and the chromosomes. Gene is the genetic material, DNA, that controls the production of a single protein (or polypeptide chain). Genes are grouped into units called chromosomes. Humans have 46 chromosomes that contain an estimated 100,000 genes, including numerous duplicates. Each chromosome has a paired mate that is referred to as the homolog. Genes on homologs control the same genetic traits and, except for genes on the X and Y chromosomes, there are at least two genes that control each inherited trait. Thus the human chromosome complement consists of 23 pairs of chromosomes. Twenty-two of these pairs are the autosomes; the remaining pair, the X and the Y chromosome, are the sex chromosomes.

TERMS COMMONLY USED

Some of the common terms used to describe genetic abnormalities:

Autosomal dominant disorders: They arise due to the defects in at least one gene out of a pair of genes on autosomes and are vertically transmitted in every generation. Each child of an affected parent is at 50% risk of inheriting the abnormal gene.

Autosomal recessive disorders: These occur when both the genes on an autosome are affected. Since two abnormal genes are required for obtaining a given clinical phenotype, their incidence is low compared to autosomal dominant disorders.

X-linked disorders: These are disorders that arise due to the defect in the gene(s) located in X-chromosome.

Deletion: Loss of part of chromosome, e.g. Cri-du-Chat syndrome.

Translocation: A portion of chromosome attached to another, e.g. translocation carrier.

Inversion: A portion of chromosome upside down.

Duplication: A chromosome is larger than normal, the extra segment being identical to a segment of the normal chromosome.

CLASSIFICATION OF CHROMOSOMAL ABERRATIONS

Choromosomal aberrations can be classified as:
1. According to number of cells involved:
   i. Involving chromosome sets.
      - Monoploidy (Haploid, 23X)
      - Euploid: A complete second set of chromosome, the total number being 92 (46 + 46)

- Polyploid: Three triploid or four tetraploid complete sets of chromosome. This is incompatible with human life.
  ii. Involving individual chromosome (Aneuploidy): Any extranumber of chromosomes that do not represent an exact multiple of total chromosome complement.
     a. Involving autosomes.
        - Monosomy: A missing chromosome pair.
        - Trisomy: Down syndrome (45+ XX or 45 + XY)
     b. Involving sex chromosomes, for example,
        - Turner's syndrome.
        - Klinefelter's syndrome.
        - Superfemale.
2. According to alteration in structure of chromosome:
   a. Deletion—loss of part of chromosome, e.g. Cri-du-Chat syndrome.
   b. Translocation—a portion of chromosome attached to another, e.g. translocation carrier.
   c. Inversion—a portion of chromosome upside down.
   d. Duplication—a chromosome is larger than normal, the extra-segment being identical to a segment of the normal chromosome.
3. According to type of chromosome abnormality:
   a. Gross chromosomal aberrations in which there is either a structural or numerical abnormality of chromosome.
   b. Single gene abnormalities which are transmitted in an autosomal dominant, autosomal recessive or X-linked pattern.
   c. Polygenic disorders in which environmental interaction may play a significant role.

Down Syndrome (Mongolism)

It is one of the most common recognizable malformation syndromes and has an incidence of approximately one in 600 newborns.

Types of Down Syndrome

There are 3 main types of Down syndrome:

Trisomy 21: Vast majority of children (95%) with Down syndrome have an extra 21 chromosome. Instead of normal 46 chromosomes, the individual has 47 chromosomes (45+XX or 45+XY). This condition is called trisomy 21.

Translocation: Less common is called translocation where the extra 21 chromosome material is attached or translocated onto another chromosome, usually on 14, 22 or 21. In at least 1/3rd of the cases, a parent may be a carrier of the translocation.

Mosaicism: It is the least occurring type. In this some cells have 47 chromosomes and others have 46 chromosomes.

Etiology

Although many theories have been developed, it is believed to be due to:
- Hormonal abnormalities
- X-rays
- Viral infection
- Immunologic problems
- Genetic predisposition
- Advancing maternal age

Clinical Features

Head: Microcephaly with prominence of forehead, shortening of anteroposterior diameter and flattening of occiput.

Face: Round flat face with characteristic flat nasal bridge, epicanthal folds and upward—slanting palpebral fissures.

Eyes: Hypoplasia of iris stroma and Brushfield spots.

Mouth

- Underdevelopment of maxilla contributing to open mouth
- Normal appearing protruded tongue
- Palate is of normal height but short and narrow
- Delayed and abnormal sequence of eruption of teeth First primary teeth may not appear until 2 years of age, and dentition may not be complete by 4 to 5 years of age.
- Defective or absent of upper incisor
- Anomalies of tooth shape
- Early shedding of deciduous dentition
- High incidence of rapid destructive periodontal disease
- Bruxism
- Malocclusion
- Poor oral hygiene
- Dental caries susceptibility is usually low in those with Down syndrome. This is due to increased pH of saliva, delayed eruption and early shedding of primary teeth
- Congenital absence of permanent teeth is common.

Limbs

- Broad and shortened hands, feet and digits
- Simian crease (transverse palmar crease)
- Decreased muscle tone and loose ligaments.
- Clinodactyly (permanent deviation of one or more finger)
- Wide space between the 1st and 2nd toes are present in majority of patient.

Nervous system

- Level of intelligence in these children (25–50 IQ) ranges from mild to severe retardation

- Generalized muscular hypotonia which becomes less pronounced with increasing age
- Hearing defects
- Congenital heart disease
- Intestinal abnormalities, e.g. blockage of esophagus, duodenum
- Increased incidence of eye problems such as cataracts, strabismus, near sightedness, far sightedness, etc.
- Thyroid dysfunctions—hypothyroidism.
- Skeletal problems such as kneecap subluxation, hip dislocation, atlantoaxial instability and severe neck problems
- Leukemia, immunologic problems, Alzheimer's disease, seizure disorders, sleep apnea and skin disorders.

Trisomy 18 (Edward's Syndrome)

- Children with this disorder are more seriously affected than in Down syndrome.
- Usually they have short life span of few months.
- It is associated with an extra 18 autosome (45 + XX).

Clinical Features

- Marked retardation in physical and mental growth and development
- Low birth weight
- Hypertonicity of muscles
- Epicanthal folds, small mouth and micrognathia
- Low set ears, prominent occiput and small eyes
- Flexion and overlapping of fingers
- Congenital heart disease.

Trisomy 13 (Patau Syndrome)

- This disorder is characterized by multiple abnormalities in various organs. 70% live born infants die within 7 months
- Characteristic clinical findings include bilateral cleft lip and palate, microophthalmia or anophthalmia (small or no eyes) superficial hemangioma of forehead or nape of neck, growth retardation, severe mental retardation, polydactyly of hand and feet, clenching of fist with the thumb under the fingers, several anomalies of external genitals and defects of the brain.

Cri-du-Chat (Cat Cry Syndrome)

- This syndrome is characterized by a deletion on the short arm of chromosome 5. Newborns with a chromosome 5 deletion exhibit cat like cry at birth due to abnormality of larynx and are mentally retarded.
- Physical changes include hypotonia, microcephaly, downward slanting of palpebral fissures, hypertelorism and epicanthic folds, cleft lip and cleft palate.

Turner's Syndrome (Gonadal Dysgenesis)

It results from complete or partial monosomy of X chromosome and is characterized primarily by hypogonadism in phenotypic female.

Clinical Features

- These women have short stature
- Webbing of neck
- Edema of hand and feet
- Exhibit a low hairline at the nape of neck
- Body hair is sparse
- The chest is broad with wide space nipples
- The aorta is frequently abnormal
- Idiopathic hypertension
- Hypoplastic 4th metacarpal
- Poor development of secondary sexual characteristics and streak gonads
- High arched palate and hypoplastic mandible
- Hearing loss.

Klinefelter's Syndrome

Defined as male hypogonadism that occurs when there are two or more X chromosomes.

Clinical Features

- Male phenotype and condition cannot be detected until after puberty
- These patients are taller than normal
- Have wide hips
- Gynecomastia
- Intelligence levels are lower than normal
- Small testis
- Absence of spermatogenesis of seminiferous tubules

GENETICS AND DENTAL CARIES

It is often seen that children living in similar environmental conditions have different susceptibility for caries. This difference can be attributed to genetic difference and this makes a person more susceptible than the other. Therefore, genetic influences may modify the overt expression of the disease in an individual.

GENETICS AND PERIODONTAL DISEASE

It is observed that about 38 to 82% of the periodontal disease is attributable to genetic factors. Several forms of early-onset periodontitis (e.g. localized prepubertal periodontitis, localized and generalized aggressive periodontitis) are found to be influenced by other genetic factors. A number of other conditions that can predispose to periodontal disease, such as leukocyte adhesion deficiencies, Chediak-Higashi syndrome, cyclic neutropenia, and Papillon-Lefevre syndrome have been associated with genetic influence.

GENETICS AND MALOCCLUSION

Factors necessary to attain and maintain normal occlusion such as skeletomuscular balance, the size of the maxilla, the size of the mandible, the arch form, anatomy of teeth and the presence or absence of teeth have genetic influence. Genetic influences on each of these traits are rarely due to a single gene and are often polygenic with potential for environmental influence.

It is thus not possible to make accurate predictions about the development of occlusion in a child by simply studying the frequency of its occurrence in parents. Although family patterns of resemblance are frequently obvious, predictions must be made cautiously because of the genetic and environmental variables that are unknown and difficult to evaluate.

GENETIC COUNSELING

Genetic disorders occur among nearly 30% of admissions to pediatric hospitals, and mortality rate is between 40 to 50%. Genetic diseases are almost always serious, are not curable and relatively few are amenable to satisfactory modes of treatment. Thus in current situation the prevention of this group of diseases remains of paramount importance. The most effective means of preventing genetic diseases remains the provision of genetic counseling for individuals at risk of having a child with a serious genetic disorder.

Definition

The American Society of Human Genetics in 1975 has defined genetic counseling as "a process of communication, the intent of which is to provide individuals and families having a genetic disease or at risk of such a disease with information about their condition and to provide information that would allow couples at risk to make informed reproductive decisions."

Indications for genetic counseling	
1.	Known or suspected hereditary disease in a patient or family
2.	Birth defects
3.	Unexplained mental retardation
4.	Advanced maternal age
5.	Exposure to a teratogen
6.	Consanguinity

Information Conveyed during Genetic Counseling

1. The magnitude of the risk
2. The burden of the disease on the patient and family
3. Possibility of modification of either the burden or the risk

> The psychological needs and issues associated with the genetic counseling process are many and complicated. There is need to cope and come to terms with emotionally traumatic information, and they need to make decisions in future reproductive plans and may also need to make fundamental alternations to their feeling about themselves and about interpersonal relationship.

Process Involved in Genetic Counseling

1. The first step in genetic counseling is to ascertain what question the counselee (the individual seeking counseling) is really asking. Since it involves communication, one must assess the receptivity, emotional and intellectual, of the individuals seeking counseling.
2. Couples should be counseled together in a quiet room.
3. The mode, in which this type of information is explained to counselees, is of utmost importance and also greatly influences the interpretation of the facts. Discussion of the options open to a couple makes the counseling process more comprehensive and relevant.
4. The information must be conveyed in a language that can be understood by the counselee. It should be believed that openness and honesty are the best way to present such information. The information communicated is heavy with emotional content and often contains medical or scientific information that is difficult for an individual to comprehend.
5. Genetic counseling must not be directive, i.e., the counselee should not be directed to whether to have children or not. Reproductive decisions are highly personal ones and should be left to individual couples rather than being made by their physicians and counselors.
6. The verbal counseling should be followed up by a letter, which enables them to read and reread the counseling and to share it with physicians, family members or other supportive individuals.

> The process of genetic counseling can be divided into 4 consecutive phases:
> - Initial phase: Information is gathered and diagnosis is made.

Contd...

Contd...

- Facts about disease, genetic implication and possible options are imparted to and discussed with the counselee.
- Counselee evaluates, assimilates and learns to cope with the given information.
- Decisions are made.

Psychological Aspects of Counseling

The responsibility of a genetic counselor does not end when he has made an accurate diagnosis. He must, in transmitting his information to the individual concerned, take into account the psychological effect of unfavorable prospects. It is not sufficient to tell the truth, but it is necessary to tell it humanely. Lack of motivation, overt anxiety and even hostility can seriously disrupt the counseling relationships. The factor most commonly found by counselors to cause difficulties in effective communication is the educational background of their client and in particular the client's knowledge of biology. The environment in which the counseling takes place can also greatly influence the process.

For a counselee to achieve the goal of psychological homeostasis and be in a position to make the important decisions that are necessary, they must have experienced the 4 phases of coping process known to follow the exposure to stressful situation.

These phases are:

1st phase : Shock
2nd phase : Denial, anger
3rd phase : Guilt, anxiety
4th phase : Depression

Awareness regarding that these phases are natural course of events and their identification can help the counselor plan his approach more successfully.

Apart from the obvious problem of finding effective treatments for genetic disorders, there is an important need to ensure that genetic advice is made as widely available as possible. There is evidence that there are many people in the population who are unaware of this. Increasing knowledge of genetics and appreciation of the risks by physicians will help to reduce this problem. There seem to be very good reasons, both ethical as well as financial, for encouraging efforts to develop and extend the preventive approach to genetic disease.

FURTHER READING

1. Bui C, King T, Proffit W, Frazier-Bowers S. Phenotypic characterization of Class III patients. Angle Orthod, 2006; 76(4):564-9.
2. Cerruti Mainardi P. Cri Du Chat syndrome. Orphanet J Rare Dis, 2006;5:1:33.
3. Dempsey PJ, Townsend GC. Genetic and environmental contributions to variation in human tooth size. Heredity. 2001;86(Pt 6):685-93.
4. Huang B, Thangavelu M, Bhatt S, J Sandlin C, Wang S. Prenatal diagnosis of 45,X and 45,X mosaicism: the need for thorough cytogenetic and clinical evaluations. Prenat Diagn. 2002;22(2):105-10.
5. Kida M, Sakiyama Y, Matsuda A, Takabayashi S, Ochi H, Sekiguchi H, Minamitake S, Ariga T. A novel missense mutation (p.P52R) in amelogenin gene causing X-linked amelogenesis imperfecta. J Dent Res 2007;86(1):69-72.
6. Li Y, Ge Y, Saxena D, Caufield PW. Genetic profiling of the oral microbiota associated with severe early-childhood caries. J Clin Microbiol 2007;45(1):81.
7. Nakashima M, Iohara K, Zheng L. Gene therapy for dentin regeneration with bone morphogenetic proteins. Curr Gene Ther 2006;6(5):551-60 (Review).
8. Schulman GS, Redford-Badwal D, Poole A, Mathieu G, Burleson J, Dauser D. Taurodontism and learning disabilities in patients with Klinefelter syndrome. Pediatr Dent 2005;27(5):389-94.
9. Semerci CN, Satiroglu-Tufan NL, Turan S, Bereket A, Tuysuz B, Yilmaz E, Kayserili H, Karaman B, Semiz S, Duzcan F, Bagci H. Detection of Y chromosomal material in patients with a 45,X karyotype by PCR method. Tohoku J Exp Med 2007;211(3):243-9.
10. Slayton R. Genetics may have a significant contribution to dental caries while microbial acid production appears to be modulated by the environment. J Evid Based Dent Pract 2006;6(2):185-6.

QUESTIONS

1. What is the difference between an autosomal dominant and autosomal recessive disorder?
2. Classify chromosomal aberrations based on the number of cells involved.
3. What is Down syndrome? Give its etiology and clinical features.
4. Write short notes on Cri-du-Chat syndrome.
5. Write in detail about Turner syndrome.
6. Explain the relation of genetics with dental caries, periodontal disease and malocclusion.
7. Define genetic counseling, explain the indications and process involved in genetic counseling.

Survey Procedures and Indices

INTRODUCTION

Survey is a non-experimental type of research that attempts to gather information about the status quo for a large number of cases by describing present conditions without directly analyzing their causes.

Surveying is far more than collecting and arraying of facts. It is a task through which many key people in a community become aware of the dental needs of the community and what can be done about them. These people are the ones who will subsequently rally popular support for the program. The real focus of any dental health survey involves the measurement of dental disease or morbidity. The teeth and their surrounding structures are so definite, easy to observe and carry with them so much of their previous disease history that the measurement of dental disease is easier than the measurement of many other forms of disease.

DEFINITION

A survey is most easily defined negatively as a "non-experimental investigation".

It is an investigation in which information is systematically collected, but in which there is no active intervention by the investigators. The purpose of most surveys is to collect information that will provide a basis for action, whether immediately or in the long-term run.

TYPES OF SURVEYS

Descriptive Survey

A descriptive survey sets out to describe a situation, e.g. the distribution of a disease in a population in relation to sex and age.

Analytic Survey

An analytic (or explanatory) survey tries to explain the situation, i.e. to study the determinative process. This is done by formulating and testing hypothesis.

The distinction between a descriptive and analytic survey is not always clear and a single survey can combine both purposes, e.g. a broad descriptive survey may be so planned, that it also provides information for the testing of a specific hypothesis.

Types of surveys:
1. Descriptive ⟶ Cross-sectional
2. Analytical ⟶ Longitudinal

Surveys whether descriptive, analytic or mixed can be usefully categorized as cross-sectional or longitudinal, depending on the time period covered by the observations.

Cross-sectional Survey

A cross-sectional (instantaneous, simultaneous, prevalence) survey provides information about the situation that exists at a single time.

Longitudinal Survey

A longitudinal (time span) survey provides data about events or changes during a period of time.

SURVEY METHODS

Health surveys can be broadly classified into four types:
1. Health interview survey (face to face survey)
2. Health examination survey
3. Health records survey
4. Questionnaire survey

Health Interview Survey (Face-to-Face Survey)

It is an invaluable method of measuring subjective phenomena, such as perceived morbidity, disability and impairment; opinions, beliefs and attitudes and some behavioral characteristics. However, the data obtained like this, may not be reliable, because of the limitation of the interview method. That is why interviews are often combined with health examination surveys.

Health Examination Survey

The information obtained through this method is more valid than health interview survey. Teams consisting of doctors, technicians and interviewers carry out this survey.

Disadvantages

- It is expensive and cannot be carried out on an extensive scale.
- The method also requires consideration—providing treatment to people found suffering from certain diseases.

Health Records Survey

It involves the collection of data from health service records. This is obviously the cheapest method of collecting data.

Disadvantages

- The data obtained is not population-based.
- Reliability is open to question.
- Lack of uniform procedures and standardization in the recording of data.

Questionnaire Survey

It is used for measuring subjective phenomena.

Advantages

- Simpler
- Economical
- Standardization (written instructions) reduce biases from differences in administration.
- Anonymity: Privacy encourages candid and honest responses to sensitive questions.

Disadvantages

- A certain level of education and skill is expected from the respondents.
- There is usually a high rate of non-response.

USES OF SURVEYS

1. Monitoring trends in oral health and disease
2. Policy development
3. Program evaluation
4. Assessment of dental needs
5. Providing visibility for dental issues

Monitoring Trends in Oral Health and Disease

When national surveys are repeated periodically under general similar conditions, broad oral health trends over time can be estimated, provided the sampling design so permits, a single survey can show how oral health varies by geographic region, social class or by race or ethnic group. The WHO's pathfinder survey protocol when repeated periodically can assess trends in health and disease and it is assumed that the results are valid enough to support national policy decisions.

Policy Development

Survey data can be used to establish oral health strategies. Scotland has successfully used survey data to develop its oral health policy. A number of American States switched their primary preventive focus from fluoride mouthrinsing to sealant application after state-wide surveys showed most carious lesions to be in pits and fissures.

Program Evaluation

Survey data are often used to evaluate programs though the principle that association does not show cause-and-effect needs to be remembered.

A survey is not a randomized controlled/[clinical] trial and inferences need to be made with caution. The success of particular programs can only be inferred from survey data, though the more localized the survey and the program, then the more plausible is the inference.

Assessment of Dental Needs

Although surveys can be used for assessment of the needs, there is a clear gap between the criteria used in surveys and those applied by dentists for patient care, e.g. Criteria for caries in surveys usually are based on cavitation, but dentists generally intervene at an earlier stage in the carious process.

Providing Visibility of Dental Issues

The visibility that oral health acquires through the mere existence of data from a national survey may be the most important of all uses of survey data.

STEPS IN SURVEYING

1. Establishing the objectives
2. Designing the investigation
3. Selecting the sample
4. Conducting the examinations
5. Analyzing the data
6. Drawing the conclusions
7. Publishing the results.

Establishing the Objectives

The investigator must be absolutely clear about the objective of the investigation before considering its design, as the latter is entirely dependent on the former. The objectives can either be stated in the form of a hypothesis which is to be tested, or the objective may be stated by describing what is to be measured. Having determined the objectives, each subsequent stage of the investigation must be carried out in a way that will enable these objectives to be met.

Designing the Investigation

Survey Protocol

It is important to prepare a written protocol for the survey, which should contain:
A. Main objective and purpose of the survey.
B. A description of the type of information to be collected and of the methods to be used.
C. A description of the sampling methods to be used.
D. Personnel and physical arrangements.
E. Statistical methods to be used in analyzing the data.
F. A provisional budget.
G. A provisional timetable of main activities and responsible staff.

Obtaining Approval from Authorities

Permission to examine population groups must usually be obtained from a local, regional or national authority. For example, if school populations are to be examined, school authorities and the parents should be approached for obtaining permission. The health authorities should also be notified, since it may be necessary to time the survey to fit in with other health related activities.

Budgeting

A budget for the survey should be prepared which should include all the resources required to carry out the survey.

Scheduling

An orderly schedule should be prepared for data collection, to prevent the waste of valuable time. The schedules should allow for some flexibility so that unexpected delays do not cause major upsets in the survey timetable. Since fatigue contributes significantly to inaccuracy and inconsistency, it is unwise to make the schedule too demanding. It is not advisable to schedule more than 15 children to be examined in an hour.

Emergency Care and Referral

All survey teams should be equipped for and ready to provide emergency care if required. It is also the responsibility of the examiner to ensure that referral to an appropriate care facility is made.

Selecting the Sample

While designing a study, it is usually impossible to examine every individual in the population under investigation. Resources in terms of time, manpower and money may not be available for the collection and analysis of vast amounts of data. For this reason, a sample must be chosen from the population.

Sampling

Sampling is the process or technique of selecting a sample of appropriate characteristics and adequate size.

Advantages of Sampling

i. It reduces the cost of the investigation, the time required and the number of personnel involved.
ii. It allows thorough investigation of the units of observation.
iii. A sample can be covered more adequately and in more depth than can a total population.

Requisites for a Reliable Sample

a. *Efficiency:* The ability of the sample to yield the desired information.
b. *Representativeness:* A sample should be representative of the parent population, so that the inferences

drawn can be generalized to that population with precision.

c. *Measurability:* The extent to which findings from the sample differ from that of the parent population should be able to be measured.

d. *Size:* A sample should be large enough to minimize sample variability.

e. *Coverage:* A sample should provide adequate coverage of the population.

f. *Feasibility:* The design should be simple enough to be carried out in practice.

g. *Economy and cost efficiency:* The sample should yield the desired information at a fixed low cost with least sampling error.

Sampling Methods

a. *Random sampling (simple random sampling):* It is a technique whereby each sampling unit has the same probability of being selected.

Basic procedure involved:

   i. Prepare a sampling frame

  ii. Decide on the size of the sample

 iii. Select the required number of units by:
   - Lottery method
   - Table of random numbers

b. *Systematic sampling:* The first unit is chosen at random and then, other units are chosen in a systematic way. For example, every third patient visiting the dentist.

c. *Stratified sampling:* The population is first divided into subgroups or strata according to certain common characteristics. Then random or systematic sampling is performed independently in each stratum:
   - Stratified random sampling;
   - Stratified systematic sampling.

Advantages

1. It eliminates sampling variation with respect to be the properties used in stratifying.

2. Cluster sampling: Here, a simple random sampling is selected, not of individual subjects, but of groups or clusters of individuals. The sampling units are clusters and the sampling frame is a list of these clusters.

3. Administratively simple

4. Less expensive than random sampling.

Disadvantage

If clusters contain similar persons, the findings cannot be generalized to the parent population.

Other Types of Sampling

1. *Multistage sampling:* It is a sub-sampling within groups chosen as cluster samples. The first stage is to select the groups or clusters. Then sub-samples are taken in as many subsequent stages as necessary to obtain the desired sample size. For example, 1st stage: choice of states within countries; 2nd stage: choice of towns within each state; 3rd stage: choice of neighborhoods within each town.

2. *Multiphase sampling:* This is used to take basic data from a large sample and details from a sub-sample.

3. *Sequential sampling:* Here, a small sample is tested in order to answer certain questions about the population. If the questions are not answered, the number of subjects or units in the sample is increased gradually until the conclusions may be drawn.

4. *Panels:* They are useful for studying trends. A sample is randomly selected and then data are collected from the sample on several occasions. For example, every person is interviewed every 6 months.

5. *Area sampling:* It is a type of random sampling in which maps rather than lists are used.

Conducting the Examinations

The three important aspects in the survey of dental disease and conditions are:
   - The examination methods and diagnostic aids
   - The diagnostic criteria
   - The indices used for measurement.

Basic Requirements for an Oral Examination

A. A chair preferably with a head rest.

B. A source of illumination, which can either be a separate unit, a lamp attached to the head of the examiner or a fiber optic light source.

C. Some methods of cleaning the teeth to remove loose debris where necessary.

D. A recorder, live or tape is necessary for receiving the information called by the examiner.

E. Some workers prefer to have the subject in a reclining position on a couch; the dentist can then remain seated at the head and no bending or chair adjustments are required to compensate for the varying size of the subjects.

F. The length of time that it takes to examine each subject depends on the extent and detail of the examination and the habits and inclination of the examiner. Extremes of thirty seconds to one and a half hours have been admitted.

G. The examination should be as automatic as possible to obviate excessive intrusion of subjective thought. Therefore it should be performed quickly. The object of epidemiological surveys is to examine subjects in fairly large numbers. Excessive time spent on each individual necessitates a reduction in the number of individuals seen. The flow of subjects through the examination unit needs careful regulation and should be discussed prior to arrival.

H. The diagnostic method chosen should be both valid and reliable. The validity of a test is its ability to measure what is intended to measure. For example, all ill individuals should be detected but no healthy subjects should be diagnosed as ill. The validity can be determined by calculating the sensitivity and specificity of the method.

> A test is **sensitive** if all cases in which the condition exists are positively diagnosed.
>
> A test is **specific** if a positive diagnosis is made only when the condition is present, e.g. false positive: where a sound surface has been diagnosed as carious. False negative: where a carious surface has been diagnosed as sound.
>
> The **reliability** of a test is its ability to give the same results if repeated. The reliability or repeatability of a diagnostic method may be measured by carrying out the examination on two occasions and comparing the results. This is sometimes known as test-retest.

Classification of Types of Inspection and Examination

The ADA has standardized four main types of examination and inspection.

Type 1: Complete examination, using mouth mirror and explorer, adequate illumination, thorough roentgenographic survey and when indicated, percussion, pulp-vitality tests, trans-illumination, study models and laboratory tests. This method can seldom be used in public health work.

Type 2: Limited examination, using mouth mirror and explorer, adequate illumination, posterior bitewing roentgenograms. This method is of great value where public health programs combine service to individual patients with population survey work and gives superior results for pure survey work where time and money permit.

Type 3: Inspection, using mouth mirror and explorer and adequate illumination. This is the most-used method in public health surveying.

Type 4: Screening, using tongue depressor and available illumination. This method identifies individuals in urgent need of treatment, but is too unreliable for most public health surveying.

Selection of the Examiners

The following precautions should be taken when selecting the examiners.

a. Keep the number of examiners to a minimum.

b. Discuss the interpretation of borderline problems carefully in advance, e.g. distinction between non-carious and carious pits or fissures.

c. Use only one make and design of explorer, making rules for discard as explorers become dull.

d. Have all members of the team examine a few cases in sequence and then exchange cases until each examiner has examined each patient, to minimize divergences of opinion or observation.

e. Type and circulate among the examiners any rules or systems which may seem pertinent.

f. The supervisor should recheck an occasional case throughout the entire survey.

g. Subtle changes in interpretation should be guarded against.

For maximum efficiency, recorders should be provided.

> Sufficient numbers of instruments should be available to avoid the need to interrupt examinations while used-ones are sterilized (A minimum of 30 sets per examiner).

> The organizer of the survey should maintain a log book in which are recorded the location of each day's examinations, the number of persons examined and information about each location.

Analyzing the Data

Once the examination procedures of a survey have been completed, the work of assembling the material and interpreting it begins. In large surveys, where detailed findings are to form the basis of clinical research, transfer to punched cards may prove advisable. In small public health surveys, tally sheets can be set up to produce frequency distributions, that is, number of cases showing the different categories of findings. From these frequency distributions, means and standard deviations can be computed.

Drawing the Conclusions and Publishing the Report

The conclusions are specifically related to the investigation that has been carried out and no extrapolation is made to the population as a whole unless the investigation was designed accordingly.

The final step in the survey procedure should be the construction of a report with or without set of recommendations. Clearness and simplicity should be sought.

The WHO outline for a formal written report is:

1. Statement of the purposes of the survey.

2. Material and methods:
   - Description of area and population served.
   - Types of information collected.
   - Methods of collecting data
   - Sampling method
   - Examiner personnel and equipment
   - Statistical analysis and computational procedure
   - Cost analysis
   - Reliability and reproducibility of results.
3. Results: They should be tabulated and illustrated appropriately.
4. Discussion and conclusions: The investigations, its findings and its conclusions are discussed.
5. Summary.

ORAL HEALTH SURVEYS (PATHFINDER SURVEYS)

Basic oral health surveys are used to collect information about the oral health status and treatment needs of a population and subsequently, to monitor changes in levels and patterns of disease.

There are special factors associated with the most common oral diseases which have enabled a practical, economic survey sampling methodology to be defined, called the "pathfinder" method.

The special considerations considering the two major oral diseases are:
- The diseases are strongly age related.
- The diseases exist in all populations, varying only in severity and prevalence.
- Dental caries is irreversible and therefore information on previous disease experience can be got.
- There is excessive documentation on variation of profiles of dental caries for population groups with different socioeconomic levels and environmental conditions.

The "pathfinder method" is a stratified cluster sampling technique, which aims to include the most important population subgroups likely to have differing disease levels. It also proposes appropriate numbers of subjects in specific index age groups in any one location. In this way, reliable and clinically relevant information for planning is obtained at minimum expense.

Classification of Pathfinder Survey

Pathfinder surveys are of two types depending on the number and type of sampling sites and age groups included:
- Pilot
- National

Pilot Survey

A pilot survey is one that includes only the most important subgroups in the population and only one or two index ages, usually 12 years and one other age group. Such a survey provides the minimum amount of data needed to commence planning. Additional data should then be collected to provide a reliable baseline for implementing of services.

National Pathfinder Survey

A national pathfinder survey incorporates sufficient examination sites to cover all important subgroups of the population that may have differing disease levels or treatment needs and at least three of the age groups or index ages. This type of survey design is suitable for the collection of data for the planning and monitoring of services in all countries whatever the level of disease, availability of resources or complexity of services. In a large country, a larger number of sampling sites is needed. However, the number and distribution of sampling sites depend upon the specific objectives of the study. Sampling sites are usually chosen so as to provide information on population groups likely to have different levels of oral disease, e.g. cities, small towns or ethnic groups. Once the different groups are decided upon, random sampling of subjects within the groups is done.

The recommended index ages and age groups are 5, 12, 15, 35–44 and 65–74 years.

5 years: Children should be examined between their 5th and 6th birthdays. This age is of interest in relation to levels of caries in the primary dentition which may exhibit changes over a shorter time span than the permanent dentition.

(In some countries, 5 years is the age at which children begin primary school).

12 years: This age is especially important as it is generally the age at which children leave primary school and is the last age at which a reliable sample may be obtained easily through the school system. Also, it is at this age, that all permanent teeth, except third molars, will have erupted. For these reasons, 12 years has been chosen as the global monitoring age for caries for international comparisons and monitoring of disease trends.

In some countries, if many children do not attend school, two or three groups of non-attenders should be surveyed from different areas, so as to compare their oral health status with that of the attenders.

15 years: At this age, the permanent teeth have been exposed to the oral environment for 3–9 years. The assessment of caries prevalence is therefore often more meaningful than at 12 years of age. This age is also important for the assessment of periodontal disease indicators in adolescents.

35–44 years: (Mean 40 years): This age group is the standard monitoring group for health conditions of adults. The full effect of dental caries, the level of severe periodontal involvement and the general effects of care provided can be monitored using data for this age group.
65–74 years (Mean 70 years): This age group has become more important with the changes in age distribution and increases in life span that are now occurring. Data for this group are needed both for planning appropriate care for the elderly and for monitoring the overall effects of oral care services in a population.

The number of subjects in each index age group to be examined ranges from a minimum of 25 to 50 for each cluster or sampling site, depending on the expected prevalence and severity of oral disease.

INDICES USED IN ROUTINE DENTAL PRACTICE

Definition
Russel AI defined index "as a numerical value describing the relative status of a population on a graduated scale with definite upper and lower limits, which is designed to permit and facilitate comparison with other populations classified by the same criteria and methods".

Criteria for Selecting an Index
1. The index must be simple to use and calculate.
2. The index should permit the examination of many people in a short period of time. The index should require minimum armamentarium and expenditure.
3. The index should have the criteria which define its components clear and readily understandable so as to promote maximum intra and inter-examiner reproducibility.
4. The index should be as free as possible from subjective interpretation.
5. The index should define clinical conditions objectively.
6. The index should be highly reproducible in assessing a clinical condition when used by one or more examiners.
7. The index should be amenable to statistical analysis.
8. The index should be strongly related numerically to the clinical stages of the specific disease under investigation.
9. The index should be equally sensitive throughout the scale, if it relates the severity of a variable.
10. The index should not cause discomfort to the patient and should be acceptable to the patient.

Oral Hygiene Index-Simplified (OHI-S Index)
The simplified oral hygiene index (OHI-S) was introduced in 1964 by John C Greene and Jack R Vermillion.
Instruments used: Mouth mirror, explorer
It has two components: The debris index and the calculus index
Teeth selected (Fig. 19.1): 16 (buccal surface), 11 (labial surface), 26 (buccal surface), 36 (lingual surface), 31 (labial surface) and 46 (lingual surface)

Criteria for Classifying Debris (Fig. 19.2)

Scores	Criteria
0	No debris or stain present
1	Soft debris covering not more than one-third of the tooth surface, or presence of extrinsic stains without other debris regardless of surface area covered
2	Soft debris covering more than one-third, but not more than two thirds, of the exposed tooth surface.
3	Soft debris covering more than two thirds of the exposed tooth surface.

Criteria for Classifying Calculus

Scores	Criteria
0	No calculus present.
1	Supragingival calculus covering not more than third of the exposed tooth surface.
2	Supragingival calculus covering more than one-third but not more than two-thirds of the exposed tooth surface or the presence of individual flecks of subgingival calculus around the cervical portion of the tooth or both.
3	Supragingival calculus covering more than two-thirds of the exposed tooth surface or a continuous heavy band of subgingival calculus around the cervical portion of the tooth or both.

Calculation

- After the scores for debris and calculus are recorded, the Index values are calculated.
- For each individual, the debris scores are totalled and divided by the number of surfaces scored. At least two of the six possible surfaces must have been examined for an individual score to be calculated.
- The score for a group or individual is obtained by computing the average of the individual scores.
- The average individual or group score is known as the Simplified Debris Index (DI-S).
- The same methods are used to obtain the calculus scores or the Simplified Calculus Index (CI-S).
- The average individual or group debris and calculus scores are combined to obtain the Simplified Oral Hygiene Index.

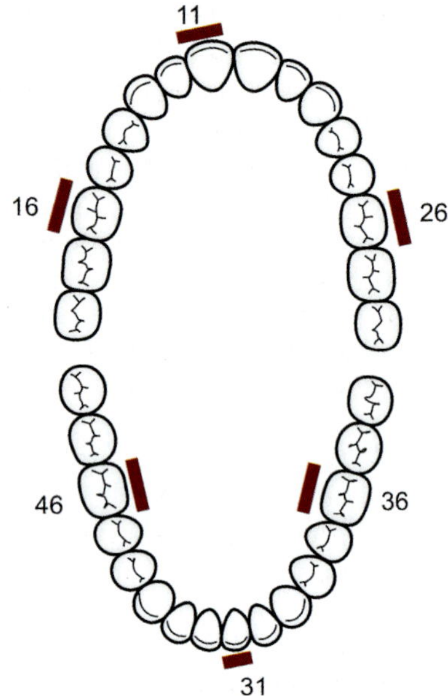

Fig. 19.1: Diagrammatic representation of the different teeth and its their surfaces to be checked

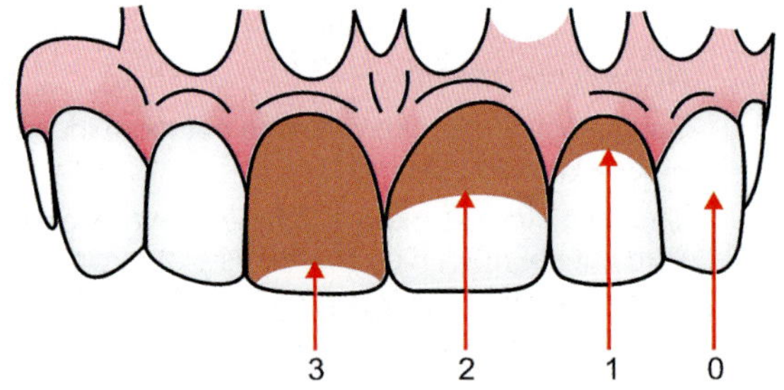

Fig. 19.2: Diagrammatic representation of the criteria used for scoring debris

The CI-S and DI-S values may range from 0 to 3:

Good: 0.0–0.6

Fair: 0.7–1.8

Poor: 1.9–3.0

The OHI-S values may range from 0 to 6:

Good: 0.0–1.2

Fair: 1.3–3.0

Poor: 3.1–6.0

Recording form for DI-S and CI-S

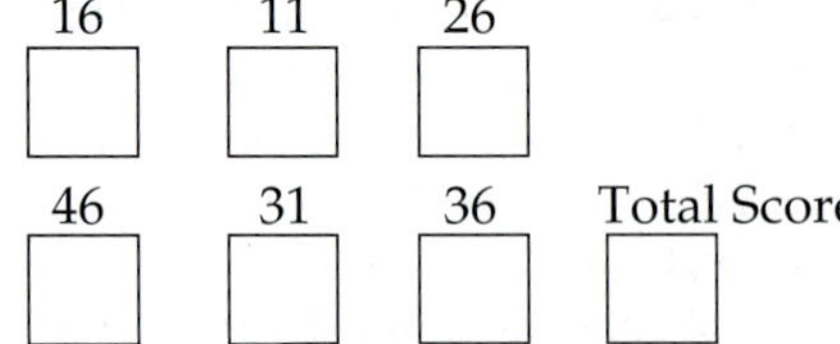

Plaque Index

This index was described by Sillness and Loe in the year 1964.

Instruments used: Mouth mirror, explorer

This index can be used both as a simplified index or a full mouth index.

Teeth selected: 16, 12, 24, 36, 32, and 44

Surfaces examined: The labial or buccal surface are divided into mesiofacial, facial and distofacial. The palatal or lingual surface is considered as a single surface. The recording format is given in Figure 19.3.

Scoring Criteria

The teeth have to be dried before examination.

Score 0: No visible plaque. When a probe is passed along the cervical portion of the tooth surface no plaque adheres to the tip of the explorer.

Score 1: No visible plaque. When a probe is passed along the cervical portion of the tooth surface a film of plaque adheres to the tip of the explorer.

Score 2: A thin to moderate accumulation of plaque is seen on the tooth surface at the cervical portion of the crown.

Score 3: Abundance of plaque is seen on the tooth surface at the cervical portion of the crown.

Individual plaque index is calculated as follows:

Plaque score for each tooth is calculated by adding the plaque scores of mesiofacial, facial, distofacial, palatal surfaces and dividing it by four. The individual scores of all the teeth are added and divided by the total number of teeth examined.

The patient can be evaluated based on the plaque index score as:

Excellent—0

Good—0.1–0.9

Fair—1.0–1.9

Poor—2.0–3.0

Gingival Index

This index was developed by Loe and Sillness in the year 1963.

In this method the severity of gingivitis is assessed.

Instruments used: Mouth mirror, periodontal probe.

This index can be used both as a simplified index or a full mouth index.

Teeth selected: 16, 12, 24, 36, 32 and 44

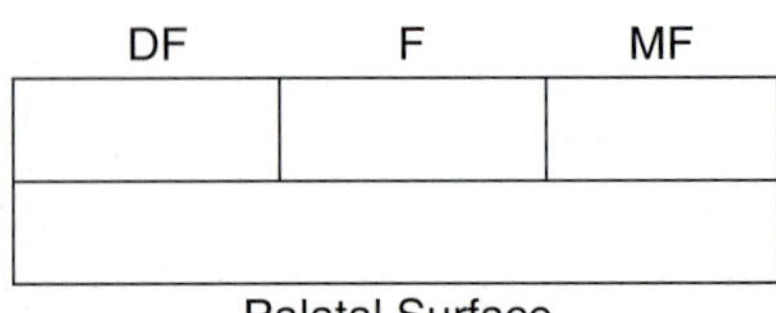

Fig. 19.3: Columns made for recording the surfaces for individual tooth

Surfaces examined: The labial or buccal gingival is divided into mesiofacial papilla, mid facial margin and distofacial papilla. The palatal or lingual gingiva is considered as a single surface. The recording format is the same as for plaque index, given in Fig. 19.3.

The gingiva is scored based on the following scoring criteria:

Score 0: Normal gingiva. No signs of gingivitis
Score 1: Mild inflammation. Slight change in color, mild edema and no bleeding on probing
Score 2: Moderate inflammation. Moderate glazing, redness, edema. Bleeds on probing
Score 3: Severe inflammation. Marked redness, hypertrophy, ulcerations. Bleeds spontaneously.

Calculation

Gingival score for each tooth is calculated by adding the gingival scores of mesiofacial, facial, distofacial, palatal surfaces and dividing it by four. The individual scores of all the index teeth are added and divided by the total number of teeth examined.

The patient can be evaluated based on the gingival index score as:

Mild gingivitis—0.1–1.0
Moderate gingivitis—1.1–2.0
Severe gingivitis—2.1 – 3.0

Decayed-Missing-Filled Index (DMF Index)

This index was introduced by Henry Klein, Carrole E Palmer and Knutson JW in 1938.

Instruments used: Mouth mirror and explorer or a CPI probe (WHO 1997)

The DMFT index is an irreversible index, which measures the total lifetime caries experience.

D describes decayed teeth

M describes missing teeth due to caries

F describes restored teeth due to caries

All the teeth in oral cavity are examined, the teeth not included are:

1. Third molars
2. Unerupted teeth/congenitally missing teeth/supernumerary teeth
3. Teeth extracted or lost for reasons other than caries
4. Teeth restored for reasons other than for caries like trauma.

Rules in Recording DMFT

1. No tooth must be counted more than once.
2. Decay, missing and filled teeth are recorded separately.
3. Recurrent caries adjacent to restorations is considered as decay.

4. List only those teeth as missing, which have been lost due to caries. Also included should be those teeth which are so badly decayed that they are indicated for extraction.
5. A tooth may have several restorations but it is counted as one.
6. Deciduous teeth are not included in a DMF count.
7. Tooth is considered erupted when occlusal surface or incisal edge is exposed to oral cavity.
8. A tooth is considered to be present even though the crown has been destroyed and only the roots are left.

WHO Modification of DMF Index (1986)

1. All third molars are included.
2. Temporary restorations are considered as 'D', decayed.
3. Only carious cavities are considered as 'D', decayed.

Calculation of DMFT Index

All the decayed, missing and filled components are added separately to get the DMF score for that patient. Values for permanent and deciduous teeth should not be added, they should be kept separate.

DMFS

A more detailed index is DMF/dmf calculated per tooth surface, DMFS/dmfs. Molars and premolars are considered as having 5 surfaces, anterior teeth 4 surfaces. Maximum value for DMFS comes to 128 for 28 teeth and 148 if third molars are included.

The rules and criteria are the same as for DMFT/dmft. Instead of calculating the number of decayed teeth, here the number of decayed surfaces is calculated. When a tooth is missing due to caries, the missing tooth is given the score of 5 for posterior tooth and 4 for anterior tooth. The decayed, missing and filled surfaces are added to get the DMFS score for that patient.

Caries Indices for Deciduous Dentition

'def' Index

This index was developed by Gruebbel AO in the year 1944. The basic principle and rules are the same as that for the DMF index.

During the developmental period, deciduous teeth are shed physiologically and some teeth might have been extracted due to caries. In this situation it might be difficult for the parent to provide the exact reason for the loss of a particular tooth. To avoid this problem, the 'm' component of the dmft/dmfs index has been replaced by the 'e' component, where 'e' denotes indicated for extraction. It includes those teeth that are missing as well as those present in the oral cavity and needs to be extracted.

'DMF' Index

This index is used in children before the age of exfoliation, 7 to 12 years. The principles and rules are the same as that for the DMF index. It can be used to determine decayed-missing-filled teeth (DMFT) or decayed-missing-filled surfaces (DMFS).

Values for permanent and deciduous teeth should never be added together.

According to the WHO (1997), codes are used to denote the dentition status			
Section 1.01	Code		Condition/status
Primary teeth	Permanent teeth		
Crown	Crown	Root	
A	0	0	Sound
B	1	1	Decayed
C	2	2	Filled, with decay
D	3	3	Filled, no decay
E	4	–	Missing, as a result of caries
–	5	–	Missing, any other reason
F	6	–	Fissure sealant
G	7	7	Bridge abutment, special crown or veneer/implant
–	8	8	Unerupted tooth (crown)/un-exposed root
T	T	–	Trauma (fracture)
–	9	9	Not recorded

0 (A). Sound crown: A crown is recorded as sound if it shows no evidence of treated or untreated clinical caries. The stages of caries that precede cavitation, as well as other conditions similar to the early stages of caries, are excluded because they cannot be reliably diagnosed. Thus, a crown with the following defects, in the absence of other positive criteria, should be coded as sound:
* White or chalky spots
* Discolored or rough spots that are not soft to touch with a metal CPI probe
* Stained pits or fissures in the enamel that do not have visual signs of undermined enamel, or softening of the floor or walls detectable with a CPI probe
* Dark, shiny, hard, pitted areas of enamel in a tooth showing signs of moderate to severe fluorosis
* Lesions that, on the basis of their distribution or history, or visual/tactile examination, appear to be due to abrasion.

Sound root: A root is recorded as sound when it is exposed and shows no evidence of treated or untreated clinical caries. (Unexposed roots are coded 8).

1 (B). Decayed crown: Caries is recorded as present when a lesion in a pit or fissure, or on a smooth tooth surface, has an unmistakable cavity, undermined enamel, or a detectably softened floor or wall. A tooth with a temporary filling, or one which is sealed (code 6 (F)) but also decayed, should also be included in this category. In case where the crown has been destroyed by caries and only the root is left, the caries is judged to have originated on the crown and therefore scored as crown caries only. The CPI probe should be used to confirm visual evidence of caries on the occlusal, buccal and lingual surfaces. Where any doubt exists, caries should not be recorded as present.

1 (B). Decayed root: Caries is recorded as present when a lesion feels soft or leathery to probing with the CPI probe. If the root caries is discrete from the crown and will require a separate treatment, it should be recorded as root caries. For single carious lesions affecting both the crown and the root, the likely site of origin of the lesion should be recorded as decayed. When it is not possible to judge the site of origin, both the crown and the root should be recorded as decayed.

2 (C). Filled crown, with decay: A crown is considered filled, with decay, when it has one or more permanent restorations and one or more areas that are decayed. No distinction is made between primary and secondary caries (i.e., the same code applies whether or not the carious lesions are in physical association with the restoration(s)).

2 (C). Filled root, with decay: A root is considered filled, with decay, when it has one or more permanent restorations and one or more areas that are decayed. No distinction is made between primary and secondary caries.

In the case of fillings involving both the crown and the root, judgement of the site of origin is more difficult. For any restoration most likely site of the primary carious lesion is recorded as filled, with decay. When it is not possible to judge the site of origin of the primary carious lesion, both the crown and the root should be recorded as filled, with decay.

3 (D). Filled crown, with no decay: A crown is considered filled, without decay, when one or more permanent restorations are present and there is no caries anywhere on the crown. A tooth that has been crowned because of previous decay is recorded in this category. (A tooth that has been crowned for reasons other than decay, e.g. a bridge abutment, is coded 7 (G)).

3 (D). Filled root, with no decay: A root is considered filled, without decay, when one or more permanent restorations are present and there is no caries anywhere on the root.

In the case of fillings involving both the crown and the root, judgement of the site of origin is more difficult.

For any restoration involving both the crown and the root, the most likely site of the primary carious lesion is recorded as filled. When it is not possible to judge the site of origin, both the crown and the root should be recorded as filled.

4 (E). Missing tooth, as a result of caries: This code is used for permanent or primary teeth that have been extracted because of caries and is recorded under coronal status. For missing primary teeth, this score should be used only if the subject is at an age when normal exfoliation would not be a sufficient explanation for absence.

Note: The root status of a tooth that has been scored as missing because of caries should be coded "7" or "9".

In some age groups, it may be difficult to distinguish between unerupted teeth (code 8) and missing teeth (code 4 and code 5). Basic knowledge of tooth eruption patterns, the appearance of the alveolar ridge in the area of the tooth space in question, and the caries status of other teeth in the mouth may provide helpful clues in making a differential diagnosis between unerupted and extracted teeth. Code 4 should not be used for teeth judged to be missing for any reason other than caries. For convenience, in fully edentulous arches, a single "4" should be placed in boxes 66 and 81 and/or 114 and 129, as appropriate, and the respective pairs of numbers linked with straight lines.

5 (-). Permanent tooth missing, for any other reason: This code is used for permanent teeth judged to be absent congenitally, or extracted for orthodontic reasons or because of periodontal disease, trauma, etc. As for code 4, two entries of code 5 can be linked by a line in cases of fully edentulous arches.

Note: The root status of a tooth scored 5 should be coded "7" or "9".

6 (F). Fissure sealant: This code is used for teeth in which a fissure sealant has been placed on the occlusal surface; or for teeth in which the occlusal fissure has been enlarged with a rounded or "flame-shaped" bur, and a composite material placed. If a tooth with a sealant has decay, it should be coded as 1 or B.

7 (G). Bridge abutment, special crown or veneer: This code is used under coronal status to indicate that a tooth forms part of a fixed bridge, i.e. is a bridge abutment. This code can also be used for crowns placed for reasons other than caries and for veneers or laminates covering the labial surface of a tooth on which there is no evidence of caries or a restoration.

Note: Missing teeth replaced by a bridge are coded 4 or 5, under coronal status, while root status is scored 9.

Implant: This code is used under root status to indicate that an implant has been placed as an abutment.

8 (-). Unerupted crown: This classification is restricted to permanent teeth and used only for a tooth space with an unerupted permanent tooth but without a primary tooth. Teeth scored as unerupted are excluded from all calculations concerning dental caries. This category does not include congenitally missing teeth, or teeth lost as a result of trauma, etc. For differential diagnosis between missing and unerupted teeth, see code 5.

8 (-). Unexposed root: This code indicates that the root surface is not exposed, i.e., there is no gingival recession beyond the CEJ.

T (T). Trauma (fracture): A crown is scored as fractured when some of its surface is missing as a result of trauma and there is no evidence of caries.

9 (-). Not recorded: This code is used for any erupted permanent tooth that cannot be examined for any reason (e.g. because of orthodontic bands, severe hypoplasia, etc.).

The D-component includes all teeth with codes 1 or 2.

The M-component comprises teeth with code 4 in subjects under 30 years of age, and teeth coded 4 or 5 for subjects 30 years and older, i.e., missing due to caries or for any other reason.

The F-component includes only teeth with code 3.

The basis for DMFT calculations is 32, i.e. all permanent teeth including wisdom teeth and for dmft calculations is 20.

Teeth coded 6 (fissure sealant) or 7 (bridge abutment, special crown or veneer/implant) are not included in calculations of the DMFT.

FURTHER READING

1. Abramson JH, Abrahmson ZH. Survey Methods in Community Medicine. 5th edition. Edinburgh: Churchill Livingstone, 1999.
2. Ainamo J, Etemadzadeh H and Kallio P. Comparability and discriminating power of 4 plaque quantifications. J Clin Periodontol 1993;20:244.
3. Dunning JM. Surveying. In : Principles of Dental Public Health. 4th edition. Cambribge: Harvard University Press; 1986;310-62.
4. Esther M Wilkins. Clinical practice of the dental hygienist, ninth edition, Lippincott Williams & Wilkins, 2005.
5. Fink A. The Survey Handbook. California: Sage Publications, 1995.
6. Jong AW. Community dental health. Mosby 1993. Third edition.
7. Litwin MS. How to Measure Survey Reliability and Validity. California: Sage Publications: 1995.
8. Marks RG, Magnusson I, Taylor M, Clouser B, Maruniak J, Clark WB. Evaluation of reliability and reproducibility of dental indices. J Clin Periodontol 1993;20:54.

9. Peter S. Essentials of preventive community dentistry. Arya Publishing House. Second edition, 2003.
10. Silness J, Roynstrand T Partial mouth recording of plaque, gingivitis and probing depth in adolescents. J Clin Periodontol 1988;15:189.
11. Slack GL. Dental public health - an introduction to community dental health. John Wright and Sons 1981, second edition.
12. Soben Peter, "Essentials of preventive & Community Dentistry" Third Edition, Arya (Medi) Publishing House, New Delhi, 2006.
13. World Health Organization. Oral Health Surveys: Basic Methods. 4th edition. Geneva. WHO; 2000.

QUESTIONS

1. Define survey. What are the different types of survey techniques?
2. Explain the differences between descriptive, analytic, cross-sectional and longitudinal survey.
3. What are the uses and different types of survey methods?
4. Enumerate the steps in surveying. Explain each one of them in detail.
5. What are the different sampling methods?
6. Write the difference between random sampling and cluster sampling.
7. Write short notes on oral health surveys.
8. Define 'Index'.
9. What are the Indices used in routine dental practice?
10. Explain the criteria for selecting an index.
11. Write in detail the method of recording oral hygiene index-simplified.
12. Explain the Plaque Index as given by Sillness and Loe.
13. Explain the scoring criteria for gingival index as given by Loe and Sillness.
14. Write in detail the DMF Index.

Dental Auxiliaries

INTRODUCTION

Socrates, in defining the ideal state, gives as a prerequisite that men should divide labor, certain men becoming expert in certain fields, others in other fields and all working as a team for the common good.

DEFINITION

A dental auxiliary is a person who is given responsibility by a dentist, so that he or she can help the dentist render dental care, but who is not himself or herself qualified with a dental degree.

The duties undertaken by dental auxiliaries range from simple tasks, such as sorting instruments, to relatively complex procedures which form part of the treatment of patients.

CLASSIFICATION OF DENTAL AUXILIARIES

They may be classified according to the training they have received, the tasks they are expected to undertake and the legal restrictions placed upon them.

WHO Classification (Suggested at the Conference Conducted by the WHO in New Delhi in 1967)

1. Non-operating Auxiliaries
   A. Clinical: This is a person who assists the professional [dentist] in his clinical work, but does not carry out any independent procedures in the oral cavity.
   B. Laboratory: This is a person who assists the professional by carrying out certain technical laboratory procedures.
2. Operating Auxiliary: This is a person who, not being a professional, is permitted to carry out certain treatment procedures in the mouth under the direction and supervision of a professional.

Revised Classification

1. Non-operating Auxiliary:
   A. Dental Surgery Assistant
   B. Dental Secretary/Receptionist
   C. Dental Laboratory Technician
   D. Dental Health Educator
2. Operating Auxiliary:
   A. School Dental Nurse [New Zealand Type]

B. Dental Therapist
C. Dental Hygienist
D. Expanded Function Dental Auxiliary

Dental Surgery Assistant

- A dental assistant is a non-operating auxiliary who assists the dentist or dental hygienist in treating patients.
- They are not legally permitted to treat patients independently.
- A dental assistant may only work under the supervision of a licensed dentist, carrying out duties prescribed by the dentist.

> The first dental assistant was hired by Dr C Edmund Kells in 1885 as a "lady in attendance" so that, female patients could respectfully come to his clinic unattended.

The duties of the dental assistants are:
- Reception of the patient.
- Preparation of the patient, for any treatment, he or she may need.
- Preparation and provision of all necessary facilities such as mouthwashes and napkins.
- Sterilization, care and preparation of instruments.
- Preparation and mixing of restorative materials, including both filling and impression materials.
- Care of the patient after treatment until he or she leaves, including clearing away of instruments and preparation of instruments for rinse.
- Preparation of the surgery for the next patient.
- Presentation of documents to the surgeon for his completion and filing of these.
- Assistance with X-ray work and the processing and mounting of X-rays.
- Instruction of the patient, where necessary, in the correct use of the toothbrush.
- Aftercare of persons who have had general anesthetics.

> *Four-Handed Dentistry (Fig. 20.1):* The term four-handed dentistry is given to the art of seating both the dentist and the dental assistant in such a way that both are within easy reach of the patient's mouth. The patient is in a fully supine position. The assistant will hand the dentist the particular instrument he needs. She will also perform additional tasks such as retraction or aspiration. The dentist can thus keep his hands and eyes in the field of operation and work with less fatigue and greater efficiency.

Dental Secretary/Receptionist

- This is a person who assists the dentist with his secretarial work and patient reception duties.

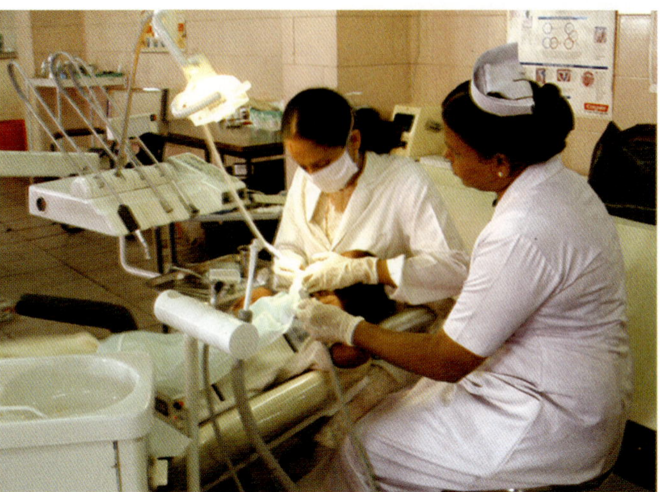

Fig. 20.1: Four-handed dentistry

Dental Laboratory Technician

- A dental laboratory technician is a non-operating auxiliary who fulfills the prescriptions provided by dentists regarding the extraoral construction and repair of oral appliances and bridgework.
- The title, "dental mechanic" is also applied to this type of auxiliary.
- His specific duties, in addition to the casting of models from impressions made by the dentist, include the fabrication of dentures, splints, orthodontic appliances, inlays, crowns and special trays.
- Dental laboratory technicians may be employed by dentists in private or public health practice, they may be self-employed and accept work from dentists in the area or they may be employed by commercial laboratories.
- Denturist is a term applied to those dental laboratory technicians, who are permitted in some states in the US and elsewhere to fabricate dentures directly for patients without a dentist's prescription.

Dental Health Educator

- This is a person who instructs in the prevention of dental disease.
- They may also be permitted to carry out certain preventive procedures such as to conduct fluoride mouth-rinsing programs to groups of school children.
- They are not, however, allowed to undertake any intra-oral procedures.

School Dental Nurse (New Zealand Type)

This is a person who is permitted to diagnose dental disease and to plan and carry out certain specified preventive and treatment measures, including some operative procedures for the treatment of dental caries and periodontal disease, in defined groups of people, usually school children, under the direction of a dentist, but not necessarily in his presence.

He or she has to refer to the dentist those patients requiring diagnosis or treatment that he or she is not able or legally entitled to carry out.

Duties of nurses

- Oral examination
- Prophylaxis
- Topical fluoride application
- Advice on dietary fluoride supplements
- Administration of local anesthetic
- Cavity preparation and placement of amalgam fillings in primary and permanent teeth
- Pulp capping
- Extraction of primary teeth
- Individual patient instruction in tooth brushing and oral hygiene
- Classroom and parent-teacher dental health education
- Referral of complex cases to a dentist in the area.
- A school dental nurse may work only in the Public Health Dental Service. A supervising dentist of the school dental service is expected to make periodic visits to ensure that she is providing an effective service.

The training for the New Zealand School Dental Nurse began in 1921, in Wellington and they began treatment in 1923.

Dental Therapist

This is a person, who is permitted to carry out, to the prescription of a supervising dentist, certain specified preventive and treatment measures including the preparation of cavities and restoration of teeth.

Dental Hygienist

- This is a person who is permitted to carry out, to the prescription of a supervising dentist, certain specified preventive and treatment measures, including some operative procedures in the treatment of periodontal disease.
- He is not permitted to carry out any operative procedures for the treatment of dental caries.

The usual functions of the dental hygienist are:

- Cleaning of mouths and teeth, with particular attention to calculus and stains.
- Topical application of fluorides, sealants and other prophylactic solutions.
- Screening or preliminary examination of patients as individuals or in groups, such as school children or industrial employees, so that they may be referred to dentists for treatment.
- Instruction in oral hygiene.
- Resource work in the field of dental health education.

> In 1905, Dr Alfred C Fones of Bridgeport, Connecticut trained Mrs Irene Newman in the procedures of dental prophylaxis. In 1906, she was at work in Dr Fones office and became the first dental hygienist. The first training school for dental hygienists came into being in November 1913.

Expanded Function Dental Auxiliary

- This is a person who is permitted to carry out certain specified preventive and treatment measures including "reversible" parts of some operative procedures in the treatment of dental caries.
- They are also called expanded function dental assistants, expanded duty dental auxiliaries or simply as auxiliaries.
- Tasks include the placing of restorations into cavities that have been prepared by a dentist.

Their functions

- Placing and removing rubber dams.
- Placing and removing temporary restorations.
- Placing and removing matrix bands.
- Condensing and carving amalgam restorations in previously prepared teeth.
- Placing of silicate and acrylic restorations in previously prepared teeth.
- Applying the final finish and polish to the previously listed restorations.

The practice of dentistry involves a personal relationship between the dentists, dental auxiliaries and the patients who elect to seek professional service from them. Because of the unique privileges granted to them, the members of the dental profession have the responsibility of providing a high standard of service to their patients and they should assume their duties freely and voluntarily.

FURTHER READING

1. Boyer EM, Cupta GC. Dentist involvement in care provided by the dental hygienist. J Dent Hyg 1990; 64(6):273-7.
2. Boyer EM. Examination services provided by dental hygienists. J Dent Hyg 1992;66(8):354-62.
3. Govan P: New scope of duties for oral hygienists. SADJ. 2001;56(2):98.
4. MacDonald L. Collaboration of health care professionals: the dental hygienists' role. Probe 1993; 27(2):62-5.

5. Nash DA. Developing a pediatric oral health therapist to help address oral health disparities among children. J Dent Educ 2004;68(1):8-20; discussion 21-2. Review.

6. Nash DA. Developing and deploying a new member of the dental team: a pediatric oral health therapist. J Public Health Dent 2005 Winter;65(1):48-55.

7. Pritzel SJ, Green TG. Working relationship between dentists and dental hygienists: their perceptions. J Dent Hyg 1990;64(6):269-72.

8. Uitenbroek DG, Schaub RM, Tromp JA, Kant JH. Attitudes of two groups of dentists towards dental hygienists. Community Dent Oral Epidemiol 1989; 17(1):11-3.

9. Wang NJ. Variation in clinical time spent by dentist and dental hygienist in child dental care. Acta Odontol Scand. 1994;52(5):280-9.

10. Wyche CJ.: Dental hygienists and dental therapists. J Dent Educ 2004;68(4):413.

QUESTIONS

1. Define dental auxiliary. Give the WHO classification of dental auxiliaries.
2. Explain the duties of dental surgery assistant.
3. Write short notes on dental laboratory technician.
4. Who is a school dental nurse?
5. What are the functions of a dental hygienist?
6. What is the role of expanded function dental auxiliary in dental clinics?

Practice Management

INTRODUCTION

Practice management, in addition to being a method to increase income, also includes creating an efficient practice that has a low stress level and where there is open communication between the dental staff and the patients.

Practice management aims at developing management skills to achieve a good practice, harmonious staff, satisfied patients and a good income.

COMPONENTS OF A SUCCESSFUL DENTAL PRACTICE

Success of dental practice depends on the office staff, patients and the entire operational system.

Personnel Systems

- A charming, friendly and professional staff is vitally important for practice success.
- The number of employees in an office varies depending upon the type of practice and patient load.
- Persons involved in patient management should be warm, empathetic with an aptitude for learning and capacity to learn and apply from past experience in new situations.
- Every new employee must be oriented on the first day of employment and a written training schedule must be given. Orientation may begin with a review of the office manual which outlines the duties, obligations and mutual expectations of the employee and employer and clarifies office policies. A training period may be necessary if the person is very new with no experience.
- Fair salaries and good benefits are necessary to avoid job dissatisfaction.
- Motivated and hardworking staff members must be recognized and encouraged and this also indirectly motivates other staff members to perform better.

Patient Systems

- As the saying goes 'First impression is the best impression' a good first appointment experience provides the foundation for an enjoyable long-term relationship with patients and parents.
- The dental receptionist should be adequately trained in the skills of communication as she is the first person to greet the new patient.
- At the first visit, patient's records are made. Communication with the parents is very important. Informal dialogues with the child will help reduce any anxiety in the child.
- It is better not to have a hard and fast rule that parents remain in the reception area. Parents can be helpful in calming the child, holding radiographic films and helping to restrain the child, who would

be less frightened than if restrained by strangers. It is important to remember to inform the parent before any procedure to avoid misunderstandings.

- Care should be taken to schedule the first appointment of very young child. Appointments should be avoided during the sleep time.
- An appointment time should be maintained to fully utilize the dentist's time throughout the day.

Operational Systems

- It is very important to schedule and document all the necessary activities necessary for the smooth functioning of the dental clinic. First most important is the efficient appointment scheduling which makes the office functioning pleasant whereas poor scheduling creates a hectic, stressful environment for patients and staff members.
- Block scheduling can also be used. In block scheduling, patients with similar treatments are given appointments in a pre-determined period. For example, more difficult and lengthy procedures such as pulpotomies, crown, composite restorations, and procedures for pre-school children are scheduled early in the day when the dentist, auxiliary personnel and patients are fresh. Less difficult procedures such as simple operative treatments, orthodontic adjustments and hygiene appointments for older children may be scheduled in the afternoons. Appointments just before lunch and in late afternoon should be reserved for the simplest procedures such as suture removals, simple extractions, eruption checks and post-trauma examinations. Sedated and difficult patients and those needing hospitalization require the dentist's undivided attention, so their treatment should be scheduled weekly at a particular time.
- Patients who miss their appointments should be separately listed and seen that they are not lost. They should be contacted periodically and invited to re-schedule.
- Computerized data management systems are available, which makes scheduling easier.

PRODUCTION AND COLLECTIONS

For the dental practice to operate profitably, high quality dental treatment must be provided in an efficient manner.

A production goal is important for any successful enterprise. It determines the amount of money that must be charged to reach the Break-Even Point (BEP) and enjoy a certain amount of profit. The BEP is the amount of money needed each year to pay all office expenses, both fixed as well as variable costs. Fixed cost includes staff salaries and benefits, occupancy costs, administrative costs, continuing education, taxes, insurance and repayment of money borrowed to finance the practice start up or purchase. Variable costs usually include laboratory fees and dental supplies, the cost of which varies depending upon patient load.

Office supplies and dental supplies account for a considerable bulk of the gross income. Proper inventory control methods help in saving quite an amount on supplies. An inventory control card should be maintained for each item purchased. The card should contain information such as name, address and phone number of each preferred vendor, an alternate vendor and a third vendor, if desired; the price of the item, the date of the pricing and the time needed for delivery. The preferred vendor is chosen not only because of the low price but also because of other factors like best availability or the fastest delivery. The alternate vendor may be more expensive but deliver at short notice. Whenever an item is ordered, the date and amount ordered must be noted. Ordering supplies on contract for 1 year at dental conventions where there are special prices from manufacturers, results in substantial savings. Therefore, inventory control and proper timing of purchases can considerably reduce the total cost of supplies, indirectly increasing the profits.

The following factors must be considered when setting fees:

1. The dentist's and assistant's time required to do the procedure.
2. The cost of operations per hour, including fixed as well as variable costs.
3. Prevailing professional fees in the area.

Fees must be reviewed annually and if necessary, raised more than the inflation rate to continue to generate adequate margin of profit. Most patients accept and may not even notice small adjustment in fees. Problems may arise, when a dentist who does not increase fees for several years, implements an increase of 20% or higher. Most patients notice and complain about such a large increase. Fee increase should not be announced to patients. However, staff members should be informed about the expenses such as laboratory fees and office supplies and utilities so as to allow them to understand the necessity of regular fee increases.

DENTAL OFFICE SETTING

Primarily, the dental office projects how the dentist feels about his office. It is important that patients should not be intimidated by the office and the dentist also needs to be comfortable in his working environment.

The dental clinic should not be looking like a 'hospital' with plain and white wall and curtains. Important is the presence of a colorful play area where children are most comfortable.

The furniture in the reception area must be durable, esthetic and comfortable. Otherwise patients may wonder if the quality of dental work is as cheap as the furnishing or, if the reception area is excessively lavish, patients may wonder if the dental work is going to be more expensive than usual.

Sound proofing is an important consideration in the pediatric dental office. Buffering the noise from the reception area is advised by having a second waiting area between the operating and reception/waiting areas. Having a "quiet room" where difficult patients can be treated is also useful. The waiting room should be carefully decorated, so that safety comes first and the area should require little or no supervision.

When equipping the dental operatory, one should purchase equipment that is functional and durable with a track record of minimum repair. It is important to have equipment that will enable the work to be performed with the greatest of ease. Another necessary equipment in the dental office is the computer. A computer is one of the easiest ways to maintain patients' record. Dental charts are legal documents and must be stored for at least 7 years after the patient leaves the practice.

Daily or monthly statistics regarding the number of patients, the type of treatment given, the fees and the expenses can be documented in a single-sheet format which allows for quick evaluation and comparison. Reader can refer the chapter on Behavior Management for more details about clinic settings.

FURTHER READING

1. Asai RG. What are my ethical obligations in enhancing my practice through marketing? J Am Dent Assoc 2007; 138(1):106-7.
2. Davidson JP. Enhance your image and your patient flow with marketing. Dent Stud 1985;63(5):14-5, 18-9, 44.
3. Lebster R. Learning the business side of dentistry. J Mich Dent Assoc 2007;89(2):1.
4. Levin RP. Improving your practice's financial performance. Dent Today 2004;23(6):102.
5. Little P. Effective website promotion. Alpha Omegan 2006;99(3):126-7.
6. McGuigan PJ, Eisner AB. Marketing the dental practice, Eight steps towards success. J Am Dent Assoc 2006; 137(10):1426-33.
7. Nacht ES. Practice management in pediatric dentistry. Dent Clin North Am 2000;44(3):697-711.
8. Stevens A. The Do's and Don'ts when building your marketing plan. Dent Stud 1985;63(5):21-3.
9. Wessberg G. A positive attitude strengthens the team. Hawaii Dent J. 2006;37(4):4.
10. Wintersteen L. Marketing with a patient focus. J Am Dent Assoc 1997;128(12):1657-9.

QUESTIONS

1. What is the need to under practice management?
2. Enumerate the components of a successful dental practice.
3. Explain the role of clinic personnel in managing dental practice.
4. Explain the role of scheduling and appointments.
5. What is Break-Even point?
6. Explain the dental office setting.

Chapter 22

General Epidemiology

CHAPTER OUTLINE

- Definition
- The Components of Epidemiology
- Aims of Epidemiology
- Principles of Epidemiology
- Epidemiologic Methods

- Descriptive Studies
- Analytical Epidemiology
- Experimental Epidemiology
- Uses of Epidemiology

INTRODUCTION

Epidemiology has its origins in the idea first expressed over 2000 years ago by Hippocrates and others, that environmental factors can influence the occurrence of disease.

Epidemiology is derived from the word epidemic (epi-among; demos = people; logos = study), which is a very old word dating back to the 3rd Century BC.

DEFINITION

"The study of the distribution and determinants of health-related states or events in specified population, and the application of this study to control health problems" (Last 1988).

COMPONENTS OF EPIDEMIOLOGY

The three components of epidemiology are studies of disease frequency, studies of the distribution and studies of the determinants. Each of these components confers an important message.

Disease Frequency

It involves the measurement of frequency of disease, disability or death, and summarizing this information in the form of rates and ratios like prevalence rate and incidence rate. These rates may yield important clues to disease etiology, which forms a vital step in the development of strategies for prevention and control of health problems.

Prevalence Rate

Disease prevalence refers to all current cases existing at a given point in time or over a period of time in a given population.

$$P = \frac{\text{Number of people with the disease or condition at a specified time}}{\text{Number of people in the population at risk at the specified time}} \times 10^n$$

Prevalence rate is often expressed as cases per 1000 or per 100 population (10^n).

Prevalence is of two types
1. Point prevalence: If the data have been collected for one point in time.
2. Period prevalence: If the data has been collected during a specified period of time.

Factors influencing prevalence rate

Uses of prevalence:
1. To estimate the magnitude of disease problems in the community and identify high risk groups.
2. For administration and planning of services.

Incidence Rate

Incidence rate is defined as "the number of new cases occurring in a defined population during a specified period of time".

Incidence rate (I) is calculated as follows:

$$I = \frac{\text{Number of people who get a disease in a specified period}}{\text{Sum of the length of time during which each person in the population is at risk}} \times 10^n$$

The numerator strictly refers only to first events of disease. The units of incidence rate must always include a dimension of time (date, month, year).

The denominator is the sum of all the disease free time periods in the defined time period of the study. This is usually calculated approximately by multiplying the average size of the study population by the length of the study period.

Interrelationships of Prevalence and Incidence

Prevalence = Incidence × Average duration of disease

Uses of incidence

1. To take action to control disease
2. For research into disease etiology and distribution
3. To determine the efficacy of preventive and therapeutic measures.

Distribution of Disease

Disease and health are not uniformly distributed in human populations. An important function of epidemiology is to study the distribution patterns in the various subgroups of the population by time, place and person. An important outcome of this study is the formulation of an etiological hypothesis. This aspect of epidemiology is known as descriptive epidemiology.

Determinants of Disease

A unique feature of epidemiology is to test etiological hypotheses and identify the underlying causes of disease.

This aspect of epidemiology is known as analytical epidemiology.

AIMS OF EPIDEMIOLOGY

- To describe the distribution and size of disease problems in human populations
- To identify etiological factors in the pathogenesis of disease
- To provide data needed for planning, implemen¬tation of and evaluation of services for the prevention, control and treatment of disease and to the setting up of priorities among these services.

PRINCIPLES OF EPIDEMIOLOGY

- Exact observation
- Correct interpretation
- Rational explanation
- Scientific construction

EPIDEMIOLOGIC METHODS

1. Descriptive studies
2. Analytical studies
3. Experimental or intervention studies

DESCRIPTIVE STUDIES

They are the first phase of an epidemiologic investigation. These studies formulate an etiological hypothesis.

Procedures in Descriptive Epidemiology

1. Defining the population to be studied
2. Defining the disease under study
3. Describing the disease by:
   - Time
   - Place
   - Person
4. Measurement of disease
5. Comparing with known indices
6. Formulation of an etiological hypothesis.

Defining the Population to be Studied

The population should be described in terms of the total number and composition such as age, sex, occupation and cultural characters.

The defined population can be the whole population or a representative sample taken from it. The defined population should be large enough, stable, without migration into or out of the area and community participation should be forthcoming.

The defined population provides the denominator for calculating rates.

Defining the Disease Under Study

To obtain an accurate estimate of disease in a population, a definition that is both precise and valid is needed to identify those who have the disease from those who do not. An operational definition is a definition by which the condition can be identified and measured in the defined population with a degree of accuracy. Once established, the definition must be adhered to throughout the study.

Describing the Disease: By Time, by Place, by Person

By time

There are three kinds of time fluctuations in disease occurrence.
   i. Short-term fluctuations
  ii. Periodic fluctuations
 iii. Long-term fluctuations

   i. Short-term fluctuations:An epidemic is an example of a short-term fluctuation in the occurrence of a disease. An epidemic is defined as "the occurrence in a community or region of cases of an illness or other health-related events clearly in excess of normal expectancy".
       Types of epidemics
       a. Common-source epidemics
          – Single exposure or point source epidemics, e.g. epidemic of food poisoning
          – continuous or multiple exposure, e.g. a well of contaminated water.
       b. Propagated epidemics: Results from person-to-person transmission of infectious agent, e.g. epidemics of hepatitis A and Polio.
       c. Slow or modern epidemics, e.g. AIDS
  ii. Periodic fluctuations
       • Seasonal trend, e.g. upper respiratory tract infections
       • Cyclic trend, e.g. mumps, automobile accidents
 iii. Long-term or secular trends, e.g. coronary heart disease, cancers.

Distribution by place
   i. International variations
  ii. National variations
 iii. Rural-urban differences
  iv. Local distributions.

   i. *International variations:* Descriptive studies have shown that the pattern of disease is not the same everywhere. There is a marked difference between the incidence of each cancer in different parts of the world. Thus, cancer of the stomach is very common in Japan, but unusual in US. Cancers of the oral cavity are exceedingly common in India as compared to industrialized countries.
  ii. *National variations:* Variations in disease occurrence also occur within countries or national boundaries. For example, the distribution of fluorosis has shown variations, with some parts of the country being more affected and others less affected or not affected at all. Such situations exist in every country.
 iii. Rural/urban variations in disease distribution are also well-known. These variations may be due to differences in population density, social class, deficiencies in medical/dental care, education or environmental factors.
  iv. *Local distributions:* Inner and outer city-variations in disease frequency are best studied with the aid of 'spot maps' or 'shaded maps'. These maps show at a glance areas of high or low frequency, the boundaries and patterns of disease distribution. For example, if the map shows "clustering" of cases, it may suggest a common source of infection or a common risk factor shared by all the cases.

Migrant studies

Migrant studies can be carried out in two ways:
a. Comparison of disease and death rates for migrants with those of their kin who have stayed at home. This permits study of genetically similar groups but living under different environmental conditions or exposures. If the disease and death rates among migrants are similar to country of adoption over a period of time, the likely explanation would be a change in the environment.
b. Comparison of migrants with the local population of the host country provides information on genetically different groups living in a similar environment. If the migration rates of disease and death are similar to the country of origin, the likely explanation would be genetic factors.

Distribution by person

a. *Age:* Age is strongly related to disease than any other single host factor. Certain diseases are more frequent in certain age groups than in others, e.g. dental caries in childhood, cancer in middle age and root caries in old age.
b. *Sex:* Sex is another host characteristic which is often studied in relation to disease. It has been found that certain chronic diseases such as diabetes, hyperthyroidism and obesity are more common

in women than in men and diseases such as lung cancer and coronary heart disease are less frequent in women.

c. *Ethnicity:* Differences in disease occurrence have been noted between population subgroups of different racial and ethnic origin.

d. *Marital status:* It has been found that mortality rates were always lower for married individuals than for the unmarried of the same age and sex.

e. *Occupation:* Man's occupation from which he earns his livelihood has an important bearing on his health status. Occupation may alter the habit pattern of employees, e.g. sleep, alcohol, smoking, drug addiction, night shifts, etc. It is obvious that persons working in particular occupations are exposed to particular types of risks, e.g. workers in coal mines are more likely to suffer from silicosis.

f. *Social class:* Epidemiological studies have shown that health and disease are not equally distributed in social classes. Individuals in upper social classes have a longer life expectancy and better health and nutritional status than those in the lower social classes. Certain diseases like coronary heart disease, hypertension and diabetes have shown a higher prevalence in upper classes than in the lower classes.

g. *Behavior:* Human behavior is increasingly looked upon as a risk factor in modem-day diseases such as coronary heart disease, cancer, obesity and accidents. The behavioral factors which have attracted the greatest attention are cigarette smoking, sedentary life, over-eating and drug abuse.

h. *Stress:* Stress has been shown to affect a variety of variables related to patients response, e.g. susceptibility to disease, exacerbation of symptoms, compliance with medical regimen, etc.

i. *Migration:* In India diseases like leprosy, filaria and malaria are considered to be rural problems. However, because of the movement of people from rural to urban areas these diseases have created serious problems in urban areas also.

Measurement of Disease

It is mandatory to have a clear picture of the amount of disease in the population. This information should be available in terms of mortality, morbidity and disability. Incidence can be obtained from "longitudinal" studies, and prevalence from "cross-sectional" studies. Descriptive epidemiology may use a cross-sectional or longitudinal design to obtain estimates of magnitude of health and disease problems in human populations.

Cross-sectional studies: Cross-sectional study is the simplest form of an observational study. It is based on a single examination of a cross-section of a population at one point in time. Cross-sectional studies are useful for chronic diseases.

Longitudinal studies: In longitudinal studies, observations are repeated in the same population over a prolonged period of time by means of follow-up examinations.

Comparing with Known Indices

The essence of epidemiology is to make comparisons and ask questions. By making comparisons between different populations and subgroups of the same population, it is possible to arrive at clues to disease etiology. We can also identify or define groups who are at increased risk for certain diseases.

Formulation of a Hypothesis

A hypothesis is a supposition arrived at from observation or reflection. An epidemiological hypothesis should specify the following:

1. The population—the characteristics of the persons to whom the hypothesis applies
2. The specific cause being considered
3. The expected outcome—the disease
4. The dose-response relationship—the amount of the cause needed to lead to a stated incidence of the effect
5. The time-response relationship—the time period that will elapse between exposure to the cause and observation of the effect.

Uses of Descriptive Epidemiology

1. Provides data regarding the magnitude of disease load and types of disease problems in the community.
2. Provides clues to disease etiology and help in the formulation of an etiological hypothesis.
3. Provides background data for planning, organizing and evaluating preventive and curative services.
4. Contributes to research by describing variations in disease occurrence by time, place and person.

ANALYTICAL EPIDEMIOLOGY

Analytical studies are the second major type of epidemiological studies.

The object is not to formulate, but to test the hypotheses.

Analytical studies comprise two distinct types of observational studies:

a. Case control study
b. Cohort study

From each of these study designs, one can determine:

i. whether or not a statistical association exists between a disease and a suspected factor; and
ii. if one exists, the strength of the association.

Case Control Study

Case control studies, often called "retrospective studies" are a common first approach to test causal hypothesis. The case control method has three distinct features:

a. Both exposure and outcome (disease) have occurred before the start of the study
b. The study proceeds backwards from effect to cause
c. It uses a control or comparison group to support or refute an inference

By definition, a case control study involves two populations—cases and controls. Cases and controls must be comparable with respect to known "confounding factors" such as age, sex, occupation, social status, etc.

There are four basic steps in conducting a case control study:

1. Selection of cases and controls
2. Matching
3. Measurement of exposure, and
4. Analysis and interpretation.

Selection of Cases and Controls

The first step is to identify a suitable group of cases and a group of controls.

Selection of cases

- Definition of a case:
  i. *Diagnostic criteria:* The diagnostic criteria of the disease and the stage of disease must be specified before the study is undertaken. Once the diagnostic criteria are established they should not be altered or changed till the study is over.
  ii. *Eligibility criteria:* The second criterion is that of eligibility. A criterion customarily employed is the requirement that only newly diagnosed (incident) cases within a specified period of time are eligible than old cases or cases in advanced stages of the disease (prevalent cases).
- Sources of cases:
  The cases may be drawn from:
  i. *Hospitals:* The cases may be drawn from a single hospital or a network of hospitals, admitted during a specified period of time.
  ii. *General population:* All cases of the study disease occurring within a defined geographic area during a specified period of time are ascertained. The entire case series or a random sample of it is selected for study.

Selection of controls

The controls must be free from the disease under study. They must be as similar to the cases as possible, except for the absence of the disease under study. Selection of an appropriate control group is an important prerequisite, for it is against this, we make comparisons, draw inferences and make judgements about the outcome of the investigation.

Sources of controls

1. *Hospital controls:* The controls may be selected from the same hospitals as the cases but with different illness than the disease under study.
2. *Relatives:* The controls may also be taken up from relatives (spouses and siblings).
3. *Neighborhood controls:* The controls may be drawn from persons living in the same locality as cases, persons working in the same factory or children attending the same school.
4. *General population:* Population controls can be obtained from defined geographic areas, by taking a random sample of individuals free of the study disease.

Matching

The controls may differ from the cases in a number of factors such as age, sex, occupation, social status, etc.

Matching is defined as the process by which we select controls in such a way that they are similar to cases with regard to certain pertinent selected variables which are known to influence the outcome of disease and which, if not adequately matched for comparability, could distort or confound the results.

A "confounding factor" is defined as one which is associated both with exposure and disease and is distributed unequally in the study and control groups. A confounding factor is one that, although associated with "exposure" under investigation, is itself, a "risk factor" for the disease.

Matching can be of two types

- *Group matching:* This may be done by assigning cases to sub-categories based on their characteristics (e.g. age, occupation) and then establishing appropriate controls.
- *Pairs matching:* For each case, a control is chosen which can be matched quite closely. Thus, if we have a 20-year old adult with a particular disease, we will search for 20-year old adult without the disease as a control. Thus, one can obtain pairs of patients and controls of the same sex, age, duration and severity of illness, etc.

Measurement of Exposure

Information about exposure should be obtained in the same manner both for cases and controls. This may be obtained by interviews, by questionnaires or by studying past records such as hospital records, employment records, etc.

Analysis

The final step is analysis, to find out:

a. Exposure rates among cases and controls to suspected factor
b. Estimation of disease risk associated with exposure (Odds ratio)

Exposure rates

Exposure rates among cases =

$$\frac{\text{Cases exposed to risk factor}}{\text{Total No. of cases (in percentage)}}$$

Exposure rates among controls =

$$\frac{\text{Controls exposed to risk factor}}{\text{Total No. of controls (in percentage)}}$$

Estimation of risk

Persons and incidence among non-exposed.

It is given the formula:

Relative risk = Incidence among exposed/incidence among non-exposed.

A typical case control study does not provide incidence which relative risk can be calculated directly, because there is no appropriate denominator or population at risk.

Bias in Case Control Studies

Bias is any systematic error in the determination of the association between exposure and disease.

Types of bias

a. *Bias due to confounding:* This bias is removed by matching in case control studies.
b. *Memory or recall bias:* When cases and controls are asked questions about their past history, it may be more likely for the cases to recall the existence of certain events or factors than the controls who are healthy.
c. *Selection bias:* The cases and controls may not be representative of cases and controls in the general population.
d. *Berksonian bias:* It is termed after Dr Joseph Berkson who had this problem. The bias arises because of the different rates of admission to hospitals for people with different diseases.
e. *Interviewer's bias:* Bias may also occur when the interviewer knows the hypothesis and also knows who the cases are. This information may lead him to question cases more thoroughly than controls.

Advantages and Disadvantages of Case Control Studies

Advantages

1. Relatively easy to carry out
2. Rapid and inexpensive (compared with cohort studies)
3. Require comparatively few subjects
4. Particularly suitable to investigate rare diseases or diseases about which little is known
5. No risk to subjects
6. Allows the study of several different etiological factors
7. Risk factors can be identified
8. No attrition problems, because case control studies do not require follow-up of individuals into the future
9. Ethical problems minimal.

Disadvantages

1. Problems of bias.
2. Selection of an appropriate control group may be difficult
3. We cannot measure incidence, and can only estimate the relative risk
4. Does not distinguish between causes and associated factors
5. Not suited for the evaluation of therapy or prophylaxis of disease
6. Another major concern is the representativeness of cases and controls.

Cohort Study

Cohort study is another type of analytical (observational) which is usually undertaken to obtain additional evidence to refute or support the existence of an association between the suspected cause and the disease.

Cohort study is known by a variety of names, prospective study, longitudinal study, incidence study, forward-looking study.

Distinguishing Features of Cohort Studies

a. The cohorts are identified prior to the appearance of disease under investigation.
b. The study groups, so defined, are observed over a period of time to determine the frequency of disease among them.
c. The study proceeds forwards from cause to effect.

The term "cohort" is defined as a group of who share a common characteristic or experience within a time period (e.g. age, occupation).

Indications for Cohort Studies

a. When there is good evidence of an association between exposure and disease.

b. When exposure is rare, but the incidence of disease high among exposed.
c. When attrition of study population can be minimized.
d. When ample funds are available.
In assembling cohorts, the following general considerations should be taken into account:
a. The cohorts must be free from the disease under study.
b. Both the groups (i.e. study and control cohorts) should be equally susceptible to the disease.
c. Both the groups should be comparable with respect to all the possible variables, which may influence the frequency of the disease.
d. The diagnostic and eligibility criteria of the disease must be defined beforehand.

Types of Cohort Studies

1. Prospective cohort studies: Is one in which the outcome has not yet occurred at the time the investigation begins.
2. Retrospective cohort studies: Is one in which the outcomes have all occurred before the start of the investigation. The investigator goes back in time to select his study groups from past medical or employment records and traces them forward.
3. A combination of retrospective and prospective cohort studies: Here the cohort is identified from past records and is assessed till date for the outcome. The same cohort is followed up prospectively into the future for further assessment of outcome.

Elements of a Cohort Study

The elements of a cohort study are:
1. Selection of study subjects
2. Obtaining data on exposure
3. Selection of comparison groups
4. Follow-up
5. Analysis

Selection of study subjects: They can be from:
a. General population: When exposure is frequent, cohorts may be assembled from the general population.
b. Special groups:
   • Select groups: These may be professional groups (e.g. doctors, nurses, lawyers) college students, volunteers, etc.
   • Exposure groups: These groups comprise individuals who are known to have experienced the exposure (e.g. radiologists exposed to X-rays).

Obtaining data on exposure: Information about exposure can be obtained by:
• Personal interviews or mailed questionnaires

• Review of records
   – Medical examinations
   – Environmental surveys.

Selection of comparison groups

a. *Internal comparisons:* In some cohort studies, no outside comparison group is required. The comparison groups are in-built. That is, single cohort enters the study, and its members may be classified into several comparison groups according to the degrees of exposure to risk.
b. *External comparisons:* When information on degree of exposure is not available, it is necessary to put up an external control, to evaluate the experience of the exposed group, e.g. smokers and non-smokers.
c. *Comparison with general population rates:* If no groups are available, the mortality experience of the exposed group is compared with the mortality experience of the general population in the same geographic area as the exposed people.

Follow-up:

It consists of:

• Periodic medical examination of each member
• Review of hospital records
• Surveillance of death records
• Mailed questionnaires, periodic home visits.

Analysis: The data obtained are analyzed to obtain:
• Incidence rates
   Among cases = no. of individuals with disease in the study group/study population
   Among controls = no. of individuals with disease in the controls/control population
• Estimation of relative risk (RR)
   RR = Incidence of disease among exposed/Incidence of disease among non-exposed
• Estimation of attributable risk (AR)
   AR = Incidence of disease among exposed minus Incidence of disease among non-exposed/Incidence of disease among exposed in percentage.

Advantages and Disadvantages of Cohort Studies

Advantages

1. Incidence can be calculated.
2. Several possible outcomes related to exposure can be studied simultaneously.
3. Provides a direct estimate of relative risk.
4. Dose-response ratios can be calculated.
5. Certain forms of bias can be minimized.

Disadvantages
1.   Involves a large number of people.
2.   Study takes a long time.
3.   Attritional problems are inevitable.
4.   Expensive.
5.   Ethical problems may arise.

EXPERIMENTAL EPIDEMIOLOGY

Experimental or intervention studies are studies carried out under the direct control of the investigator. These studies involve some action, intervention or manipulation such as the deliberate application or withdrawal of a suspected cause or changing one variable in the causative chain in the experimental group while making no change in the control group and observing and comparing the outcome of the experiment in both the groups.

Aims of Experimental Studies
a.   To provide "scientific proof' of etiological (or risk) factors which may permit the modification or control of those diseases
b.   To provide a method of measuring the effectiveness and efficiency of health services for the prevention, control and treatment of disease and improve the health of the community.
Experimental studies may be conducted in animals or human beings.
Experimental studies are of two types:
1.   Randomized controlled trials (those involving a process of random allocation).
2.   Non-randomized or "non-experimental" trials (those departing from strict randomization for practical purposes, but in such a manner that non-randomization does not seriously affect the basis of conclusions).
In modern usage, experimental epidemiology is often equated with randomized controlled trials.

Randomized Controlled Trials (RCTs)
The basic steps in conducting a RCT include the following:
1.   Drawing up a protocol
2.   Selecting reference and experimental populations
3.   Randomization
4.   Manipulation or intervention
5.   Follow-up
6.   Assessment of outcome

1.   *Drawing up a protocol:* The protocol specifies the aims and objectives of the study, criteria for the selection of study and control groups, size of the sample, the procedures for allocation of subjects into the study and control groups, treatments to be applied, standardization of working procedures and schedules, up to the stage of evaluation of outcome of the study.
Once a protocol has been evolved, it should be strictly adhered to throughout the study.
2.   *Selecting reference and experimental populations:*
   a.   Reference or target population: It is the population to which the findings of the trial, if found successful, is expected to be applicable. A reference population may be as broad as mankind or it may be geographically limited or limited to persons in specific age, sex or social groups.
   b.   Experimental or study population: The study population is derived from the reference population. It is the actual population that participates in the experimental study. Ideally, it should be randomly chosen from the reference population, so that it has the same characteristics as the reference population.
   When an experimental population has been defined, its members are invited to participate in the study.
   The participants or volunteers must fulfill the following three criteria:
   –   They must give "informed consent". That is they must agree to participate in the trial after having been fully informed about the purpose, procedures and possible dangers of the trial.
   –   They should be representative of the population to which they belong.
   –   They should be qualified or eligible for the trial. In other words, the participants must be fully susceptible to the disease under study.
3.   *Randomization:* Randomization is a statistical procedure by which the participants are allocated into groups usually called "study" and "control" groups, to receive or not to receive an experimental preventive or therapeutic procedure or intervention. Randomization is an attempt to eliminate "bias" and allow for comparability. By random allocation, every individual gets an equal chance of being allocated into either group.
   Randomization is best done using a table of random numbers.
4.   *Manipulation:* Having formed the study and control groups, the next step is to intervene or manipulate the study (experimental) group by deliberate application or withdrawal or reduction of the suspected causal factor as laid down in the protocol.
5.   *Follow-up:* This involves examination of the experimental and control group subjects at defined intervals of time, in a standard manner under the same given circumstances till final assessment of outcome.

Some losses to follow-up are inevitable due to factors such as death, migration and loss of interest. This is known as attrition.

6. *Assessment:* The final step in assessment of the outcome of the trial is in terms of:
   a. *Positive results:* That is, benefits of the experimental measure such as reduced incidence or severity of the disease.
   b. *Negative results:* That is, severity and frequency of side effects and complications, including death.

Bias may arise from errors of assessment of the outcome due to the human element. These may be from three sources:

a. Bias on the part of the participants, who may subjectively feel better or report improvement if they knew they were receiving a new form of treatment.
b. Observer bias that is the investigator measuring the outcome of a therapeutic trial may be influenced it he knows beforehand the particular procedure or therapy to which the patient has been subjected to.
c. Bias in evaluation, that is, the investigator may subconsciously give a favorable report of the outcome of the trial.

In order to reduce these problems, a technique known as "blinding" is adopted.

Blinding

Blinding can be done in three ways:

a. *Single blind trial:* The trial is so planned that the participant is not aware whether he belongs to the study group or control group.
b. *Double blind trial:* The trial is so planned that neither the doctor nor the participant is aware of the group allocation and the treatment received.
c. *Triple blind trial:* The participant, the investigator and the person analyzing the data are all 'blind".

Ideally, of course, triple blinding should be used but double blinding is the most frequently used method.

USES OF EPIDEMIOLOGY

1. *To study historically the rise and fall of disease in the population:* The first use of epidemiology relates to this aspect, that is, study of the history of disease in human population. Health and disease pattern in a community is never constant. There are fluctuations both over short and long periods of time. Epidemiology provides a means to study disease profiles and time trends in human populations. Thus, useful projections into the future can be made and emerging health problems can be identified.

2. *Community diagnosis:* Refers to the identification and quantification of health problems in a community. This helps in laying down priorities in disease control and prevention. It can also serve as a benchmark for the evaluation of health services. It can also be a source of new knowledge about disease distribution, causation and prevention.

3. *Planning and evaluation:* Planning is essential for a rational allocation of the limited resources. Epidemiologic information about the distribution of health problems overtime and place provides the basis for planning health services.
   Evaluation is done to find out whether the measures undertaken to prevent a disease are effective in reducing the frequency of this disease.

4. *Evaluation of individual's risks and chances:* Making a statement about the degree of risk in a population is one of the important tasks in epidemiology. Relative risk and attributable risk need to be calculated for a factor related to the cause of the disease.

5. *Syndrome identification:* Syndromes are identified by observing frequently associated findings in individual patients.

6. *Completing the natural history of disease:* In epidemiology, disease patterns in the community are studied in relation to agent, host and environmental factors and this facilitates the filling up of the gaps in the natural history of disease.

7. *Searching for causes and risk factors:* By relating disease to interpopulation differences and other attributes of the population examined, epidemiology tries to identify the causes of disease.

FURTHER READING

1. Abramson JH, Abramson ZH. Survey Methods in Community Medicine, 5th ed. Edinburgh; Churchill Livingstone 1999.

2. Downer MC. Caries experience and sucrose availability: an analysis of the relationship in the United Kingdom over fifty years. Community Dent Health 1999;16:18-21.

3. Duffy SW, Jonsson H, Agbaje OF, Pashayan N, Gabe R. Avoiding bias from aggregate measures of exposure. J Epidemiol Community Health. 2007;61(5):461-3.

4. Edwards P, Roberts I, Clarke M, Diguiseppi C, Pratap S, Wentz R, Kwan I, Cooper R. Methods to increase response rates to postal questionnaires. Cochrane Database Syst Rev 2007;18:(2).

5. Eisenberg JN, Lewis BL, Porco TC, Hubbard AH, Colford JM Jr : Bias due to secondary transmission in estimation of attributable risk from intervention trials. Epidemiology 2003;14(4):442-50.

6. Gunning-Schepers LJ, Barendregt JJ. Timeless epidemiology or history cannot be ignored. J Clin Epidemiol 1992;45(4):365-72.

7. Kunz R, Vist G, Oxman A. Randomisation to protect against selection bias in healthcare trials. Cochrane Database Syst Rev 2007;18:(2).

8. Park K. Park's Textbook of Preventive and Social Medicine. 18th ed. India: M/s Banarsidas Bhanot; 2005.

9. Smith FG, Smith JE. Key topics in clinical research. BIOS Scientific Publishers.

10. Sreebny LM. Sugar availability, sugar consumption and dental caries. Community Dent Oral Epidemiol 1982;10(1):1-7.

11. World Health Organization. Health research methodology. A guide for training in research methods. 2nd ed. Manila: World Health Organization. Regional office for the Western Pacific; 2001.

QUESTIONS

1. Define epidemiology. What are the components of epidemiology?
2. What is disease frequency?
3. Explain prevalence rate.
4. What is incidence rate?
5. What are the aims and principles of epidemiology?
6. What are the different epidemiologic studies?
7. Explain the difference between the longitudinal and cross-sectional studies.
8. Explain analytical and experimental epidemiology.
9. What is the difference between case control and cohort study?

Medical Emergencies in Dental Clinic

INTRODUCTION

Life-threatening emergencies are the most dreaded phrase in dental practice. This is especially true in the pediatric dental clinic where even the parents are involved. In the unlikely and unfortunate event of an emergency, the instinctive reaction of the dentist is to put the patient in the supine position and then often panic and confusion take over. This loss of clear thinking can be traced back to a lack of practical training and the lack of a simple protocol to be followed in the event of a life-threatening emergency. This chapter attempts to present a simple and systematic way of handling life-threatening medical emergencies in the pediatric dental clinic.

There are three aspects to be considered during the discussion of an emergency in the dental clinic:
1. Equipping for an emergency
2. Precautions against an emergency
3. Management during an emergency

EQUIPPING FOR AN EMERGENCY

Emergency is a real possibility in dental practice and this fact has to be accepted by the clinician. This is especially true in a pediatric dental practice where drugs to induce various grades of sedation are administered. So rather than hoping that emergencies don't happen, the dentist should be ready for the impending emergency. He should start by
a. Equipping himself.
b. Equipping the office.

Equipping Himself

- The practicing clinician and his staff should be up-to-date in delivering basic life support (BLS) care to sustain the child till emergency medical service arrives.
- A thorough understanding of the pharmacology of important emergency drugs, their dosage during emergencies and the preferred route of administration during emergencies is very essential.
- It is also very important to learn and practice how to administer drugs via the desired parenteral route, i.e. SC, IM or IV.
- Investing in emergency equipment without knowing how to use them is unwise. So learning to operate emergency equipment like the oxygen cylinder is of paramount importance.

Equipping the Office

The emergency equipment and drugs required in a pediatric dental setup varies depending on the expertise and the training undergone by the clinician. But, some equipment and drugs are indispensable in pediatric dental practice.

These include:

- A dental chair which can easily be changed into supine position.
- A high volume suction to clear oral secretions.
- An oxygen cylinder attached to a positive pressure/demand valve with a clear face mask capable of delivering 5 L/min for at least 30 minutes. (Size E)
- Pocket mask for emergency ventilation.
- Spirit of ammonia
- Adrenaline (1:1000)—for severe immediate allergic and severe asthmatic reactions.
- Diphenhydramine—for allergic reactions of slower onset.
- Hydrocortisone sodium succinate—to treat acute adrenal insufficiency.
- Diazepam—for continuous epileptic seizures (Status Epilepticus).
- Flumazenil—for reversal of sedation induced by benzodiazepines.
- Nitroglycerin—a vasodilator to treat angina.
- A sugar source—in cases of hypoglycemia.
- Dextrose 50%—for unconscious hypoglycemic patients to be given IV.
- Glucagon—for unconscious hypoglycemic patients to be given IM when IV access cannot be established.
- Prearranged emergency medical service which can be called on short notice.

PRECAUTIONS AGAINST AN EMERGENCY

With the emergency training and equipment now in order, a few precautionary steps taken for every child coming for treatment significantly reduce the chances of an emergency. These include:

a. Recording ASA Classification for the child
b. Recording physical signs
c. Careful use of drugs.

Recording ASA Classification for the Child

The American Society of Anesthesiologists (ASA) proposed a classification indicating the systemic status of a patient. For every child to undergo dental treatment, record a systematic medical history. Based on their medical history, put every child under their respective ASA category which is as follows:

- ASA I: A normal healthy patient without systemic disease.
- ASA II: A patient with mild systemic disease.
- ASA III: A patient with severe systemic disease that limits activity but is not incapacitating.

- ASA IV: A patient with an incapacitating systemic disease that is a constant threat to life.
- ASA V: A moribund patient not expected to survive 24 hours with or without an operation.
- ASA E: Emergency operation of any variety, with E preceding the number to indicate the patient's physical status.

(ASA V and E do not hold good for a dental OPD).

An ASA classification alerts the clinician to the possibility of an emergency in say an ASA II, III or IV child and can prepare in advance for the same or do the treatment in a hospital setting.

Recording Physical Signs

- Record a baseline blood pressure, pulse rate and respiratory rate for all children or at least the ASA II, III and IV categories. In case of an intraoperative deteriorating condition, fresh values can be recorded and compared with baseline values.
- The weight of every child should also be recorded. This will help to calculate the dosage of the emergency drug to be given.

Careful Use of Drugs

- Drugs especially local anesthetics and sedatives should be used in the correct dosage calculated based on the weight of the child and following the proper protocol.
- Local anesthetics should be administered very slowly at the rate of 1 ml/min.

MANAGEMENT DURING AN EMERGENCY

In spite of all the precautions, life-threatening emergencies do occur and most often happen when least expected. It may be comforting to know that dentists are not expected to diagnose an emergency. That is the responsibility of the physician. The dentist is only expected to sustain the patient with basic life support (BLS) and treat the physical signs till the patient is stable or till he can be shifted to an emergency medical centre. An uncomplicated approach will make the whole scenario much simpler.

The golden rule is that regardless of the emergency in children, start by assessing and maintaining basic life support, i.e. P, A, B, C.

P Position of the patient on the dental chair.
A Airway should be open and patent.
B Breathing should be maintained, i.e. sufficient oxygen should be reaching the patient's lungs.
C Circulation of blood in carotid artery is assessed to see if the heart is beating and adequately perfusing the brain.

Once the PABC (Basic Life Support/Cardiopulmonary Resuscitation) has been assessed.

D Definitive therapy, i.e. use of drugs or dialing emergency is done depending on the physical signs and the presenting emergency situation.

PABC Assessment and Management (BLS/CPR)

P: Position

Any clinical management of a medical emergency on the dental chair calls for a stoppage in the dental procedure. This has to be followed by proper positioning of the child. There are primarily three positions during an emergency.

1. Supine (Horizontal) position with the brain at the same level as the heart and the feet elevated slightly (Fig. 23.1).

    This position is used during unconsciousness or impending unconsciousness. The head down or the Trendelenburg position should be avoided because gravity pushes the abdominal viscera into the diaphragm reducing the effectiveness of breathing.

2. Erect/semi-supine position: This position is used in case of signs of respiratory distress. This position makes it easier for the child to breathe.

A: Airway

The idea is to obtain a patent and open airway so that enough oxygen reaches the lungs. First, all the secretions in the oral cavity are cleared using a high volume suction. If the patient is conscious, proceed to assess B-Breathing.

If the patient is unconscious, the tongue tends to fall back and block the airway. The airway can be opened using the head tilt-chin lift maneuver (Fig. 23.2). The jaw thrust maneuver can also be used to open the airway.

It is especially useful in cases of cervical spine injuries seen during road traffic accidents. Now proceed to assess breathing.

In case of foreign body obstruction, the airway has to be cleared using back blows or Heimlich maneuver which will be described later in the chapter.

B: Breathing

First, 'Look, Listen, Feel is done. Here, the operator keeps his ears 1 inch away from the child's nose and listens and feels the breath sounds. At the same time he observes the child's chest for its rise and fall. The listening and feeling of the breath sounds is more crucial than observing the rise and fall of the chest because the child may only be trying to breathe without adequate ventilation (Fig. 23.3). Not more than 10 seconds should be used for this exercise.

If the child is conscious and is breathing adequately, then monitor the vital signs and administer supplemental oxygen if required.

If the child is unconscious, but is breathing adequately then administer supplemental oxygen if required with the head tilt-chin lift to ensure open airway. Monitor the vital signs and proceed to assess C-Circulation.

If the child is not breathing or is breathing inadequately (gasping), then administer oxygen under positive pressure or assist ventilation using a well-fitting a pocket mask. Maintaining a head tilt-chin lift, deliver a breath over a period of 1 second and check for visible chest rise. Give two full ventilations with the pocket mask with the head tilted for an open airway before proceeding to assess circulation. The mouth-to-mouth or mouth-to-nose techniques are not described because pockets masks are now easily available and should be stocked in every dental practice. Bag valve mask devices like the ambu bag can be used in case of two trained rescuers.

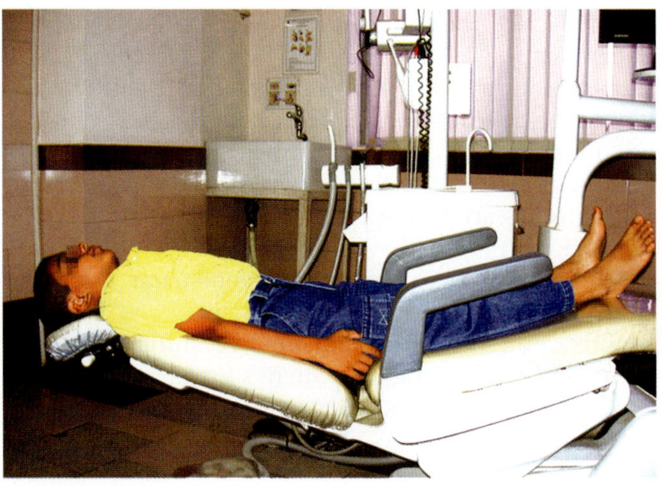

Fig. 23.1: Supine position with legs elevated

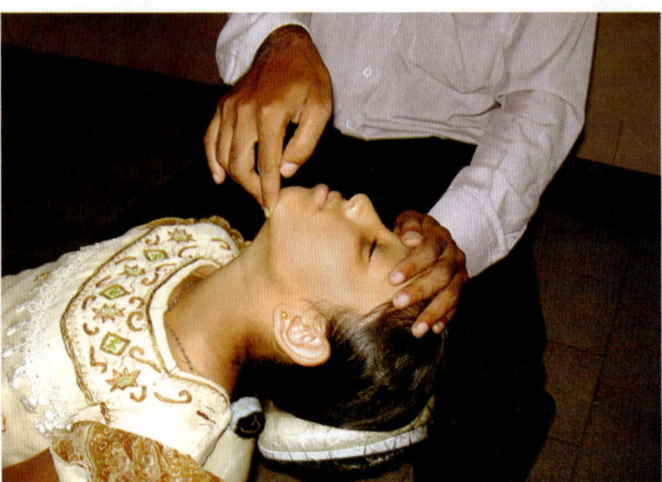

Fig. 23.2: Head tilt-chin lift maneuver

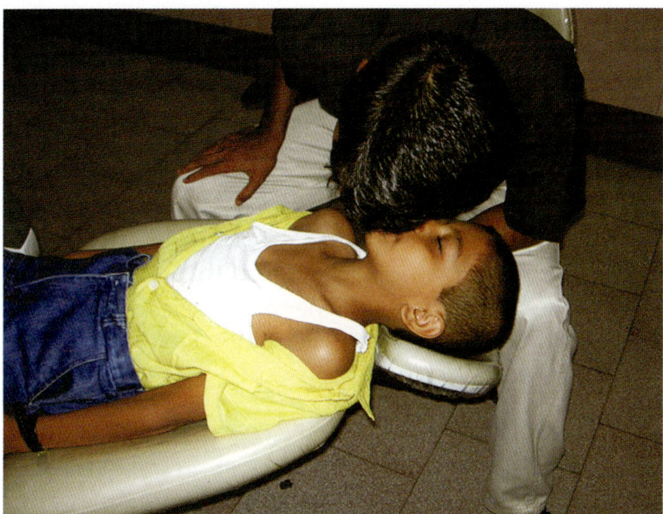

Fig. 23.3: Look, listen and feel

C: Circulation

The purpose of assessing circulation is to ensure that the heart is beating and enough oxygenated blood is reaching the vital organs especially the brain. This is especially crucial in the child as the child is prone to hypoxia very quickly because of its higher respiratory rate and higher BMR.

The best way to assess circulation in an emergency is to palpate the carotid artery because the carotid artery is easy to locate and it is the artery supplying blood to the brain. The carotid artery is palpated between the Adams apple and the sternocleidomastoid muscle (Fig. 23.4). No more than 10 seconds should be used to palpate the carotid artery.

It should be noted that the carotid artery should not be palpated with the thumb because the thumb has a pulsating artery of its own.

If the carotid pulse is felt, then airway and breathing are maintained and the vital signs are monitored. One rescue breath every 5–6 seconds for pubescents and one rescue breath every 3–5 seconds for the child is recommended. Definitive therapy is started if required.

If the carotid pulse is not felt, then external cardiac compression is started immediately. Shift the child to a hard surface or if the place in the clinic is inadequate, place a hard board under the back of the child on the dental chair.

The anatomic area for compression is the mid nipple line. The operator has to keep his arms locked straight, place the heel of one hand over the mid nipple line and lock it with the other hand. Now the chest is compressed firmly at the rate of 100 compressions/minute. The compression depth should be at least 2 inches. For every 30 compressions, 2 ventilations are given (30:2). In children when there are two rescuers, the compressions ventilations ratio is 15:2. Continue this cycle till the child is shifted to an emergency.

For children less than 7 years old only the heel of one hand is used for compression (Fig. 23.5).

It should be noted in the preceding paragraphs that assessment and maintenance of ABC (Airway, Breathing and Circulation) differs between the conscious and the unconscious child. Once the PABC has been assessed and stabilized, i.e., the basic life support is maintained, D-Definitive therapy can be started.

D: Definitive Therapy

Definitive therapy comprises:
- Drug administration if indicated
- Monitoring vital signs.
- Dialing emergency medical service if the condition is deemed serious.

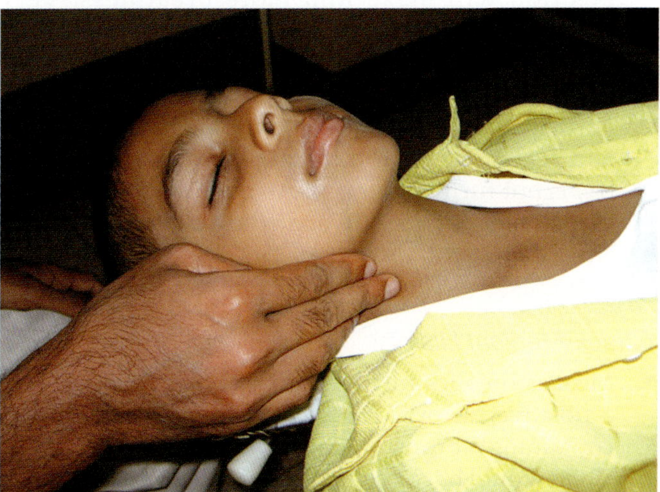

Fig. 23.4: Palpating carotid artery

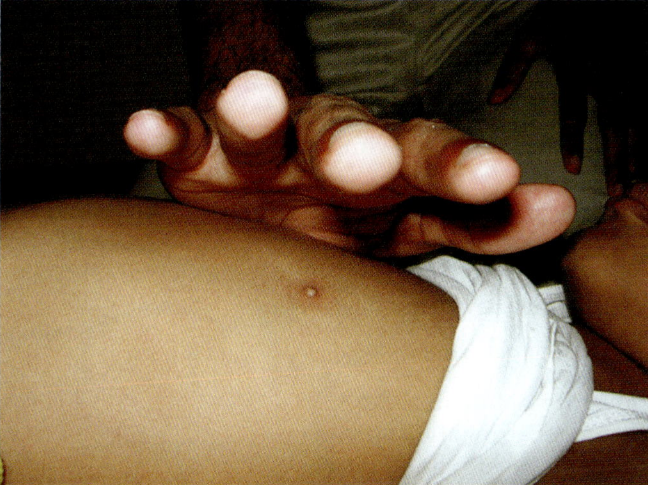

Fig. 23.5: Heel of one hand for children less than 7 years

Definitive Therapy is not necessarily in this order and should change according to the presenting situation.

So in summary, the management of any emergency should comprise the following steps:

- Note the physical signs occurring at the time.
- Assess PABC according to the individual situation.
- Check the medical history of the child to see if the presenting emergency is due to an underlying medical condition.
- Start definitive therapy (D).

Changes in the 2010 AHA guidelines for CPR

- The exception to the above mentioned protocol will be in case of a witnessed cardiac arrest. According to the American Heart Association 2010 guidelines, the management sequence is now CAB, i.e. Circulation, Airway and Breathing instead of the traditional ABC. This holds good for both adults and pediatric patients (children and infants). The rationale is that starting CPR with 30 compressions rather than 2 ventilations will prevent the delay in starting the first compression.
- AHA 2010 guidelines also no longer endorse "LOOK LISTEN and FEEL" in witnessed cardiac arrest as it is considered time consuming.
- AHA 2010 guidelines minimize the importance of even pulse checks citing that even trained health care providers find it difficult to accurately assess the presence or absence of a carotid pulse in case of an emergency. It recommends no more than 10 seconds for a pulse check if it has to be done. In case of laymen rescuers, 2010 AHA guidelines for CPR recommends immediate activation of the emergency response system followed by cycles of 30 chest compressions and 2 breaths for any collapsed victim (witnessed) who is unresponsive and not breathing or breathing in gasps (not breathing normally). According to the guidelines chest compressions delivered to patients subsequently found not to be in cardiac arrest rarely lead to significant injury.
- In the case of an unwitnessed cardiac arrest, the cause of the arrest would be unknown to the rescuer. The cause could be asphyxial (respiratory). In such a case AHA 2010 guidelines recommend traditional ABC sequence including rescue breathing before activating the emergency response system.

Commonly occurring emergencies in dental clinic

- Acute Asthmatic Attack
- Acute Adrenal Insufficiency
- Hypersensitivity Reactions
- Foreign Body Obstruction
- Local Anesthesia Overdosage
- Syncope
- Seizures
- Hypoglycemic Attack
- Hyperventilation

MANAGEMENT OF EMERGENCY SITUATIONS

The management for some of the emergencies encountered in the pediatric dental clinic is described in the following section:

Acute Asthmatic Attack

The goal of management during an acute asthmatic episode on the dental chair should be to relieve the bronchospasm associated with the attack.

Presenting Signs and Symptoms

- Child complains of a thickness in the chest.
- Followed by a coughing spell with or without sputum production.
- Characteristic expiratory wheeze is heard.
- Dyspnea, i.e. labored breathing using accessory muscles of respiration like sternocleidomastoid and scalenus to lift the entire rib cage.
- Sits up fighting for air.
- Tachypnea, i.e. very rapid respiration.
- Very anxious child.
- Cyanosis of mucous membrane and nail beds will follow.
- Eventual loss of consciousness if not managed.

PABC Assessment

- Position (P) the child erect/semi-erect as supine position will make him more breathless. Very often just removing the child from the treatment environment ceases the attack.
- Child is usually conscious and breathing with a partially obstructed airway. Clear all dental materials and secretions from the oral cavity so that Airway (A) is not further blocked. Assess Breathing (B) and Circulation (C) quickly according to the presenting situation.
- Administer oxygen.

Check Medical History

- Most asthmatics are aware of their condition and give a positive history. They generally carry an inhaler containing a bronchodilator.
- Child would have been classified under ASA category II or III at the end of medical history thus already

having alerted the clinician to the possibility of an attack.

Definitive Therapy

- 2 puffs of a bronchodilator generally a β_2 adrenergic agonist such as salbutamol, or albuterol through an aerosol inhaler. These drugs act on the β_2 receptors in the bronchial smooth muscle and relax the bronchoconstriction.
- The drug in the aerosol inhaler has to be inhaled slowly over approximately 5–6 seconds and then the breath is held for 10 seconds and slowly exhaled.
- The child can also use his own bronchodilator.
- The onset of action is rapid and improvement is noted in 15 seconds.
- If the physical signs and symptoms are not relieved, dial medical assistance and in the meanwhile administer 0.15 mg of 1:1000 adrenaline SC or IM.

Acute Adrenal Insufficiency

This condition can manifest in children receiving or who have received corticosteroid therapy continuously for two weeks or longer, within two years of dental treatment *(Rule of Twos)*. In these children, normal release of increased amounts of endogenous glucocorticosteroids during stressful situations is prevented resulting in an acute adrenal attack.

Presenting Signs and Symptoms

- Mental confusion.
- Intense pain in the abdomen, lower back and legs.
- Nausea and vomiting.
- Loss of consciousness if not managed.

PABC Assessment

- Place child in supine position with legs elevated slightly.
- Assess ABC quickly. Administer oxygen.

Check Medical History

- Parents would have given a positive history of corticosteroid therapy satisfying the rule of twos.
- Child would have been classified under ASA category II or III at the end of medical history thus already having alerted the clinician to the possibility of an attack.

Definitive Therapy

- Dial medical assistance.
- Administer 2 ml of 100 mg hydrocortisone sodium succinate IV preferably or IM.
- Monitor vital signs especially for hypotension.

Hypersensitivity Reactions

Of the four basic types of hypersensitivity reactions, Type 1 or Immediate hypersensitivity reaction is of particular importance in the practice of dentistry. Type 1 or Immediate hypersensitivity may range from mild skin reactions to life-threatening generalized anaphylaxis. The speed with which the signs and symptoms of allergy appear and the rate of progressive involvement of systems determines the intensity of management.

The various clinical manifestations of Type 1 or immediate hypersensitivity reactions include:

Delayed Onset Skin Reaction

These signs appear after 60 minutes or more have elapsed since the introduction of the antigenic stimuli most likely the administration of the drug.

Presenting signs and symptoms

- Localized areas of erythema.
- Urticaria, i.e. elevated areas of skin which are erythematous, indurated and frequently pruritic.
- Angioedema (Swollen tissue).

PABC assessment

- Since the patient is not in distress except slight etching, position of the child is based on comfort if the signs appear in the midst of treatment.
- ABC is quickly assessed. Generally, at this juncture ABC is adequately maintained by the child.

Check medical history

- Would most likely be ASA I in the absence of any other significant medical history. Positive histories of allergic adverse drug reactions (ADR) especially to local anesthetics may not always be reliable as the patient may have actually experienced syncope or an overdosage reaction.

Definitive therapy

- Diphenhydramine 25 mg, IM or chlorphenaramine 5 mg, IM is the dosage for children.
- This has to be followed by oral diphenhydramine 25 mg or oral chlorphenaramine 5 mg, every 4–6 hours for 2–3 days.

Rapid Onset Skin Reaction

The signs appear less than 60 min after the introduction of the antigenic stimuli. Although these skin reactions are not in themselves dangerous, they may be the first indication of more serious manifestations to follow.

Presenting signs and symptoms, PABC assessment and medical history

- Similar to delayed skin reactions.

Definitive therapy

- It is same as above. But, in this case the child has to be kept under observation for at least an hour to see if signs of respiratory and cardiovascular system involvement appear in which case adrenaline administration becomes essential as will be described in the subsequent section.
- Child should also be sent for a medical evaluation to ascertain the cause of the reaction.

Respiratory Signs with or without Skin Signs

The respiratory signs may be a sequel to the skin signs or may occur independently. Allergic reactions affecting the respiratory tract are more serious and require more aggressive intervention.

The allergic reactions of the respiratory tract can manifest in two ways either independently or progressively, i.e.
- Bronchospasm—affecting the lower respiratory tract.
- Laryngeal edema—affecting the upper respiratory tract.

Bronchospasm: Signs and symptoms are due to constriction of bronchial smooth muscle and similar to an asthmatic attack.

Presenting signs and symptoms

- Wheezing
- Dyspnea
- Use of accessory muscles of respiration.

PABC assessment

- Position child in an upright or semi-erect position.
- Clear all the secretions and materials from the oral cavity.
- Breathing may be inadequate and may range from mild dyspnea to cyanosis. Administer oxygen 6 liters/minute.
- Circulation is usually adequate at this juncture.

Check medical history

- The child would have been classified ASA I in the absence of any other significant medical history especially asthma.
- The diagnosis of an allergic reaction over asthma will be established if the respiratory signs are preceded by the skin reaction. In any case, epinephrine will be the drug of choice to relieve the Bronchospasm.

Definitive therapy

- Dial emergency medical assistance.
- Administer 0.15 ml, 1:1000 epinephrine IM/SC. Repeat after 5 minutes if signs progress because epinephrine gets metabolized quickly.
- Monitor vital signs.
- Administer diphenhydramine, 2 mg/kg, IM to prevent recurrence.
- Observe in office for one hour or hospitalize for further observation.
- Prescribe oral antihistamines, i.e. oral diphenhydramine 25 mg or oral chlorphenaramine 5 mg, every 4–6 hours for 2–3 days.

Laryngeal Edema

Involvement of the larger airways in an allergic reaction usually first manifest at the most narrow portion of the air passage, i.e. the larynx. The signs and symptoms are due to angioedema of the vocal cords causing partial or total airway obstruction.

Presenting signs and symptoms

- Characteristic high pitched crowing sounds (Stridor) in cases of partial obstruction or no sound in cases of total obstruction even in the cases of exaggerated chest movements.
- Cyanosis
- Loss of consciousness if not managed.

PABC assessment

- Position child in an upright or semi-erect position.
- Clear all the secretions and materials from the oral cavity.
- Obtain patent airway by head tilt-chin lift maneuver.
- Breathing will be labored. Administer oxygen 6 liters/minute.
- Quickly assess circulation.

Check medical history

- The child would have been classified ASA I in the absence of any other significant medical history.

Definitive therapy

- Dial emergency medical assistance.
- Administer 0.15 ml, 1:1000 epinephrine IM. Repeat after 5 minutes if signs progress.
- Monitor vital signs.
- If laryngospasm is not still relieved, an emergency cricothyrotomy may have to be performed. The technique of cricothyrotomy is beyond the scope of the chapter.

- On clinical recovery with administration of epinephrine (noted as improved breath sounds, absence of cyanosis and less exaggerated chest movements) administer diphenhydramine, 2 mg/kg, IM and corticosteroid 100 mg IM.
- Corticosteroids inhibit edema and capillary dilatation by stabilizing the basement membrane.
- These additional drugs are not administered during the emergency because they are of no immediate value as their onset of action is slow.
- It is wise to hospitalize the patient after such a severe attack.

Generalized Anaphylaxis

This life-threatening reaction occurs within seconds or minutes following parenteral administration. A wide range of clinical manifestations involving multiple systems quickly progressing from skin reactions, gastrointestinal manifestations and respiratory distress followed by signs and symptoms of the cardiovascular system like hypotension, unconsciousness finally cardiac arrest.

Presenting signs and symptoms

- Typically begins with the patient complaining of a feeling of impending doom.
- Skin manifestations like urticaria, erythema and pruritus appear on the face and the trunk.
- Nausea, vomiting, abdominal cramping and urinary incontinence may appear.
- Symptoms of respiratory embarrassment follow with dyspnea, wheezing and stridor.
- Cyanosis of nail beds and mucosa is seen.
- Disordered CVS function manifests as tachycardia and palpitations.
- The patient becomes unconsciousness.
- Cardiac arrest follows if not managed immediately.

PABC assessment

- Position the patient supine with legs elevated on a back board on the dental chair or shift the patient onto the floor.
- A hard surface is necessary for external cardiac compression in case of a cardiac arrest.
- Open the airway with head tilt-chin lift.
- Ask the assistant to prepare the oxygen cylinder while the doctor quickly progresses to definitive therapy.
- Generalized anaphylaxis is the only emergency where priority to drug administration of epinephrine is given over the usual sequence of PABC because epinephrine can be life-saving in this situation.

- Oxygen 5–6 liters/minute can be administered any time during the incident.

Check medical history

- The child would have been classified ASA I in the absence of any other significant medical history.

Definitive therapy

- Administer 0.15 ml, 1:1000 epinephrine IM preferably from a preloaded syringe because time is crucial here.
- Epinephrine can be injected sublingually to the floor of the mouth because of the increased perfusion in the area.
- Dial emergency medical care.
- Repeat adrenaline after 5 minutes if the clinical picture fails to improve.
- Monitor vital signs. Record blood pressure and heart rate at the carotid artery every 5 minutes.
- Start chest compression if cardiac arrest occurs.
- Once and if clinical improvement is noticed, i.e. increased BP, decreased bronchospasm and return of consciousness, administer diphenhydramine and corticosteroids IM to prevent recurrence.
- Hospitalize the patient for further observation.

Foreign Body Obstruction

The extensive use of stainless steel crowns, endodontic instruments, conscious sedation and the small oral cavity of the child are factors which make foreign body obstruction a potential problem in the practice of pediatric dentistry.

When an object is lost in the oropharynx, the chances are high that the child will either swallow the object into the esophagus or the object will be retrieved by spontaneous coughing. The object may also be small, thereby bypassing the larynx into the trachea and the right bronchus. In these cases, no signs and symptoms of respiratory obstruction appear. Chest radiographs are taken to determine the location of the foreign object.

If the object on the radiograph is seen in the abdomen, it passes uneventfully from the stomach and the intestines through the fecal matter more than 90% of the time. Parents should be asked to locate the object in the fecal matter over the next week. Potential complications can be GI blockage, peritoneal abscess and intestinal perforations.

If the object on the radiograph is seen in the bronchus, then the object has to be removed by the medical specialist using bronchoscopy.

Airway obstruction by the object can be complete or partial.

Partial Airway Obstruction

Presenting signs and symptoms

- Child will reflexly cough forcefully.
- Wheezing may be seen between coughs.
- Child is able to breathe, though with some difficulty.
- No signs of cyanosis appear.

PABC assessment and management

- In case of partial airway obstruction as judged by the presenting signs and symptoms, the child should be positioned (P) in a left lateral decubitis position with the head down (Fig. 23.6). The child will cough spontaneously which may be adequate to throw out the aspirated object and clear the airway (A). Once a patent airway is obtained the signs and symptoms cease on their own.

Total Airway Obstruction

Presenting signs and symptoms

- Patient grasps the throat (Universal sign of choke)
- Inability to speak
- Inability to cough
- Inability to exchange air in spite of respiratory movements
- Cyanosis
- Loss of consciousness if not managed
- Cardiac arrest finally.

PABC assessment and management

The management differs depending on if the child is conscious or unconscious. The goal is to remove the foreign body from the airway. Once a clear and patent airway is obtained, the other signs and symptoms cease on their own.

i. Conscious child

The abdominal thrust or the Heimlich maneuver is used to expel the foreign body. It acts like an artificial cough that produces a rapid increase in intrathoracic pressure thus helping expel the foreign body. It is done as follows (Fig. 23.7):
- Stand behind the child and wrap under the child's arms.
- Place fist slightly above the umbilicus with the thumb side against the abdomen.
- Grasp the fist with the free hand.
- Thrust inwards and backwards repeatedly till the foreign body is expelled or till the chills loses consciousness.

ii. Unconscious child (Fig. 23.8)

- Put the child in the supine position (P) with legs elevated slightly.
- Stand next to the child's hips.
- Place heel of one hand slightly above umbilicus, but below the xiphoid. Place second hand on top of the first hand.
- Perform five thrusts in an inward and upwards direction.
- This should be followed by a finger sweep in the child's mouth. The idea of a finger sweep is to move the dislodged object into the mouth where it can be removed with a large diameter powerful suction.
- If the foreign object is still not dislodged and the patient's condition continues to deteriorate, then a surgical procedure called cricothyrotomy should

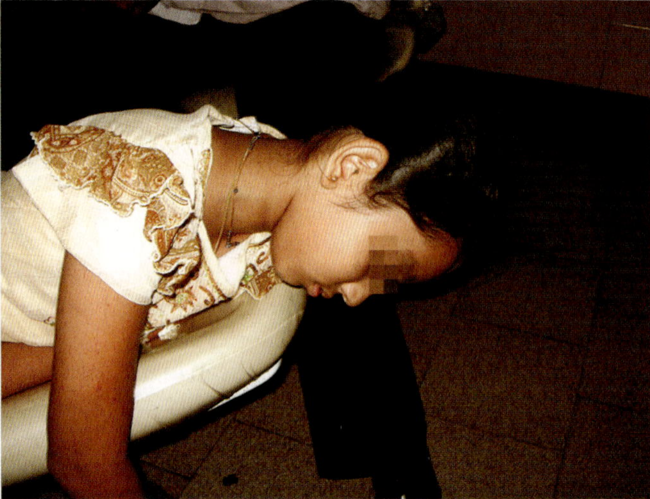

Fig. 23.6: Left lateral decubitus position

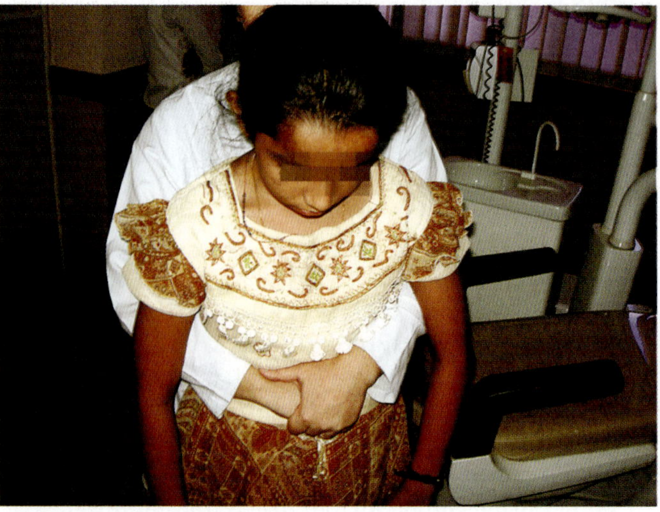

Fig. 23.7: Heimlich maneuver

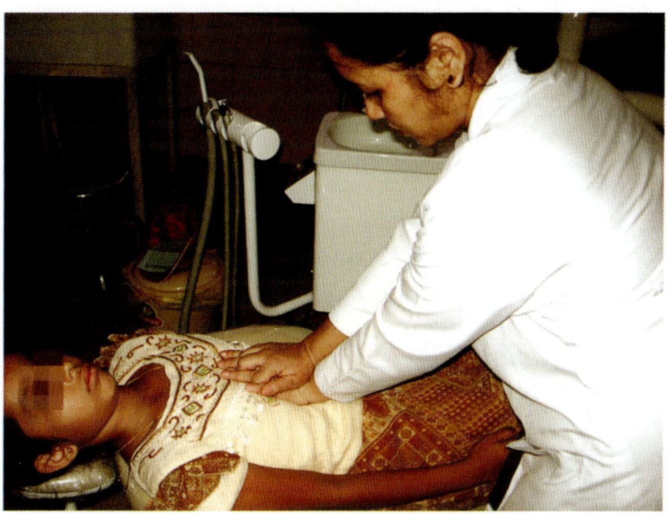

Fig. 23.8: Heimlich maneuver in an unconscious child

be considered. This requires proper training and is beyond the scope of this chapter.

Local Anesthesia (LA) Overdosage

Local anesthetics are the most commonly used drugs in dentistry. Their overdosage is caused by a high blood level of the drug when the drug's entry into the blood exceeds its rate of removal. Most of the LA overdose reactions are self-limiting. The blood level of the drug decreases continuously because of redistribution and biotransformation of the drug in the body. Maintenance of ABC and oxygen are probably the only measures indicated.

Simple measures to prevent an LA overdose reaction are:

- Calculating the proper dose for each individual (for example, 4.4 mg/kg body weight for 2% Lidocaine with 1:100,000 adrenaline).
- Aspiration before injecting
- Slow rate of injection (1 ml/minute)
- Proper systemic history: For example, patients with congestive cardiac failure are more prone to overdose reactions because of a reduced blood volume for drug distribution and reduced blood flow to the liver secondary to a reduced cardiac output. The amount of LA given should be reduced for this patient.

The LA overdose reactions can be mild reactions or severe reactions depending on the rate of absorption of the drug and the blood level of the drug. Clinically LA overdose reactions are manifested depending on the severity as a phase of excitation (Slurred speech, confusion, convulsions) followed by a proportional phase of depression (drowsiness, shallow breathing, unconsciousness).

Mild Overdosage Reaction

Mild overdosage reaction of rapid onset is seen within 5–10 minutes of administration. The causes can be intravascular injection or administration of a large dose.

Presenting signs and symptoms

- Confused, talkative.
- Slurred speech
- Ringing ears
- Facial muscle twitching
- Blurred vision
- Dizziness

PABC assessment and management

- Position (P) is based on patient comfort usually supine.
- ABC is usually adequate. A lower $PaCO_2$ elevates the seizure threshold. So the patient should be asked to hyperventilate by deep breathing of room air or breathe oxygen via a full face mask. This will decrease the $PaCO_2$ thus preventing the development of seizures.

Check medical history

- Patient would have been classified under ASA category I in the absence of other systemic conditions. It should be noted that some conditions like congestive cardiac failure and pulmonary diseases (show increase in $PaCO_2$) are more prone to LA overdosage reactions.

Definitive therapy

- Monitor the vital signs. No other drug treatment is indicated. The reactions are self-limiting with time.

Mild LA overdose reactions can also have a late onset usually above 10 minutes after administration. The management of these reactions is essentially the same as above.

Severe Overdose Reaction

Severe overdose reaction of rapid onset is usually manifested seconds after LA administration. It sometimes occurs during the process of injection. Intravascular injection is the likely cause.

Presenting signs and symptoms

- Signs and symptoms appearing almost immediately.
- Generalized tonic clonic seizures.
- Loss of consciousness.

PABC assessment and management

- Shift the patient to supine position with legs elevated.

- Assess ABC quickly. Administer oxygen as quickly as possible. The seizure threshold is lowered if the patient becomes acidotic. Good ventilation helps in termination of the seizure along with adequate oxygenation of the brain.

Check medical history

- Patient would have been classified under ASA category I in the absence of other systemic conditions. Check if any previous episodes of seizures have been noted in the systemic history. It should be noted that some conditions like congestive cardiac failure and pulmonary diseases (show increase in $PaCO_2$) are more prone to LA overdosage reactions.

Definitive therapy

- If loss of consciousness was the only sign, proper positioning will return consciousness rapidly and syncope was probably the cause.
- If patient does not regain consciousness after adequate positioning or if seizure develops immediately after LA administration, then dial emergency medical care as a precautionary measure.
- Monitoring vital signs with adequate ventilation is usually sufficient because anesthetic blood level will gradually fall below the seizure threshold and seizures will cease. Prevention of injury due to seizures is the primary aim of seizure management.
- Drug administration like diazepam for seizure management during LA overdose reactions is unnecessary in most cases because the period of excitement will be followed by a period of depression (Shallow breathing, hypotension, bradycardia, drowsiness and loss of consciousness). This phase of depression will be magnified by the administration of a depressant drug like diazepam.
- Generally adequate maintenance of PABC will gradually return the consciousness and BP/heart rate return to base line levels.

Severe LA overdose reactions can also have a late onset usually above 10 minutes after administration. If manifestations appear at home, the patient should be shifted to a hospital immediately and instructions given to the hospital staff. The management of these late onset reactions is essentially the same as above.

Syncope

It is a benign and self-limiting common faint, but potentially life-threatening if not managed properly. It refers to a sudden transient loss of consciousness secondary to a period of cerebral ischemia. Children very rarely manifest syncope because they do not hide their fears. They yell and cry and move about thus increasing the cerebral blood flow.

Simple ways of preventing syncope are:
- Do not wave needle in front of the patient.
- Administer LA in supine position.
- See that the clinic is not hot and humid.
- Check that patient is not on an empty stomach.
- Use mild sedatives if required.

Physical Signs and Symptoms

- Pale color
- Heavy perspiration primarily on the forehead
- Dizziness
- Nausea
- Hyperpnea
- Cold hands and feet
- Loss of consciousness with pupillary dilatation (deathly appearance).

The individual thus exhibits several warning symptoms for several minutes (Pre-syncope) before losing consciousness.

PABC Assessment and Management

- P: As soon as presyncopal signs appear, patient is placed in supine position with legs elevated. Patient can also be encouraged to vigorously move his legs so that muscles can pump blood back into the heart.
- If the patient has already lost consciousness, the ABC should be assessed and maintained.
  - A: Maintain airway by head tilt-chin lift
  - B: Look, Listen and Feel for breathing. Administer oxygen if necessary.
  - C: Check the carotid pulse. The carotid pulse may be weak during the syncope period.

Check Medical History

- The child would have been classified ASA I in the absence of any other significant medical history.

Definitive Therapy

- Monitor vital signs.
- Loosen clothing and belt.
- A respiratory stimulant like spirit of ammonia can be helpful because it stimulates breathing and muscular movement as it has a noxious odor.
- A cold towel can be placed on the patient's forehead.
- A glucose drink can be given after consciousness is regained.
- Medical assistance is rarely required because consciousness rapidly returns on proper positioning.

Seizures

Among the various types of seizures (convulsions), the one with the most dramatic appearance is a generalized form of epilepsy called the generalized tonic clonic seizure (grandmal epilepsy) and will be discussed here. These seizures are not life-threatening as is commonly believed. They are self-limiting in most cases and prevention of injury and adequate ventilation are of primary concern. Drugs are generally not indicated. Only if the Generalized Tonic-Clonic Seizure (GTCS) persists for more than 5 minutes continuously, then the condition is called Status Epilepticus which is a serious condition requiring immediate IV administration of an anticonvulsant.

Presenting Signs and Symptoms

- Aura is a typical sign exhibited by each individual minutes before an attack. It may be manifested as increased anxiety or depression. The patient cannot warn the dentist about the aura because he has already become amnesic at the onset of this stage. If a friend or a relative notices this typical aura during dental treatment, he should warn the dentist and treatment should be stopped immediately.
- This is followed by a loss of consciousness. This is called as the preictal phase, i.e. the phase before convulsions.
- This is followed by the tonic-clonic convulsions. It is called as the ictal phase. It lasts for about 2–5 minutes.
- Bleeding from the mouth and frothing may be seen in the ictal stage.
- This is followed by the post-ictal phase where the tonic-clonic movements cease and consciousness gradually returns.
- Urinary or fecal incontinence may occur in the post-ictal phase because of sphincter relaxation.

PABC Assessment and Management

- On warning of the aura, cease treatment and position (P) patient in the supine position.
- Remove all dental equipment and appliances from the mouth of the patient before loss of consciousness.
- Maintain airway (A) by head tilt-chin lift on the headrest of the dental chair. Also suction the secretions by placing a flexible suction between the cheek and teeth.
- Administer oxygen if possible to aid in breathing (B). Circulation is usually adequate.

Check Medical History

- Check the patient's systemic history to see if the patient has a history of epilepsy or any other condition like diabetes which manifests convulsions during a hypoglycemic attack.
- The patient would have categorized as ASA II if he had a previous history of seizures, ASA III if seizures occur once a month and ASA IV if seizures are seen weekly.

Definitive Therapy

- Prevention of injury to the patient is the primary goal.
- Remove instruments like handpieces, burs and other instruments from the vicinity of the patient.
- Loosen clothes to aid in breathing.
- Gently restrain the patient's extremities allowing for minor movement. Care should be taken not to fix the extremities during convulsions as this may result in fractures.
- The ictal phase may last up to 5 minutes.
- With cessation of seizures, a period of generalized depression sets in. PABC is maintained along with oxygen administration. Vital signs are monitored and the patient is reassured.
- Should the seizures continue after 5 minutes or appear at very short intervals then the condition is serious and is called status epilepticus.
- In this case dial medical assistance. The dentist can administer an anticonvulsant like diazepam (0.3 mg/kg) IV slowly if trained. If not maintain basic life support till patient is shifted or till emergency medical help arrives.

Hypoglycemic Attack

Hypoglycemic attack may be seen in a diabetic patient undergoing dental treatment. Diabetes mellitus can be type I, i.e. insulin dependent diabetes mellitus (IDDM) or type II, i.e. NIDDM. Type I is genetic. Here insulin is totally absent and the patient requires exogenous insulin for glucose metabolism. In type II, insulin in the body may be adequate but the receptors in the tissues may be insensitive to the insulin.

Dental treatment modifications are required more with a type I diabetes patient. He may miss or avoid a meal before his dental appointment after taking his usual dose of insulin resulting in a hypoglycemic attack. The patient should be asked to take his usual dose of insulin along with his normal meal before the appointment. If the daily insulin dose of the patient is i.e. > 40 units daily, then a medical consultation should be arranged before the dental appointment. Antibiotic coverage is also recommended for such patients before undergoing surgical procedures. The type II diabetic patient is less prone to acute fluctuations in blood glucose level and generally tolerates all dental procedures well.

Any known diabetic who has become unconscious should be treated for hypoglycemia rather than hyperglycemia because hypoglycemia can rapidly result in serious neurologic damage or death if not treated immediately. In contrast, complications from hyperglycemia tend to develop over a long period of time.

Presenting Signs and Symptoms

- Weakness
- Dizziness
- Moist skin
- Altered level of consciousness, i.e. bizarre behavior or changes in personality.
- Loss of consciousness and GTCS if not managed.

Conscious Patient

PABC assessment and management:

- Position (P) is determined by patient comfort.
- ABC is assessed. Generally adequate at this stage.

Check medical history

- The patient would have generally given a positive history of diabetes. The patient would have been classified as ASA II, III or IV depending on the blood glucose level and depending on whether he is a well-controlled or poorly controlled diabetic. If the patient is a ASA I, syncope can be a possible reason and proper positioning should lead to rapid recovery.

Definitive therapy

- Give the patient an oral carbohydrate like orange juice, sugar or a candy. It should be repeated every 5 minutes till recovery.

Unconscious Patient

PABC assessment and management

- Position (P) patient in a supine position with legs elevated slightly.
- Assess and maintain ABC. Administer oxygen if necessary. But the underlying problem of low blood sugar has to be corrected for consciousness to be regained.

Check medical history

The patient would have generally given a positive history of diabetes. The patient would have been classified as ASA II, III or IV.

Definitive therapy

- Dial emergency medical care.

- Administer Glucagon 1 mg IM. Leads to elevation of the blood glucose level by breaking down glycogen stores in the liver. The recovery usually takes 20–40 minutes.
- If trained, the dentist can administer 50% dextrose solution IV. If not, it can be done by the emergency personnel.
- If glucagon or dextrose is not available immediately, a thick paste of concentrated glucose (cake cream), honey or syrup can be placed in the buccal fold safely. Even though the onset of action is slow, it is better than no treatment.
- Once conscious, the individual is administered oral source of carbohydrates.

Hyperventilation

Hyperventilation means an increase in the rate and depth of respiration primarily because of anxiety associated with dental treatment. It is like an athlete breathing after a 100 meter sprint. In the dental clinic, it is most commonly seen in the 15–40 years age group because this age group tends to suppress their fears unlike children who tend to cry and move around or adults above 40 who are able to adjust and accept the dental treatment. More commonly seen in girls than boys. Hyperventilation does not lead to unconsciousness, but only causes a change in the level of consciousness like dizziness and lightheadedness. In this condition, due to rapid and deep breathing the body loses more carbon dioxide (hypocapnea) increasing the blood pH and resulting in respiratory alkalosis. Hypocapnea produces vasoconstriction of the cerebral blood vessels thus resulting in dizziness.

Presenting Signs and Symptoms

- Very anxious patient with cold hands and pale sweaty forehead.
- Rapid breaths especially before LA administration.
- Palpitation (pounding of heart).
- Lightheaded as the carbon dioxide level falls.
- Tingling or paresthesias of hands and cramps.
- Syncope if not managed.

PABC Assessment and Management

- The goal of the treatment is to lessen the anxiety and to correct the respiratory problem.
- Terminate the dental procedure and reassure and calm the patient.
- Upright position is the preferred position (P) as the supine position makes breathing difficult.
- Have the patient breathe slowly and regularly at a rate of 4–6 breaths per minute. This will increase the carbon dioxide level in the body.

- ABC is generally adequate as the patient rarely loses consciousness.

Check Medical History

- The anxiety of the patient should be noted during the initial contact. Sedation for treatment can be very useful. The ASA status would generally be I.

Definitive Therapy

- The goal of treatment is to increase the blood $PaCO_2$ level. This can be achieved by asking the patient to cup his hands in front of his mouth and rebreathe his CO_2 rich exhaled air rapidly.
- This will also serve to warm the cold hands of the patient which will further decrease his anxiety.
- Oxygen even though not harmful is neither indicated nor useful in a hyperventilated patient.

In conclusion, a dentist treating children has a moral responsibility towards the overall well-being of the child. The dentist has to make efforts to upgrade his knowledge and be fully prepared to face any emergency during the course of the treatment. Only then can he confidently tell the parents that – "Your child is in good hands".

FURTHER READING

1. Agostini FG, Flaitz CM, Hicks MJ. Dental emergencies in a university-based pediatric dentistry postgraduate outpatient clinic: a retrospective study. ASDC J Dent Child 2001;68(5-6):316-21, 300-1.
2. Aragon CE, Burneo JG. Understanding the patient with epilepsy and seizures in the dental practice. J Can Dent Assoc 2007;73(1):71-6. Review.
3. Atherton GJ, Pemberton MN, Thornhill MH. Medical emergencies: the experience of staff of a UK dental teaching hospital. Br Dent J 2000;188(6):320-4.
4. Ayed AK, Jafar AM, Owayed A. Foreign body aspiration in children: diagnosis and treatment. Pediatr Surg Int 2003;19(6):485-8.
5. Boren E, Teuber SS, Naguwa SM, Gershwin ME. A critical review of local anesthetic sensitivity. Clin Rev Allergy Immunol 2007;32(1):119-28.
6. Bouillon R. Acute adrenal insufficiency. Endocrinol Metab Clin North Am 2006; 35(4):767-75.
7. Hahner S, Allolio B. Management of adrenal insufficiency in different clinical settings. Expert Opin Pharmacother 2005;6(14):2407-17.
8. Hass DA. Management of Medical Emergencies in the Dental Office: Conditions in Each Country, the Extent of Treatment by the Dentist Anesth Prog. 2006 Spring; 53(1):20-4.
9. Hodges ED, Durham TM, Stanley RT. Management of aspiration and swallowing incidents: a review of the literature and report of case. ASDC J Dent Child 1992; 59(6):413-9. Review.
10. Kennedy BT, Haller JS. Treatment of the epileptic patient in the dental office. NY State Dent J. 1998;64(2):26-31.
11. Kong JS, Teuber SS, Gershwin ME. Aspirin and nonsteroidal anti-inflammatory drug hypersensitivity. Clin Rev Allergy Immunol 2007;32(1):97-110.
12. Lambrianidis T, Beltes P. Accidental swallowing of endodontic instruments. Endod Dent Traumatol 1996; 12(6):301-4.
13. Malamed SF. Emergency medicine in pediatric dentistry: preparation and management. J Calif Dent Assoc. 2003; 31(10):749-55.
14. Malamed SF. Medical emergencies in the Dental office, 6th edition. St Louis, Missouri, Mosby: An imprint of Elsevier, 2007.
15. Part 1: Executive summary 2010 American heart association guidelines for cardiopulmonary resuscitation and emergency cardiovascular care. Circulation 2010; 122:S640-S656.
16. Pinto A, Scaglione M, Pinto F, et al. Tracheobronchial aspiration of foreign bodies: current indications for emergency plain chest radiography. Radiol Med (Torino). 2006;111(4):497-506. Epub 2006.
17. Sapir S, Shapira Y, Amir E. Emergencies evolving from local anesthesia in the pediatric dental clinic: prevention and treatment. Refuat Hapeh Vehashinayim 2003; 20(4):28-34, 87.
18. Tiwana KK, Morton T, Tiwana PS. Aspiration and ingestion in dental practice: a 10-year institutional review. J Am Dent Assoc 2004;135(9):1287-91.
19. Willmore LJ. Epilepsy emergencies: the first seizure and status epilepticus. Neurology 1998;51(5 Suppl 4): S34-8.

QUESTIONS

1. What are the main considerations for managing emergency in dental clinic?
2. Explain the precautions to be taken for preventing an emergency.
3. What is PABC assessment and management?
4. What are 2010 AHA guidelines for CPR?
5. Write in detail management of Acute Asthmatic Attack in dental clinic.
6. What are hypersensitivity reactions?
7. Write in detail the management of foreign body obstruction of airway.
8. What would be your steps in the managing local anesthesia overdosage?

Index

Page numbers followed by *f* refer to figure and *t* refer to table